Bioinformatics and Drug Discovery

METHODS IN MOLECULAR BIOLOGY™

John M. Walker, SERIES EDITOR

METHODS IN MOLECULAR BIOLOGY™

Bioinformatics and Drug Discovery

Edited by

Richard S. Larson

Department of Pathology
University of New Mexico School of Medicine
Albuquerque, NM

HUMANA PRESS ✳ TOTOWA, NEW JERSEY

© 2006 Humana Press Inc.
999 Riverview Drive, Suite 208
Totowa, New Jersey 07512

www.humanapress.com

This publication is printed on acid-free paper. ∞
ANSI Z39.48-1984 (American Standards Institute)

Permanence of Paper for Printed Library Materials.

Production Editor: Amy Thau

Cover design by Patricia F. Cleary

Cover illustration:Figure 27 from Chapter 11, "Nuclear Magnetic Resonance-Based Screening Methods," by Laurel Sillerud and Richard Larson (background image).
Representative data of clustering analysis (left) and principal component analysis (center) from microarray data. Docking of small peptide to protein target ICAM-1 (right) is shown (foreground image, courtesy of Richard Larson).

For additional copies, pricing for bulk purchases, and/or information about other Humana titles, contact Humana at the above address or at any of the following numbers: Tel.: 973-256-1699; Fax: 973-256-8341; E-mail: orders@humanapr.com; or visit our Website: www.humanapress.com

Printed in the United States of America. 10 9 8 7 6 5 4 3 2 1

eISBN: 1-59259-964-8

ISSN:1064-3745

Library of Congress Cataloging-in-Publication Data

Bioinformatics and drug discovery / edited by Richard S. Larson.
  p. ; cm. -- (Methods in molecular biology ; 316)
 Includes bibliographical references and index.
 ISBN 1-58829-346-7 (alk. paper)
 1. Drug development. 2. Bioinformatics. 3. High throughput screening
(Drug development) 4. Combinatorial chemistry.
 [DNLM: 1. Drug Design. 2. Computational Biology--methods. 3. Drug
Evaluation, Preclinical. 4. Genetic Techniques. 5. Microarray Analysis. 6.
Pharmacogenetics--methods. QV 744 B6136 2005] I. Larson, Richard S. II.
Series: Methods in molecular biology (Clifton, N.J.) ; v. 316.
 RM301.25.B56 2005
 615'.19--dc22
                                        2005010943

Preface

Recent advances in drug discovery have created new, powerful technologies that have a prominent bioinformatic component. One of the chief difficulties in using these technologies is their requirement for interdisciplinary expertise in the physical sciences, life sciences, and/or computer science. As a result, these new methodologies can present a challenge when establishing a research laboratory.

The purpose of *Bioinformatics and Drug Discovery* is to facilitate the employment of these new, powerful technologies in the process of drug discovery. This volume describes the pipeline of methods and techniques that are used in modern drug discovery. These technologies prominently use bioinformatics for analysis of their output. In *Bioinformatics and Drug Discovery*, the systematic process of drug discovery—from gene identification to protein modeling to identification of drug candidates—is described first. The next part of the book focuses on target identification, including microarray analysis and bioinformatic techniques used to analyze genes as potential drug targets. In addition, examples of how this analysis can be used clinically are also described. The latter part of the book discusses protein modeling and cheminformatics, including virtual screening and *in silico* protein design for identification of drug candidates. Because these technologies are just emerging, the authors of each chapter have provided an extended introduction that describes the theory and application of the technology and techniques described. In the second part of each chapter, every effort has been made to incorporate detailed procedures, including software and its use, related to these technologies.

Bioinformatics and Drug Discovery is directed to those interested in the different aspects of drug design that include academicians (biologists, chemists, and biochemists), clinicians, and scientists at pharmaceutical companies. All the chapters in *Bioinformatics and Drug Discovery* have been written by well-established investigators who use the methods on a regular basis. In all, this book is designed to provide readers not only with the planned insightful overview of key topics, but also with the customary ample supply of unfailing reproducible step-by-step procedures for techniques described.

Richard S. Larson

Contents

Contributors

FATIMA AL-SHAHROUR • *Department of Bioinformatics, Centro de Investigacion Principe Felipe, Valencia, Spain*

FRANCISCO AZUAJE • *Computer Science Research Institute, University of Ulster, Northern Ireland, UK*

STEVEN H. BROWN • *Department of Veterans Affairs, Department of Biomedical Informatics, Vanderbilt University, Nashville, TN*

JEFFREY R. BUCHHALTER • *Department of Child and Adolescent Neurology, Mayo Clinic College of Medicine, Rochester, MN*

CHRISTIAN G. BOLOGA • *Division of Biocomputing, Department of Biochemistry and Molecular Biology, University of New Mexico, Albuquerque, NM*

QIONG CHENG • *Biological and Chemical Sciences and Engineering, DuPont Central Research and Development, Wilmington, DE*

JENNIFER M. COMMINS • *Bioinformatics and Pharmacogenomics Laboratory, National University of Ireland, Maynooth, County Kildare, Ireland*

BASSIL I. DAHIYAT • *Xencor, Monrovia, CA*

T. GREGORY DEWEY • *Keck Graduate Institute of Applied Life Sciences, Claremont, CA*

JOAQUIN DOPAZO • *Department of Bioinformatics, Centro de Investigacion Principe Felipe, Valencia, Spain*

ALEXANDER V. DUBANOV • *Institute of Biomedial Chemistry, RAMS, Moscow, Russia*

PETER L. ELKIN • *Department of Internal Medicine, Mayo Clinic College of Medicine, Rochester, MN*

JOHN D. ELLIOTT • *MMPD CEDD, GlaxoSmithKline, King of Prussia, PA*

JOHN R. ENGEN • *Department of Chemistry, University of New Mexico, Albuquerque, NM*

JAWED FAREED • *Department of Pathology, Loyola University Medical Center, Maywood, IL*

CAROLINE S. FINNERTY • *Bioinformatics and Pharmacogenomics Laboratory, National University of Ireland, Maynooth, County Kildare, Ireland*

DARREN R. FLOWER • *Edward Jenner Institute for Vaccine Research, Compton, Berkshire, UK*

THOMAS K. HARRIS • *Department of Biochemistry and Molecular Biology, Miller School of Medicine, University of Miami, Miami, FL*

CASEY S. HUSSER • *Department of Anesthesiology, Mayo Clinic College of Medicine, Rochester, MN*

OMER IQBAL • *Department of Pathology, Loyola University Medical Center, Maywood, IL*

ALEXIS S. IVANON • *Institute of Biomedial Chemistry, RAMS, Moscow, Russia*
ANTHONY G. JOHNSON • *CVU CEDD, GlaxoSmithKline, King of Prussia, PA*
SUMA KAVETI • *Lerner Research Institute Proteomics Core, Cleveland Clinic Foundation, Cleveland, OH*
RICHARD S. LARSON • *Department of Pathology, Cancer Research and Treatment Center, University of New Mexico School of Medicine, Albuquerque, NM*
KAREN E. LEE • *Department of Facilities and Systems Support Services, Mayo Clinic College of Medicine, Rochester, MN*
JAMES O. MCINERNEY • *Bioinformatics and Pharmacogenomics Laboratory, National University of Ireland, Maynooth, County Kildare, Ireland*
SCOTT A. NESS • *Department of Molecular Genetics and Microbiology, University of New Mexico School of Medicine, Albuquerque, NM*
ELIOT H. OHLSTEIN • *CVU CEDD, GlaxoSmithKline, King of Prussia, PA*
MARIUS M. OLAH • *Division of Biocomputing, Department of Biochemistry and Molecular Biology, University of New Mexico, Albuquerque, NM*
TUDOR I. OPREA • *Division of Biocomputing, Department of Biochemistry and Molecular Biology, University of New Mexico, Albuquerque, NM*
GAYLE K. PHILIP • *Bioinformatics and Pharmacogenomics Laboratory, National University of Ireland, Maynooth, County Kildare, Ireland*
O. SCOTT RAFFO • *Department of Anesthesiology, Mayo Clinic College of Medicine, Rochester, MN*
ANNE M. ROMANIC • *CVU CEDD, GlaxoSmithKline, King of Prussia, PA*
AMNON SHABO • *Healthcare and Life Sciences Group, IBM Research Lab, Haifa, Israel*
LAUREL O. SILLERUD • *Department of Biochemistry and Molecular Biology, University of New Mexico, Albuquerque, NM*
VLADLEN S. SKVORTSOV • *Institute of Biomedial Chemistry, RAMS, Moscow, Russia*
ALEXANDER V. VESELOVSKY • *Institute of Biomedial Chemistry, RAMS, Moscow, Russia*
SIQUN WANG • *Life Sciences and Chemical Analysis, Agilent Technologies Inc., Wilmington, DE*
XIWEI WU • *Keck Graduate Institute of Applied Life Sciences, Claremont, CA*

1

New Strategies in Drug Discovery

Eliot H. Ohlstein, Anthony G. Johnson, John D. Elliott, and Anne M. Romanic

Summary

Gene identification followed by determination of the expression of genes in a given disease and understanding of the function of the gene products is central to the drug discovery process. The ability to associate a specific gene with a disease can be attributed primarily to the extraordinary progress that has been made in the areas of gene sequencing and information technologies. Selection and validation of novel molecular targets have become of great importance in light of the abundance of new potential therapeutic drug targets that have emerged from human gene sequencing. In response to this revolution within the pharmaceutical industry, the development of high-throughput methods in both biology and chemistry has been necessitated. Further, the successful translation of basic scientific discoveries into clinical experimental medicine and novel therapeutics is an increasing challenge. As such, a new paradigm for drug discovery has emerged. This process involves the integration of clinical, genetic, genomic, and molecular phenotype data partnered with cheminformatics. Central to this process, the data generated are managed, collated, and interpreted with the use of informatics. This review addresses the use of new technologies that have arisen to deal with this new paradigm.

Key Words: Target validation; drug discovery; experimental medicine.

1. Introduction

The Human Genome Project was initiated on October 1, 1990, and the complete DNA sequence of the human genome was completed in 2001 (www.nhgri.nih.gov [1,2]). Central to the drug discovery process is gene identification followed by determination of the expression of genes in a given disease and understanding of the function of the gene products. It is of interest that the identification, in the early 1980s, of the gene believed to be responsible for cystic fibrosis took researchers approx 9 yr to discover, whereas the gene responsible for Parkinson's disease was identified within a period of several

From: *Methods in Molecular Biology, vol. 316: Bioinformatics and Drug Discovery*
Edited by: R. S. Larson © Humana Press Inc., Totowa, NJ

weeks *(3)*. This quantum leap in the ability to associate a specific gene with a disease can be attributed primarily to the extraordinary progress that has been made in the areas of gene sequencing and information technologies.

Selection and validation of novel molecular targets have become paramount in light of the abundance of new potential therapeutic drug targets that have emerged from human gene sequencing. The development of high-throughput methods in both biology and chemistry is therefore necessary. In addition, it has become increasingly challenging to translate successfully basic scientific discoveries into clinical experimental medicine and novel therapeutics. Consequently, a new paradigm for drug discovery has emerged. The integration of clinical, genetic, genomic, and molecular phenotype data partnered with cheminformatics is involved in this process. Central to this process, the data that are generated are managed, collated, and interpreted with the use of informatics. In this review, we address the use of new technologies that have arisen to deal with this new paradigm.

2. Target Validation

Several thousand molecular targets have now been cloned and are available as potential novel drug discovery targets. These targets include G protein-coupled receptors, ligand-gated ion channels, nuclear receptors, cytokines, and reuptake/transport proteins *(4)*. The sheer volume of information being produced has shifted the emphasis from the generation of novel DNA sequences to the determination of which of these many new targets offer the greatest opportunity for drug discovery. Thus, with several thousand potential targets available, target selection and validation have become the most critical component of the drug discovery process and will continue to be so in the future.

An example of the new paradigm of target selection comes as a result of the pairing of the orphan G protein-coupled receptor GPR-14 with its cognate neuropeptide ligand urotensin II. Urotensin II is the most potent vasoconstrictor identified to date; it is approximately one order of magnitude more potent than endothelin-1 *(5)*. Thus, GPR-14/urotensin II represents an attractive therapeutic target for the treatment of disorders related to or associated with enhanced vasoconstriction, such as hypertension, congestive heart failure, and coronary artery disease, to name but a few.

In general, most tissues express between 15,000 and 50,000 genes in different levels. In diseased tissue, gene expression levels often differ from those observed in normal tissues, with certain genes being over- or underexpressed, or new genes being expressed or completely absent. Localization of this differential gene expression is one of the first crucial steps in identifying an important potential molecular target for drug discovery. In addition to the traditional techniques of Northern analysis, a number of newer methods are used to localize gene expression. The techniques that typically yield the highest quality data are *in situ* hybridization (ISH) and immunocytochemistry, both of which are labor intensive. For example, ISH or immunohistochemical localization of a prospective molecular target to a particular tissue or subcellular region is likely to yield valuable information concerning gene function. Examples of the success of this approach include the case of the orexin peptides and receptors whose hypothalamic regional localization suggested an involvement in feeding *(6)*.

Each of these localization techniques has its advantages and disadvantages. ISH can be initiated immediately following gene sequencing and cloning; however, gene detection is only at the transcriptional mRNA level. Immunocytochemistry, on the other hand, offers the ability to measure protein expression but requires the availability of antibodies having the requisite affinity and selectivity, which may often take several months to generate. With either of these techniques, target localization within the cell is possible at the microscopic level but is dependent on the availability of high-quality normal and diseased human tissues, which may often represent a limiting factor.

The localization of a gene in a particular tissue does not necessarily shed light on all of the functions of that gene. As an example, the discovery of orexin as a putative regulator of energy balance and feeding was initially concluded as a result of localization in the dorsal and lateral hypothalamic regions of the brain *(6)*. However, subsequently this gene product was discovered to be a major sleep-modulating neurotransmitter that may represent the gene responsible for narcolepsy *(7)*.

Technologies, such as microarray gridding (GeneChip™) and TaqMan® polymerase chain reaction (PCR) that would appear destined to play a more prominent role in the high-throughput localization of genes, and the identification of their regulation in disease, have emerged *(8)*. Microarray gridding and Spotfire® data analysis are already evolving into procedures that allow the comprehensive evaluation of differences in gene expression patterns in normal, diseased, or pharmacologically manipulated systems *(8, 9)*. For genes expressed in low abundance, more sensitive techniques may be required, and reverse transcriptase (RT)-PCR-based TaqMan technology offers the ability to detect changes in gene expression with as little as two copies per cell. TaqMan technology also has the potential to be developed into a robust methodology for high-throughput tissue localization.

3. Functional Genomics

The term *functional genomics* is now being used to describe the post-Human Genome Project era and encompasses the many efforts needed to elucidate gene function. Traditionally, functional genomics pertains to the use of genetically manipulated animals, such as knockout or knockin mice or transgenic mice, to study a particular gene's function in vivo. Although these traditional methods are still a valuable tool in understanding gene function, more recently developed methods, such as RNA interference and mRNA silencing, offer an alternative that allows relatively faster methods of gene modification and function analysis in vivo *(10,11)*.

Indeed, the phenotyping of genetically manipulated animals is informative in determining the biological function of a particular gene. However, in reality, the discipline of functional genomics has its foundation in the physiological and pharmacological sciences. Although the evaluation of genetically manipulated animals requires a thorough understanding of physiology and pharmacology, the experimental approach involves many new technologies. These methods include in vivo imaging (i.e., magnetic resonance imaging, micropositron emission tomography, ultrafast computed tomography, infrared spectroscopy), mass spectrometry (MS), and microarray hybridization, all of which enhance the speed and accuracy at which functional genomics is achieved.

4. Proteomics, Metabolomics, and Lipomics

As high-throughput drug discovery has progressed through the genome, it is now moving toward assessing the proteome and metabolome. It is recognized that mRNA expression does not always correlate with protein expression *(12)*, and many factors such as alternative splicing, posttranslational modification (e.g., glycosylation, phosphorylation, oxidation, reduction), and mRNA turnover may account for this. Because modified proteins can have different biological activities, research and new technologies are now more focused on protein expression.

The term *proteome* refers to all the proteins produced by a species, much as the genome is the entire set of genes *(13)*. However, unlike the genome, the proteome can vary according to cell type and the functional state of the cell *(14,15)*. Proteomic analysis allows a point-in-time comparison of the protein profile, such as before and after therapeutic intervention. It can also be used to compare protein profiles in diseased and nondiseased tissues.

Microarrays are currently the major tool in the assessment of gene expression via cDNA and RNA analysis; however, they are also used to screen libraries of proteins and small molecules. Just as DNA microarrays allow the detection of changes in genes in various diseases, protein, peptide, tissue, and cell microarrays can be used to detect changes in proteins, phospholipids, or glycation of proteins in disease. Protein arrays are also used to examine enzyme–substrate, DNA–protein, and protein–protein interactions *(16,17)*. The practical application of proteomics depends on the ability to identify and analyze each protein product in a cell or tissue *(18)*. Because proteins cannot be amplified like DNA or RNA and proteins also tend to be degraded more readily, sensitive and rapid analyses are necessary to account for the small sample sizes and instability of proteins. Although this field is still developing, a MS and ProteinChip-surface-enhanced laser desorption/ionization technologies using slides with various surface properties (e.g., ion exchange, hydrophobic interaction, metal chelation) to bind and selectively purify proteins from a complex biological sample are being utilized *(18,19)*. An important challenge encountered with protein microarrays is maintaining functionality of the protein, such as posttranslational modifications and phosphorylation. Another important consideration is the retention of both secondary and tertiary structures. The use of immobilizing coatings, such as aluminum, gold, or hydrophilic polymers, on slides or imprinting the proteins on porous polyacrylamide gels is being explored to address these issues *(17)*. For example, proteomic analysis has been used successfully to identify serum biomarkers. ProteinChip-surface-enhanced laser desorption/ionization technology, in conjunction with bioinformatics tools, has been utilized to identify a proteomic pattern in serum that is diagnostic for ovarian cancer *(20)*. It is anticipated that proteomics and bioinformatics will facilitate the discovery of new and better biomarkers of disease.

Metabolomics is the study of the metabolome, which is the entire metabolic content of the cell or organism at any given moment *(21)*. Although metabolomics generally focuses on biofluids, such as serum and urine, investigators are now evaluating the cell as well. Metabolic profiling has been used regularly to characterize toxicity and disease states, such as inborn errors of metabolism. Additionally, blood and urine are screened routinely for metabolites such as cholesterol and glucose in patients to test for cardiovascular disease and diabetes. However, a recent advance in metabolomics is the analysis of small molecules within a sample to find new markers for disease or metabolic patterns as indicators for drug toxicity. Techniques such as nuclear magnetic resonance spectroscopy, MS, and chromatographic analysis of cell extracts are used in metabolomic research *(22,23)*. These techniques have been especially useful in generating lipid metabolome data (i.e., lipomics) to study the effects of dietary fats and lipid-lowering drugs on cardiac, plasma, adipose, and liver phospholipid metabolism *(22–27)*. Metabolic changes during tumor proliferation have also been studied using metabolomics. For example, the tumor metabolome is characterized by high glycolytic and glutaminolytic capacities and high phosphometabolite levels to allow tumor cells to proliferate over broad ranges in oxygen and glucose supply *(28)*. It is anticipated that metabolics will provide insight into the metabolism of tumor cells that might be helpful in understanding and modifying tumor cell proliferation.

5. High-Throughput Screening, Cheminformatics, and Medical Chemistry

During the last decade, the pharmaceutical industry has sought to expand its collections of compounds for the purpose of high-throughput screening (HTS) against novel molecular targets *(29)*. Many hit structures have been identified through HTS, and both the average potency and quality of these molecules continue to improve *(30)*. Although it is possible that a sustainable chemical lead can be identified from HTS, it has been more commonly the case that "hits" emerging from HTS require substantial chemical optimization to provide molecules with the desired level of potency, selectivity, and suitable pharmacokinetic (PK) properties *(31)* to support a fully fledged drug discovery program. Furthermore, the data available from an HTS effort are still of limited utility from the point of view of generating structure–activity relationships (SARs) capable of directing medicinal chemistry efforts. Combinatorial chemistry in some of its earliest incarnations was seen as a means of rapidly synthesizing massive numbers of molecules for HTS. However, in recent years this has evolved into the synthesis of more focused, smaller arrays of molecules directed both at enhancement of the properties of early hits emerging from HTS and at optimization of lead molecules in the progression toward development of candidates *(32,33)*. This change of emphasis has been enabled by significant developments in the areas of high-throughput purification and characterization.

In rising to the challenge of providing HTS data on collections of a million or more compounds, the scientist involved in HTS has sought increasing use of automation, as well as miniaturization, to reduce the demands on precious protein reagents and chemical supplies. Traditional radioligand-binding assays are giving way to more rapid and easily miniaturizable homogeneous fluorescence-based methods. The increased efficiency of ultra-HTS offers the potential to screen discrete collections of a million or more single compounds, at multiple concentrations, and thereby generate SAR information to "jump-start" a medicinal chemical lead optimization effort. Historically, medicinal chemical endeavors have involved the analysis of detailed biological data from hundreds or perhaps thousands of compounds. It is not surprising that the prospect of such an explosive growth of information from both screening- and program-directed combinatorial chemistry has driven the evolution of cheminformatics *(34)*, in much the same way that genomic sequencing gave rise to the science of bioinformatics.

The successful medicinal chemical drug discovery effort of the future will rely on a hybrid approach of parallel and iterative (single-molecule) synthesis. As HTS collections are built up through parallel synthesis, lead structures will be amenable to high-throughput follow-up. Iterative analog preparation will, however, continue to play a key role. In particular, as a research program nears candidate selection, a greater level of iterative synthesis will likely become necessary to "fine-tune" the properties of the lead molecules. The lead optimization phase of the drug discovery process also relies heavily on SARs developed around absorption, distribution, metabolism, and excretion data, and physiochemical properties that improve the overall developability of the series (e.g., solubility, permeability, P450 activity, and human ether-a-go-go-related gene potassium channel activity). It is anticipated that the greater attention given to the evaluation of developability characteristics in candidate molecules will lead to reduced attrition, improving the likelihood that a compound will enter clinical development and be successful in getting to market in a time- and cost-effective manner.

6. Pharmacogenomics, Toxicogenomics, and Predictive Toxicology

Just as it is possible that a compound can affect gene expression in a positive manner, so too can it affect gene expression in a negative, toxic manner. In addition, a drug might not affect gene expression in a given subpopulation that is representative of the larger group. In an attempt to identify how genes are expressed following drug treatment or to determine toxicity issues associated with a compound, DNA arrays can be used for what are termed *pharmacogenomic* and *toxicogenomic* studies *(35)*. Pharmacogenomics refers to the identification of genes that are involved in determining drug responsiveness and that may cause differential drug responses in different patients. These studies include the evaluation of allelic differences in gene expression, and the evaluation of genes responsible for drug resistance and sensitivity *(35,36)*. Toxicogenomics refers to the characterization of potential genes involved in toxicity and the adverse effects of drugs *(35,37)*. Toxicogenomics allows for a gene profile of candidate biomarkers of toxicity and carcinogenicity. *Predictive toxicology* is a term used for the application of toxicogenomics and the evaluation of compounds *in silico* against a panel of genes associated with toxicity *(38)*. Models of SAR are used to predict potential toxic effects based on chemical structures and their properties *(39)*. Predictive toxicology also takes into account computer-based predictions of adsorption, distribution, metabolism, and excretion and PK properties in addition to toxicology, all of which contribute to the lead optimization process.

7. Experimental Medicine

With the identification of many new targets for drug development, it is increasingly important to test rapidly and accurately the effects of new chemical entities in the early phase of development in relevant in vivo models, including humans. For example, drug candidates aimed at inflammation can be tested in a human blister model *(40, 41)*. In this model, suction is applied to the forearm of healthy volunteers following preexposure to ultraviolet-B light. The resulting blister is used to evaluate secreted inflammatory mediators and changes in gene expression within 48 h of insult. Cell counts, prostaglandin (PG)E_2 (measured by enzyme-linked immunosorbent assay), PGD_2 (measured by gas chromatography), and gene expression of cyclo-oxygenase-2, and PGE and PGD synthases (measured by real-time PCR) are assessed. This model allows the rapid analysis of effects of drugs on cellular infiltration, soluble mediator formation in blister fluid, and steady-state gene expression in cellular infiltrates. These markers (e.g., new transcription factors, cytokines, and other mediators) can be followed in both the inflammatory and resolution phases of human inflammation. In addition, coupled with DNA array technology, this model may be useful in defining new targets for the treatment of inflammation. Furthermore, toxicity and efficacy profiles of new and existing drugs can be studied. For example, a gene chip of the subset of human genes identified in blister fluid can be used to identify surrogate markers of toxicity and efficacy in modulating gene expression in drug evaluation.

Inflammation also plays an important role in the initiation and progression of atherosclerosis. To this end, identification of relevant signaling pathways that mediate plaque inflammation may provide therapeutic targets for the improvement of clinical outcomes in high-risk individuals. For example, inhibition of p38 mitogen-activated protein kinase (MAPK) attenuates inflammatory responses and matrix-degrading activities in human atherosclerotic plaque, suggesting a potential therapeutic strategy for the regression and stabilization of atherosclerosis. Signaling mechanisms involving p38 MAPK as well as other inflammatory responses can be characterized by TaqMan real-time RT-PCR in human carotid atherosclerotic plaques and nonatherosclerotic vessels. In addition, the biological effects of the p38 MAPK pathway can be assessed in an ex vivo organ culture system *(42)*. In these studies, a selective p38 MAPK inhibitor is added to the organ culture system and a variety of analyses are conducted. Current analyses of human plaque specimens include a panel of markers, such as interleukin (IL)-1β, IL-6, IL-8, monocyte chemoattractant protein-1, tumor necrosis factor-α, and matrix metalloproteinases. Other analyses include the evaluation of phosphorylated p38 MAPK, extracellular signal-regulated kinase 1/2, and c-Jun NH_2-terminal kinase.

These and other in vivo and ex vivo human experimental platforms are of tremendous value and can be used to validate the efficacy and assess the toxicity of drugs early in development. Because these studies are conducted in the clinical setting, the field of experimental medicine offers great potential in identifying new therapeutic targets particularly relevant to human disease.

Pharmacogenomics, also referred to as pharmacogenetics, involves the study of variability in pharmacokinetics (absorption, distribution, metabolism, or elimination) or pharmacodynamics (relationship between drug concentrations and pharmacological effects or the time course of such effects) owing to hereditary factors in different populations. There is evidence that genotype may impact the incidence of adverse events for a given drug. The aim is to identify genetic polymorphic variants that represent risk factors for the development of a particular clinical condition, or that predict a given response to a specific therapeutic. More important, the rate-limiting step in revealing biologically relevant phenotype–genotype associations is the collection of human DNA

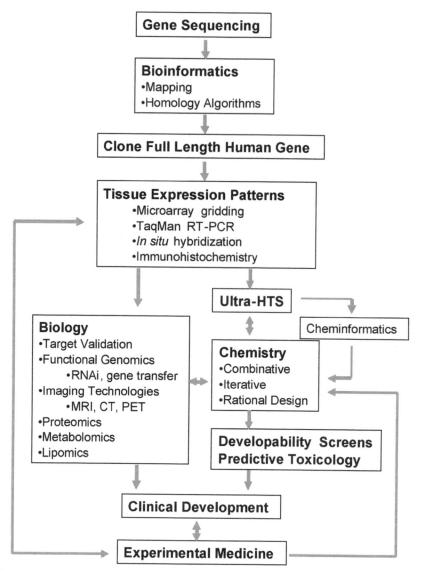

Fig. 1. Progression of molecular targets to novel therapeutics under a new paradigm for drug discovery.

samples from carefully phenotyped individuals *(43)*. Two general approaches may be used to investigate genetic variation in drug handling or response: (1) the hypothesis-driven method is based on *a priori* hypotheses and involves selecting specific sections of DNA known to encode the drug target, drug-metabolizing enzymes, disease or genetic regions associated with mechanisms of action, or adverse effects; and (2) the genome-wide scan investigates a large number of single nucleotide polymorphisms (SNPs) covering the entire genome with the aim of identifying a collection of SNPs that are associated with differential drug handling or response.

In addition to investigating variability in efficacy, pharmacogenetics allows detection of susceptibility to relatively uncommon but severe adverse events that otherwise would not be detected until large numbers of patients had been exposed to a given drug. For example, 4% of individuals with human immunodeficiency virus treated with the antiretroviral Abacavir develop a specific hypersensitivity reaction *(44)*. Lai et al. *(45)* identified a 250,000-bp region of extended linkage disequilibrium that was associated with this hypersensitivity reaction. Several SNPs were predictive in that individuals with these SNPs (e.g., human leukocyte antigen B57) taking Abacavir had a 97% chance of experiencing the adverse event, although only 50% of the individuals who experienced the adverse event while taking Abacavir actually carried the variants (i.e., 97% specific, 50% sensitive). More important, these approaches may generate a large amount of data and statistical methods must adjust for multiple testing while attempting to tease out gene–gene and gene–environment interactions from gene–disease or gene–response to treatment associations.

8. Conclusion

The tremendous impact of unraveling the mysteries of the genome is currently being felt across all areas of drug discovery, and major challenges for the pharmaceutical industry are in the areas of drug target selection and validation. **Figure 1** shows the progression of new molecular targets into novel drugs under this new paradigm for drug discovery. One can already anticipate the future availability of genetic structure and susceptibility to disease at the individual level. With such information available early in a research program, the drug discovery scientist is faced with the unprecedented opportunity to address the individual variability to drug therapy and safety prior to advancing a compound into clinical trials. The exponential growth of attractive novel molecular targets for potential drug therapy has heavily taxed the core disciplines of drug discovery, and automated methods of compound synthesis and biological evaluation will play an even more dominant role in the future of the pharmaceutical industry.

References

1. Vanter, J. C., et al. (2001) The sequence of the human genome. *Science* **291,** 1304–1351.
2. Lander, E. S., et al. (2001) Initial sequencing and analysis of the human genome. *Nature* **409,** 860–921.
3. Venkatesh, T. V., Bowen, B., and Lim, H. A. (1999) Bioinformatics, pharma and farmers. *Trends Biotechnol.* **17,** 85–88.
4. Stadel, J. M., Wilson, S., and Bergsma, D. (1997) Orphan G protein-coupled receptors: a neglected opportunity for pioneer drug discovery. *Trends Pharmacol. Sci.* **18(11),** 430–437.
5. Ames, R. S., Sarau, H. M., Chambers, J., et al. (1999) Human urotensin-II, the most potent vasoconstrictor identified, is a ligand at the novel receptor GPR-14. *Nature* **401,** 282–286.
6. Sakurai, T., Amemiya, A., Ishii, M., et al. (1998) Orexins and orexin receptors: a family of hypothalamic neuropeptides and G protein-coupled receptors that regulate feeding behavior. *Cell* **92,** 573–585.

7. Lin, L., Faraco, J., Li, R., et al. (1999) The sleep disorder canine narcolepsy is caused by a mutation in the hypocretin (orexin) receptor 2 gene. *Cell* **98,** 365–376.

8. Debouck, C. and Metcalf, B. (2000) The impact of genomics on drug discovery. *Annu. Rev. Pharmacol. Toxicol.* **40,** 193–207.

9. Ahlberg, C. (1999) Visual exploration of HTS databases: bridging the gap between chemistry and biology. *Drug Discov. Today* **4,** 370–376.

10. Laatsch, A., Ragozin, S., Grewal, T., Beisiegel, U., and Joerg, H. (2004) Differential RNA interference: replacement of endogenous with recombinant low density lipoprotein receptor–related protein (LPR). *Eur. J. Cell Biol.* **83,** 113–120.

11. Pederson, T. (2004) RNA interference and mRNA silencing, 2004: how far will they reach? *Mol. Biol. Cell* **15,** 407–410.

12. Gygi, S. P., Rochon, Y., Franza, B. R., and Aebersold, R. (1999) Correlation between protein and mRNA abundance in yeast. *Mol. Cell. Biol.* **19,** 1720–1730.

13. Kvasnicka, F. (2003) Proteomics: general strategies and application to nutritionally relevant proteins. *J. Chromatogr.* **787,** 77–89.

14. Marshall, T. and Williams, K. M. (2002) Proteomics and its impact upon biomedical science. *Br. J. Biomed. Sci.* **59,** 47–64.

15. Panisko, E. A., Conrads, T. P., Goshe, M. B., and Veenstra, T. D. (2002) The postgenomic age: characterization of proteomes. *Exp. Hematol.* **30,** 97–107.

16. Gerhold, D. L. (2002) Better therapeutics through microarrays. *Nat. Genet.* **32,** S547–S551.

17. MacBeath, G. and Schreiber, S. L. (2000) Printing proteins as microarrays for high-throughput function determination. *Science* **289,** 1760–1763.

18. Witzmann, F. A. and Grant, R. A. (2003) Pharmacoproteomics in drug development. *Pharmacogenom. J.* **3,** 69–76.

19. He, Q. Y., Yip, T. T., Li, M., and Chiu, J. F. (2003) Proteomic analysis of arsenic-induced cell transformation with SELDI-TOF ProteinChip technology. *J. Cell Biochem.* **88,** 1–8.

20. Petricoin, E. F., Ardekani, A., Hitt, B. A., et al. (2002) Use of proteomic patterns in serum to identify ovarian cancer. *Lancet* **359,** 572–577.

21. Adams, A. (2003) Metabolomics: small molecule "omics." *Scientist* **17,** 38–40.

22. Watkins, S. M. and German, J. B. (2002) Toward the implementation of metabolomic assessments of human health and nutrition. *Curr. Opin. Biotechnol.* **13,** 512–516.

23. Watkins, S. M. (2004) Lipomic profiling in drug discovery, development and clinical trial evaluation. *Curr. Opin. Drug Discov. Dev.* **7,** 112–117.

24. Watkins, S. M., Hammock, B. D., Newman, J. W., and German, J. B. (2001) Individual metabolism should guide agriculture toward foods for improved health and nutrition. *Am. J. Clin. Nutr.* **74,** 283–286.

25. Watkins, S. M., Lin, T. Y., Davis, R. M., et al. (2001) Unique phospholipid metabolism in mouse heart in response to dietary docosahexaenoic or α-linolenic acids. *Lipids* **36,** 247–254.

26. Watkins, S. M., Reifsnyder, P. R., Pan, H., German, J. B., and Leiter, E. H. (2002) Lipid metabolome-wide effects of the PPAR-γ agonist rosiglitozone. *J. Lipid Res.* **43,** 1809–1811.

27. Fitzgerald, D. A. (2001) Drug discovery: lipid profiling for studying the metabolome. *Gen. Eng. News* **21,** 32–36.

28. Mazurek, S. and Eigenbrodt, E. (2003) The tumor metabolome. *Anticancer Res.* **23,** 1149–1154.

29. Doherty, A. M., Patt, W. C., Edmunds, J. J., et al. (1995) Discovery of a novel series of orally active non-peptide endothelin-A (ETA) receptor-selective antagonists. *J. Med. Chem.* **38,** 1259–1263.

30. Mullin, R. (2004) Drug discovery: as high-throughput screening draws fire, researchers leverage science to put automation into perspective. *Chem. Eng. News* **82,** 23–32.
31. Anonymous. (2000) Computational chemistry. *Nat. Biotech.* **18,** IT50–IT52.
32. Lee, A. and Breitenbucher, J. G. (2003) The impact of combinatorial chemistry on drug discovery. *Curr. Opin. Drug Discov. Dev.* **6,** 494–508.
33. Dolle, R. E. (2004) Comprehensive survey of combinatorial library synthesis: 2003. *J. Comb. Chem.* **6,** 623–679.
34. Lipinski, C. A., Lombardo, F., Dominy, B. W., and Feeney, P. J. (1997) Experimental and computational approaches to estimate solubility and permeability in drug discovery and development settings. *Adv. Drug Deliv. Rev.* **23(1–3),** 3–25.
35. Chin, K. V. and Kong, A. N. T. (2002) Application of DNA microarrays in pharmaco-genomics and toxicogenomics. *Pharm. Res.* **19,** 1773–1778.
36. Sengupta, L. K., Sengupta, S., and Sarkar, M. (2002) Pharmacogenetic applications of the post genomic era. *Curr. Pharm. Biotechnol.* **3,** 141–150.
37. Tugwood, J. D., Hollins, L. E., and Cockerill, M. J. (2003) Genomics and the search for novel biomarkers in toxicology. *Biomarkers* **8,** 79–92.
38. Wilson, A. G. E., White, A. C., and Mueller, R. A. (2003) Role of predictive metabolism and toxicity modeling in drug discovery—a summary of some recent advancements. *Curr. Opin. Drug Discov. Dev.* **6,** 123–128.
39. Helma, C. and Kramer, S. (2003) A survey of the predictive toxicology challenge 2000–2001. *Bioinformatics* **19,** 1179–1182.
40. Cooper, S., Parisis, K., Day, R. O., and Williams, K. M. (2000) The skin suction blister: a human model of inflammation. *Proc. Aust. Soc. Clin. Exp. Pharmacol. Toxicol.* **8,** 140–147.
41. Follin, P. (1999) Skin chamber technique for study of in vivo excudated human neutro-phils. *J. Immunol. Methods* **232,** 55–65.
42. Zhang, L., Mazurek, T., Zalewski, A. (2005) Regulation of inflammatory responses and matrix degrading activities by p38 MAPK in advanced human atherosclerotic plaque, in press.
43. Roses, A. D. (2004) Pharmacogenetics and drug development: the path to safer and more effective drugs. *Nat. Rev. Genet.* **5,** 645–656.
44. Hetherington, A., Hughes, A. R., Mosteller, M., et al. (2002) Genetic variations in HLA-B region and hypersensitivity reactions to abacavir. *Lancet* **359,** 1121–1122.
45. Lai, E., Bowman, C., Bansal, A., Hughes, A., Mosteller, M., and Roses, A. D. (2002) Medicinal applications of haplotype-based SNP maps: learning to walk before we run. *Nat. Genet.* **32,** 353.

2

Basic Microarray Analysis

Strategies for Successful Experiments

Scott A. Ness

Summary

Microarrays offer a powerful approach to the analysis of gene expression that can be used for a wide variety of experimental purposes. However, several types of microarray platforms are available. In addition, microarray experiments are expensive and generate complicated data sets that can be difficult to interpret. Success with microarray approaches requires a sound experimental design and a coordinated and appropriate use of statistical tools. Here, the advantages and pitfalls of utilizing microarrays are discussed, as are practical strategies to help novice users succeed with this method that can empower them with the ability to assay changes in gene expression at the whole-genome level.

Key Words: Microarrays; Affymetrix; GeneChips; genomics; gene expression; transcription; clustering; normalization; data analysis; hybridization.

1. Introduction

The large-scale genome-sequencing projects have identified most or all of the genes in humans, mice, rats, yeast, and a number of other commonly used experimental systems. At the time of this writing, the publicly available human genome information available from the National Center for Biotechnology Information includes more than 2.8×10^9 nucleotides of finished, annotated DNA sequence. Although the exact number of genes continually fluctuates as annotation and gene prediction programs change and improve, the current number of human genes is nearly 43,000 (Human genome build 34, version 3). (Information about the current human genome build is available at www.ncbi.nlm.nih.gov.) Microarrays provide a means of measuring changes in expression of all the genes at once. This ability provides researchers with enormous potential to perform experiments that were impossible just a few years ago and also offers unique challenges in experimental design and data analysis.

From: *Methods in Molecular Biology, vol. 316: Bioinformatics and Drug Discovery*
Edited by: R. S. Larson © Humana Press Inc., Totowa, NJ

Microarray experiments and the laboratories that perform them can be divided into several categories. First are the laboratories that specialize in microarray technology and that perform experiments with hundreds of microarray samples. Such research groups are often responsible for developing new methods of microarray data analysis and include dedicated groups of biostatisticians and computer programmers working to improve the statistical methods and computer programs for analyzing complex data sets generated by very large microarray experiments. A second class of laboratories has performed dozens of microarray experiments and has already become familiar with the data analysis tools necessary to accomplish their goals. Such laboratories generally make use of commercial software for data analysis or "freeware" packages written by the aforementioned large groups. This chapter is geared toward the third group: the laboratories that are considering their first microarray experiments and that need help with experimental design and data analysis. New users are most likely to rely on a core facility to actually perform the microarray experiments. For that reason, I do not discuss the details of manufacturing, manipulating, hybridizing, and scanning the microarrays here. Instead, the goal is to outline the potential benefits and pitfalls that arise with microarray experiments in order to help new users avoid common mistakes and reap the most benefit from experiments that can be very expensive and time-consuming. In addition, the commercial microarray platform offered by Affymetrix (Santa Clara, CA) is the most dominant and readily available means for new users to begin performing microarray experiments. Consequently, this chapter focuses on the Affymetrix platform and its use in the academic laboratory, although most or all of the discussion also applies to custom spotted arrays produced by local microarray facilities. There is a wide variety of uses for microarrays, including detection of single nucleotide polymorphisms, analysis of alternative RNA splicing, and analysis of transcription factors binding to promoters (ChIP on a Chip). However, here the discussion is limited to the use of microarrays for gene expression analysis, the most common use of the platform and the most likely way that new users will be tempted to use microarray technology.

2. When Is a Microarray the Best Approach?

Microarray experiments are extremely powerful and provide researchers with a new and exciting means of tackling important problems on a genomewide scale. Most microarrays contain probes for 10,000–40,000 different genes, allowing researchers to assess simultaneously changes in expression of nearly all the genes in the genome. However, they are also complex, time-consuming, and often very expensive experiments, and they generate large and complicated data sets that require substantial effort to analyze and validate. For these reasons, researchers should not be lured into performing microarray experiments without spending some time considering other options or without considerable thought regarding appropriate experimental design. New users should consult extensively with their local microarray core facility before beginning to prepare samples for microarray analysis. Every microarray facility can tell stories about users who approached them with samples only to find out that unsuitable preparation or storage had resulted in RNA that was too degraded for high-quality analysis. Proper preparation and storage of the RNA is crucial to the success of microarray experiments.

This is especially true for samples derived from patients or tissues that are difficult or impossible to replace. The microarray facility should be able to guide users to the best methods for preparing samples and storing the RNA to ensure that their experiments will succeed. Because of these limitations, some experiments are better suited for microarray analysis than others.

2.1. For Better or Worse: What Can Microarrays Do?

Microarray technology has proven to be extremely powerful for following changes in gene expression that occur as synchronized cells progress through the cell cycle *(1,2)* or when tissue culture cells are treated with a drug *(3,4)* or are infected with a virus expressing a recombinant transcription factor *(5,6)*. In such situations, all the cells in the population are responding in parallel and relatively synchronously, and the microarrays, which measure the average change in gene expression in the population of cells being studied, can detect changes in gene expression that occur simultaneously in all the cells. Because of variations in measurements, microarrays are best at detecting changes that are relatively robust—a twofold or greater change is a common benchmark—in genes that are expressed at relatively high levels. Cells from different individuals, such as different patients, can display markedly different gene expression patterns, so microarrays perform best when the samples are closely related, such as tissue culture cells or treated vs untreated cells from a single patient or animal. Because different cell types display complex differences in gene expression patterns, heterogeneous samples, such as solid tumors or tissue samples, give complex microarray results. Optimum results are obtained from homogeneous samples, such as cell lines or purified cell populations, when they are available.

Some experiments are poorly suited for microarray analysis or need a modified design to make them work. For example, many researchers would like to transfect tissue culture cells with a plasmid expressing a molecule of interest and then use microarrays to measure subsequent changes in gene expression. The problem with this approach is that transfections are often inefficient and generally only yield 5–10% of cells expressing the molecule of interest. Because microarrays measure the average changes in gene expression in all the cells in the culture, a gene would have to be induced at least 20-fold in the transfected cells to show up as twofold induced when averaged over the entire cell population. A better design would be to transfect the cells with a plasmid that expresses the protein of interest as well as green fluorescent protein or some other marker that would allow the transfected (e.g., green fluorescent protein-positive) cells to be purified by flow cytometry before performing the microarray analysis. Alternatively, recombinant adenoviruses or some other method of expressing the protein of interest in nearly 100% of the cells in the culture could be used in place of transfection *(5,6)*. The goal is to compare the changes in gene expression in one nearly homogeneous population with those in another.

Changes in gene expression patterns have been used to provide evidence that particular biochemical, signaling, or transcription factor pathways are activated or inhibited in different cell types *(7,8)*. Microarrays can detect subtle changes in gene expression induced by a variety of extracellular or environmental stimuli *(9,10)*. However, such results can be quite complicated. In general, microarray experiments should be designed with some hypothesis in mind, rather than just as a "fishing" experiment. By testing a hypothesis, it will be possible to design positive and negative controls that will greatly facilitate the data analysis. This is discussed in more detail under **Heading 4**.

3. Choosing a Microarray Platform

The first choice a new user will have to make is which type of microarray to use. Essentially, microarrays are thousands of spots or probes immobilized on a solid surface such as glass or silicon that can be hybridized simultaneously to fluorescently labeled experimental samples, referred to as targets. In the simplest scenario (**Fig. 1**), mRNA from each sample is used as template in a complementary (c)DNA synthesis reaction that includes dinucleotide triphosphates labeled with fluorescent tags, usually Cy3 or Cy5. The resulting fluorescent target cDNA is hybridized to the microarray, which contains cDNA or oligonucleotide probes for each gene of interest. Usually, a separate microarray is used for each experimental sample. After washing, a laser scanner is used to measure the fluorescence at each spot, and the data are converted into a spreadsheet format showing the relative intensity or expression of each gene. Several variations on this theme provide increased sensitivity or reproducibility. For example, in the Affymetrix GeneChip system, the target samples are labeled with biotin and are detected with fluorescent streptavidin. However, even from this simple description of microarray technology, it is apparent that the most important parameters in the assay are the quality of the samples, the efficiency of the labeling with fluorescent nucleotides, and the quality and reproducibility of the gene-specific probes on the microarray.

3.1. Glass Slide Arrays

The first microarrays were produced by using modified writing pens to spot samples of DNA directly onto glass microscope slides. After chemical or ultraviolet (UV) cross-linking to fix the DNA to the glass, the fluorescently labeled cDNAs were applied in a drop of hybridization buffer, covered with a standard cover slip, and allowed to hybridize overnight. This is still the basic process for most microarrays produced in core facilities, although the machines that make the arrays have become highly automated and new chemistries and surfaces have been developed to make the glass slides more efficient at binding the DNA and to decrease the background in the hybridization. There are also differences in what types of DNA probes are attached to the glass.

3.1.1. cDNA Arrays

The first laboratories that made extensive use of microarrays spotted libraries of cDNA clones, either polymerase chain reaction (PCR)-amplified inserts or whole plasmids, directly onto glass slides. The use of relatively long (>300 bp) cDNAs has advantages and disadvantages. The biggest advantage is that the hybridization is quite robust Thus, point mutations or even small deletions that might occur in some individuals will have little or no impact on the results of the hybridization. This feature makes cDNA arrays quite useful for studies of large sets of human patients who might have minor differences in some of their genes. Another advantage of using cDNAs is the relatively low

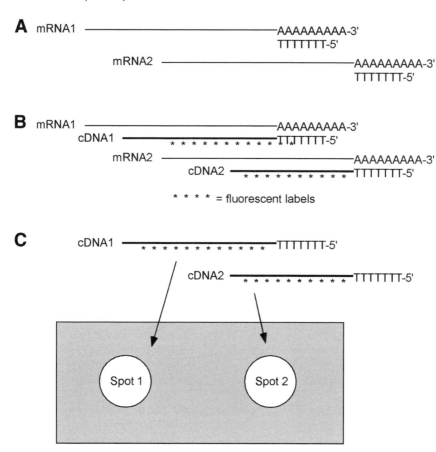

Fig. 1. Basic steps in microarray analysis. (**A**) Starting RNA. Purified mRNA is annealed with a primer (oligo-dT), ready for the reverse transcription reaction. At this point, control RNAs are often added ("spiked in") to give an internal control for the efficiency of the following steps. (**B**) Labeled cDNAs. In the simplest case, reverse transcription is performed using fluorescently tagged (e.g., Cy3 or Cy5), dinucleotide triphosphates (dNTPs), resulting in the generation of fluorescent cDNA. In the Affymetrix system, the dNTPs are biotinylated, and later detection is performed with fluorescent streptavidin. (**C**) Target hybridization. The fluorescently labeled cDNAs, referred to as "targets," are hybridized to gene-specific "probes." Each target anneals to its corresponding probe spot on the microarray. The probes can be spotted cDNAs or oligonucleotides, or oligonucleotides that were synthesized directly on the microarray surface. Although only two spots are shown, a single microarray can have probes for up to 50,000 different genes and more than a million spots per square inch. After hybridization, a laser scanner is used to detect the specific fluorescence at each spot. If all goes well, fluorescence intensity is proportional to the concentration of the relevant mRNA in the original sample.

cost. A single miniprep or PCR reaction can generate enough purified DNA to produce many thousand microarrays. Owing to their long lengths, the spotted cDNAs are likely to detect all the transcripts, such as different versions produced through alternative promoter use or alternative RNA splicing, which could be an advantage. Major disadvantages are the cost and effort required to assemble large libraries of purified cDNAs or PCR products, all of which must be correctly identified, subjected to nucleotide sequencing, and annotated. There have been problems with collections of cDNAs provided by commercial suppliers, which contain a large fraction of clones that are improperly identified or contaminated with other plasmids that interfere with PCR amplification. In addition, cDNAs can contain repeated sequences and may hybridize to closely related transcripts (gene families) and so may not provide enough specificity for many applications. Because cDNAs vary in length and G-C content, it is difficult to ensure that all will hybridize equally well or give the same amount of background signal. These disadvantages make cDNAs difficult to work with and have contributed to their waning popularity.

3.1.2. Oligonucleotide Arrays

The most common type of glass slide microarrays use custom oligonucleotides, usually 40 to 60 mer, instead of cDNAs. The oligonucleotides, if designed properly, can overcome problems of specificity and G-C content associated with using cDNAs. There are generally fewer problems with improper identification or labeling when ordering custom oligonucleotides from commercial suppliers, although one must still trust the supplier to synthesize and purify them correctly and to put the correct oligonucleotides in each tube. The major drawbacks of using oligonucleotides are the relatively high cost of purchasing 10,000 or more custom oligonucleotides and the huge amount of bioinformatics support required to design all the necessary bits of DNA specific for each gene with matched G-C content and free of hairpins that could affect hybridization efficiency. Depending on how the oligonucleotides are designed, they might still suffer from some of the specificity problems associated with cDNAs. Complete sets of oligonucleotides are now available from commercial suppliers, greatly simplifying their use by microarray core facilities producing homemade microarrays. Nevertheless, because of the cost, it is rare for such collections to contain intentionally more than one oligonucleotide representing each gene.

3.1.3. Advantages and Disadvantages of Glass Slide Microarrays

The biggest advantage of using homemade or in-house-produced glass slide microarrays is the relatively low cost, generally less than $100 per array. However, such arrays are limited to 20,000 or fewer spots per array, so more than one array is necessary to screen an entire mammalian genome. It is also rare to have more than one spot for any gene on each array. Thus, if there are any discrepancies in the production of the arrays, such as some spots that get too little DNA or that are misshaped or smeared, there are no backup spots from that gene to confirm the hybridization results. Unfortunately, not all spots are identical on any spotted array, which makes the data subject to more variability and also makes multiple hybridizations absolutely essential. As a consequence, most users hybridize their samples to several identical arrays in order to have multiple measurements and to be able to perform statistics for each spot. This increases the cost substantially. Thus, if a single array costs $80, two arrays are necessary to rep-

Table 1
Comparison of Microarray Platforms

	Glass slide arrays	Affymetrix GeneChips
Typical cost per array	$80	$450
Arrays per 40,000 genes	2	1
Measurements per gene on each array	1	12
Arrays needed per sample to achieve at least three measurements per gene	6	1
Array cost per sample	$480	$450
Typical amount of total RNA needed per array	10 µg	0.1–1 µg
Total amount of RNA needed from each sample	>30 µg	<1 µg
Total arrays needed for a three-sample experiment (untreated, control-treated, experimental-treated) performed in duplicate	36	6
Total array cost	$2880	$2700

resent 40,000 human genes, and each sample is hybridized to three independent arrays in order to generate statistically significant measurements, each biological sample would require a total of six arrays, or a total cost of $480 just for the arrays. Thus, the apparent cost savings by using homemade arrays often disappears when the problems associated with such arrays are considered in the bigger picture (**Table 1**).

3.2. Affymetrix GeneChips

The most common commercial microarray platform is the GeneChip system from Affymetrix. GeneChips are made by synthesizing matched sets of short oligonucleotide pairs, one that matches perfectly (perfect match) and one with a single mismatch, on a silicon-based substrate using a photolithographic process similar to methods used in the computer chip industry. The newest GeneChips contain at least 12 pairs of probe sets for each gene; contain probe sets for more than 50,000 human, mouse, or rat genes; and generally cost academic users about $450 apiece. Having multiple probe sets for each gene ensures that even if part of the GeneChip surface becomes damaged or obscured by background, enough probe sets will still be readable to salvage the experiment. Multiple probe sets also allow statistical analyses to be performed, so both an expression level and a p value of expression can be reported for each gene. The Affymetrix system includes detailed protocols that rely on commercially available kits, automated fluidics stations for washing the arrays after hybridization, and an automated scanner and software package for analyzing the arrays. The complete system is expensive but produces very high-quality data and is relatively user-friendly, so it is the platform of choice for mainstream microarray facilities and for novice microarray users. The analysis kits from Affymetrix can be used with very small amounts of total RNA, even less than 20 ng, and new kits and specially designed GeneChips offer the ability to analyze samples extracted from paraffin-embedded clinical samples, making the analysis of gene expression in archived samples a possibility. The key feature of the Affymetrix system is the high-density GeneChips, which are available for several mammalian species and several other common experimental organisms. Researchers studying gene expression in unrepresented organisms will need an alternative approach or will have to contract with Affymetrix (for a substantial fee) to produce customized GeneChips for their unique needs.

As shown in **Table 1**, for users who wish to screen more than 20,000 genes (which requires two spotted glass slide microarrays but only one Affymetrix GeneChip) and to have high-quality data (which requires at least three glass slide microarrays but only one GeneChip), experiments with Affymetrix GeneChips can be less expensive than using glass slide microarrays.

4. Types of Microarray Experiments

Most microarray experiments can be classified as one of three types. The first is the comparison of a single cell line, micro-organism, or animal strain before or after some defined treatment. The second type is a comparison of organisms (micro-organisms, cell lines, or inbred animals) that are isogenic except for one or a limited number of genetic changes, such as a single overexpressed or mutated gene. The third type is the comparison of normal or tumor tissues from multiple individuals, such as breast tumors or leukemia samples from different patients. Each of these types of experiments can be addressed with great success using microarray assays, provided that certain pitfalls can be avoided.

4.1. Treatment Comparisons

Treating a cell line or micro-organism with a specific treatment condition such as UV light or a drug that blocks a signal transduction cascade generates immediate and rapid changes in gene expression that can be detected with microarray assays. This is the simplest type of microarray experiment to analyze, because all the cells should behave similarly and relatively synchronously following the treatment. Nevertheless, there are several things to consider about such an experiment, such as the time course or duration of the treatment and the dose, etc., that can have dramatic effects. For example, the gene expression changes that occur 2 h after UV treatment of a human tissue culture cell line could be completely different from the changes observed 8 h after treatment. In addition, cells that are synchronized in the cell cycle could show significant differences compared with cells that are growing asynchronously or are density arrested. Thus, new users are encouraged to spend some time thinking about exactly what type of gene expression changes are expected, and in what type of cells those changes would be best detected.

An example from our laboratory illustrates this point. We developed recombinant adenovirus vectors expressing the c-Myb transcription factor. The c-Myb virus or a control virus was used to infect human MCF-7 mammary cells, primary lung epithelial cells, or primary lung fibroblasts. After 16 h, microarray assays were used to detect changes in gene expression. In each case, the c-Myb transcription factor caused specific changes in gene expression. However, the genes that were affected were completely different in each of the three cell types, suggesting that c-Myb transcriptional activity was strongly affected by cellular context (5). In this case, if we were trying to identify genes that were regulated by c-Myb, we would have obtained completely different results in each cell type. Similarly, UV light or drug treatments could cause different gene expression changes in different cell types. Thus, it is crucial to study induced gene expression changes in the most relevant cell type available.

4.2. Analysis of Genetic Differences

A second type of experiment involves comparing otherwise isogenic organisms that differ at a single genetic locus, through either overexpression or mutation. Such experiments are especially common with yeast, cell lines, and genetically altered mice, or with cell lines derived from mouse knockout strains. These experiments differ from the ones described in **Subheading 4.1.** because the gene expression changes are at steady state. For example, researchers might use microarrays to compare the gene expression patterns in cells that differ by a mutation at a single genetic locus. However, if the cells compensate for the loss of one gene by upregulating other genes, the observed results could be quite complex. In this case, although the gene expression changes are a result of the mutation, the genes that are affected may be regulated by pathways that have nothing to do with the gene that was mutated, but are affected through secondary compensatory pathways. A better design might be to reexpress transiently the wild-type gene in the mutant cells to follow short-term changes in gene expression that are more directly affected by the gene of interest. This example points out that interpreting microarray data can be quite complicated, because gene expression pathways are influenced by so many regulatory interactions. Microarray experiments are relatively easy to perform, but poor experimental design may yield results that are difficult or impossible to interpret.

4.3. Comparison of Patient Samples

Microarray assays offer a rapid and sensitive means of comparing the gene expression profiles in tumors from different individuals and offers the promise of being used as a clinical tool to identify tumors that might respond better to a particular treatment or for identifying patients with better or worse prognoses. Such information could be extremely valuable for helping clinicians make decisions about which therapeutic options are most appropriate. Many investigators have access to dozens or even hundreds of clinical samples and see microarrays as a means of analyzing them for common patterns of gene expression. Several laboratories have been successful at identifying patterns of gene expression that correlate with clinical outcome or define classes of tumors, similar to other cytogenetic markers *(7,11,12)*. However, these studies invariably require quite complex data and statistical analyses including methods, such as hierarchical clustering, support vector machines, and other advanced approaches *(13,14)*. For this reason, novice users should consult with experts in complex data analysis before beginning such a study. In addition, successful clinical studies require balanced cohorts designed by qualified biostatisticians to avoid common pitfalls and artifacts (*see* **Subheading 5.5.**).

5. Planning and Experimental Design

Microarray experiments generate large and complicated data sets that pose special problems for statistical analysis and researchers trying to interpret the results. This section discusses the most common problems faced by novice users beginning microarray experiments and approaches for eliminating them.

5.1. The Problem With Statistics

Most statistical methods depend on the comparison of replicates to estimate experimental variability in order to determine whether an observed difference is statistically significant. In general, such methods work better as the number of replicates increases. Thus, the best types of data for normal statistical analyses have relatively few variables (rows) and many replicate measurements (columns). However, microarray experiments generate data of exactly the opposite type, with many thousands of variables (genes) and, because of the high cost, very few replicates. As a consequence, the usual statistical methods have trouble dealing with microarray data. For example, it is impossible to use a t-test statistic on data that have fewer than three replicates. Yet, few researchers can afford to perform more than two or three replicates of microarray experiments that may cost $1000 per sample. Some specialized data analysis methods have been developed to get around the problems posed by microarray data. These methods often analyze the variation in other genes as pseudoreplicates in order to calculate the levels of variation among the genes in a data set. An example of such a method is the Cross-Gene Error Model used by the popular microarray analysis software program GeneSpring (Silicon Genetics, Redwood City, CA), which calculates a trust score for each gene based on its level of expression and the variation among other genes in the data set expressed at similar levels. These specialized data analysis methods can be quite effective and work best when the samples being compared are similar, such as from the same tissue culture cell line. The cross-gene methods have more difficulty when the samples being compared display more dramatic differences in gene expression patterns, such as when tumors from different patients are compared.

One of the problems with microarray data analysis is that the results of the experiments are generally reported only as fold change. This is necessary because different genes are expressed at widely different levels. If one tried to analyze microarrays using only raw expression-level scores, one would end up paying attention only to the genes that were expressed at high levels. However, in biological terms, the most highly expressed genes are often the least interesting, sometimes called "housekeeping" genes. The more interesting regulatory genes are often expressed at moderate or low levels. Thus, fold change measurements are necessary in order to emphasize the changes in gene expression, instead of the total abundance of individual transcripts. Unfortunately, reporting only fold change measurements introduces serious problems when discussing genes that are expressed at low levels. For example, using Affymetrix GeneChips, it is not uncommon for replicate measurements of a single gene in two identical samples to vary by as much as 1000 raw fluorescence units. An error of 1000 U is an inconsequential 5% change for a gene expressed at a level of 20,000 fluorescent units. However, for a gene expressed at approx 200 U, a 1000-U variation represents a sixfold change. Consequently, it is much more difficult to measure statistically significant changes in gene expression for genes that are expressed at low levels. In publications, the raw fluorescence-level numbers for individual genes are almost never reported, making interpretation of the fold change measurements difficult. However, the relative change in total fluorescence units must be considered when determining the significance of an observed fold change.

5.2. Why Replicates Are Absolutely, Positively Required

One of the most common questions raised by new users, especially after calculating the high cost of a proposed microarray experiment, is: are replicates really necessary? After all, publications almost never show replicates of Northern or Western blots, two conventional methods of analyzing changes in gene expression. Why are replicates required for microarray experiments?

The differences are that Northern and Western blots seldom try to measure changes in gene expression that are as low as twofold and do not use statistical filters to identify gene products of interest. When microarray assays are used to measure gene expression patterns in two independent samples that should be identical, the data usually have a correlation coefficient higher than 0.97. This is a very high correlation coefficient for biological studies. However, it means that for any filter used to analyze the microarray data, up to 3% of the genes that pass through the filter will do so solely owing to apparently random fluctuation in the measurements. For an experiment measuring 40,000 genes, this noise could contribute to the improper identification of up to 1200 genes, a number far too large to be tolerated. However, if the fluctuation is random, different genes should be improperly identified in each sample. Thus, by performing duplicate analyses and requiring that genes pass through the filter in both replicates, the number of genes improperly identified should be only $0.03 \times 0.03 = 0.009$, or only 36 genes out of 40,000. Applying the filters to independent triplicate samples should eliminate all but one or two "false-positives," or improperly identified genes. For these reasons, new users should be counseled that replicate microarray assays are absolutely required. If costs are a concern, duplicate assays will generally suffice, but independent triplicate assays, if possible, are best.

5.3. Hybridization and Analysis Controls

Before starting a microarray experiment, it is important to consider the controls that should be included. Microarrays should be designed to allow the inclusion of "spiked" control mRNAs in the samples to be analyzed. These are most often a set of bacterial or artificial mRNAs generated by in vitro transcription, and mixed in predefined ratios representing low-, medium-, and high-abundance transcripts, that can be added to all the experimental samples and that hybridize to their own special spots on the array. Spiked controls are an excellent means of following the efficiency of the entire microarray analysis process, from reverse transcription through labeling to hybridization, detection, and quantitation. For Affymetrix GeneChips, premade sets of control RNAs are available as a kit. Including such controls is highly recommended because it requires very little additional effort or cost and adds significantly to the quality of the data.

5.4. The "Day Effect"

Microarrays are quite capable of detecting systematic problems in the analysis or preparation of samples. This is sometimes referred to as the "day effect," detected when techniques, such as Principle Component Analysis, are applied to large data sets containing samples that were analyzed on different days. The samples analyzed on the same day often correlate with each other better than samples analyzed on different days. The causes of the day effect are unknown but presumably have to do with batches of enzymes or reagents that differed or other systematic variations. Whatever the reason, the implication is that the samples analyzed on the same day will appear to be more similar to each other than they should, and the samples analyzed on different days will appear to be more different than they should. This has important implications for experimental design. For example, because of the day effect, it would be inappropriate to analyze all the control and untreated samples on one day, and all the treated or experimental samples on a different day. Instead, if it is impossible to analyze all the samples together, it is better to divide the samples into manageable groups, keeping both control and experimental samples in each group. For example, for a small experiment with three samples—untreated, vehicle alone, and drug-treated—it is recommended that the entire experiment be performed in duplicate, but on different days. Each set of three microarrays is analyzed together on different days, and then the data sets are compared and the analyses performed. This practice will ensure that some controls and some experimental samples are analyzed on different days, so any correlation observed between replicates will be owing to the experimental manipulations, not the systematic variations that cause the day effect.

5.5. Importance of Balanced Cohorts

A common use of microarrays is the analysis of clinical samples, with the intention of identifying patterns of gene expression that are predictive of a particular outcome. For example, researchers analyze a group of breast tumors in order to identify patterns in the microarray data that correlate with and can predict poor prognosis. However, this type of study is particularly prone to problems with experimental design related to unbalanced cohorts. In a typical study, researchers might have access to 60 tumor samples, of which 80% have good prognosis and 20% have poor prognosis. They choose two-thirds of the samples, or 40, to use as a training set and save the other 20 as the test or validation set. Microarray analysis identifies genes whose expression patterns can distinguish between the good and poor prognosis samples in the training set. When the expression patterns of those genes are analyzed in the test samples, they predict the outcome with 80% accuracy, so the experiment appears to be a success. However, if the researchers failed to balance the cohorts, they may have been misled. Because 80% of the original samples had good prognosis, a random selection of any sample would have an 80% chance of being in the good prognosis group. If the microarray analysis fails to perform better than random chance, it has not really worked. A better design would be to choose a balanced cohort, 50% with good and 50% with poor prognosis, to use as the training set. In this type of experiment, it is essential to get help from a qualified biostatistician before beginning, in order to obtain results that are valid and meaningful.

6. Basics of Microarray Data Analysis

Microarray experiments can produce complex data sets, and analyzing them can be difficult and time-consuming. The details of microarray data analysis methods are beyond the scope of this chapter. However, even if an expert performs the actual data analysis, it is important for the researchers to understand the basics of data analysis so that they can interpret the analysis summaries provided to them and ask the right questions of the expert analyst.

The analysis of microarray results has three phases. The initial analysis checks quality scores and controls in order to judge whether the labeling, hybridization, and scanning of the microarrays worked as planned and to identify problematic results that should be eliminated from the larger data set used for the final analysis. The second step is scaling and normalization, which adjusts the data obtained from individual arrays so that they can be compared. The normalization step is particularly important and dramatically affects the outcome. Choosing the correct normalization method is critical to obtaining the best results. Once the data are normalized, the third step, applying a variety of statistical tests and filters to identify genes whose expression change in the various samples is employed. There are many methods for performing this analysis, which indicates that there is no best or standard approach. Indeed, the statistical methods used for microarray data analysis are a major area of biostatistics research. For novice users, the experts in the core facility will likely choose the particular statistical methods that they are comfortable with and prefer to use, so a description of all possible methods or software packages currently in use is beyond the scope of this chapter. However, a description of some of the types of filters that can be applied to simple microarray data sets is useful to understand how the data are structured and to identify some of the pitfalls that can occur in microarray data analysis.

6.1. Initial Data Analysis

The first steps in the analysis of microarray data are to check the quality of the data obtained from each array or GeneChip; validate that all the wet-lab steps, such as reverse transcription, probe labeling, hybridization, and scanning were successful and efficient; and eliminate any data sets that are of low quality. For the novice user, these steps will usually be carried out by the core facility, which should provide the user with a report describing the overall quality of the data. The exact measurements used for judging data quality will depend on the microarray platform used and the types of controls present on the microarray. The Affymetrix GeneChip system includes a number of standard controls and quality measures that provide excellent examples of how data quality can be monitored.

6.1.1. Interpreting Affymetrix Quality Scores

Affymetrix GeneChips contain a number of control probe sets that measure the expression of housekeeping genes, such as β-actin and glyceraldehyde-3-phosphate dehydrogenase. Unlike most probe sets, which are skewed toward the 3'-end of the mRNA, in order to be less dependent on the quality of the reverse transcription reaction, the GeneChips contain several probe sets for the housekeeping controls, located at the 5'-

end, -middle, and 3'-end of the transcripts. By comparing the hybridization signals from these probe sets the researcher can get an excellent indication of the quality of the mRNA and the reverse transcription reaction used during the labeling process. For example, because the reverse transcription reaction begins at the 3'-end, if it was inefficient the probe sets from the 3'-ends of the housekeeping genes would give much stronger hybridization signals than the probe sets from the 5'-ends. In general, the ratio of the signals from the 3'-end to the 5'-end probe sets should be less than three. In addition, the housekeeping gene probe sets should have robust signals, as expected for transcripts expressed at high levels.

6.1.2. Percent Present

A second type of quality score provided by the Affymetrix system is the Percent Present statistic. Affymetrix GeneChips contain 12 or more perfect match probes and an equal number of mismatch probes for each gene. The analysis software measures the difference in the hybridization signals for the perfect match and mismatch probe pairs and then uses a statistical algorithm to determine whether the differences are significant. Based on this calculation, each gene is labeled "Present," "Marginal," or "Absent." This statistical flag is independent of the expression level and depends only on how much agreement there is among the individual probe sets for each gene. The software also calculates the fraction of genes labeled "Present" and reports this fraction as the Percent Present. In practice, the Percent Present can vary significantly, depending on the type of sample (e.g., primary cells vs transformed cell lines) being analyzed. However, within one experiment analyzing similar samples, all of the GeneChips should give a similar Percent Present. An abnormally low Percent Present is an indicator that an RNA sample was of poor quality or that the labeling or hybridization reactions were flawed.

6.1.3. Interpretation of Scaling Factors

Affymetrix also permits data from individual GeneChips to be scaled, which is similar to per-chip normalization (*see* **Subheading 6.2.1.**). Although scaling is not absolutely necessary, it does provide an additional quality statistic, the scaling factor. Scaling works by multiplying all the gene expression values by some constant, the scaling factor, which adjusts the average expression to some preset number, usually 500 or a similar integer. If scaling is used, the scaling factor provides an excellent quality measure. Poor-quality data sets invariably have larger scaling factors, because the labeling or hybridization was affected for all the genes represented on the GeneChip. Ideally, all the samples being analyzed as a group should have similar scaling factors. If Affymetrix scaling is used, there is no need to use additional per-chip normalization, discussed in **Subheading 6.2.1.**

6.2. Scaling and Normalization

Proper scaling and normalization of microarray data is extremely important and dramatically affects the results of the analysis. The two basic types of normalization are scaling, or per-chip normalization, which adjusts the average intensity of an entire microarray sample, and per-gene normalization, which is used to compare the relative expression of a single gene within a group of samples.

6.2.1. Per-Chip Normalization

Scaling, or per-chip normalization, is a means of adjusting the overall fluorescence of each microarray to the same average intensity, analogous to adjusting the sensitivity of the scanner so that each sample has the same overall brightness. This type of adjustment makes sense for samples that are similar, and that are expected to have similar numbers of genes expressed, mostly at similar levels. However, it may not make sense for samples that are dramatically different, such as a comparison of resting cells vs proliferating cells, because the latter may have many more genes expressed. By default, most samples are subjected to scaling or per-chip normalization. However, the details of the experiment should be considered carefully to determine whether per-chip normalization is appropriate. In particular, if samples have dramatically different levels of expression of the housekeeping genes, which contribute greatly to the average fluorescence, it might be better not to subject the samples to per-chip normalization.

6.2.2. Per-Gene Normalization

The absolute level of expression among different genes varies dramatically, from thousands to less than one transcript per cell. As a result, it is difficult to compare changes in the level of expression of specific genes among samples. As discussed in **Subheading 5.1.**, a 1000-fluorescent unit change in expression of a high-abundance transcript may represent a small change, as little as 5%, but could represent a manyfold change in expression of a gene that is expressed at low levels. Per-gene normalization is used to overcome this problem by comparing the relative expression of each gene across the various samples in an experiment, expressed as fold change. As a consequence, genes that display similar patterns of up or down changes in expression across samples can be identified despite the absolute differences in their expression levels.

The big problem with per-gene normalization is deciding what to normalize each sample to. By default, most microarray data analysis programs calculate the mean expression level for each gene, then normalize each sample against that mean, or control value. This approach works but can result in some strange results. Take the example described in **Subheading 5.4.** of a small microarray experiment containing just three conditions—untreated, vehicle treated, and drug treated—performed in duplicate. The entire experiment would consist of six microarrays, two independent measurements for each condition (**Fig. 2A**). Now, consider a gene expressed at or near zero in the untreated and vehicle-treated conditions. The software never reports an expression value of zero, so assume that the average value in the untreated and vehicle-treated samples is a low number, e.g., 200. If this gene is strongly induced by the drug treatment its expression level could go up to an average of 2000 U. Using the default per-gene normalization described above, the mean intensity across all six samples would be 800. The fold change reported for the untreated and vehicle-treated samples would be 0.25 and the fold change for the drug-treated samples would be 2.5. This gene would just barely pass

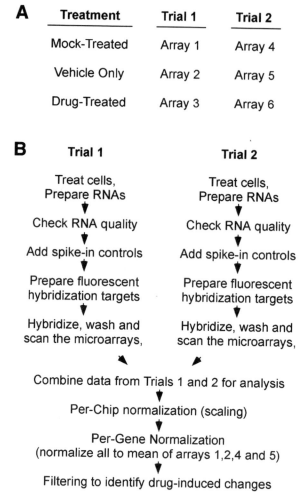

Fig. 2. Design and analysis strategy for a simple microarray experiment. (**A**) Simple micro-array experiment design. A six-microarray experiment is designed to test the effect of drug treatment on tissue culture cells. Duplicate samples of the drug-treated cells will be compared with duplicates of vehicle-treated or mock-treated samples. Each sample will be analyzed with its own microarray, making a total of six assays. (**B**) Flow chart of simple microarray experiment. RNA samples from the two trials are collected and analyzed separately, and then the data are combined for the analysis. Keeping the samples separate helps to avoid day effects and other systematic problems. The data are normalized to the mean of the four control samples (mock treated or vehicle treated) to identify drug-induced changes in gene expression in the two treated samples.

a filter designed to find genes induced more than 2.5-fold by the drug. However, comparison of the raw scores shows that the average expression actually changed from 200 to 2000, which is a 10-fold change! In this case, the default normalization scheme was inappropriate. The data should have been normalized to the untreated or the vehicle-treated samples, rather than to the average of all the samples. As the example illustrates, choosing the correct normalization scheme is extremely important and affects the results and the genes that will be identified by the analysis.

In general, if the experiment has true control samples, such as the untreated and vehicle-treated samples in the example described in **Fig. 2A**, per-gene normalization should use those samples as the controls. The result will be fold-change data that reflect the change relative to the controls, a much more logical type of result than a fold change relative to the mean of all the samples. On the other hand, when no true controls are available, such as when comparing the gene expression profiles of a number of tumor samples from different patients, normalization to the mean of all the samples may be the only available choice. In either case, it is important for the researcher to understand how the data were normalized in order to interpret the fold-change results.

6.3. The Simplest Analysis: Filtering to Identify Regulated Genes

After normalization, a variety of techniques can be used to identify genes with altered expression in one or more of the experimental conditions. This section focuses on filtering, the simplest method to identify interesting genes and one of the most useful for novice microarray users. Filtering is direct and related to the experimental design, so it is relatively easy to set up and understand. However, filtering is best used for addressing specific biological questions in relatively simple experiments. The filtering approach rapidly becomes cumbersome as the experimental design becomes more complicated and is not suitable for experiments with more than three or four types of experimental conditions. Nevertheless, a basic discussion of data analysis using filtering can point out the strengths and weaknesses in microarray data analysis and prepare users for adopting more advanced techniques, if they are necessary.

6.3.1. The Analysis Strategy

To illustrate the concepts and pitfalls of data analysis by filtering, consider the example experiment described in **Fig. 2A**, with two biological replicates each for untreated, vehicle-treated, and drug-treated samples, or a total of six microarrays. This experiment has a simple experimental design (**Fig. 2A**). Nevertheless, it is important to predict what types of results are expected in order to design the appropriate filters.

6.3.2. Filter on Flags

The first criterion is that only those genes that can actually be detected above background levels should be considered for further analysis. If a gene is expressed at such low levels that it cannot be distinguished from background in any of the samples, there is no sense in applying a filter to see whether its expression has increased. This may seem obvious but it is actually a major concern in microarray experiments that utilize normalized data, because once the data are normalized, all the information about absolute expression levels are lost. Thus, it is a common error to identify genes that are up- or downregulated based on fold change without paying attention to whether the genes are actually expressed at a level that is significant and above background. For several reasons, this problem is a special concern for users of glass spotted arrays. First, absolute background levels are difficult to measure using glass spotted arrays. This is because the background hybridization in the areas spotted with DNA can be much greater than in the areas without DNA, because background levels can vary from probe to probe, depending on the G-C content, and because such arrays often suffer from high background and "smearing," all of which complicate background measurements. Second, glass spotted arrays often have only one spot per gene, so there is no way to do statistical calculations to determine whether an expression measurement is significantly different from background. Finally, signals using glass spotted arrays are often weak, so most spots are detected in the near-background range. Sometimes it is possible to increase the sensitivity of the scanner to alleviate this problem, but detection of low- and even medium-abundance mRNAs can nevertheless be quite difficult.

The Affymetrix GeneChip system has incorporated a number of measures to enable more accurate background detection and to permit statistical measures to be applied to determine whether each gene is expressed above background. On the Affymetrix arrays, at least 12 perfect match probes and an equal number of corresponding single nucleotide mismatch probes represent each gene. By comparing the hybridization signals for the perfect and mismatch probes, which in each case differ by only one nucleotide, a fairly accurate estimate of the difference between specific and nonspecific signals can be determined. The 12 or more independent measurements allow statistical tests to be made, and the size of the corresponding p value is used to calculate a Present/Marginal/Absent call. This "flag," or qualitative measure that accompanies the raw expression score, is a measure of whether the genes are statistically different from background. The flag allows the data to be filtered to exclude genes that cannot be accurately measured. In general, it is advisable to filter Affymetrix data to exclude genes that are flagged "Absent" in all the samples, which is often one-third or more of the genes on the array. It is also possible to be more selective. In our example experiment (**Fig. 2A**), if one was interested only in genes that were "off" in the controls and "on" in the drug-treated samples, one could filter for genes that were flagged "Absent" in the untreated and vehicle-treated samples and also flagged "Present" in the drug-treated samples. However, such a specific use of flags is generally unwarranted because it could be too selective.

6.3.3. Filter on Fold Change

The most basic type of filtering is the comparison of fold change. Microarray data are generally filtered to identify genes that are at least twofold different in the experimental conditions. In our example experiment, one would try to identify genes that were at least twofold up- or downregulated in the drug-treated samples compared with both the vehicle and the untreated samples.

The best approach is to combine filters to achieve the most specific result possible. For example, to identify genes that are upregulated by the drug treatment, a filter should be designed to find only genes that are flagged "Present" and also twofold or more upregulated in both of the drug-treated samples, because it makes no sense to study genes that are apparently upregulated but cannot be detected in a statistically significant manner. Whether the genes are flagged "Present" or "Absent" in the controls is irrelevant.

For downregulated genes, the measurements must be flagged "Present" in all the controls but expressed at 0.5-fold or less in both of the drug-treated samples. It is not logical to find genes that appear to be downregulated unless they were actually expressed above background in the controls.

6.3.4. Other Filters

Numerous additional filters can be applied to microarray data. To be most conservative, some users will wish to limit their analysis only to genes that are most robustly expressed, and that can be most easily detected by other methods, such as Northern blots. For that purpose, it may be useful to filter on the raw expression level, essentially setting a cutoff for minimum expression above which a gene must be expressed to be considered further. The cutoff is somewhat arbitrary and depends on the data set and the settings used for the scanners and for the normalization. Nevertheless, this approach can help identify the genes that will be simplest to study in subsequent validation experiments, at the expense of eliminating some of the most interesting genes that are expressed at lower levels, closer to the background level.

6.4. More Advanced Analysis: Clustering

Microarray data can be extremely complex, and many methods of data analysis are available. In fact, the development of new and improved methods for analyzing microarray data is a major area of research among bioinformatics specialists. The most common of these methods involves various supervised and unsupervised clustering methods that have been developed primarily for the analysis of large data sets, especially those that compare numerous samples from different individuals, such as a series of tumor vs normal samples. These methods are generally not too useful for novice microarray users performing simple experiments; their description is beyond the scope of this article, but they are discussed in **Chapter 4**. Nearly all the advanced methods use statistical tests to group genes or patients in clusters, based on their expression profiles, and do better with larger numbers of samples. However, as a general rule, it is best to filter the data first in order to limit the analysis to the smallest possible set of genes that are informative. It makes little sense to include thousands of genes that cannot be detected above background in the data set being subjected to statistical clustering. Once the data are limited to the genes that are truly flagged "Present" and that change twofold or more in the experimental samples, clustering methods may be able to divide the genes into interesting groups, especially if the experiment includes several different types of samples, such as treatments with different drugs or a time course of drug treatments.

7. Conclusion

Microarray technologies have empowered novice users with the ability to assay changes in gene expression at the whole-genome level. There is little doubt that microarray results will lead to new and entirely unexpected results, and pursuing such experiments will be worthwhile for many investigators. However, there are several concerns that should be heeded. Microarray experiments are expensive and they can be quite labor-intensive. In addition, the data that they produce are quite complex. Novice users should seek out advice from their core facilities or collaborators to make sure that they have designed the most efficient experiment that is compatible with microarray assays. A poorly designed experiment is the most common reason that microarray experiments fail to yield results that are interpretable. In most cases, clear thinking and a discussion with an experienced microarray user, a core facility leader, or a biostatistician will lead to much better experimental design and much better data.

Acknowledgments

I thank Dr. G. G. Pickett for helpful comments on the manuscript. I am supported by grants from the USPHS/National Cancer Institute (#RO1 CA58443) and by the University of New Mexico Health Sciences Center. I am codirector of the Keck-UNM Genomics Resource, a microarray and gene expression analysis facility supported by a grant from the W. M. Keck Foundation as well as the State of New Mexico and the UNM Cancer Research and Treatment Center.

References

1. Ishida, S., Huang, E., Zuzan, H., et al. (2001) Role for E2F in control of both DNA replication and mitotic functions as revealed from DNA microarray analysis. *Mol. Cell Biol.* **21,** 4684–4699.
2. Spellman, P. T., Sherlock, G., Zhang, M. Q., et al. (1998) Comprehensive identification of cell cycle–regulated genes of the yeast Saccharomyces cerevisiae by microarray hybridization. *Mol. Biol. Cell* **9,** 3273–3297.
3. Frueh, F. W., Hayashibara, K. C., Brown, P. O., and Whitlock, J. P. Jr. (2001) Use of cDNA microarrays to analyze dioxin-induced changes in human liver gene expression. *Toxicol. Lett.* **122,** 189–203.
4. Liang, G., Gonzales, F. A., Jones, P. A., Orntoft, T. F., and Thykjaer, T. (2002) Analysis of gene induction in human fibroblasts and bladder cancer cells exposed to the methylation inhibitor 5-aza-2'-deoxycytidine. *Cancer Res.* **62,** 961–966.
5. Lei, W., Rushton, J. J., Davis, L. M., Liu, F., and Ness, S. A. (2004) Positive and negative determinants of target gene specificity in Myb transcription factors. *J. Biol. Chem.* **279,** 29,519–29,527.
6. Rushton, J. J., Davis, L. M., Lei, W., Mo, X., Leutz, A., and Ness, S. A. (2003) Distinct changes in gene expression induced by A-Myb, B-Myb and c-Myb proteins. *Oncogene* **22,** 308–313.
7. Ferrando, A. A., Neuberg, D. S., Staunton, J., et al. (2002) Gene expression signatures define novel oncogenic pathways in T cell acute lymphoblastic leukemia. *Cancer Cell* **1,** 75–87.
8. Monks, A., Harris, E., Hose, C., Connelly, J., and Sausville, E. A. (2003) Genotoxic profiling of MCF-7 breast cancer cell line elucidates gene expression modifications underlying toxicity of the anticancer drug 2-(4-amino-3-methylphenyl)-5-fluorobenzothiazole. *Mol. Pharmacol.* **63,** 766–772.
9. Karyala, S., Guo, J., Sartor, M., et al. (2004) Different global gene expression profiles in benzo[a]pyrene- and dioxin-treated vascular smooth muscle cells of AHR-knockout and wild-type mice. *Cardiovasc. Toxicol.* **4,** 47–74.
10. Verheyen, G. R., Nuijten, J. M., Van Hummelen, P., and Schoeters, G. R. (2004) Microarray analysis of the effect of diesel exhaust particles on in vitro cultured macrophages. *Toxicol. In Vitro* **18,** 377–391.

11. Sotiriou, C., Neo, S. Y., McShane, L. M., et al. (2003) Breast cancer classification and prognosis based on gene expression profiles from a population-based study. *Proc. Natl. Acad. Sci. USA* **100,** 10,393–10,398.

12. Valk, P. J., Verhaak, R. G., Beijen, M. A., et al. (2004) Prognostically useful gene-expression profiles in acute myeloid leukemia. *N. Engl. J. Med.* **350,** 1617–1628.

13. Benito, M., Parker, J., Du, Q., et al. (2004) Adjustment of systematic microarray data biases. *Bioinformatics* **20,** 105–114.

14. Segal, M. R., Dahlquist, K. D., and Conklin, B. R. (2003) Regression approaches for microarray data analysis. *J. Comput. Biol.* **10,** 961–980.

3

From Microarray to Biological Networks

Analysis of Gene Expression Profiles

Xiwei Wu and T. Gregory Dewey

Summary

Powerful new methods, such as expression profiles using cDNA arrays, have been used to monitor changes in gene expression levels as a result of a variety of metabolic, xenobiotic, or pathogenic challenges. This potentially vast quantity of data enables, in principle, the dissection of the complex genetic networks that control the patterns and rhythms of gene expression in the cell. Here we present a general approach to developing dynamic models for analyzing time series of whole-genome expression. The parameters in the model show the influence of one gene expression level on another and are calculated using singular value decomposition as a means of inverting noisy and near-singular matrices. Correlative networks can then be generated based on these parameters with a simple threshold approach. We also demonstrate how dynamic models can be used in conjunction with cluster analysis to analyze microarray time series. Using the parameters from the dynamic model as a metric, two-way hierarchical clustering could be performed to visualize how *influencing genes* affect the expression levels of *responding genes*. Application of these approaches is demonstrated using gene expression data in yeast cell cycle.

Key Words: Gene expression; time series; gene network; linear dynamic model; singular value decomposition; clustering.

1. Introduction

An emerging problem in bioinformatics is identifying the relationships among the various components of a system and inferring how one component influences another. To do this, the detailed information about molecular species must not be considered in isolation but, rather, in relation to all of the other components of the system. These relationships are often most easily represented by network structures or graphs. Thus, systems biology invariably means network analysis. To this end, systems-wide investigations

From: *Methods in Molecular Biology, vol. 316: Bioinformatics and Drug Discovery*
Edited by: R. S. Larson © Humana Press Inc., Totowa, NJ

have focused on specific functional network structures, such as metabolic, signaling, and gene regulatory networks. These networks, when refined, will ultimately provide predictive models of biological function. Other networks, such as protein–protein interaction maps or ortholog networks, are used to represent and cope with the correlations and relationships inherent in these large data sets. In this chapter, we discuss how to analyze cDNA microarray data to obtain network models of gene expression. As discussed, these methods are more akin to the correlative networks than to true gene regulatory networks.

To infer gene expression networks from microarray data, we consider time-series data taken on a population of cells at set time points after some stimulus. This stimulus is often an environmental alteration that will elicit a cellular response. Examples might be the addition of a drug or blocking agent or the change of media to alter growth conditions. Systems-level gene expression profiles can be measured for each time point using cDNA or oligomeric chips. The time progression of these gene profiles can then be analyzed using linear models to yield gene expression networks. These gene expression networks must be considered phenomenological, reflecting dynamic observations from the data and an inherently incomplete modeling of the data. These networks describe how the mRNA level of one gene influences the mRNA level of another. These are not true gene regulatory networks in the strict sense because they are correlative, and not necessarily causal, networks. This chapter describes how to proceed from data to linear model to gene expression network. It also describes methods for visualizing these networks and a clustering technique for classifying genes according to their network connectivity.

2. Methods

2.1. Source of Data

The Stanford Microarray Database (SMD; http://genome-www.stanford.edu/microarray/) serves as a microarray research database for the entire scientific community, by making freely available all of its source codes and providing full public access to data published by SMD users, along with many tools to explore and analyze those data *(1)*. Time-series expression data for cell cycle in yeast were downloaded from the SMD.

2.2. Calculation of λ-Matrix and Adjacency Matrix

All calculations were done in Matlab (Mathworks, Natick, MA). Λ Matrix was calculated as $\Lambda = \mathbf{A}(t)\,\mathbf{VE}^{-1}\,\mathbf{U}^{T}$ (*see* **Subheading 3.2.** for details). Generalized matrix inversion of the lead matrix was achieved with the singular value decomposition (SVD) routine implemented in Matlab. Entries in the diagonal matrix E were examined and entries with very small values (typically $<10^{-2}$) were set to 0. Entries in the E^{-1} matrix were calculated by inverting each of the nonzero diagonal entries in the E matrix and leaving others as zero. The computation time is within minutes with a data set of about 6000 genes and 20 time points at a 16-CPU supercomputer running an IRIX operating system. Choice of the thresholds ε (*see* **Subheading 3.3.** for a definition of this threshold) is arbitrary at this time and depends only on the size of the network that one desires. Large threshold results in a small network, and lowering the threshold "grows" the network. When a threshold is applied to the lambda matrix in Matlab, a logical matrix with entries of 0 or 1 (called "adjacency matrix") will be produced. The size of the network N can be easily examined by summing over all the entries in the adjacency matrix.

2.3. Network Visualization

The adjacency matrix is transformed into a graph file with Graphviz format within Matlab. Graphviz is a set of programs for graph visualization and editing developed by AT&T Labs-Research. It is freely available at www.research.att.com/sw/tools/graphviz/download.html. The *dot* program in Graphviz was used in the current study to generate gene networks. The networks produced are directed graphs with hierarchy layout, which can be converted by the *dot* program into many common graphic formats for easy visualization with the graphic viewer of one's choice. Visualization of the networks within Web browsers is also possible via the WebDot server (www.graphviz.org/web dot/). Nodes in the network can contain hyperlinks to outside databases, such as gene annotation databases, for easy exploration. Refer to the online documentations of these tools for details.

2.4. Clustering of Dynamic Parameters

The elements of the Λ-matrix, λ_{ij}, show the influence of the expression level of the jth gene on the production of the ith gene. Positive entries suggest a positive influence (either direct or indirect), and negative entries suggest an inhibition. We are interested in those genes that influence other genes strongly and identifying these by applying a threshold to the entries in the transition matrix. For λ_{ij} entries whose absolute value is above a fixed threshold, we identify the ith gene as the *responding gene* and the jth gene as the *influencing gene*. The threshold values are chosen somewhat arbitrarily and will dictate the number of *influencing genes* that will ultimately be identified. The new transition matrix Λ' consists of $\lambda_{i,j}$ for *influencing genes* vs all of the genes in the data set (*responding genes*). Average linkage hierarchical clustering with Pearson correlation as distance measurement was then applied to the Λ' matrix using J-Express v2.1 (Molmine AS, Norway). Results of the cluster analysis are displayed using a color-coded dendrogram. As a convention, red indicates a positive entry in Λ' matrix, and green indicates a negative entry. The brighter the color (red or green), the larger the absolute entry in transition matrix.

3. Networks From Linear Models

3.1. Motivation for Linear Models

Dynamic linear models are ones in which the change in time of one of the variables is linearly related to the other variables. In our example, the expression levels of a set of genes at a given time will influence the production of a given gene at a later time. The rate of production of the responding gene as measured by the mRNA level will be linearly proportional to the amount of mRNA of the influencing genes. If one considers the simple case of a transcription factor and its target genes, this model would predict that the rate of mRNA production of the target gene would be proportional to the mRNA concentration of the transcription factor. In general, one does not know if the linear model is an accurate one and, indeed, one would anticipate that some genes would show very nonlinear responses with complex feedback loops.

Considering the complexity and inherent nonlinearity of biological phenomena, why should one even consider simple linear models? There are several answers to this question. First, linear models are appealing because they are simple and are computationally easy to handle. Even though they may not represent the underlying phenomena, they nevertheless are a good starting point. Before one moves to more complicated models, it is important to establish where the simple models fail. This is especially true when dealing with limited data with large statistical errors, as found in most microarray studies. Second, the linear model may act as a first approximation to a more complicated nonlinear expression. Any nonlinear function can be "linearized" through a power series expansion, and the linear model can be considered the first term in such an expansion. At this stage of sophistication and data quality, we are primarily seeking phenomenological connections, rather than quantitative mathematical connections. For such "datamining" goals, linear models serve an extremely useful purpose. The initial goal is to understand connections between genes rather than to establish a full-blown mathematical description of gene regulation, so linear models provide an excellent starting point.

There are many variations on linear models, and the choice of a specific model will often depend on the experimental conditions or experimental design *(2–7)*. In our work, we used a form that is perhaps the simplest one. It is a linear finite difference model and is described by **Eq. 1**:

$$a_i(t) = \sum_{j=1}^{M} \lambda_{i,j} \, a_j(t-1) \tag{1}$$

In **Eq. 1**, $a_i(t)$ is the experimentally measured mRNA concentration for the ith gene at time t. **Equation 1** relates the mRNA concentration at time t to the linear combination of all other mRNA concentrations at the previous time, $t - 1$. The transition coefficients $\lambda_{i,j}$ are the respective elements of the $M \times M$ transition matrix (referred to as the Λ matrix) and are the model parameter *(5)*. These coefficients are unitless and show how strongly weighted each contribution from the previous time will be to the production of the ith gene. This model is sometimes referred to as an autoregression model because all the variables at a later time are dependent only on the values of these same variables at an early time.

The goal of the data analysis is to determine the values for $\lambda_{i,j}$. In **Subheading 3.2.**, we show how to calculate $\lambda_{i,j}$ and use these parameters to determine the gene expression network.

A second form of the linear model uses differential equations rather than difference equations to analyze expression time series *(3,7)*. The differential form follows a series of coupled equations given by

$$\dot{a}_i(t) = \sum_{j=1}^{M} W_{i,j} \, a_j(t) + b_i(t) + \xi_i(t) \tag{2}$$

in which $a_i(t)$ is the expression level of the ith gene at time t after some exposure or treatment, the overdot represents a time derivative, $W_{i,j}$ is a matrix of first-order rate constants showing the influence of the *j*th gene on the production of the *i*th gene, $b_i(t)$ is an external forcing function, $\xi_i(t)$ and is a noise term. The sum is over all *m* different genes that are measured.

Although these models may appear quite different, they can be directly related to each other. **Equation 2** can be solved in closed form using standard methods. Such solutions can be substituted into **Eq. 1** and a complicated relationship between $\lambda_{i,j}$ and $W_{i,j}$ is obtained. In our work, we chose to deal with the finite difference form because it required no data manipulation such as calculation of time derivatives (*see* **Heading 4.**) and no assumptions on the nature of the noise or the driving forces. Under the current technology, the noise and driving forces are not experimentally accessible quantities.

3.2. Calculation of Parameters of Linear Model

Our data set consists of the measurement of *M* gene expression levels or concentrations at *N* different times. A single measurement is expressed as $a_i(t_k)$, indicating the mRNA level of the *i*th gene at time t_k in which the indices *i* can range from 1 to *M* and *k* ranges from 1 to *N* (*see* **Heading 4.** for a discussion of units). The data are ordered in an $M \times N$ matrix as follows:

$$M \text{ genes} \downarrow \quad \begin{bmatrix} a_1(t_1) & a_1(t_2) & \cdots & a_1(t_N) \\ a_2(t_1) & a_2(t_2) & \cdots & a_2(t_N) \\ \vdots & \vdots & \vdots & \vdots \\ a_M(t_1) & a_M(t_2) & \cdots & a_M(t_N) \end{bmatrix} \overset{N \text{ times} \rightarrow}{}$$

in which each column is the measured values of all the genes at a given time point, and each row is the value of a given gene at all time points. Our goal is to use this data set to calculate the $\lambda_{i,j}$ of the linear model in **Eq. 1**. Rather than use **Eq. 1** directly, it is easier to write it as the equivalent matrix equation of the following form:

$$\begin{bmatrix} a_1(t_2) & a_1(t_3) & \cdots & a_1(t_N) \\ a_2(t_2) & a_2(t_3) & \cdots & a_2(t_N) \\ \vdots & \vdots & \vdots & \vdots \\ a_M(t_2) & a_M(t_2) & \cdots & a_M(t_N) \end{bmatrix} = \Lambda \bullet \begin{bmatrix} a_1(t_1) & a_1(t_2) & \cdots & a_1(t_{N-1}) \\ a_2(t_1) & a_2(t_2) & \cdots & a_2(t_{N-1}) \\ \vdots & \vdots & \vdots & \vdots \\ a_M(t_1) & a_M(t_2) & \cdots & a_M(t_{N-1}) \end{bmatrix} \quad (3)$$

in which the data matrix on the left-hand side of **Eq. 3** has the column with the first time point removed and is an $M \times (N-1)$ matrix called the lead matrix. The $M \times (N-1)$ matrix on the right-hand side has the column with the last time point removed and is called the lag matrix. The Λ matrix is an $M \times M$ containing the elements $\lambda_{i,j}$ as in **Eq. 1**. The Λ matrix is called the transition matrix because it is used to calculate the transition from the previous time to the next time point. It can also be said to "propagate" the data matrix from the past to the present.

Equation 3 can be written more succinctly as

$$\mathbf{A}(t) = \Lambda \cdot \mathbf{A}(t-1) \quad (4)$$

in which $\mathbf{A}\,(t)$ is the time lead matrix and $\mathbf{A}\,(t-1)$ is the time lag matrix. The Λ-matrix can be solved by inverting $\mathbf{A}\,(t-1)$ and multiplying both sides of **Eq. 4** by the inverse:

$$\Lambda = \mathbf{A}\,(t)\cdot\mathbf{A}\,(t-1)^{-1} \qquad (5)$$

Computationally, all that is needed to calculate the Λ-matrix is a matrix inversion routine, a common tool in any matrix algebra software package. However, standard methods cannot be used on this problem for two main reasons. First, most methods invert square matrices. In our case, we have a very lopsided matrix with M being on the order of thousands of genes and N being on the order of 10. A second problem is that $\mathbf{A}\,(t-1)$ is potentially a singular matrix. In any given experiment, it is conceivable that two genes have identical profiles as a result of being under identical gene control. The consequence of this is that two of the rows in the data matrix could be identical. Matrices with identical columns or rows are called singular and their inverse is undefined. To solve **Eq. 5**, methods described as "generalized matrix inversion" techniques must be used *(8)*.

We have used a matrix method known as SVD to calculate the matrix inverse in **Eq. 5** *(5)*. This is mathematically the same method used in the well-known tool of principal component analysis used in multivariate statistics. The SVD method is derived from a theorem in matrix algebra that states that any matrix can be "decomposed" into the product of three matrices. This gives

$$\mathbf{A}\,(t-1) = \mathbf{U}\mathbf{E}\mathbf{V}^{\mathrm{T}} \qquad (6)$$

in which $\mathbf{U}$ is an $M\times M$ orthogonal matrix of singular vectors, $\mathbf{E}$ is an $M\times(N-1)$ diagonal matrix of eigenvalues, and $\mathbf{V}$ is an $(N-1)\times(N-1)$ orthogonal matrix of singular vectors *(see* **Heading 4.** for a discussion of SVD). The singular vector matrices create an abstract vector space in which the original data matrix is represented. There is often a temptation to ascribe some biological significance to the vectors derived from SVD of a data matrix. This is difficult because SVD is a mathematical device, not a scientific theory, and there is no *a priori* reason that the matrices should have significance in biological terms. An SVD can be performed on any matrix regardless of its origin or the type of data that it represents. However, one can get a very generic interpretation of the singular vectors in terms of the eigenvectors of the correlation matrices. To calculate correlations between genes averaged over the time series, one uses $\mathbf{U}$ and $\mathbf{E}$. Correlations in time points averaged over all genes can be calculated using $\mathbf{V}$ and $\mathbf{E}$. Thus, the eigenvectors in $\mathbf{U}$ capture gene correlations, and the eigenvectors in $\mathbf{V}$ capture time correlations.

An SVD on the data matrix $\mathbf{A}\,(t-1)$ is performed using a routine in MatLab giving $\mathbf{A}\,(t-1) = \mathbf{U}\mathbf{E}\mathbf{V}^{\mathrm{T}}$. The inverse of $\mathbf{A}\,(t-1)$ is now given by

$$\mathbf{A}\,(t-1)^{-1} = \mathbf{V}\mathbf{E}^{-1}\,\mathbf{U}^{\mathrm{T}} \qquad (7)$$

in which the properties of orthogonal matrices have been used. SVD provides a way of handling the redundant data in singular matrices *(see* **Heading 4.**). When a singularity occurs, one of the eigenvalues in $\mathbf{E}$ will be zero. When taking the inverse of $\mathbf{E}$ in **Eq. 7**,

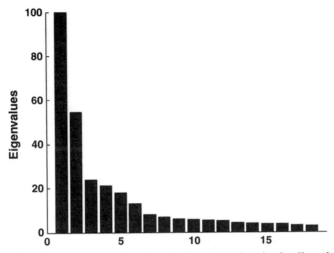

Fig. 1. Bar plot showing eigenvalues from α-factor synchronized cell-cycle data set *(1)*. Singular value decomposition was conducted in Matlab. Note how the first two eigenvalues dominate.

one truncates the eigenvalues to include only nonzero eigenvalues in $\mathbf{E}$ so that the inverse of zero is never needed; that is, all zeros in $\mathbf{E}$ are set to zero in $\mathbf{E}^{-1}$. Because of experimental error in the measurements, two rows are never exactly the same. Consequently, $\mathbf{E}$ contains very small eigenvalues that are not exactly zero. Typically, to remove the singularity, one still truncates $\mathbf{E}$ to eliminate the small eigenvalues. This procedure acts as a filter and removes noise from the data set.

Figure 1 shows an example of eigenvalues calculated from an SVD of a microarray data set. As can be seen, the first few eigenvalues are much larger than all of the other ones. In our experience, only three to five eigenvalues are significant and the others can be removed by truncation. A general rule of thumb is that when the eigenvalue is comparable to the error in the measured quantity in the data matrix, it should be truncated. For the case when $\mathbf{E}$ is truncated at two eigenvalues, designated $\mathbf{E_t}$, the inverse is given by

$$\mathbf{E_t}^{-1} = \begin{bmatrix} \dfrac{1}{\varepsilon_1} & 0 & 0 & \cdots \\ 0 & \dfrac{1}{\varepsilon_2} & 0 & \cdots \\ 0 & 0 & 0 & \cdots \\ \vdots & \vdots & \vdots & \ddots \end{bmatrix} \tag{8}$$

in which all values in the matrix are zero except for the first two diagonal entries. Using the truncated eigenvalue matrix, the calculated transition matrix Λ is then given by

$$\Lambda = \mathbf{A}(t)\,\mathbf{V}\mathbf{E}_t^{-1}\,\mathbf{U}^T \tag{9}$$

This represents the first step in calculating a gene expression network from expression time-series data. The next section describes how to construct a network from the calculated transition matrix.

3.3. Networks From Time-Series Data

Once **Eq. 9** is calculated, phenomenological networks of gene interactions can be derived from the transition matrix. The Λ transition matrix can be viewed as a weighted graph showing the influence of one expression level on another. This is the starting point for the description of the genetic circuitry. Rather than work with these weighted graphs, we consider a simpler approach in which Λ is converted into an adjacency matrix for digraphs, indicating the connectivity but not the strengths of the influence. We describe the operation (*adj*) as

$$\Gamma(\varepsilon) = adj(\Lambda) \tag{10}$$

in which the entries in Λ are set equal to 1 if the absolute values are above a certain threshold, ε, and are set equal to 0 below this threshold (this can be achieved with a command "ADJ = abs(Λ) $\geq \varepsilon$" in Matlab, in which ADJ is the adjacency matrix). For high values of the threshold, the resulting $\Gamma(\varepsilon)$ matrix will be a sparse adjacency matrix with a small network. As the value of ε is lowered, one can "grow" the network to include more nodes (genes). This threshold parameter is an adjustable parameter of the model. For example, for a yeast cell-cycle data set, the values in the transition matrix range from -0.0543 to 0.2239. A threshold of 0.04 results in a network with 102 edges. **Figure 2** gives an example of the type of network obtained with this methodology. This network derived from the analysis of the α-factor synchronized cell-cycle data in yeast is a network characterized by central hubs connecting a large number of nodes of low connectivity.

3.4. Gene Expression Networks and Classification of Genes

These gene regulatory networks obtained in **Subheading 3.3.** can also be used as a classification scheme by combining cluster analysis with dynamic modeling to show how dynamic characteristics of a biological system, such as the cell cycle, can be explored (*9*). By choosing a model parameter as a metric, one can extend the level of inference of the cluster analysis to include inferences implicit in the model. Conversely, cluster displays provide a facile method for visualizing genomewide parameters obtained from specific models.

Using the linear model parameter $\lambda_{i,j}$ as a metric, two-way clustering can be performed that shows how *influencing genes* affected the expression levels of *responding genes*. The application of this unsupervised method to the cell-cycle data in yeast shows strikingly strong clustering of cell-cycle-regulated genes. **Figure 3** shows a two-way clustering of $\lambda_{i,j}$ obtained from an analysis of yeast cell-cycle data. The two-way clustering is about *j*, the *influencing genes*, and about *i*, the *response genes*. The striking observation is that the blocks crossing clusters in columns (*influencing genes*) and rows (*responding genes*) can infer the relationship between cell-cycle phases. For example, if

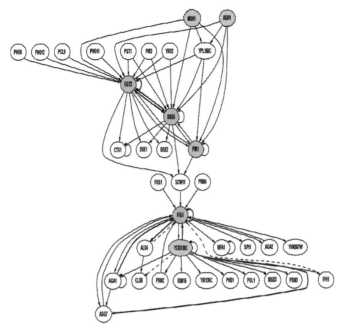

Fig. 2. Network generated from yeast cell-cycle data set. The nodes are genes labeled with standard gene names, and the edges indicate the phenomenological influence of one gene on another. Solid lines indicate positive influence (induction). Dashed lines indicate negative influence (inhibition). Bold solid lines indicate a strong influence (absolute value of entry of ≥0.08). Dark gray nodes are genes with more than four edges coming into and going out from them. Light gray nodes are genes with more than four edges going out from them. (Reprinted with permission from ref. *9*.)

one looks down the column representing S phase in **Fig. 3**, one can see that S phase genes influence S and M phase genes positively (red in image) but influence genes in M/G1 and G1 phase negatively (green in image).

A schematic presentation of interaction between genes among different cell cycles, as well as alpha pheromone and heat-shock-activated genes, is shown in **Fig. 4**. The influences are defined by the mean value of clustered blocks in **Fig. 3**. We found that genes in one cell-cycle phase activate genes in the next phase (solid lines) and sometimes inhibit genes in the previous phase (dashed lines). Genes responding to α-pheromone activate genes in S/G2 and G2/M, driving the cells into the cell cycle. Similar observations can be found with heat-shock-activated genes, which activate genes in M/G1 phase to drive the cells into the cell cycle. Interestingly, it is well-known that α-pheromone arrests cells in G1 phase, whereas low temperature arrests cdc-15 strains in late mitosis. Cells tend to reenter the cell cycle in the next phase beyond which they are arrested. The serial regulation of genes forms a connected regulatory network that is a

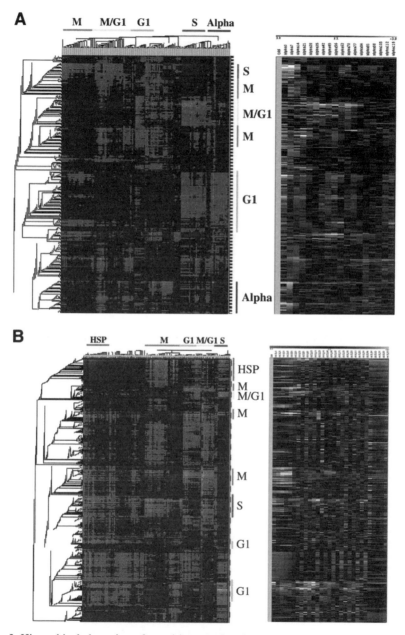

Fig. 3. Hierarchical clustering of transition matrix: (**A**) α-data set; (**B**) cdc-15 data set. The clustering result of the λ-matrix is shown on the left. Influencing genes are across the top and responding genes are along the side. Expression profiles of genes in the same order as in clustering are shown on the right. Genes with similar expression profiles are grouped together and are labeled with the cell-cycle phases. α-Labels α-pheromone-regulated genes, and HSP labels genes from heat-shock-activated proteins. (Reprinted with permission from ref. *9*.)

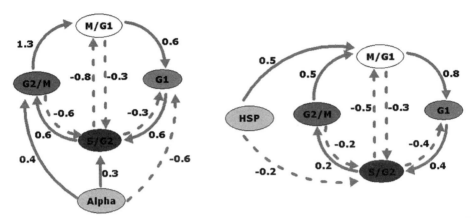

Fig. 4. Interaction of expression levels among cell-cycle phases: (**A**) α-Data set; (**B**) cdc-15 data set. Cell-cycle genes for different phases are shown, as well as α-pheromone-activated genes (α) and heat-shock-activated genes (HSP). Solid lines indicate positive influence or induction, and dotted lines indicate negative influence or inhibition. Numbers along the edges are the mean value of transition matrix entries of each clustered block and correspond to the influence between cell-cycle phases. (Reprinted with permission from ref. *9*.)

cycle, as discovered by Simon et al. *(10)*. Note that our result was obtained in an unsupervised fashion without any prior knowledge of chronological characteristics of the cell cycle. These results show how linear models can be used not in a fully quantitative capacity but, rather, in a qualitative, descriptive fashion. Considering the quality of the data and the phenomenological nature of the model, this is perhaps a more appropriate use of these models than as tools for quantitative prediction of expression levels.

4. Notes

Two main types of gene expression data are obtained from either two-colored cDNA microarray or Affymetrix Genechips. We briefly describe how these data were handled in our laboratory. The main analysis tools are libraries or packages within well-established programming and analysis languages Matlab and R. This permits easy exploitation of numerous data manipulation and statistical analysis tools available in these environments and facilitates tailoring analysis methods to the particular question and data collected to address it. Bioconductor is a collection of open-source R packages that support extensive microarray analysis *(11)* and has been used primarily as the analysis tool in our laboratory. Gene filtering and selection can greatly reduce the number of parameters, hence the speed of calculation.

The preprocessing steps specific for two-colored cDNA microarray are as follows:

a. Format new data for two-colored cDNA microarray in tab-delimited text files or comparables. Spot intensity, background intensity, and spot quality are commonly reported in these files, which can be imported into Matlab with the standard command *importdata*.

b. Examine data set for poor-quality spots that cause incorrect ratio estimates. Quality assurance methods consider spot shape, size, and uniformity; percentage of pixels with intensity larger than local or global background intensity; signal-to-noise ratio, defined by $[Spot_{intensity} - Background_{intensity}) / \sigma_{background}])$; or a weighted combination of these above. This quality-filtering step is sometimes included in the software packages for image analysis such as QuantArray (Perkin-Elmer, Boston, MA) and GenePix (Axon, Union Ciy, CA). Otherwise, it is straightforward to implement in Matlab or R.

c. Perform normalization to correct the possible bias or artifacts. Intensity-dependent location normalization implemented in the *marrayNorm* package within Bioconductor is probably a good choice for within-slide normalization. Normalization involving multiple slides is less developed, but scale normalization using the median absolute deviation (MAD) has been proposed *(12)* and included in the *marrayNorm* package. We recommend examining the MAD plot before and after normalization to ensure the effectiveness of this step.

d. Combine results from replicates, such as replicated spots, replicated slides with the same biological sample or different biological samples, and dye-swap slides. Averaging is a common practical method to combine the results from replicates. However, statistical evaluation of the replicates such as correlation or coefficient of variance (CV) should be applied to exclude outliers.

e. Conduct filtering to remove genes that are "uninteresting" from the analysis. Commonly used filters include fixed cutoff of fold change at more than a certain number of measurements, CV for replicated measurements, and statistical tests such as a *t*-test and a nonparametric test. These methods are either built-in functions or easy to implement in Matlab and R. Multiple comparison issues need to be considered to control the false-positive rate.

The preprocessing steps specific for Affymetrix GeneChips are as follows:

a. Conduct probe-level analysis. Affy package in Bioconductor implements a variety of preprocessing algorithms for Affymetrix GeneChip data, including data importing, background subtraction, normalization, photomultiplier correct, and summarization methods. Different algorithms have been compared to a benchmark developed by Cope et al. *(13)*. For the user's convenience, commands *mas5*, *li.wong*, and *justRMA* include all these preprocessing steps with some predefined parameters. Recent study indicates that Robust Multi-Array Average has many advantages over other algorithms *(14)* and, hence, is the choice in our laboratory.

b. Conduct gene filtering. Any gene with too low or too high intensity should not be considered as an acute measurement. A common practice is to reset any gene with intensity lower than 100 to 100 and any gene with intensity higher than 16,000 to 16,000.

c. Conduct gene selection. Common selection criteria include max(intensity)/min(intensity) with more threshold (>3), max(intensity)/min(intensity) with more threshold (>300), and a certain percentage of genes with the largest CV. Note that the choice of thresholds is very heuristic and depends on the properties of the data set.

With cDNA microarray data, the data are a ratio of expression levels. This ratio is dictated by the choice of the "reference" sample in the hybridization reaction. For time-series data, this reference is most often the sample at time $t - 0$, which is the mRNA extract from the experimental population before any stimulus occurs. In this case, the experimentally measured quantity is the ratio

$$a_i(t_j) = \frac{[mRNA_i(t_j)]}{[mRNA_i(0)]}$$

in which the brackets stand for concentration and the subscript i indicates the gene. This ratio is unitless, which means that the model parameters $\lambda_{i,j}$ are also unitless. However, since all ratios have the same denominator, the zero time concentration, the change in ratio over time will be proportional to the change in mRNA concentration. For Affymetrix data, one does not measure a ratio but, rather, an average quantity that is proportional to the concentration. If these concentrations are used directly instead of ratios, the genes with high concentration tend to dominate the model. We have calculated ratios for the Affymetrix data to avoid this problem. We have also avoided linear models that use the time derivative (i.e., the differential form of **Eq. 2**), because the time points are so widely separated that the approximation $da_j(t_k)/dt \approx [a_j(t_k) - a_j(t_{k-1})]/(t_k - t_{k-1})$ will be extremely inaccurate.

Using SVD, any matrix can be decomposed into a product of three matrices giving $\mathbf{A} = \mathbf{UEV^T}$. The matrices $\mathbf{U}$ and $\mathbf{V}$ are orthogonal matrices. This means that the transpose (created by exchanging rows and columns) is equal to the matrix inverse. Thus, $\mathbf{U}^{-1} = \mathbf{U^T}$ and $\mathbf{V}^{-1} = \mathbf{V^T}$. This gives $\mathbf{UU^T} = \mathbf{VV^T} = \mathbf{1}$, in which $\mathbf{1}$ is the unit matrix (diagonal 1s and 0s elsewhere). This property of the SVD makes it very simple to do matrix inversion. The matrix $\mathbf{A}$ is inverted by SVD according to

$$\mathbf{A}^{-1} = (\mathbf{UEV}^T)^{-1} = (\mathbf{V}^T)^{-1}\,\mathbf{E}^{-1}\,\mathbf{U}^{-1} = \mathbf{VE}^{-1}\,\mathbf{U^T}$$

in which the orthogonal property has been used to convert inverses into transposes. The matrix $\mathbf{E}$ is not a unitary matrix. It is a diagonal matrix of eigenvalues:

$$\mathbf{E} = \begin{bmatrix} \varepsilon_1 & 0 & \cdots & 0 \\ 0 & \varepsilon_2 & 0 & \vdots \\ \vdots & 0 & \ddots & 0 \\ 0 & \cdots & 0 & \varepsilon_N \end{bmatrix}$$

The inverse of a diagonal matrix is

$$\mathbf{E}^{-1} = \begin{bmatrix} \varepsilon_1^{-1} & 0 & \cdots & 0 \\ 0 & \varepsilon_2^{-1} & 0 & \vdots \\ \vdots & 0 & \ddots & 0 \\ 0 & \cdots & 0 & \varepsilon_N^{-1} \end{bmatrix}$$

SVD can also be used to calculate the gene and time covariance. The gene covariance matrix, $\mathbf{C_g}$, is

$$\mathbf{C_g} = \mathbf{AA^T} = (\mathbf{UEV^T})(\mathbf{UEV^T})^T = \mathbf{UEV}^T\,\mathbf{VE}^T\,\mathbf{U}^T = \mathbf{UEE}^T\,\mathbf{U}^T$$

Thus, the gene covariances are contained in matrix $\mathbf{U}$ and $\mathbf{E}$. The time covariance matrix, $\mathbf{C_t}$, is given by

$$\mathbf{C_t} = \mathbf{A^T A} = (\mathbf{UEV^T})^T(\mathbf{UEV^T}) = \mathbf{VE}^T\,\mathbf{U}^T\,\mathbf{UEV^T} = \mathbf{VE}^T\,\mathbf{EV}^T$$

showing that the time covariance is contained in $\mathbf{V}$ and $\mathbf{E}$.

Acknowledgments

We gratefully acknowledge funding from the W. M. Keck Foundation, and National Institutes of Health grant 1R01 GM63912-01.

References

1. Gollub, J., Ball, C. A., Binkley, G., et al. (2003) The Stanford Microarray Database: data access and quality assessment tools. *Nucleic Acids Res.* **31,** 94–96.
2. Bhan, A., Galas, D. J., and Dewey, T. G. (2002) A duplication growth model of gene expression networks. *Bioinformatics* **18,** 1486–1493.
3. Chen, T., He, H. L., and Church, G. M. (1999) Modeling gene expression with differential equations. *Pac. Symp. Biocomput. 1999,* 29–40.
4. D'Haeseleer, P., Wen, X., Fuhrman, S., and Somogyi, R. (1999) Linear modeling of mRNA expression levels during CNS development and injury. *Pac. Symp. Biocomput. 1999,* 41–52.
5. Dewey, T. G. and Galas, D. J. (2001) Dynamic models of gene expression and classification. *Funct. Integr. Genomics* **1,** 269–278.
6. Yeung, M. K., Tegner, J., and Collins, J. J. (2002) Reverse engineering gene networks using singular value decomposition and robust regression. *Proc. Natl. Acad. Sci. USA* **99,** 6163–6168.
7. de Hoon, M. J., Imoto, S., Kobayashi, K., Ogasawara, N., and Miyano, S. (2003) Inferring gene regulatory networks from time-ordered gene expression data of Bacillus subtilis using differential equations. *Pac. Symp. Biocomput. 2003,* 17–28.
8. Compton, L. A. and Johnson, W. C. Jr. (1986) Analysis of protein circular dichroism spectra for secondary structure using a simple matrix multiplication. *Anal. Biochem.* **155,** 155–167.
9. Wu, X. and Dewey, T. G. (2003) Cluster analysis of dynamic parameters of gene expression. *J. Bioinf. Comput. Biol.* **1,** 447–458.
10. Simon, I., Barnett, J., Hannett, N., et al. (2001) Serial regulation of transcriptional regulators in the yeast cell cycle. *Cell* **106,** 697–708.
11. Dudoit, S., Gentleman, R. C., and Quackenbush, J. (2003) Open source software for the analysis of microarray data. *Biotechniques* **34(Suppl.),** 45–51.
12. Yang, Y. H., Dudoit, S., Luu, P., et al. (2002) Normalization for cDNA microarray data: a robust composite method addressing single and multiple slide systematic variation. *Nucleic Acids Res.* **30,** e15.
13. Cope, L. M., Irizarry, R. A., Jaffee, H. A., Wu, Z., and Speed, T. P. (2004) A benchmark for Affymetrix GeneChip expression measures. *Bioinformatics* **20,** 323–331.
14. Irizarry, R. A., Hobbs, B., Collin, F., et al. (2003) Exploration, normalization, and summaries of high density oligonucleotide array probe level data. *Biostatistics* **4,** 249–264.

4

Microarray Analysis in Drug Discovery and Clinical Applications

Siqun Wang and Qiong Cheng

Summary

DNA microarray analyzes genome-wide gene expression patterns and is used in many areas including drug discovery and clinical applications. This chapter summarizes some of these applications such as identification and validation of anti-infective drug target, study mechanisms of drug action and drug metabolism, classification of different types of tumors, and use of molecular signatures for prediction of disease outcome. A step-by-step protocol is provided for sample preparation, sample labeling and purification, hybridization and washing, feature extraction, and data analysis. Important considerations for a successful experiment are also discussed with emphasis on drug discovery and clinical applications. Finally, a clinical study is presented as an example to illustrate how DNA microarray technology can be used to identify gene signatures, and to demonstrate the promise of DNA microarray as a clinical tool.

Key Words: Microarray analysis; expression profiling; drug discovery; molecular signature; clinical diagnosis.

1. Introduction

Microarray refers to an analysis tool for biological molecules arrayed on a surface, and later extended to nonsurface-based, such as the bead-based technique. Depending on the type of biological molecules interrogated, microarrays can be classified as DNA arrays, protein arrays, carbohydrate arrays, cell arrays, and tissue arrays. DNA microarrays can be further categorized as olignonucleotide arrays, cDNA arrays, and bead-based arrays. The first microarray was developed as a cDNA array *(1)* and cDNA arrays are still widely used today. The majority of commercial array products on the market is oligonucleotide based, and currently they provide probe densities up to a half million per square inch. These oligonucleotide arrays can be manufactured by first synthesizing the oligonucleotides and then spotting them on surfaces. Alternatively, they can be manufactured by *in situ* synthesis of oligonucleotides using Agilent's *SurePrint®* inkjet

From: *Methods in Molecular Biology, vol. 316: Bioinformatics and Drug Discovery*
Edited by: R. S. Larson © Humana Press Inc., Totowa, NJ

technology, Affymetrix's photolithographic technology, or NimbleGen's digital mask technology. Some specialized arrays are commercially available. Studying single nucleotide polymorphism of the human p53 tumor suppressor gene could be facilitated by the high-density oligonucleotide array of the p53 gene (Affymetrix GeneChip P53 assay). Studying regulation of p53 as a transcriptional factor could be facilitated by the cDNA-based p53 target gene array (Panomics Human TranSignal™ p53 Target Gene Array). Other commercial microarrays are designed for global gene expression profiling. They are usually designed for organisms with biological, pharmaceutical, or economical significance. The whole-genome arrays of organisms such as human, rat, mouse, yeast, arabidopsis, and rice will undoubtedly provide value and convenience to the pharmaceutical, agricultural, as well as academic researchers.

Microarrays have found many applications in drug discovery and clinical diagnosis and prognosis. DNA microarrays can be used to study pathogenesis to identify potential new targets for anti-infective drugs. They were used to identify Group A *Streptococcus* genes whose expression is specifically induced in a contact-mediated manner following interaction with human cells *(2)*. They were also used to identify bacterial virulence factors by comparing strain-specific differences between pathogenic and nonpathogenic strains *(3)* or strains of different serotypes *(2)*. Microarrays can also be used to study the mechanism of drug action and drug metabolism by examining the effect of drugs on host gene expressions *(4)*. Novel genes may be identified from the microarray that are involved in mediating resistance to drugs *(5)*. Such target genes might potentially be therapeutically valuable, or be predictive biomarkers of drug response. Gene expression profiling was used to classify different types of diffuse large B-cell lymphoma *(6)*. It was also used to predict the clinical outcome of breast cancer *(7,8)*. Molecular signatures associated with tumor metastasis were identified by microarray analysis *(9,10)*. Pending regulatory approval, Roche plans to introduce AmpliChip™ CYP450 Array for use in clinics to detect genetic variations in genes encoding P450 enzymes, which is the main mechanism for the body to metabolize most drugs. It is hoped that one day by examining variance in certain DNA markers, physicians will be able to predict patients' responses to many common drugs.

This chapter describes methods for DNA microarray analysis with emphasis on drug discovery and clinical applications. We provide step-by-step protocols for sample preparation, sample labeling and purification, hybridization and washing, feature extraction, and data analysis. We also discuss important factors for a successful experiment. Finally, we describe a clinical study as an example to illustrate how DNA microarray technologies can be used to identify a group of gene signatures, which is a powerful predictor of disease outcome.

2. Materials

1. *RNAlater*™ (product no. 7020; Ambion).
2. Trizol® reagent (product no. 15596-026; Invitrogen).
3. Total RNA Isolation Mini Kit (product no. 5185-6000; Agilent).
4. Low RNA Input Fluorescent Linear Amplification Kit (product no. 5184-3523; Agilent).
5. RNeasy mini kit (cat. no. 74104 for 50 columns or 74106 for 250 columns; Qiagen).

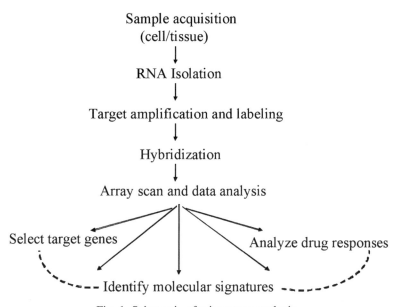

Fig. 1. Schematic of microarray analysis.

6. DNA microarrays, e.g., Agilent Human 1A(2) microarray (product number G4110B).
7. Hybridization rotator rack (product no. G2530-60020; Agilent).
8. Hybridization chamber (product no. G2534A; Agilent).
9. Hybridization oven (product no. G2505-80081 or G2505-80082; Agilent).
10. Wash solution 1 (6X saline sodium citrate [SSC], 0.005% Triton X-102).
11. Wash solution 2 (0.1X SSC, 0.005% Triton X-102).
12. 10X SSC: 87.6 g/L NaCl and 44 g/L Na citrate.
13. Cyanine 3-CTP (10 mM) (cat. no. NEL580; Perkin-Elmer/NEN), cyanine 5-CTP (10 mM) (cat. no. NEL 581; Perkin-Elmer/NEN), DNase/RNase-free distilled water (cat. no. 10977015; Invitrogen).
14. 100% Ethanol (cat. no. E193; Amresco).
15. Scanner, e.g., Agilent high-throughput high-sensitivity scanner (product no. G2565BA).
16. Data analysis softwares, e.g., Feature Extraction from Agilent (product no. G2567AA), Rosetta Resolver gene expression analysis software platform, or Spotfire DecisionSite platform.

3. Methods

Microarray analyzes genomewide gene expression levels under different conditions. A microarray experimental work flow (**Fig. 1**) starts with the sample acquisition. Depending on the design of the experiments, the samples may be obtained from different sources in different forms. RNA needs to be isolated from these samples. The RNA is amplified and labeled for hybridization with probe DNAs on the microarray. Following hybridization and washing, the array is scanned and ready for data analysis. Analysis results may lead to a variety of applications, such as selecting target genes for drug discovery and identifying molecular signatures for clinical diagnosis.

3.1. Sample Acquisition

Diverse biological samples have been used in microarray experiments and each may require special considerations. One of the most critical objectives for sample acquisition is to maintain the integrity and ratio of the original RNA population. Addition of reagents such as *RNAlater* can help minimize RNA degradation during sample acquisition. *RNAlater* contains a high concentration of salt, which precipitates and inactivates the RNase enzymes instantly. It has been shown to work with most types of cell lines and tissues from humans or animals, as well as from plant and bacterial samples. Flash-freezing samples in liquid nitrogen followed by storage at −70°C can also help maintain the integrity of the RNA population. Here we describe two types of samples that are most prevalent in the drug discovery and clinical applications.

3.1.1. Solid Tissue Samples

Solid tissue samples are probably the most common samples used today in microarray experiments for clinical applications. They can range from animal tissues of various disease models to human tissues from biopsies, pathological samples, and postmortem dissections. Although relative pure samples can be obtained with surgical procedures, this process is labor-intensive and requires experience and delicacy in execution. For genomics and proteomics studies, it is increasingly important to obtain pure populations of cells, such as cancer cells free from supporting stroma or neurons from a particular nucleus in the brain. Introduction of the computer-guided laser microdissection (LMD) technique makes the sample retrieval process easy for most laboratory personnel. A specific cell or a group of morphologically similar cells can be selected and excised from their surroundings under a microscope using the LMD technique. The extraction process can be either positive, in which case the cells are "lifted" or "dropped" to a microcentrifuge tube directly or with the help of an adhesive membrane, or negative, in which case a laser is used to destroy the surrounding tissue and leave the interested cells untouched. Several manufacturers offer products in this area, such as PixCell® from Arcturus Engineering, P.A.L.M.® MicroBeam from PALM Microlaser Technologies, μCUT from Molecular Machines and Industries, Leica AS LMD from Leica Microsystems, LaserScissors® Pro300 Workstation from Cell Robotics, and Clonis™ from Bio-Rad's microscopy division. With the capability of obtaining cells in such small numbers, the next challenge is how to isolate and process a small amount of RNA for the subsequent experiments. Advancements in sample preparation and labeling have enabled scientists to look at the expression of a few hundred cells with total RNA quantities in the nanogram or even subnanogram range.

3.1.2. Liquid Samples

Blood or other body fluids are commonly used liquid samples because they can be obtained with less invasive procedures. These samples can usually be concentrated via a procedure such as centrifugation or filtration. However, sometimes there is a need to separate a subset of a cell population, such as CD8+ T-cells from CD4+ T-cells. This is particularly relevant in drug development in monitoring drug response or disease process. Fluorescence-activated cell sorting is the predominant method used to separate specific cell populations according to a specific cellular marker, when the monoclonal antibodies are available. Separation methods based on magnetic beads provide another way to achieve a similar goal with relatively lower cost. The desired cell types can also be enriched by cell lysis such as antibody-dependent cell cytotoxicity to deplete a specific subset of a cell population. Cells in fluidic samples can also be applied to a surface and extracted by LMD as described in **Subheading 3.1.1.**

3.2. Preparation of Samples

Generally, RNA extraction methods can be classified as liquid-phase extraction exemplified by the Trizol methodology or solid-phase extractions such as with many silica-based column purification kits. Care should always be taken to minimize RNA degradation during extraction of samples.

3.2.1. Liquid-Phase Extraction

The phenol-based liquid extraction method has been the classic method to isolate biological molecules such as DNA and RNA. It is simple to use and requires minimum investment. Following is a protocol using the phenol-based Trizol reagent from Invitrogen. It can be easily scaled up or down for various applications.

1. Conduct homogenization as follows:
   a. Tissues: Homogenize tissue samples in 1 mL of Trizol reagent/50–100 mg of tissue using a glass-Teflon® or power homogenizer (Polytron, or Tekmar's Tissumizer®, or equivalent). The sample volume should not exceed 10% of the volume of Trizol reagent used for homogenization.
   b. Cells grown in monolayer: Lyse the cells directly in a culture dish by adding 1 mL of Trizol reagent to a 3.5-cm-diameter dish and passing the cell lysate several times through a pipet. The amount of Trizol reagent added is based on the area of the culture dish (1 mL/10 cm^2) and not on the number of cells present. An insufficient amount of Trizol reagent may result in contamination of the isolated RNA with DNA.
   c. Cells grown in suspension: Pellet cells by centrifugation. Lyse the cells in Trizol reagent by repetitive pipetting. Use 1 mL of reagent per 5–10×10^6 of animal, plant, or yeast cells, or per 1×10^7 bacterial cells. Washing cells before the addition of Trizol reagent should be avoided because this increases the possibility of mRNA degradation. Disruption of some yeast and bacterial cells may require the use of a homogenizer.
   Optional: An additional isolation step may be required for samples with a high content of proteins, fat, polysaccharides, or extracellular material, such as muscles, fat tissue, and tuberous parts of plants. Following homogenization, remove insoluble material from the homogenate by centrifuging at 12,000*g* for 10 min at 2–8°C. The resulting pellet contains extracellular membranes, polysaccharides, and high-molecular-weight DNA, and the supernatant contains RNA. In samples from fat tissue, an excess of fat collects as a top layer and should be removed. In each case, transfer the cleared homogenate solution to a fresh tube and proceed with chloroform addition and phase separation as described in **step 2**.
2. To perform phase separation, incubate the homogenized samples for 5 min at 15–30°C to permit the complete dissociation of nucleoprotein complexes. Add 0.2 mL of chloroform/ 1 mL of Trizol reagent. Cap the sample tubes securely. Shake the tubes vigorously by hand for 15 s and incubate them at 15–30°C for 2–3 min. Centrifuge the samples at no more than 12,000*g* for 15 min at 2–8°C. Following centrifugation, the mixture separates into a

lower red, phenol-chloroform phase; an interphase; and a colorless upper aqueous phase. RNA remains exclusively in the aqueous phase. The volume of the aqueous phase is about 60% of the volume of Trizol reagent used for homogenization. To reduce viscosity, shear the genomic DNA with two passes through a 26-gage needle prior to addition of chloroform.

3. To perform RNA precipitation, transfer the aqueous phase to a fresh tube, and save the organic phase if isolation of DNA or protein is desired. Precipitate the RNA from the aqueous phase by mixing with isopropyl alcohol. Use 0.5 mL of isopropyl alcohol/1 mL of Trizol reagent used for the initial homogenization. Incubate the samples at 15–30°C for 10 min and centrifuge at no more than 12,000g for 10 min at 2–8°C. The RNA precipitate, often invisible before centrifugation, forms a gel-like pellet on the side and bottom of the tube.

   For isolation of RNA from small quantities of tissue (1–10 mg) or cell (10^2–10^4) samples, add 5–10 μg RNase-free glycogen (Invitrogen cat. no. 10814) as carrier to the aqueous phase prior to precipitating the RNA with isopropyl alcohol. The glycogen remains in the aqueous phase and is coprecipitated with the RNA. It does not inhibit first-strand synthesis at concentrations up to 4 mg/mL and does not inhibit PCR.

4. To perform the RNA wash, remove the supernatant. Wash the RNA pellet once with 75% ethanol, adding at least 1 mL of 75% ethanol/1 mL of Trizol reagent used for the initial homogenization. Mix the sample by vortexing and centrifuge at no more than 7500g for 5 min at 2–8°C.

5. To redissolving the RNA, at the end of the procedure, briefly dry the RNA pellet (air-dry or vacuum dry for 5–10 min). Do not dry the RNA by centrifuging under vacuum. It is important not to let the RNA pellet dry completely because this will greatly decrease its solubility. Partially dissolved RNA samples have an $A_{260/280}$ ratio less than 1.6. Dissolve RNA in RNase-free water or 0.5% sodium dodecyl sulfate (SDS) solution by passing the solution a few times through a pipet tip, and incubating for 10 min at 55–60°C. Avoid SDS when RNA will be used in subsequent enzymatic reactions. RNA can also be redissolved in 100% formamide (deionized) and stored at −70°C.

3.2.2. Solid-Phase Extraction

Most of the columns on the market are based on either silica or membrane technologies. These technologies utilize the binding or insolubility of DNA or RNA in organic solvents, such as ethanol or isopropanol. The precipitated nucleotides are then washed and eluted with low-ionic-strength buffers or water for subsequent use. We describe here the generation of very pure RNAs in a short time using a new membrane-based technology from Agilent (product cat. no. 5185-6000).

1. Collect the sample and then process it immediately or flash freeze it in liquid nitrogen. Store the flash-frozen sample at −70°C.

2. Obtain a weight for the sample, and then place the sample (fresh or still frozen) in a suitable tube containing prepared lysis solution. Use 20 μL of lysis solution/mg of sample to be homogenized.

3. Immediately and vigorously homogenize using a conventional rotor-stator homogenizer at 15,000 rpm (this is 50% of the speed for an Omni International TH homogenizer) for 30 s. To reduce foaming, move the probe from side to side rather than up and down. Larger volumes (more than 10 mL) or fibrous tissues may require slightly longer homog-

enization times. If the homogenate will not be processed immediately, store it at −70°C. To process frozen homogenate, thaw it at 37°C for 15–20 min.

4. Centrifuge up to 600 µL of homogenate (equivalent to 30 mg of tissue) through a mini prefiltration column (natural) for 3 min at full speed (for a typical microcentrifuge, approx 16,000g). This step ensures complete homogenization of the tissue and removes cellular contaminants. Mini prefiltration columns cannot be reused. If processing more than 600 µL, use a new prefiltration column.

5. Add an equal volume of 70% ethanol to the filtrate and mix until the solution appears homogeneous. For certain tissues, the resultant mixture may appear opalescent. This poses no problem.

6. Add ethanol/lysis mixture (up to 700 µL) to the mini isolation column (blue), and then centrifuge for 30 s at 16,000g. Discard the flow-through, and replace the RNA-loaded column in the collection tube. If the homogenate/ethanol mixture volume exceeds 700 µL, add aliquots successively onto the mini isolation column, and then centrifuge and discard the flow-through as just described.

7. Add 500 µL of the previously prepared wash solution (to which ethanol has been added) to the mini isolation column, and then centrifuge for 30 s at 16,000g. Discard the flow-through, and then replace the mini isolation column in the same collection tube.

8. Repeat **step 7** one more time.

9. Spin the mini isolation column for 2 min at 16,000g. It is important to completely dry the mini isolation column to ensure that residual ethanol is not carried over during the elution.

10. Transfer the mini isolation column into a new 1.5-mL RNase-free final collection tube. Add 20–50 µL of nuclease-free water. Wait 1 min and then centrifuge for 1 min at 16,000g. If more concentrated RNA samples are desired for downstream application, the elution volume may be decreased (to as low as 10 µL). However, if the final RNA concentration exceeds 3–5 µg/µL, quantitative recovery of the RNA may be compromised.

It is recommended that the quality and the quantity of the RNA samples be determined before moving on to the next steps. Methods such as ultraviolet (UV) spectroscopy, gel electrophoresis, or capillary electrophoresis (e.g., Agilent's Bioanalyzer lab-on-chip system) can be applied for the determination. The RNAs purified with the Agilent Total RNA Isolation Mini Kit (product no. 5185-6000) usually contain up to 1000-fold less genomic DNA compared to silica-based column purification techniques.

3.3. Sample Labeling and Purification

RNA can be labeled directly or indirectly using fluorescent-based techniques. Direct labeling using dye-coupled nucleotides can be performed during reverse transcription or amplification into cDNA. The indirect labeling method incorporates modified nucleotides first and then couples with dyes either covalently or noncovalently. Biotin streptavidin interaction has been the choice for noncovalent coupling of a dye to the nucleotides. Aminoallyl-modified nucleotides have been the choice for covalent linking to a monofunctionalized NHS ester dye. Eukaryotic mRNAs with polyA tails can be preferentially labeled with oligo dT primers. Prokaryotic mRNAs with no or very short polyAs can be labeled with random primers such as random hexamers *(11,12)* or random ninemers *(13)*. We describe next a direct labeling protocol, based on a method originally developed in Eberwine's laboratory *(14)*, to generate fluorescently labeled cRNA molecules

Table 1
Master Mix

Component	Volume/reaction (μL)	Volume for 6.5 reaction (μL)
5X First-strand buffer	4.0	26
0.1 *M* DTT	2.0	13
10 m*M* dNTP mix	1.0	6.5
MMLV RT	1.0	6.5
RNaseOUT	0.5	3.3
Total volume	8.5	55.3

DTT, dithiothreitol; MMLV RT, Moloney murine leukemia virus reverse transcriptase; dNTP, dinucleotide phosphate.

by in vitro transcription. In this protocol, mRNA is first converted into cDNA by reverse transcription. A coliphage T7 promoter is incorporated into these cDNA molecules via a poly-dT/T7 hybrid primer. The cDNA molecules can be transcribed in vitro by T7 RNA polymerase with dye-coupled ribonucleotides (as either uracil triphosphate or cytosine triphosphate [CTP]). This method can generate fluorescently labeled cRNA molecules from limited samples such as biopsy or rare tissue source. It can use as little as 50 ng total RNA to generate fluorescently labeled cRNA in 8–10 h.

3.3.1. Linear Amplification With Low-RNA Input (Agilent Product No. 5184-3523)

1. Add 50–500 ng of total RNA in a volume of 10.3 μL or less to an Eppendorff tube. The total concentration should be at least 5 ng/μL.
2. Add 1.2 μL of T7 promoter primer containing both the poly dT to bind to the mRNA and the promoter sequence for the T7 RNA polymerase. If the total RNA input is greater than 500 ng, add 5 μL of T7 promoter primer.
3. Bring the total volume up to 11.5 μL using nuclease-free water.
4. Denature the primer and the template by incubating the reaction at 65°C in a heating block for 10 min.
5. Place the tube on ice and incubate for 5 min.
6. Make a master mix as outlined in **Table 1**.
7. Add 8.5 μL of cDNA mix to each sample tube.
8. Incubate the samples at 40°C in a circulating water bath for 2 h for the reverse transcription reaction.
9. Move the samples to a heating block or water bath set to 65°C, and incubate for 15 min to inactivate the murine Moloney leukemia virus reverse transcriptase.
10. Move the samples to ice. Incubate on ice for 5 min.
11. Spin the samples briefly in a microcentrifuge to bring down the condensations.
12. Add either 2.4 μL of cyanine 3-CTP (10 m*M*) or 2.4 μL of cyanine 5-CTP (10 m*M*) to each sample tube.
13. Immediately prior to use, gently mix the components in **Table 2** by pipetting in the order indicated at room temperature.
14. Add 57.6 μL of transcription master mix to each sample tube. Mix gently by pipetting.
15. Incubate the samples in a circulating water bath at 40°C for 2 h.

Table 2
Linear Amplification Components

Component	Volume/reaction (µL)	Volume for 6.5 reaction (µL)
Nuclease-free water	15.3	99.4
4X Transcription buffer	20	130
1 *M* DTT	6.0	39
NTP mix	8.0	52
50% PEG	6.4	41.6
RNaseOUT	0.5	3.3
Inorganic pyrophosphatase	0.6	3.9
T7 RNA polymerase	0.8	5.2
Total volume	57.6	374.4

DTT, dithiothreitol; PEG, polyethylene glycol; NTP, neuclotide triphosphate.

3.3.2. Purification of Amplified cRNA (Qiagen product no. 74104)

1. Add 20 µL of nuclease-free water to the cRNA sample, to obtain a total volume of 100 µL.
2. Add 350 µL of buffer RLT and mix thoroughly.
3. Add 250 µL of ethanol (96–100% purity) and mix thoroughly by pipetting.
4. Transfer 700 µL of cRNA sample to an RNeasy column in a new collection tube and add 500 µL to buffer RPE to the column. Centrifuge the sample for 30 s at 14,000*g*. Discard the flow-through and the collection tube.
5. Transfer the RNeasy column to a new collection tube and add 500 µL of buffer RPE to the column. Centrifuge the sample for 30 s at 14,000*g*. Discard the flow-through and the collection tube.
6. Again, add 500 µL of buffer RPE to the column. Centrifuge the sample for 60 s at 14,000*g*. Discard the flow-through and the collection tube.
7. Elute the cleaned cRNA sample by transferring the RNeasy column to a new 1.5-mL collection tube. Add 30 µL of nuclease-free water directly onto the RNeasy filter membrane. Wait 60 s before centrifuging for 30 s at 14,000*g*. The flow-through contains the purified cRNA and needs to be saved in the collection tube.
8. Again, add 30 µL of nuclease-free water directly onto the RNeasy filter membrane. Wait 60 s before centrifuging for 30 s at 14,000*g*. The total final flow-through volume should be approx 60 µL. Proceed immediately to hybridization or store the labeled target at −80°C until needed. Discard the RNeasy column.

3.4. Hybridization and Washing

Hybridization and washing steps are prone to human handling and environmental conditions, which would affect the quality of the microarray data. Manual hybridization requires minimum investment and is suitable for most daily operations in laboratories where throughput is not very high. The use of cover slips has been the common hybridization method for glass slide-based microarrays. It requires no specific setup other than a well-sealed humidified chamber. However, the cover slip method is cumbersome and introduces large variations. Recent improvement has been made in the use of a hybridization chamber, where it is possible to perform hybridization more evenly

Table 3
Hybridization Mix

22K Microarrays	11K Microarrays
0.75 µg of cyanine 3-labeled, linearly amplified cRNA	0.50 µg of cyanine 3-labeled, linearly amplified cRNA
0.75 µg of cyanine 5-labeled, linearly amplified cRNA	0.50 µg of cyanine 5-labeled, linearly amplified cRNA
50 µL of 10X control targets	50 µL of 10X control targets
Nuclease-free water to volume	Nuclease-free water to volume
Total volume per tube: 215 µL	Total volume per tube: 215 µL

with a larger volume of hybridization buffer. To increase reproducibility and through-put of the array experiments, automated hybridization and washing are recommended.

3.4.1. Manual Hybridization and Washing

Microarrays from Agilent (1 × 3 in. glass slide-based) are used to illustrate the pro-cedures for hybridization and washing. 11K microarrays contain 11,000 features/array and two arrays/slide. 22K microarrays contain 22,000 features/array and one array/slide. Many homemade arrays can be processed similarly.

3.4.1.1. STEP 1: HYBRIDIZATION MIX

1. Use 1.5-mL nuclease-free microcentrifuge tubes for this step. Either fluorescently labeled cRNA or cDNA can be used for hybridization. Prepare a target solution following **Table 3**.
2. The 2X target solution can be quick frozen on dry ice and stored in the dark at –80°C for up to 1 mo. When using frozen solution, thaw, vortex, and centrifuge for 5–10 s before use. For each microarray, prepare 1X hybridization solution as shown in **Table 4**.
3. Mix well by careful pipetting. Take care to avoid introducing bubbles. Do not vortex. Spin briefly in a microcentrifuge to drive the sample to the bottom of the tube. Use immediately; do not store.

3.4.1.2. STEP 2: HYBRIDIZATION

An agilent hybridization chamber (cat. no. G2534A) was used for the hybridization step.

1. Based on the type of Agilent oligonucleotide microarray being used, either 11K or 22K formats, choose the appropriate gasket slide from the gasket slide kit. Only handle these slides with powder-free gloves and by their edges when removing them from the packag-ing. Load a clean gasket slide into the chamber base with the label facing up and aligned in the rectangular section of the chamber base. Ensure that the gasket slide is flush with the chamber base and is not ajar. Slowly draw up the entire amount of solution from one tube, avoiding any bubbles in the solution. For each 11K microarray, approx 200 µL of hybridization solution will be used. Remember that there are two microarrays per slide. For each 22K microarray, approx 440 µL of hybridization solution will be used. Slowly dispense the solution onto the microarray gasket slide in a "drag and dispense" manner as

Table 4
1X Hybridization Solution

Per tube, for 22K Microarrays	Per tube, for 11K Microarrays
1. Add 215 µL of 2X target solution.	1. Add 100 µL of 2X target solution.
2. Add 9 µL of 25X fragmentation buffer.	2. Add 4 µL of 25X fragmentation buffer.
3. Mix well by gentle vortexing. Incubate at 60°C in a water bath in the dark for 30 min.	3. Mix well by gentle vortexing. Incubate at 60°C in a water bath in the dark for 30 min.
4. To each tube, add the following volume of hybridization buffer to terminate the fragmentation reaction: 225 µL of 2X hybridization buffer (from *in situ* hybridization kit) Total volume per microarray: 449 µL	4. To each tube, add the following volume of hybridization buffer to terminate the fragmentation reaction: 100 µL of 2X hybridization buffer (from *in situ* hybridization kit) Total volume per microarray: 204 µL

outlined in the Agilent microarray hybridization chamber user guide (G2534-90001). Do not move the chamber base or the gasket slide once the hybridization solution has been dispensed.

2. Remove the appropriate Agilent oligo microarray from its packaging using clean and powder-free gloves. Handle the oligo micrrray only by the ends of the slide, to avoid damaging the microarray surface. Flip the oligo microarray so that the numeric side is facing up as it is lowered onto the gasket slide. Lower carefully and align with the four guideposts on the chamber base. Once aligned and slightly above the gasket slide, let the oligo microarray slide drop to complete the sandwiched slide pair. Quickly assess that the slides are completely aligned and that the oligo microarray is not ajar (ends/sides can get caught on the upper part of the chamber base). Realign quickly if necessary.

3. Correctly place the chamber cover onto the sandwiched slides, and then slide on the clamp assembly until it comes to a stopping point in the middle of the chamber base and cover pair. Tighten the thumbscrew by turning it clockwise until it is fully hand-tight. Hold the chamber assembly in your hand vertically, and slowly rotate it clockwise two to three times to allow the hybridization solution to wet the gasket.

4. Inspect the sandwiched slides and note the bubble formation. A large mixing bubble should have formed. If stray, small bubbles are present and do not move when the chamber is rotated, gently tap one corner of the assembled chamber on a hard surface and rotate it vertically again. Determine whether the stray or stationary bubble(s) moved. If not, repeat by gently tapping another corner and proceed with vertical chamber rotation and inspection again. It is critical that the stray or stationary bubbles be dislodged before loading into the hybridization rotator rack and oven.

5. Continue loading and assembling the rest of the Agilent microarray hybridization chambers as specified in the Agilent microarray hybridization chamber user guide or as briefly detailed in **steps 3** and **4**.

6. Once all the chambers are fully assembled, load them into the hybridization rotator rack. If all the available positions on the hybridization rotator rack are not being loaded, be sure to balance the loaded hybridization chambers on the rack so that there are an equal number of empty positions on each of the four rows on the rack. Set the hybridization rotator to

rotate at a speed setting of 4 on an Agilent–recommended hybridization oven (e.g., Agilent product no. G2505-80081 or G2505-80082). Hybridize at 60°C for 17 h.

3.4.1.3. Step 3: Washing

1. Before incubation has finished, prepare three staining dishes:
   a. Add wash solution 1 (6X SSC, 0.005% Triton X-102) at room temperature to the first wash staining dish (large volume, approx 250 mL, to facilitate disassembly of hybridization chambers).
   b. Add a slide rack and a magnetic stir bar to the second wash staining dish. Cover the rack with room temperature wash solution 1. Place this dish on a magnetic stir plate.
   c. Place the third wash staining dish in another container filled with ice (a Pyrex loaf pan is well-suited for this purpose). Add a magnetic stir bar. Add 4°C wash solution 2 (0.1X SSC, 0.005% Triton X-102) to a depth sufficient to cover a slide rack. Be sure to replenish the ice in the outer container, which will keep the solution as cold as possible.
   Be sure to have all wash solution dishes prepared before hybridization chamber disassembly. The washing steps should be done as efficiently as possible. Do not wash slides in the slide rack immersed in wash solution by placing on an orbital rotator/shaker. This does not provide adequate mixing to facilitate robust washing.
2. Remove a maximum of two hybridization chambers from the oven at a time to avoid chamber cooldown before disassembly in the wash dish. Determine whether bubbles formed during hybridization, and if all bubbles are rotating freely. Place the hybridization chamber assembly on a flat surface and loosen the thumbscrew, turning counterclockwise. Slide off the clamp assembly and remove the chamber cover. With gloved fingers, remove the "sandwiched slides" from the chamber base by grabbing the slides from their ends. Keep the oligo microarray slide (numeric bar code facing up) while quickly transferring the sandwiched slides to the first wash staining dish. Without letting go of the sandwiched slides, submerge the slides into the first wash staining dish containing wash solution 1. With the sandwiched slides completely submerged in the wash solution, pry the two slides apart from only the bar code end. Do this by slipping one of the blunt ends of a pair of tweezers between the slides and then gently turning the tweezers upward or downward. Let the gasket slide drop to the bottom of the wash staining dish. Remove the oligo microarray slide quickly, and place in the slide rack contained in the second wash staining dish containing wash solution 1. Minimize exposure of the slide to air.
3. Complete the chamber disassembly and oligo microarray slide removal steps for the second chamber assembly. Once the second chamber has been disassembled and the slide is removed, proceed to retrieve a maximum of two more hybridization chambers from the hybridization oven and repeat **step 2**.
4. After all the slides have been collected in the slide rack, set the magnetic stir plate to medium speed. Wash the slides for 10 min at room temperature. Transfer the slide rack to the third staining dish containing wash solution 2, which is on ice. Place the entire dish on a magnetic stirring plate set to medium speed. Wash the slides for 5 min.
5. The slide rack containing slides must stay immersed in wash solution 2 during the individual slide-drying process. Dry each slide, one slide at a time. Remove one slide from the slide rack. Using a nitrogen-filled air gun, quickly blow drops of solution from the slide surface. Repeat this procedure for each individual slide in the slide rack.
6. Take care to avoid allowing drops of solution to travel back over the slide once the microarray has been dried. To measure fluorescence intensities, load the slides into a microarray scanner, or store in the dark under nitrogen until ready to scan.

3.4.2. Automated Hybridization and Washing

Automation holds the promise of increasing the throughput and reproducibility of microarray experiments, which are particularly important for applications such as molecular diagnostics. Several instruments are currently available, such as, the HS series hybridization station from Techan, the Ventana Discovery System from Amersham, and the GenTAC Hybridization Station from Genomic Solutions. However, cost and validation of the technology could prevent easy integration into the laboratory work flow.

3.5. Scanning and Data Analysis

After hybridization and washing, the data for gene expression are collected with a scanner and analyzed with the aid of bioinformatic software.

3.5.1. Image Scanning and Feature Extraction

Many different scanners are available. Depending on the requirement of the performance and throughput, available models include Axon's relatively low-cost "personal scanner" (GenePIX 4100A) or Agilent's high-throughput, high-sensitivity scanner (G2565BA). It is worthwhile to point out that the quality of the scanner, such as the dynamic range as well as the signal to noise, can impact the sensitivity of the microarray experiment.

Scanners usually are equipped with software for extraction and conversion of fluorescence or chemiluminescence intensities to relative numbers. For example, the Agilent Feature Extraction 7.1 can accurately determine the positions of each spot on the Agilent microarrays based on auto-grid and auto-spotfinding algorithms. One can also interactively position a grid and subgrids over non-Agilent or Agilent microarrays and locate the spots based on the grids one defines. The software can efficiently and rapidly convert data extracted from these features into quantitative log ratios. It also calculates the error associated with each log ratio and p values for statistical analysis, which helps to identify random and systematic errors during printing or processing.

3.5.2. Data Analysis and Hypothesis Building

One of the major bottlenecks for microarray experiments is the data analysis. Reduction of the vast amount of data generated from the microarrays to some biologically meaningful results is very challenging. Although it is critical to design an experiment correctly, postexperiment data analysis is also extremely important for a successful experiment. Some software with more comprehensive and robust features, such as the Resolver from Merck Rosetta, could help with the data analysis. Rosetta Resolver can input data generated from different array platforms and compile large amounts of array data. It can also include multivariables simultaneously for statistical analysis and allow comparisons between samples, experiments, and laboratories after data normalization. Although the simple "unsupervised" hierarchical clustering ranking can provide quite useful information, more valuable insight is often obtained after a "supervised" ranking process, i.e., combining the biological information with the statistical analysis. In addition, Rosetta Resolver can map the expression data to biological pathways in other databases to facilitate the hypothesis-building process. The hypothesis needs to be tested further with other experimental methods.

4. Notes

The procedures described here using the Agilent *in situ*-synthesized oligonucleotide array could be applied with slight modifications to other types of arrays in a variety of applications. The most critical factor in a successful array experiment is the sample acquisition because most biological samples are limited and mRNA species are inherently unstable. Care should be taken to minimize RNA degradation during sample acquisition and extraction. RNA quality should be verified by methods such as UV spectroscopy or electrophoresis.

For study infectious diseases, the samples for the microarray experiment would usually be different microbes (virulent strain vs avirulent strain, wild-type strain vs mutant strain). Care should be taken to grow the microbes under the same conditions to minimize nonrelevant expression differences between the strains. Comparison of the gene expression patterns between the different strains would facilitate identification of drug targets, which may be used for development of antibiotics and vaccines. To identify molecular signatures for a disease, the samples for the microarray experiment would usually be different tissue samples (normal tissue vs abnormal tissue, or tissue samples from different subgroups of patients). The differentially expressed genes between tissue samples (molecular signatures) need to be validated with clinical phenotypes including traditional pathological classification. These molecular signatures could be used as prognostic markers to identify disease susceptibility for early treatment. To study drug response and drug metabolism, the samples for the microarray experiment would usually be cells that are treated or not treated with the drug. Expression analysis of these samples would allow prediction of toxicity and side effects of the drug even prior to clinical trials. In the future, personalized treatment could be applied based on the genetic background of the individual and the predicted responses to the drugs.

Internal controls can be included through the entire work flow for normalization to allow comparisons between samples, experiments, and data from different laboratories. Internal controls, or spike-ins, are usually selected from sequences with minimum homology to the genes being studied. For example, bacterial and viral genes have been used as controls for human and other mammalian arrays. These controls provide useful information on the reliability and sensitivity of the experiments and also a calibration for the experimental data *(15)*. Other types of controls include probe sets for manufacturing quality control such as the eQC probe sets for Agilent arrays and the ICT-LIZ probe sets for ABI arrays.

In a two-color hybridization system, bias may be introduced by differences of the two fluorophores such as Cy3 and Cy5. The bias could be owing to the differences in quantum yield, enzyme incorporation efficiency, as well as sensitivity to the environmental factors. It is highly recommended that a dye-swap experiment *(16)*, in which duplicate microarrays are hybridized with reciprocal dye combinations, be carried out to avoid bias and test the correlation between the two sets of dyes. Successful protocols should give a high correlation (in our experience usually about 0.9), whereas lower correlation coefficients suggest that the amount of dye in the labeling reaction needs to be balanced.

The statistical confidence of the data depends on the system's noise, which includes noise in the biological replicates (which is usually the largest); noise in the sample preparation; noise in the labeling, amplification, and hybridization procedures; and noise in scanning, such as laser stability of the scanner and array manufacturing. Noises or errors in replicate samples, sample preparation, or processing are random errors. Noises in array manufacturing or scanning are systematic errors. It is recommended that the level of these noises be defined and incorporated into the analysis process. As a result of this type of analysis (e.g., error modeling), a calculated confidence level could be associated with the data.

Expression data obtained from DNA microarray experiments usually needs to be validated by other experimental methods. Northern blot and real-time reverse transcriptase polymerase chain reaction are alternative methods to measure transcriptional expression as the DNA microarrays. In some cases, mRNA levels do not directly correlate with protein levels in the cell. Proteomics enabling simultaneous monitoring of all proteins in a cell is complementary to DNA microarrays.

As an example to illustrate microarray applications, we describe here in more detail two consecutive studies carried out by clinicians and scientists at Netherlands Cancer Institute and Rosetta Inpharmatics *(7,8)*. This example shows how the microarray technology described in this chapter was used to profile breast cancer patients and identify gene signatures for prediction of disease outcome. A total of 98 breast cancer samples were selected according to their original tumor size, metastasis, and patient age. Total RNA was extracted first with phenol (RNAzolB) and subsequently treated with DNase followed by purification with RNeasy columns. This two-step procedure usually yields higher-quality RNA samples than the use of either phenol or the column alone. Individual tumor RNA samples were labeled with one fluorescent dye and mixed with the same amount of reverse-colored Cy-labeled product from a pool consisting of an equal amount of cRNA from each patient. The labeled cRNAs were fragmented and hybridized to an oligonucleotide DNA array containing 25,000 human genes synthesized by Agilent's ink-jet technology. Two hybridizations were carried out using the swapped fluorescent dyes for labeling RNA samples. Fluorescent intensities of the 25,000 genes were quantified and normalized. Approximately 5000 genes were significantly up- or downregulated. An unsupervised hierarchical clustering algorithm allowed the investigators to classify the 98 tumors into two distinct groups based on the expression profile of the 5000 genes. In group A, only 34% of the patients developed a distant metastasis within 5 yr (good-prognosis group), whereas in group B, 70% of patients developed progressive disease (poor-prognosis group).

To search for a minimal set of genes to be used as prognostic signature, the investigators performed a three-step supervised clustering for 78 sporatic lymph node-negative patients. First, they determined the correlation of the expression of each of these 5000 genes with the disease outcome. Two hundred thirty-one genes were selected as significantly associated with the disease (correlation coefficient r value <-0.3 or >0.3). Second, they ranked these 231 genes according to the magnitude of the correlation or the absolute value of the correlation coefficient. Third, they evaluated the contribution of the 231 genes by adding a group of 5 genes at a time from the top of this rank list and cross validated this new set of genes with a scheme of "leave one out." Briefly, the investigators generated the gene rank list from these 231 predictive genes using 77 of the 78 tumor samples (left one out). The new list was used to predict the outcome of the one cancer that was left out in the first place. They measured both false-positive and false-negative rates for each of the set of the predictive genes by adding 5 genes at a time until all 231 genes had been used. This exercise was carried out for each of the 78 tumors, and the investigators found that minimum false rates were achieved when they used a group of 70 genes. With this set of 70 genes, 65 of the 78 tumors can be correctly classified.

This set of 70-gene prognosis signature was applied to classify a larger group of 295 patients with primary breast cancer. It is gratifying that prediction of both long-term survival and distal metastasis using this set of prognosis signature genes was more accurate than using the standard classification methods based on clinical and histopathological criteria by the multivariable Cox regression analysis. This example not only confirms the value of this 70-gene signature in predicting the outcome of breast cancer, but also demonstrates the promise of using gene expression profiling for clinical diagnosis.

References

1. Schena, M., Shalon, D., Davis, R. W., and Brown, P. O. (1995) Quantitative monitoring of gene expression patterns with a complementary DNA microarray. *Science* **270,** 467–470.
2. Graham, M. R., Smoot, L. M., Lei, B., and Musser, J. M. (2001) Toward a genome-scale understanding of group A Streptococcus pathogenesis. *Curr. Opin. Microbiol.* **4,** 65–70.
3. Israel, D. A., Salama, N., Arnold, C. N., et al. (2001) Helicobacter pylori strain-specific differences in genetic content, identified by microarray, influence host inflammatory responses. *J. Clin. Invest.* **107,** 611–620.
4. Hooper, L. V., Wong, M. H., Thelin, A., Hansson, L., Falk, P. G., and Gordon, J. I. (2001) Molecular analysis of commensal host-microbial relationships in the intestine. *Science* **291,** 881–884.
5. Longley, D. B., Harkin, D. P., and Johnston, P. G. (2003) 5-fluorouracil: mechanisms of action and clinical strategies. *Nat. Rev. Cancer* **3,** 330–338.
6. Alizadeh, A. A., Eisen, M. B., Davis, R. E., et al. (2000) Distinct types of diffuse large B-cell lymphoma identified by gene expression profiling. *Nature* **403,** 503–511.
7. van 't Veer, L. J., Dai, H., van de Vijver, M. J., et al. (2002) Gene expression profiling predicts clinical outcome of breast cancer. *Nature* **415,** 530–536.
8. van de Vijver, M. J., He, Y. D., van't Veer, L. J., et al. (2002) A gene-expression signature as a predictor of survival in breast cancer. *N. Engl. J. Med.* **347,** 1999–2009.
9. Woelfle, U., Cloos, J., Sauter, G., et al. (2003) Molecular signature associated with bone marrow micrometastasis in human breast cancer. *Cancer Res.* **63,** 5679–5684.
10. Ramaswamy, S., Ross, K. N., Lander, E. S., and Golub, T. R. (2003) A molecular signature of metastasis in primary solid tumors. *Nat. Genet.* **33,** 49–54.
11. Arfin, S. M., Long, A. D., Ito, E. T., et al. (2000) Global gene expression profiling in Escherichia coli K12: the effects of integration host factor. *J. Biol. Chem.* **275,** 29,672–29,684.

12. Xiang, C. C., Kozhich, O. A., Chen, M., et al. (2002) Amine-modified random primers to label probes for DNA microarrays. *Nat. Biotechnol.* **20,** 738–742.
13. Schut, G. J., Zhou, J., and Adams, M. W. (2001) DNA microarray analysis of the hyperthermophilic archaeon Pyrococcus furiosus: evidence for a new type of sulfur-reducing enzyme complex. *J. Bacteriol.* **183,** 7027–7036.
14. Van Gelder, R. N., von Zastrow, M. E., Yool, A., Dement, W. C., Barchas, J. D., and Eberwine, J. H. (1990) Amplified RNA synthesized from limited quantities of heterogeneous cDNA. *Proc. Natl. Acad. Sci. USA* **87,** 1663–1667.
15. Hughes, T. R., Mao, M., Jones, A. R., et al. (2001) Expression profiling using microarrays fabricated by an ink-jet oligonucleotide synthesizer. *Nat. Biotechnol.* **19,** 342–347.
16. Foreman, P. K., Brown, D., Dankmeyer, L., et al. (2003) Transcriptional regulation of biomass-degrading enzymes in the filamentous fungus Trichoderma reesei. *J. Biol. Chem.* **278,** 31,988–31,997.

5

Ontology-Driven Approaches
to Analyzing Data in Functional Genomics

Francisco Azuaje, Fatima Al-Shahrour, and Joaquin Dopazo

Summary

Ontologies are fundamental knowledge representations that provide not only standards for annotating and indexing biological information, but also the basis for implementing functional classification and interpretation models. This chapter discusses the application of gene ontology (GO) for predictive tasks in functional genomics. It focuses on the problem of analyzing functional patterns associated with gene products. This chapter is divided into two main parts. The first part overviews GO and its applications for the development of functional classification models. The second part presents two methods for the characterization of genomic information using GO. It discusses methods for measuring functional similarity of gene products, and a tool for supporting gene expression clustering analysis and validation.

Key Words: Gene ontology; clustering; expression data; similarity; functional genomics.

1. Introduction

One fundamental requirement of the drug discovery paradigm in the postgenome era is the capacity to analyze and combine large amounts of data originating from genomics and proteomics. Such a framework relies not only on the application of powerful bioinformatics tools to classify data patterns, but also on the automated incorporation of formal and usable knowledge representations for making data mining a more meaningful process. Drug discovery requires advanced pattern discovery platforms for facilitating a better understanding of spatial and temporal properties of molecules and processes, such as those observed in gene and protein expression and protein–protein interactions. These technologies help scientists to understand how biological systems may be both monitored and engineered. The former goal is concerned with the task of identifying biomarkers. The latter is relevant to the problem of discovering potential drug targets.

From: *Methods in Molecular Biology, vol. 316: Bioinformatics and Drug Discovery*
Edited by: R. S. Larson © Humana Press Inc., Totowa, NJ

Outcomes originating from genomics and proteomics can now be accessed through diverse data repositories, which may also provide annotations and vocabularies used to describe the structure and function of genes and their products. This type of prior information becomes an important source of background knowledge, which can be exploited to facilitate cross-database queries and to support the validation of bioinformatics and experimental results for drug discovery.

An *ontology* is a structured and controlled representation of background knowledge. It consists of taxonomies and rules that define properties and relationships between concepts. In a biological context, a concept may be represented as an annotation term. These representations are designed to be understandable by both humans and computers.

Ontologies represent an important step in supporting the unification of databases. They facilitate information search tasks across databases, because they offer a framework to store and query different repositories using the same query terms. The most relevant bioontologies may be accessed through the Open Biomedical Ontologies (OBO) Web site. These ontologies have been created and accepted by the OBO group as authoritative biological knowledge resources (http://obo.sourceforge.net/). It includes ontologies representing generic knowledge across different organisms, or associated with several biological domains and specific model organisms.

Gene ontology (GO) *(1)* website is one of the Open Biomedical Ontologies resources and offers controlled vocabularies and shared hierarchies for supporting the annotation of molecular attributes across model organisms. However, the relevance of ontologies, such as GO, goes beyond information search and retrieval applications. It has been suggested that they may significantly facilitate large-scale applications for functional genomics. For example, it has been suggested that the GO can be used for implementing advanced functional prediction systems *(1)*.

Assessment of gene or protein similarity is at the center of important tasks in functional genomics. One key strategy to exploit the information encoded in an ontology such as GO may consist of processing it to measure the similarity between gene products. This type of similarity information is sometimes referred to as semantic similarity, because it takes into account information relevant to the definition of concepts and their interrelationships within a specific problem domain. Another important problem comprises the application of GO knowledge to automatically describe gene clusters in terms of functional categories.

There are two major classification schemes for studying proteins *(2)*. Structural classification measures similarity based on protein sequence and tertiary structure. Functional classification assesses similarity in terms of functional features such as biochemical pathways and cellular localization. Such a scheme does not comprise structural similarity features or models. The methods discussed in this chapter emphasize the application of ontology-driven information for functional classification applications.

This chapter introduces techniques for incorporating GO information into functional classification tasks. It discusses the problem of measuring gene product similarity within GO and describes a technique for functionally characterizing gene clusters using information automatically extracted from GO. **Heading 2** provides an overview of GO and some of its applications in functional classification. **Heading 3** introduces the problem of measuring semantic similarity in a taxonomy. It describes methods to measure similarity based on GO annotations, as well as potential significant relationships with gene expression correlation. **Heading 4** introduces FatiGO, a data-mining tool for labeling gene clusters on the basis of their most characteristic GO terms. Finally, **Heading 5** discusses the advantages and limitations of the methods proposed.

2. GO for Functional Classification Applications

GO defines a structured and controlled vocabulary to annotate molecular attributes across model organisms *(1)*. It allows users to access annotation and specialized query information resulting from different model organisms. For instance, different databases such as the *Saccharomyces* Genome Database (SGD) and the Database of the *Drosophila* Genome (FlyBase) provide annotations defined by this ontology. Such annotation files also offer useful information about the evidence for the knowledge represented. This information is stored in the form of evidence codes. There are different types of GO evidence codes, such as TAS (Traceable Author Statement) and IEA (Inferred from Electronic Annotation). The evidence code TAS refers to annotations supported by articles or books written by experts in the field. By contrast, IEA annotations are based on results automatically derived from sequence similarity searches, which have not been reviewed by curators.

GO actually comprises three ontologies, sometimes referred to as "aspects" or "taxonomies": molecular function, biological process, and cellular component. The first taxonomy refers to information on what a gene product does. Biological process is related to a biological objective to which a gene product contributes. Cellular component refers the cellular location of the gene product. **Figure 1A** depicts a partial view of the first level of terms included under molecular function. The reader is referred to **ref. 1** and its Web site for further information on the design and implementation principles of GO (www.geneontology.com).

GO vocabularies (one for each ontology) and their relationships are represented in the form of directed acyclic graphs. Thus, a taxonomy in GO may be seen as a network in which each term or concept may represent a "child node" of one or more "parent nodes." There are two types of child-to-parent relationships: is–a and part–of. The first type is defined when a child is an instance of a parent. For example, from the molecular function ontology, drug binding is a child of binding. The second type is used to describe when a child node is a component of a parent. For example, from the biological process ontology, cell aging is part of cell death. **Figure 1B** illustrates a partial view of the type of directed acyclic graphs found in GO.

In the area of drug discovery, ontologies have been traditionally used to improve database search applications owing to their ability to describe unambiguously molecules, processes, and compounds. Pharmaceutical companies are developing joint projects to integrate GO annotations and other relevant resources for analyzing genomic data, including gene expression data *(3)*. Some of them are also contributing to the development of new ontologies, such as specialized tissue-type ontologies, which eventually will become publicly available *(3)*. For additional information on ontology design and current collaborative projects in this area, the reader is referred to **refs. 3** and *4*.

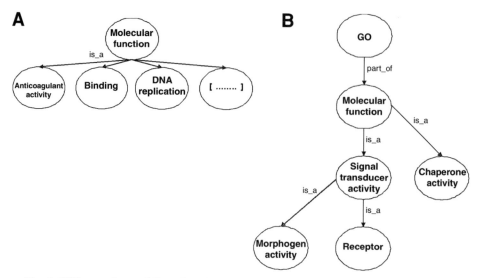

Fig. 1. Different views of Gene Ontology. (**A**) Partial view of first level of molecular function ontology; (**B**) typical example of a directed acyclic graph in GO. Dashed lines indicate the
presence of several terms not included here.

Recent research advances go well beyond information annotation and retrieval applications. For example, King et al. *(5)* have predicted known and novel gene–phenotype
associations in yeast. Their model processes phenotypic annotations extracted from the
Munich Information Center for Protein Sequences database and gene annotations based
on more than 3000 GO terms. Decision trees and a cross-validation procedure are implemented to infer these associations. Hvidsten et al. *(6)* have combined a series of gene
expression data with annotations originating from GO biological process ontology. They
propose a supervised classification system, based on rough set theory, to assign biological process categories to genes represented by expression patterns. King et al. *(7)* have
applied decision trees and Bayesian networks to predict new GO terms–gene associations using existing annotations from the SGD and FlyBase. These models allow the
calculation of the probability that a gene, *g*, is annotated using a particular annotation
term, *c*, taking into account the known annotation profile of *g* and its similarity relationship with other annotation patterns observed in the database. King et al. *(7)* processed
terms originating from all the GO taxonomies. An evaluation of these predictions showed
that 41 gene–annotation associations were accepted to be true, and 42 were both novel
and likely significant, out of 100 predictions semiautomatically validated. Laegreid et
al. *(8)* have also applied supervised learning methods to predict GO annotation terms.
However, they use temporal gene expression patterns as the inputs to the prediction
model. They also focus on the prediction of GO biological process terms. These investigators established significant associations between these ontology categories and expression patterns extracted from a fibroblast serum response data set, which was generated

by Iyer et al. *(9)*. Validation based on literature search and homology information confirmed the relevance of some of the process roles assigned to uncharacterized genes.

The following section introduces the problem of measuring semantic similarity in a taxonomy, as well as an application of GO-driven similarity assessment for gene expression data analysis, which is not addressed by the previously discussed research.

3. Gene Product Similarity Assessment and GO

To understand the problem of measuring semantic similarity between gene products based on their annotations, it is first necessary to describe approaches to calculating the similarity between annotation terms in an ontology. The similarity between ontology terms may be calculated on the basis of different types of taxonomical interrelationships.

Given a pair of terms, $c1$ and $c2$, a method for measuring their similarity consists of calculating the distance between the nodes associated with these terms in the ontology. The shorter this distance, the higher the similarity. If there are multiple paths, one may use the shortest or the average distance. This approach is commonly referred to as the "edge" or "node counting" method. A variation of this method defines weights for the links according to their position in the taxonomy *(10)*. It stresses the idea that differences between upper-level terms are stronger than between lower-level terms. Artificial intelligence researchers have studied the constraints exhibited by this type of model *(11)*. One of its major limitations is that it heavily relies on the idea that nodes and links in an ontology are uniformly distributed. This is not an accurate assumption in ontologies exhibiting variable link densities.

An alternative approach to measuring semantic similarity applies information-theoretic principles *(11)*. It has been demonstrated that this type of approach is less sensitive and in some cases not sensitive to the problem of link density variability *(12)*.

Let C be the set of terms in GO. One key approach to assessing the similarity between terms, $c \sim C$, is to analyze the amount of information they share in common. In GO or any other taxonomy this information may be represented by the set of parent nodes, which subsume the terms under consideration. For example, in **Fig. 1B** the terms "Morphogen activity" and "Receptor" are subsumed by the terms "Signal transducer activity" and "Molecular function." Thus, one may say that the terms "Morphogen activity" and "Receptor" shared those attributes (parents) in common.

For each term, $c \, L \, C$, $p(c)$ is the probability of finding a child of c in the taxonomy. Thus, as one moves up to the root node of GO (i.e., the terms "molecular function," "biological process," and "cellular component") $p(c)$ monotonically approaches a value equal to 1. This together with the principle of information theory allows the quantification of the information content of a term as equal to $-\log(p(c))$.

Information content allows measurement of the semantic similarity between terms based on the assumption that the more information two terms share in common, the more similar they are. In this situation, the information shared by two terms may be calculated using the information content of the terms subsuming them in the ontology. Such a semantic similarity model was proposed by Resnik *(12)* and is mathematically defined as follows:

$$Sim(c_i, c_j) = \max_{c \in S(c_i, c_j)} \ [-\log(p(c))] \tag{1}$$

in which $S(c_i, c_j)$ comprises the set of parent terms shared by both terms c_i and c_j, and max represents the maximum operator. The value of this metric can vary between 0 and infinity. For example, in **Fig. 1B** "Signal transducer activity" and "Molecular function" belong to $S(c_1, c_2)$, in which c_1 and c_2 are "Morphogen activity" and "Receptor," respectively. Nevertheless, "Signal transducer activity," which provides the minimum $p(c)$ and the maximum $-\log(p(c))$, also represents the most informative term. Thus, **Eq. 1** provides the information content of the lowest common ancestor of two terms.

Lin *(13)* proposed an alternative information-theoretical method. It takes into account not only the parent commonality of two query terms, but also the information content associated with them. Thus, given terms c_i and c_j, their similarity may be defined as follows:

$$sim(c_i, c_j) = \frac{2 \times \max\limits_{c \in S(c_i, c_j)} \ [\log(p(c))]}{\log(p(c_i)) + \log(p(c_j))} \tag{2}$$

in which $p(c_i)$ and $p(c_j)$ are as previously defined. The values generated by **Eq. 2** vary between 0 and 1. This technique may be seen as a normalized version of Resnik's method. For additional information on these and related techniques for semantic similarity assessment, the reader is referred to **refs.** *11* and *13*.

Based on **Eqs. 1** or **2** it is then possible to calculate the semantic similarity between gene products based on their annotations. Given a pair of gene products, g_i and g_j, that are annotated by a set of terms A_i and A_j, respectively, in which A_i and A_j comprise m and n terms, respectively, the semantic similarity $SIM(g_i, g_j)$ may be defined as the average interset similarity between terms from A_i and A_j. Thus, this method allows integration of similarity contributions originating from all of the terms used to describe g_i and g_j. This is formally defined as follows:

$$SIM(g_i, g_j) = \frac{1}{m \times n} \times \sum_{c_k \in A_i, c_p \in A_j} sim \ (c_k, c_p) \tag{3}$$

Lord et al. *(14)* have investigated the relationship between semantic similarity and protein sequence similarity. They have suggested that semantic similarity metrics, such as those based on **Eqs. 1–3**, are correlated with sequence similarity. Such a relationship seems to be stronger when similarity is computed using the molecular function ontology. Their results are based on the analysis of the Swiss-Prot-Human database. They conclude that semantic similarity may support more powerful gene sequence search and retrieval tasks.

This chapter discusses the incorporation of ontology-driven similarity for functional classification applications. The following section illustrates how this approach may be applied to support gene expression analysis.

3.1. Linking GO-Driven Similarity and Expression Data

The results presented here aim to establish associations between GO terms and gene products included in the SGD. One important goal is to formulate quantitative relationships between the semantic similarity of pairs of gene products and gene expression correlation. The analyses may consider only non-IEA annotations owing to their reliability and quality, as explained under **Heading 2**. As a way of illustration, this integration process is based on data that characterize mRNA transcript levels during the cell cycle of *Saccharomyces cerevisiae (15)*. Semantic similarity analyses were performed on 225 genes that show significant and periodic transcriptional fluctuations during five cell-cycle phases: early G1, late G1, S, G2, and M phases *(15)*. These phases may also be seen as gene clusters on the basis of their expression patterns. Each gene is described by 17 expression values, which are associated with 17 time points. The total number of gene pairs generated by this data set is 25,200. Thus, 25,200 pairs of semantic similarity values and 25,200 expression correlation values were calculated. Gene expression correlation is calculated using the well-known Pearson correlation coefficient. Graphic analyses and analysis of variance (ANOVA) between groups of genes/samples may be implemented to visualize potential relationships among semantic similarity, expression correlation, and cell-cycle phases. Significant quantitative relationships between ontology-driven similarity and expression correlation for a particular data set may justify the application of this type of tool in predictive and evaluation tasks.

Figure 2 depicts mean expression correlation values between pairs of gene products against semantic similarity based on the molecular function ontology. The axis of abscissas is divided into a number of similarity intervals, and the axis of ordinates shows the mean expression correlation values for these intervals and their ±0.95 confidence intervals. Graphs can be generated for the three GO taxonomies independently. The similarity values included in **Fig. 2** are based on Resnik's similarity measure (**Eq. 1**). In general, for different sizes of similarity intervals and types of ontology, high similarity values are associated with high expression correlation values, and low expression correlation is associated with weak semantic similarity. By augmenting or reducing the number of similarity intervals, it is possible to observe this global trend in terms of extreme values: lowest/highest similarity/correlation values for all types of ontologies. However, on the basis of the data available and for different numbers of similarity intervals, it is not possible to define a pattern to describe accurately the type and shape of the possible existing relationship for all of the similarity–correlation intervals. In this case, it is only possible to argue that there may exist a nonlinear relationship between these two functional features, in which the strongest and weakest semantic similarities may be linked to the highest and lowest expression correlation values, respectively. This response is significantly stronger in the case of the lowest expression correlation values.

Figure 3 illustrates results based on the semantic similarity measure proposed by Lin (**Eq. 2**) that were obtained for the molecular function ontology. These results are, in general, consistent with the results produced by Resnik's method. The results also suggest that the strongest and weakest semantic similarities may be linked to the highest and lowest expression correlation values, respectively. The same conclusion is obtained for all three of the GO taxonomies under study, whose graphic representations have not been included here owing to space constraints.

This type of analysis may be seen as an exploratory study of key functional properties reflected in GO. Once potential significant relationships have been identified, one may apply this similarity approach to supporting functional genomics analyses, such

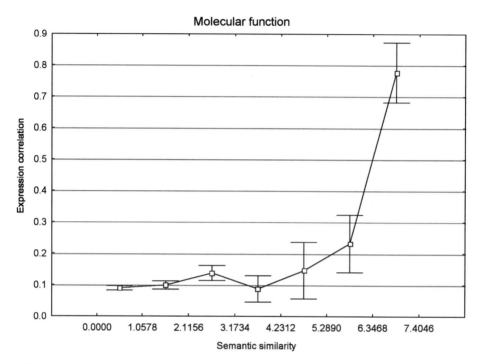

Fig. 2. Relationship between expression correlation and semantic similarity using gene ontology molecular function taxonomy. The axis of abscissas is divided into similarity intervals. The axis of ordinates shows the mean expression correlation values for each similarity interval and their ±0.95 confidence intervals. Semantic similarity is based on Resnik's measure (**Eq. 1**).

as quality assessment of gene clusters. Fundamental descriptions may be implemented by applying standard statistical tests such as ANOVA. **Figure 4** summarizes an ANOVA performed to describe relationships among semantic similarity, expression correlation, and the five cell-cycle phases studied by Cho et al. *(15)*. This one-way ANOVA procedure was applied to semantic similarity data originating from each ontology using Resnik's approach. The results suggest that there may exist significant differences among cell-cycle phases on the basis of the semantic similarity exhibited by pairs of gene products included in these categories. This type of assessment may also determine relevant properties, which may provide the basis for further analyses. **Figure 4** indicates, e.g., that early G1 phase represents one of the most compact clusters in terms of semantic similarity based on molecular function (**Fig. 4A**). This may suggest that many of the genes involved in this cluster are strongly linked to similar molecular functions. Phases G2 and M exhibited the lowest mean similarity values, which reflects a relatively low degree of semantic compactness for all of the GO taxonomies. This indicates that

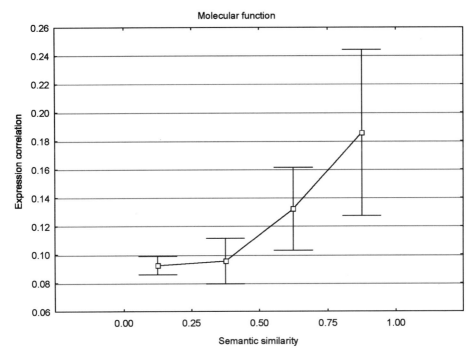

Fig. 3. Linking expression correlation and semantic similarity using gene ontology molecular function taxonomy. Semantic similarity is based on Lin's measure (**Eq. 2**).

the genes assigned to these phases may be mostly associated with diverse molecular roles, processes, and localization sites.

Semantic similarity methods may also provide the basis for predicting functional attributes from patterns of GO annotations. This task may be particularly useful for generating hypotheses about uncharacterized genes. **Figure 5** illustrates a framework for predicting GO terms from annotation sets obtained from a database such as SGD. It proposes a k-nearest neighbor method that applies semantic similarity to retrieve the most relevant genes or annotation patterns for a given query gene product, g_q. These annotation sets may originate from one or different GO taxonomies. This approach assumes that if two genes are functionally similar, then it is likely that they will share a similar set of annotation terms. Thus, a gene is represented by a structure of annotation terms, A_i. The maximum size, p, of such a list of possible annotations may be restricted to a subset of relevant GO terms in order to allow the generation of estimates with an adequate statistical confidence level. For example, a user may define a term as relevant if such a term is linked to a significant number of genes in the database. Once this selection has been performed, it is possible to construct a training data set, which describes each gene with up to p annotation terms. Each element of A_i indicates whether or not an annotation term has been used to characterize a gene, g_i.

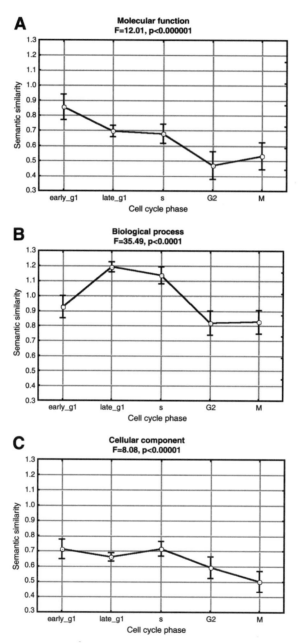

Fig. 4. Linking expression correlation and semantic similarity based on gene ontology. One-way analysis of variance using Resnik's semantic similarity as the dependent variable and cell-cycle phase as categorical predictor (factor). (**A**) Results generated by molecular function taxonomy; (**B**) results generated by biological process taxonomy; (**C**) results generated by cellular component taxonomy.

The symbols "0" and "1" may depict the absence and presence of a term in each A_i, respectively. The symbol "?" indicates undetermined annotations in the training data set, or terms whose presence/absence in g_q is to be estimated. In this hypothetical example, each gene can be described by a maximum number of five terms. The query gene, g_q, has been associated with the first and third terms, and it is accepted that there are no associations between this gene and the fifth term. Unknown or possible associations exist between g_q and the second and fourth terms. The semantic k-nearest neighbor model may be applied to predict gene–term associations, which are considered as unknown or plausible. The first step consists of calculating semantic similarity values between g_q and all of the genes included in the training data set of size m. The most similar k genes are then retrieved and used to estimate the presence or absence of terms in A_q. This prediction may be achieved by implementing, e.g., a voting strategy to calculate the probability, P, of correctly assigning a particular annotation term to g_q. This value together with other reliability indicators may be generated based on the annotation information available in the set of k genes. A prediction will not, of course, take into account the contribution of unknown annotations from the training data set. The value of k may be manually chosen or automatically estimated using statistical or machine learning criteria. In the example shown in **Fig. 5**, this method assigns the fourth term to g_q with a confidence P value equal to 0.9.

4. A Statistical Framework for Finding GO Terms Differentially Represented in Sets of Genes

Here we show how to use GO terms to transform data generated by means of different high-throughput techniques in genome-scale experiments into biologically relevant information. Results from functional genomics, such as DNA microarray data, allow organization of genes in groups that coexpress across sets of experiments, or production of lists of genes sorted on the basis of their differential expression in the different experimental conditions. These arrangements are a consequence of the biological roles that genes are playing in the cell. If a sufficient number of genes have GO annotations, relevant information on the biological properties of the system studied can be obtained.

We use a procedure to extract relevant GO terms for a group of genes with respect to a reference group. Terms are considered to be relevant by means of the application of a test that takes into account the multiple-testing nature of the statistical contrast performed. The procedure has been implemented as a Web-based application, FatiGO (*[16]*; http://fatigo.bioinfo.cnio.es/), which can deal with thousands of genes from different organisms. The utility of these approaches is proven by the fact that after the publication of FatiGO in the GO consortium Web page, approx 1 yr ago, a number of tools have been implemented based on the same idea of mapping biological knowledge on sets of genes. For example, Onto-Express (*17*) generates tables that correlate groups of genes to biochemical and molecular functions. MAPPFinder (*18*) is a searchable Web interface that identifies GO terms overrepresented in the data. Other tools are available, such as FunSpec (*19*), which evaluates groups of yeast genes in terms of their annotations in diverse databases, or GoMiner (*20*), which performs a test on the distribution of GO terms in groups of genes. Many of these tools are stand-alone applications with

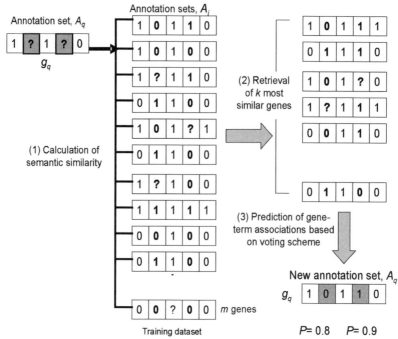

Fig. 5. A framework proposed for predicting gene-term associations based on a semantic similarity *k*-nearest neighbor approach. Symbols "0" and "1" indicate the absence and presence of a term, respectively, in an annotation set, A_i. The symbol "?" represents undetermined annotations in the training data set, or terms whose association with g_q is to be estimated. In this hypothetical example, each gene can be described by a maximum number of five terms, and associations between g_q and the second and fourth terms are predicted.

user-friendly interfaces. However, they exhibit scalability constraints as well as limitations in processing large amounts of data. Moreover, important issues, such as the multiple-testing nature of the statistical contrasts, are not well addressed.

Here we show how GO information associated with genes can be used to check the validity of their arrangements obtained by means of functional genomics experiments. Moreover, it can be applied to gain insight into the biological roles that these genes are playing in the cell. We show how to use GO terms to define biologically meaningful clusters of genes.

4.1. Finding Significantly Over- and Underrepresented GO Terms in a Set of Genes

After experimentally identifying a set of relevant genes, the question is: What makes these genes different from the rest? The FatiGO tool can be used to find GO terms that are over- and underrepresented in a set of genes with respect to a reference group. A GO level first must be chosen taking into account that deeper terms in the GO hierarchy are more precise. Nevertheless, the number of genes with annotations decreases at deeper

GO levels. GO level 3 constitutes a good compromise between information quality and the number of genes annotated at this level *(21)*, although in many cases, levels 4 and 5 may generate good results (for additional information, visit http://fatigo.bioinfo.ochoa. fib.es/help/FatiGO.html). If a gene is annotated at deeper levels than the selected level, FatiGO climbs up the GO hierarchy until the term for the selected level is reached. The use of these parent terms reduces the number of terms to be tested and increases the number of genes annotated with a given GO term (i.e., the sizes of the classes to be tested), making it easier to find relevant differences in distributions of GO terms among clusters of genes. The information is not lost and can be recovered later.

FatiGO collects two lists of GO terms at the defined level for the two sets of genes to be compared. A Fisher's exact test for 2 ↔ 2 contingency tables is applied in order to find GO terms that are significantly over- or underrepresented in both data sets. A *p* value, adjusted for multiple testing, is provided for each resulting term. Multiple testing is an important issue that is not very often properly addressed *(22)*. An increase in the rate of false positives (i.e., terms identified as over- or underrepresented that, in reality, are not significant) may occur if the multiple-testing nature of the statistical contrast is not taken into account.

FatiGO returns adjusted *p* values based on three different procedures that account for multiple testing:

1. The step-down minP method of Westfall and Young *(23)*, which provides control of the familywise error rate (i.e., the probability of making a type I error rate over the family of tests).
2. The False Discovery Rate (FDR) method of Benjamini and Hochberg *(24)*, which offers control of the FDR only under independence and specific types of positive dependence of the test's statistics.
3. The FDR method of Benjamini and Yekutieli *(25)*, which offers strong control under arbitrary dependency of test statistics.

4.2. Using FatiGO for Validation of Experimental Results of Functional Genomics

It has long been noted that genes coexpressing across different experimental conditions may be playing related functional or biological roles in the cell *(26)*. Finding biologically relevant clusters can be a complex task when thousands of genes are involved in the study. The distribution of GO annotations can be used to locate these clusters. A large number of genes, which is a disadvantage with traditional one-gene-at-a-time approaches, is in this case an advantage: the more genes available, the higher the possibility of obtaining GO terms showing a significant differential distribution.

As an example we have used the data obtained for the transcriptional program of sporulation in yeast *(27)*. After being processed and log2 transformed, gene expression profiles were clustered using the SOTA (the Self-Organizing Tree Algorithm) method *(28)*, a hierarchical clustering procedure based on a neural network implemented in the GEPAS (the Gene Expression Pattern Analysis Suite) package (http://gepas.bioinfo. cnio.es) *(29)*. After clustering them using correlation metrics with a resource threshold of 90%, which ensures an accurate, low-resolution classification, 31 clusters were obtained; **Figure 6** shows the results. The content of GO terms in the gene annotations from the clusters obtained can be explored with FatiGO. In one of the clusters, 55.56% of the genes were annotated in the GO as sporulation. This percentage is clearly higher than the 13.82% observed for the distribution of this term in the rest of genes. Metabolism is underrepresented, although the differences observed were not significant. Obviously, metabolism genes are not being activated during the sporulation of yeast. By exploring deeper GO levels, it is possible to observe "sporulation (*sensu fungi*)" at level 4 and "sporulation (*sensu saccharomyces*)" at level 5. The rest of the clusters did not present any significant GO terms. Despite the fact that other sporulation genes are present in other clusters, FatiGO found the cluster in which the representation of this term is significant.

4.3. GO-Driven Use of Experimental Results to Define Relevant Groups of Genes

An important aim in data mining is to superimpose biological information (GO terms in this case) over gene clusters in a similar manner to the example shown in the previous section. It is worth noting that data do not necessarily appear in the form of discrete subsets, or clusters. For example, in the case of the study of genes differentially expressed among experimental conditions, the data consist of lists of genes ranked by differential expression. Thus, to understand which genes differ among tissues, diseases, and so on, gene expression profiles are typically examined using an appropriate statistical model (and correcting for multiple testing), and only those genes that show significant differences among the classes studied are selected. A threshold based on conventional levels (e.g., type I error rate of 0.05), beyond which the genes can be considered differentially expressed among classes, is fixed based exclusively on expression values. Then, the GO terms associated with the genes differentially expressed are used to identify the biological processes that account at the molecular level for the differences among the classes studied (**Fig. 7**). FatiGO can then be used to obtain the terms that are significantly over- or underrepresented in these genes. The usual way of proceeding is to select genes that, in the absence of information other than their gene expression levels, can be considered to be differentially expressed (beyond a level that can be reached by chance, given a p value). Nevertheless, there is actually more information available on the genes: a number of them do have GO annotations. Imagine that we are comparing, for example, diabetic vs control patients. If after applying the proper statisti-

---

Fig. 6. *(Opposite page)* Clustering of gene expression profiles *(27)* obtained for transcriptional program of sporulation in yeast. The hierarchical clustering obtained by the Self-Organizing Tree Algorithm method using Pearson correlation coefficient and a 90% of variability threshold *(28)* generated 31 clusters. Exploration with FatiGO shows that in one of the clusters 56% of the genes were annotated in Gene Ontology as sporulation genes, a percentage that is clearly different from the distribution of this term in the rest of the genes. Metabolism is clearly underrepresented, although the differences observed were not significant. The p values are, from left to right, unadjusted p value, stepdown min p adjusted p value, false discovery rate (FDR) (independent) adjusted p value, and FDR (arbitrary dependent) adjusted p value.

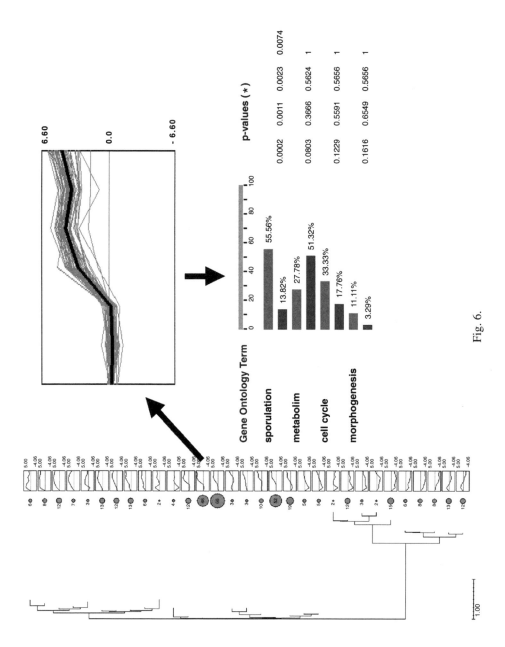

Gene Ontology Term		p-values (*)	
sporulation	55.56%	0.0002	0.0011	0.0002
	13.82%		0.0011	0.0023	0.0074
metabolim	27.78%	0.0803	0.3666	0.5624	1
	51.32%			
cell cycle	33.33%	0.1229	0.5591	0.5656	1
	17.76%			
morphogenesis	11.11%	0.1616	0.6549	0.5656	1
	3.29%			

Fig. 6.

81

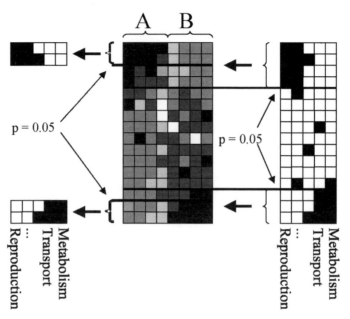

Fig. 7. Two forms of using biological information to describe a list of genes ranked by differential expression between experimental conditions A and B (highly expressed in A on the top and highly expressed in B on the bottom). (**Left**) Gene expression profiles are examined and, using an appropriate statistical model, only those genes that show significant differences (conventional levels, e.g., type I error rate of 0.05, are used for establishing a threshold) between A and B are selected. The information associated with genes over the threshold is then analyzed using, e.g., FatiGO. (**Right**) The arrangement of genes is used to study the distribution of gene ontology terms that reflect the biological processes that account for the differences between classes A and B.

cal contrast a gene is found with an expression value slightly lower than the threshold (e.g., with a *p* value of 0.06 and a threshold equal to 0.05), prior knowledge would also represent a crucial factor to consider for making a decision. If the gene were involved in a pathway of sugar processing, we probably would consider it to be differentially expressed, no matter that, strictly speaking, it did not reach the threshold. On the other hand, if the gene had to do with a completely unrelated process, such as the formation of microtubules, it will be immediately discarded.

Such an intuitive way of processing information may also be included in the algorithm. Differences in the expression of genes across distinct experimental conditions are owing to the fact that they are involved in distinct biological processes that are active in the distinct classes studied. The information carried by GO annotations on biological processes and molecular functions can be exploited to help in the selection of genes differentially expressed (*see* right side of **Fig. 7**). The study of differential representation of GO terms across groups of genes, arranged by differential expression values, is illustrated in **ref. 30**. Gene expression data from different organs were compared to look for characteristic differences among them. The approach used here involves three sequential steps. In the first step, the microarray data are analyzed to sort genes according to their differences across organs using the following ANOVA model:

$$y_{ijkl} = \mu + d_{yei} + mouse_j + organ_k + error_{ijkl} \qquad (4)$$

in which y_{ijkl} is the log2(Experimental/Control) ratio usually applied in microarray data analysis, i is the dye index ($i = 1$, meaning Cy3, and $i = 2$, meaning Cy5 on the experimental channel data), j is the index for mouse (i.e., $j = \{1, 2, 3, 4, 5, 6\}$), k is the index for organ (e.g., $k = 1$ for kidney and $k = 2$ for testis), l is the index for replicate (i.e., $l = \{1, 2, 3, 4\}$ for each tissue within mouse), m is a common intercept term, and $error_{ijkl}$ is the random error term. The greater the differences between the two organs (testis and kidney in this example), the greater the organ coefficient (the t-statistic associated with this coefficient, which is the coefficient divided by its standard error, was used). Therefore, genes that are more expressed in the kidney will have a large positive t-statistic, and those that are more expressed in the testis will have a very small (very large in absolute value, but with negative sign) t-statistic. In the second step, a window is used to define groups of genes: those within the window and the remaining set of genes. Finally, in the third step, the relative frequency of GO terms between the two groups obtained from the second step is examined. A Fisher exact test, with correction for multiple testing, is used by FatiGO to assess which of the GO terms differs significantly between the groups of genes (for details, *see* **ref. *31***). The arrangement of genes is traversed by a sliding window to which steps two and three are sequentially applied. For each sliding window, the frequency of GO terms in the genes included in the window vs the frequency of terms in the genes outside the window is compared. In other words, whether there are significant differences (adjusted for multiple testing) in the representation of GO terms in the two groups is determined (**Fig. 8**). Over- and underrepresented GO terms in genes are differentially expressed when comparing the testis and kidney in mice. The left side of the x-axis in **Fig. 8** corresponds to higher levels of expression in testis, and the right side refers to the kidney, as measured by the statistics. The y-axis represents the percentage of over- or underrepresentation of GO terms with respect to the remaining genes. Terms in black correspond to the third GO level of biological process and those in gray to the fourth level.

5. Conclusion

This chapter described two techniques that incorporate GO information into functional genomics data analysis. The automated integration of prior knowledge into a biological data-mining process is fundamental in order to achieve higher levels of validity and understandability. It can support the assessment of outcomes through consistency and significance procedures. Moreover, this type of procedure may be applied to predict functional similarity and statistically characterize groups of genes. Although applications have been illustrated in gene expression analysis problems, these methods can also be adapted to other types of ontologies and genomic data.

The method described under **Heading 3** may allow the study of relationships between GO-driven semantic similarity and gene expression correlation, which could be exploited, e.g., to describe gene clusters in terms of their intracluster similarity. It can also be applied

Azuaje et al.

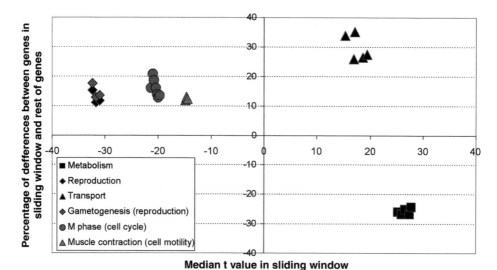

Fig. 8. Over- and underrepresented gene ontology (GO) terms in genes differently expressed when comparing testis and kidney in mice. The left side of the *x*-axis corresponds to higher levels of expression in testis, and the right side to the kidney, as measured by the statistics. The *y*-axis represents the percentage of over- or underrepresentation of GO terms with respect to the remaining genes. Terms in black correspond to the third GO level and those in gray to the fourth level.

to estimate key functional properties of uncharacterized or partially characterized gene products based on existing annotation patterns. Unlike predictive models based on traditional machine learning techniques *(6,7)*, which measure similarity purely on the basis of the presence (or absence) of annotation terms, a GO-driven semantic similarity approach explicitly takes into account taxonomical relationships among GO annotation terms. Semantic similarity information could also be applied to support annotation tasks. For instance, groups of gene products could be annotated using their lowest common ancestor rather than multiple annotations. These models may also contribute to the assessment of differences in annotations across genes, within a database or across multiple model organisms.

The method implemented in FatiGO constitutes a rigorous statistical framework for the assessment of GO terms differentially represented by two sets of genes. This simple but powerful tool can be used in different ways. The obvious, immediate use of this framework is validation of experimental results in which two or more partitions (either discrete or continuous) of genes can be obtained. In this case, experimental information is used to define partitions, and the GO terms are used to understand the biological reasons for which the genes in these partitions account for the differences in the experimental conditions studied.

Nevertheless, this rationale can be reversed, and biological information (GO terms) can directly be used to define the partitions of genes and simultaneously explain the molecular basis of the differences among the experimental conditions studied. In addition to GO terms, other different types of information could be used in the proposed framework to understand, from different points of view, phenotypic or experimental differences.

The inclusion of information from different sources for studying functional genomic data, as has been exemplified here, will most likely become an active research field in the near future. Very recently, although with a different approach, information on whether genes belong or not to metabolic pathways was used as additional evidence to detect differentially expressed genes beyond the threshold defined using exclusively gene expression measurements *(32)*.

Acknowledgments

We thank Oliver Bodenreider for helpful advice on ontologies. This work was supported by grant BIO2001-0068 from the Ministerio de Ciencia y Tecnología. F.A. was partly supported by a visiting fellowship from the US National Library of Medicine.

References

1. The Gene Ontology Consortium. (2001) Creating the gene ontology resource: design and implementation. *Genome Res.* **11,** 1425–1433.
2. Ouzounis, C., Coulson, R., Enright, A., Kunin, V., and Pereira-Leal, J. (2003) Classification schemes for protein structure and function. *Nat. Rev. Genet.* **4,** 508–519.
3. Harris, M. and Parkinson, H. (2003) Standards and ontologies for functional genomics: towards unified ontologies for biology and biomedicine. *Compar. Funct. Genomics* **4,** 116–120.
4. Bard, J. (2003) Ontologies: formalising biological knowledge for bioinformatics. *BioEssays* **25,** 501–506.
5. King, O., Lee, J., Dudley, A., Jansen, D., Church, G., and Roth, F. (2003) Predicting phenotype from patterns of annotation. *Bioinformatics* **19(Suppl. 1),** 183–189.
6. Hvidsten, T., Laegreid, A., and Komorowski, J. (2003) Learning rule-based models of biological process from gene expression time profiles using Gene Ontology. *Bioinformatics* **19,** 1116–1123.
7. King, O., Foulger, R., Dwight, S., White, J., and Roth, F. (2003) Predicting gene function from patterns of annotation. *Genome Res.* **13,** 896–904.
8. Laegreid, A., Hvidsten, T., Midelfart, H., Komorowski, J., and Sandvik, A. (2003) Predicting gene ontology biological process from temporal gene expression patterns. *Genome Res.* **13,** 965–979.
9. Iyer, V., Eisen, M., Ross, D., et al. (1999) The transcriptional program in the response of human fibroblast to serum. *Science* **283,** 83–87.
10. Zhong, J., Zhu, H., Li, Y., and Yu, Y. (2002) Conceptual graph matching for semantic search, in *Conceptual Structures: Integration and Interfaces* (Priss, U., Corbett, D., and Angelova, G., eds.), Springer Verlag, London, UK, pp. 92–106.
11. Budanitsky, A. and Hirst, G. (2001) Semantic distance in WordNet: an experimental, application-oriented evaluation of five measures, in *Workshop on WordNet and Other Lexical Resources,* Pittsburgh.
12. Resnik, P. (1995) Using information content to evaluate semantic similarity in a taxonomy, in *Proceedings of the 14th International Joint Conference on Artificial Intelligence,* Montreal, Canada (Mellish, C. S., ed.), Morgan Kaufman, San Mateo, CA, pp. 448–453.

13. Lin, D. (1998) An information-theoretic definition of similarity, in *Proceedings of the 15th International Conference on Machine Learning,* Montreal, Canada (Mellish, C. S., ed.), Morgan Kaufman, San Mateo, CA, pp. 296–304.

14. Lord, P., Stevens, R., Brass, A., and Goble, C. (2003) Investigating semantic similarity measures across the Gene Ontology: the relationship between sequence and annotation. *Bioinformatics* **19,** 1275–1283.

15. Cho, R., Campbell, M., Winzeler, E., et al. (1998) A genome-wide transcriptional analysis of the mitotic cell cycle. *Mol. Cell* **2,** 65–73.

16. Al-Shahrour, F., Diaz-Uriarte, R., and Dopazo, J. (2003) FatiGO: a web tool for finding significant associations of Gene Ontology terms with groups of genes. *Bioinformatics* **20,** 578–580 (epub).

17. Khatri, P., Draghici, S., Ostermeier, G. C., and Krawetz, S. A. (2002) Profiling gene expression using onto-express. *Genomics* **79,** 1–5.

18. Doniger, S. W., Salomonis, N., Dahlquist, K. D., Vranizan, K., Lawlor, S. C., and Conklin, B. R. (2003) MAPPFinder: using Gene Ontology and GenMAPP to create a global gene-expression profile from microarray data. *Genome Biol.* **4,** R7.

19. Robinson, M. D., Grigull, J., Mohammad, N., and Hughes, T. R. (2002) FunSpect: a web-based cluster interpreter for yeast. *BMC Bioinformatics* **3,** 1–5.

20. Zeeberg, B. R., Feng, W., Wang, G., et al. (2003) GoMiner: a resource for biological interpretation of genomic and proteomic data. *Genome Biol.* **4(4),** R28.1–R28.8.

21. Mateos, A., Herrero, J., Tamames, J., and Dopazo, J. (2002) Supervised neural networks for clustering conditions in DNA array data after reducing noise by clustering gene expression profiles, in *Methods of Microarray Data Analysis II* (Lin, S. and Johnson, K., eds.), Kluwer, Boston, MA.

22. Slonim, D. K. (2002) From patterns to pathways: gene expression data analysis comes of age. *Nat. Genet. (Suppl. The Chipping Forecast)* **32,** 502–508.

23. Westfall, P. H. and Young, S. S. (1993) *Resampling-Based Multiple Testing,* John Wiley & Sons, New York.

24. Benjamini, Y. and Hochberg, Y. (1995) Controlling the false discovery rate: a practical and powerful approach to multiple testing. *J. R. Stat. Soc. B* **57,** 289–300.

25. Benjamini, Y. and Yekutieli, D. (2001) The control of the false discovery rate in multiple testing under dependency. *Ann. Stat.* **29,** 1165–1188.

26. Eisen, M., Spellman, P. L., Brown, P. O., and Botstein, D. (1998) Cluster analysis and display of genome-wide expression patterns. *Proc. Natl. Acad. Sci. USA* **95,** 14,863–14,868.

27. Chu, S., DeRisi, J., Eisen, M., Mulholland, J., Botstein, D., Brown, P. O., and Herskowitz, I. (1998) The transcriptional program sporulation in budding yeast. *Science* **282,** 699–705.

28. Herrero, J., Valencia, A., and Dopazo, J. (2001) A hierarchical unsupervised growing neural network for clustering gene expression patterns. *Bioinformatics* **17,** 126–136.

29. Herrero, J., Al-Shahrour, F., Diaz-Uriarte, R., et al. (2003) GEPAS, a web-based resource for microarray gene expression data analysis. *Nucleic Acids Res.* **31,** 3461–3467.

30. Pritchard, C. C., Hsu, L., and Nelson, P. S. (2001) Project normal: defining normal variance in mouse gene expression. *Proc. Natl. Acad. Sci. USA* **98,** 13,266–13,271.

31. Diaz-Uriarte, R., Al-Shahrour, F., and Dopazo, J. (2003) Use of GO terms to understand the biological significance of microarray differential gene expression data, in *Methods of Microarray Data Analysis III* (Lin, S. and Johnson, K., eds.), Kluwer, Boston, MA; in press.

32. Mota, V. K., Lindgren, C. M., Eriksson, K. F., et al. (2003) PGC-1-responsive genes involved in oxidative phosphorylation are coordinately downregulated in human diabetes. *Nat. Genet.* **34,** 267–273.

6

Gene Evolution and Drug Discovery

James O. McInerney, Caroline S. Finnerty,
Jennifer M. Commins, and Gayle K. Philip

Summary

Mutation and selection are the principle forces governing gene and protein sequence. Mutation is the major source of variation, and selection removes variation. Although many mutations are likely to be neutral with respect to natural selection, much of the extant sequence that is functionally important has experienced selective pressures in the past. By examining the history of DNA sequences, we can infer the functional importance of particular residues and the selective pressures that have influenced their evolution. In this chapter, we review the most interesting approaches for inferring the evolutionary history of DNA and protein sequences and indicate how these analyses can be useful in the drug discovery process.

Key Words: Orthologs; paralogs; maximum parsimony; phylogenetic tree; adaptive evolution; transcription factors; purifying selection.

1. Introduction

Proteins do not have to be of the same sequence if they are to carry out the same function. In fact, we have known for many years that there can be considerable variation in sequence among proteins with similar functions. However, given further consideration, we might ask: Why shouldn't this be the case? It might seem to make much more sense for nature to have settled on a particular protein sequence when it had optimized the desired function. What we see instead is a variety of related protein sequences that are responsible for a variety of similar functions and activities. We call these proteins "homologs." The origin of the word *homolog* dates back to the British paleontologist and first director of the British Museum of Natural History, Richard Owen. He defined homologs to be the "… same organ under every variety of form and function" *(1)*. This definition still holds today; we see that homologous proteins can differ in their substrate specificities, specific activities, level of expression, or some other basic property. Usually, however, homologs will have some residual similarity in their form and function.

From: *Methods in Molecular Biology, vol. 316: Bioinformatics and Drug Discovery*
Edited by: R. S. Larson © Humana Press Inc., Totowa, NJ

One of the issues that makes the task of understanding proteomic data difficult is the problems associated with orthology and paralogy. Orthologs are those homologs that have been created by speciation, whereas paralogs can trace their common ancestor to a duplication event. Duplication events often result in functional specialization of the paralogs. With two copies of a particular protein in the same genome, we may have functional redundancy, in which the same function is carried out by both genes. However, analyses of gene and protein evolution can be a profitable exercise and can result in quite a bit of insight. In this chapter, we introduce some of the methods that are used to analyze gene evolution and emphasize the benefits of carrying out such analyses.

The majority of DNA sequence evolution is thought to occur in a way that is consistent with the neutral theory of molecular evolution. That is to say that most mutations do not have an appreciable impact on the fitness of the individual and, therefore, the likelihood of these mutations becoming fixed in a population that is quite small. Recently, however, this notion has been under siege *(2)*. Developments in the methodology used to measure selective pressures on genes have begun to reveal that positive selection for change is quite a strong force.

1.1. Why Analyze Gene Evolution?

In their seminal paper, Zuckerkandl and Pauling *(3)* suggested that cellular macro-molecules could be read as documents that have recorded the history of organisms. The logic, therefore, was that these molecules could be used to infer the phylogenetic relationships among organisms. In the intervening four decades, analyses of molecular evolution have been used to develop a much larger range of hypotheses. In particular, analyses of molecular evolution have been used to infer gene duplication events *(4)*, gene losses *(5)*, and horizontal gene transfers *(6)*. These are the some of the most important mechanisms by which genomes evolve and, certainly, these events can result in substantial differences among closely related genomes. The most important thing to get right when making these inferences is the phylogenetic tree uniting the species of interest. Unless this tree is correct, the inferences will not be robust.

1.2. Evolutionary Rate Variation and Its Meaning

The notion of a molecular clock goes back to the same article by Zuckerkandl and Pauling *(3)*, and it suggested that evolutionary change was more or less constant. This suggestion was based on the observation that hemoglobin proteins appeared to have changed over time in a way that seemed to calibrate well with the fossil record. Therefore, it was suggested that it might follow a Poisson process. We now know that the molecular clock is not universal and that the rate of sequence change can be different for different sites in a molecule, different molecules in the same genome, different chromosomes in the same cell (mitochondria, chloroplasts, and nuclear genes), and even the same orthologs in different lineages. This does not mean that the molecular clock idea is not a good one. We can often see that the rate of molecular evolution is rather clocklike. It is simply the case that this is not a universal truth.

The significance of rate variation is that if we understand evolutionary rate variation, we can make predictions concerning the causes of this variation. We suspect that the rate

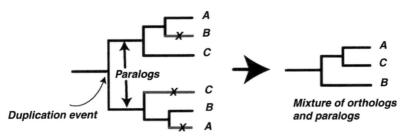

Fig. 1. On the left is the true evolutionary history of a homologous family of sequences. In this family, there have been a duplication event and two subsequent speciation events. In addition, there have been three independent gene losses, indicated by the line with the crosses. The resulting phylogenetic tree of the remaining sequences is shown on the right.

of mutation might be relatively constant in close relatives. However, selective pressures on different regions of the genome or differences in long-term effective population size or the generation time of the organism in which the molecule is found will ultimately lead to differences in the rates at which we see substitutions accumulate.

2. Methods

2.1. Identification of Orthologs and Paralogs

Orthologous proteins are those that have arisen as a result of speciation events. Paralogous proteins arise as a result of a duplication event. This should mean that identification of orthologs should be easy. Unfortunately, this is not always the case. Gene duplication is often subsequently reversed by a loss of one of the paralogs. Indeed, gene loss is quite common and differential gene loss in different lineages is also a relatively common event. Therefore, two sequences might appear to be orthologous, particularly when there is only a single homolog in each of the species in the study (*see* **Fig. 1**).

There have been a number of studies in which ortholog identification has been carried out using a database search algorithm such as BLAST (*7*) or FastA (*8*). The procedure has been to use a "reciprocal best-hit" approach. Using this approach, two sequences are deemed to be orthologous if they are each others' top hit in two database searches in which each one has been used as the query sequence. There are two problems with this type of approach. The first problem relates to gene loss in different lineages, which is outlined in **Fig. 1**. As can be seen, a duplication event has given rise to paralogous genes. Subsequent loss of paralogs has meant that gene sequences that appear to be orthologous are not.

The second problem is outlined in **Fig. 2**, where one can see differences in evolutionary rates in different paralogs. The result of these differences in evolutionary rate is that sequence A' and sequence C are quite similar to each other. They are not orthologs (however, A' and C' are orthologs), but there is a strong possibility that the reciprocal best-hit method would identify these as orthologs. Therefore, it is our opinion that orthology should always be inferred by the careful examination of phylogenetic trees derived from multiple sequence alignments, rather than the analysis of pairwise alignments and simple database searches.

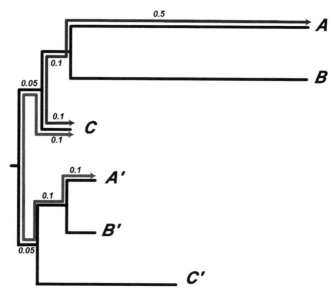

Fig. 2. Phylogenetic tree uniting a number of sequences that display evolutionary rate het-erogeneity. In this case, the similarity between sequence C and its true ortholog, sequence A, is much less than the similarity between sequences C and its paralog in species A, the sequence denoted as A'.

2.2. Methods of Phylogenetic Tree Reconstruction

Unfortunately, as each software program was developed, the developers tended to invent their own file formats or variants on existing formats. Sometimes this was neces-sary and sometimes this was simply a matter of convenience. However, over time a number of file formats have become much more common and some other formats have almost disappeared. The most sophisticated of these formats is probably the NEXUS file format *(9)*. Basically, this format is infinitely extendable and uses a system of "blocks." Examples of commonly used blocks include the DATA block, the TAXA block, the CHARACTERS block, and the TREE block. These sections of the input file always begins with "#NEXUS." An example of a NEXUS block is shown in **Table 1**.

As one can see, this file defines the number of taxa as 4 and the number of characters (aligned positions) as 22. The datatype is described as protein, and two different sym-bols should be used in the data set to indicate missing data (usually parts of the mole-cule that have not been sequenced yet) and insertion/deletion events (or gaps). There is only one block in this input file, a "data" block, which begins with the word *begin* and ends with the word *end*.

As stated previously, there are a number of file formats commonly used by phylo-genetic analysis software; however, they all have the same central requirement—an alignment of homologous nucleotides or amino acids, with each position of the align-ment being carefully checked to ensure that it is accurate. Correct alignment is not some-thing that can be guaranteed with absolute certainty. Therefore, in those instances in

Table 1
Example Data Block in NEXUS Format

```
#NEXUS
begin data;
dimensions      ntax=4 nchar=22;
format          datatype=protein missing=? gap=-;
matrix
                Taxon_1 GARFIELDTHEFASTFA-TCAT
                Taxon_2 GARFIELDTHEFASTCA-T---
                Taxon_3 GARFIELDTHEVERYFASTCAT
                Taxon_4 --------THE----FA-TCAT
     ;
end;
```

which there is no strong evidence that the alignment is correct, the researcher should consider removing the unreliable positions.

2.3. Maximum Parsimony

Maximum parsimony is based on the assumption that the optimal tree (or trees) is the one that requires the fewest evolutionary changes, i.e., has the minimum number of inferred character state changes *(10)*. In constructing the tree, the only sites considered parsimony-informative are those where at least two sequences have one character state at a site, and at least two others have a different identical character state. All other characters, whether variable or invariable, do not contain enough information to discriminate between alternative tree topologies.

The objective of maximum parsimony is to identify the phylogenetic hypothesis that minimizes the number of substitutions that need to be reconstructed in order to explain the distribution of the character states in the given alignment. Usually, all substitutions are treated equally; however, it is possible to reweight certain substitutions if there is evidence that particular kinds of substitutions are more frequent than others or if particular sites in the alignment are more likely to change than others (say, e.g., the third positions of codons, where, on average, change is more rapid than at first or second positions).

Maximum parsimony is implemented in PAUP* by choosing the Parsimony criterion. PAUP* can be purchased from http://paup.csit.fsu.edu *(11)*.

2.4. Distance Matrix Methods

One may wish to construct a phylogenetic tree using a distance matrix approach. In this type of situation, we usually make an observation of the degree of similarity between two sequences and then estimate the number of substitutions that have occurred since these two sequences last shared a common ancestor. The reason that the observed distance between these two sequences is not the same as the actual number of substitutions that have occurred since they shared a common ancestor is that there are superimposed substitutions or multiple substitutions at a single site. If there were no superimposed substitutions in any sequences in the analysis, then it would be possible to construct a perfectly "additive" tree, where the distances based on the alignment could be accurately mapped onto a unique phylogenetic tree. If we could accurately reconstruct all the substitutions that have occurred in the evolutionary time frame under consideration, then we could also construct an additive tree. Unfortunately, researchers are usually in a situation in which they do not know how many substitutions have occurred and are usually trying to estimate this quantity.

The usual method of trying to estimate the number of substitutions since the common ancestor is to assume that superimposed substitutions are negligible initially, but as sequences diverge, the probability of a superimposed substitution increases. As a result, a log-normal correction is usually used in order to estimate the true extent of substitution. The general form of the equation is

$$d = \ln(f(D)) \tag{1}$$

in which d is the estimated distance between two sequences, ln is the log-normal correction, f is some treatment of the various parts of the substitution process, and D is the observed distance between the two sequences. An example of a distance matrix transformation is the one devised by Jukes and Cantor (*12*):

$$d = -\frac{3}{4} \ln \left(1 - \frac{4}{3} D\right) \tag{2}$$

This type of correction tends to have only a small effect on distances that are small, but the correction becomes much more pronounced when distances become larger.

2.5. Maximum Likelihood

Maximum likelihood (ML) methods evaluate phylogenetic hypotheses in terms of the probability that a proposed model of the evolutionary process and the proposed unrooted tree will give rise to the observed data. The tree topology found to have the highest ML value is considered to be the preferred tree, which is called the ML tree (*13*). The likelihood function can be described by the following equation:

$$L = P(\chi \mid \tau, \upsilon, \theta) \tag{3}$$

in which, χ is the alignment, τ is the tree, υ is the branch lengths, and θ is the substitution process.

The ML method requires a probabilistic model for the process of nucleotide substitution. For a given model of nucleotide evolution, formulae are derived that describe the probability that an initial nucleotide will be transformed into a specified nucleotide during an evolutionary time period. The likelihood for each nucleotide position is then equal to the prior probability of finding the initial nucleotide at that position multiplied by the probability of transformation. The likelihood of the divergence of two sequences during the time period is then the product of the likelihoods at each position, and the overall likelihood for a tree is the product of the likelihoods along the branches. This procedure is essentially for finding the branch lengths that give the larg-

Table 2
Example MrBayes Block

```
begin mrbayes;
set autoclose=yes;
  lset aamodel=jones;
  mcmc ngen=500000 printfreq=500 samplefreq=100 nchains=4
savebrlens=yes;
end;
```

est value for the likelihood function. Likelihood models generally tend to account for variation in transition/transversion ratios, base composition, and substitution rate differences among lineages and across sites.

Since ML methods compute the probabilities for all possible combinations of ancestral states, they are very time-consuming. ML is implemented by a number of programs including the PAML package *(14)*, PAUP* for DNA sequences alone, and TREE-PUZZLE for creating ML trees from protein sequences (obtain from www.tree-puzzle.de/) *(15)*.

2.6. Bayesian Inference

Bayesian analysis searches for the best set of trees based on the notion of posterior probabilities. Thus, it seeks the tree that maximizes the probability of the trees given the data and the model for evolution *(16)*. The Bayesian approach is implemented by the MrBayes program, available from http://morphbank.ebc.uu.se/mrbayes.html *(17)*.

MrBayes requires an execution file to be created, which is simply a NEXUS-formatted alignment file with a block of MrBayes commands added after the data block. It executes a series of statements, each ending with a semicolon between the commands `begin mrbayes;` and `end;`.

Starting the MrBayes program and typing the word *help* will give a complete list of the available commands. Typing `help <command>` explains the various commands in more detail and allows one to include commands relevant for their data.

In **Table 2**, the *mcmc* command starts the Markov chain Monte Carlo analysis and tells MrBayes to run for 500,000 generations, printing every 500th generation to the screen, sampling every 100th Markov chain; to run four simultaneous Monte Carlo chains; and to save the branch length information on the tree file. Setting `autoclose=yes;` tells MrBayes to continue to the next statement by closing the chains after the mcmc command.

2.7. Summarizing Results When Multiple Phylogenetic Trees Are Recovered

It may be necessary to compare trees derived from different analyses, or from the same sequences using different methods. Thus, consensus trees can be generated to summarize the results. Strict consensus trees only report branching patterns that occur in all trees, whereas majority consensus trees report branching patterns that are supported by a majority of input trees. Both methods are implemented in PAUP*.

2.8. Visualizing Trees

Once generated, trees can be displayed in TreeView, a program that runs on both Apple MAC OS X computers and Microsoft Windows-compatible personal computers. It is available free from http://taxonomy.zoology.gla.ac.uk/rod/treeview.html *(18)*.

3. Adaptive Evolution of Proteins

3.1. Background

The source of all biological novelties is mutation. However, the likelihood of these novelties becoming dominant in a population is dependent on two other issues: random genetic drift and selection *(19)*. Random genetic drift, in turn, is related to the long-term effective population size of the species. Therefore, in populations with relatively small long-term effective population sizes, the likelihood of a beneficial mutation becoming fixed in the population is dependent on whether or not the novelty is sufficiently advantageous to overcome random genetic drift. In sufficiently large populations, drift is negligible and, therefore, the novelty has a much better chance of becoming fixed in the population.

For an organism to survive an environmental change, it is necessary for some mutation to have already occurred. Still, the organism may be ill adapted, and the adaptation must be fine-tuned for the subsequent survival of that genetic line. A mutation can be fixed or reversed by the need to survive the pressures of the internal and external environments, by way of positive and negative selection, respectively *(19)*.

Positive selection is said to have occurred when a characteristic benefits the organism so that the new genotype is fitter than the wild-type and is, therefore, more likely to contribute to subsequent generations. Positive selection can be described as either directional or nondirectional *(20)*. Nondirectional selection occurs when there is selection for several genotypes in a population. This is observed where the environment is constantly changing, allowing the organism to change its molecular traits relatively frequently. This mutation is said to be variable, and an example can be seen in the major histocompatibility complex (MHC) genes *(21)*.

MHC is a multigene family that produces cell-surface glycoproteins that play a key role in the immune system by presenting peptides to T-cells. Positive selection is known to be driving the evolution of MHC genes. Within this gene family, the presence of many variants is necessary so that MHC will be able to recognize the different antigens that it presents to the T-cells. Directional selection describes selection in a single genotype; that is, if a mutation occurs and is found to be advantageous, it is actively preserved and remains invariable in the population *(20)*. Examples of this are found in the Adh loci of *Drosophila (22)* and Lysozyme genes of Colubine monkeys *(23)*.

Until quite recently, the most convincing evidence of adaptive evolution has come from the comparison of silent and replacement substitution rates in protein-coding genes *(24)*. Silent (synonymous) substitutions occur when a nucleotide substitution does not result in an amino acid change, and replacement (nonsynonymous) substitutions occur

Table 3
Some Available Methods for Use in Detection of Adaptive Evolution

Method	Brief description	Reference
Lineage variation	Variation in *dN/dS* ratio between lineages	*27*
Site variation	Variation in *dN/dS* ratio between sites	*28*
Relative rate test	Comparison of ratio of *dN/dS* within and between closely related species	*22*
Relative rate ratio test	Deviation of *dN/dS* from neutrality	*20*

when the amino acid is changed. The respective rates of these substitutions are the number of silent substitutions per silent site (*dS*) and replacement substitutions per replacement site (*dN*). The ratio of these two rates to each other (ω or *dN/dS*) defines the type, if any, of selection that is occurring at the protein level *(24)*. When the value of ω exceeds unity, this may be because of positive selection for replacement substitutions; when it is less than unity, this may be because of purifying selection on new mutations; and when it is at unity, it may be because the molecule is evolving at the neutral rate.

There are problems that hamper the detection of adaptive evolution. The rates of substitution differ among and between different proteins, and also different sites on the same family of proteins may change at different rates and in different ways. Mutation saturation is another problem, in which multiple changes have occurred at a particular site. In some severe cases, this can cause the data to become essentially random, and all the information about any evolutionary history to be lost. Traditional methods that average ω across entire alignments may be overlooking regions of hypervariability that may be contained within a relatively conserved sequence. Therefore, methods of analysis need to be able to deal with the complexities of sequence evolution and to recover any underlying evolutionary signal. To identify proteins that may have been influenced by positive selection, it is necessary to identify the amino acid changes that are responsible for the adaptation of organisms to specific environments *(24)*.

Many methods are available for the detection of adaptive evolution in proteins (**Table 3**). Only two such methods are discussed here. The first method is implemented in a software program called CRANN *(25)*. This method is based on the neutral mutation substitution rate test proposed by Li *(26)* and the relative rate test *(22)*. The second method *(2)* uses a likelihood ratio test (LRT) for variable selective pressures at individual sites.

3.2. Relative Rate Ratio Test

The relative rate ratio test was developed in order to detect adaptive evolution in protein-coding DNA sequences *(20)*. It is available to download in multiple formats from http://bioinf.may.ie/crann. This program requires a set of protein-coding DNA sequences aligned so that the first residue of the alignment corresponds to the first position of a codon and a phylogenetic tree that can be read from a file or inferred using data from the alignment; this tree is assumed to be correct. Hypothetical ancestral sequences are reconstructed at the internal nodes of the submitted phylogenetic tree using the principal of maximum parsimony *(10)* applied at the codon level. This program incorporates many methods, of which only two are mentioned here.

Synonymous and nonsynonymous substitution rates are defined in the context of comparing two DNA sequences, with *dS* and *dN* as the numbers of synonymous and nonsynonymous substitutions per site, respectively *(29)*. Therefore, their ratio measures the strength and nature of selective restraints. If a codon change is neutral, it will be fixed at the same rate as a synonymous mutation. If the change is deleterious, purifying selection will reduce its fixation rate. Only if the change offers a selective advantage is it fixed at a higher rate than a synonymous mutation. With this in mind, we can conclude that an ω value greater than 1 is convincing evidence for diversifying selection *(2)*.

The relative rate ratio test works under the same principles as the relative rate test, but with the exception that it considers whether the number of nonsynonymous substitutions observed was greater than expected from the neutral model.

3.2.1. Materials

To carry out an analysis, it is necessary to download the platform-specific software bundle from http://bioinf.nuim.ie/software/. The program requires a FastA formatted protein-coding nucleotide sequence file, containing sequences of interest and an appropriate outgroup. The data set must be aligned and homologous. There is also the choice of providing a tree file. This should be a nested parenthesis tree (PHYLIP format).

3.2.2. Method

The software reconstructs the phylogenetic relationships between the sequences in the input file and uses this phylogenetic tree to reconstruct all the ancestral sequences at every internal node on the tree. The alternative of forcing a particular tree topology on the data is also a valid approach. The output from this analysis is a list of internal branches on the tree and the number of substitutions that occurred in the clade circumscribed by this internal branch. The substitutions are divided into four categories: those substitutions that caused an amino acid replacement that subsequently changed elsewhere (replacement variable [RV]), those substitutions that caused an amino acid replacement and nowhere else in the clade was this amino acid changed (replacement invariable [RI]), those substitutions that were silent and subsequently changed elsewhere (silent variable [SV]), and those substitutions that were silent and for which there was never another change at that site (silent invariable [SI]). We expect that the ratio of SI to SV should be the same as the ratio of RI to RV in the case of neutrality. Deviations from this ratio (the significance of which can be judged according to a G-test) indicate the presence of selection on the replacement substitutions.

3.3. Likelihood Ratio Test for Codon Substitution Rate Heterogeneity

PAML is a package of programs used for phylogenetic analysis of DNA and protein sequences using ML. It can be downloaded from http://abacus.gene.ucl.ac.uk/software/ paml.html. Within this package, the program that researchers are most interested in for the purpose of detection of adaptive evolution is codeml. This program implements the codon substitution model of Goldman and Yang *(30)* for protein-coding DNA sequences, and it also implements models for amino acid sequences *(2)*. Continuous-time Markov process models are used to describe substitutions between codons or amino acids, with substitution rates assumed to be either constant or variable among sites.

A model that employs a discrete approximation to the γ distribution is used to model the rate variation among sites. The rates for sites come from several categories used to approximate the continuous γ distribution. It is assumed in some cases that selective pressures vary across different sites in protein sequences, and, therefore, models have been developed that incorporate heterogeneous selective pressures at different sites *(2)*. Sites are given a probability of belonging to a particular site class. This probability is permitted to vary across the tree. Heterogeneous models that allow the ω ratio to vary among sites and/or among lineages are thus employed to cater for the variable pressures being exerted on the protein.

Twice the difference of the log likelihood score is approximately χ^2 distributed. Therefore, nested models of sequence evolution can be compared with each other. The number of degrees of freedom is calculated as the difference in the number of free parameters. LRTs are carried out to aid in determining the significance of the positive selection detected. The presence of a null hypothesis, which, in general, will have fewer free variables than the alternative hypothesis, allows the use of LRTs to determine whether any significant levels of positive selection are present, and the output will give the exact sites in the sequences where the adaptive evolution has been detected *(24)*.

The identification of amino acid sites or evolutionary lineages potentially under positive selection is carried out using the reconstruction of ancestral codon sequences *(31)*. This is completed using an empirical Bayes approach, which is used to estimate the probability of a site being in a particular class *(32)*. The sites placed in categories with an estimated ω value greater than unity are most likely to be under positive selection.

3.4. Models That Are Available in Codeml

Four categories of analysis are available. The simplest model assumes that there is a single, average ω value for all comparisons. Some models assume that there are branch-specific differences in the ω value. Some models assume that there are site-specific differences in the ω value, and some models assume that there are differences across sites and across branches simultaneously.

Within these categories, there are further divisions or nesting of models. The null hypothesis in each case is compared with the models, which represent the alternative hypothesis, (by way of LRTs) to determine whether there are significances in the results obtained. As with many other statistical tests, there are a number of degrees of freedom that allow basic models to be compared with those that are more complex. Some of the models that are available are presented next, along with a brief description of each, and the comparisons that are permitted for use with LRTs.

3.4.1. Nonspecific Models

The simplest model of sequence evolution is the one-ratio model. In this scheme, one ω value is assumed over the entire data set. This is equivalent to the model proposed by

Goldman and Yang *(30)*. The resulting output from this model is an estimated average ω value for the entire data set.

The free-ratio model is a little-used model that allows for the consideration of all sites and all branches individually rather than partitioning the data into more manageable groupings. The model has many parameters that are free to vary and, therefore, there may be a large number of degrees of freedom when comparing the model to simpler models.

3.4.2. Branch-Specific Models

Branch-specific models allow ω to vary at different positions on the tree. These models have been designed to address the issue of whether or not there are variable selective pressures at different parts of the tree. One or more internal branches on the tree can be labeled to identify where the partition is to be applied.

3.4.3. Site-Specific Models

One could envison a situation in which we assume in advance that all sites in the alignment have their own ω value and it reflects the selective pressures that these sites experience. However, this is unwieldy for several reasons, including the number of degrees of freedom required if we were to compare such a model to a more restrained model. In practice, we assume that there are a number of classes of sites in the alignment. The sites in a particular class have similar ω values. We manipulate the models so that these ω values are either free to vary or we can constrain these ω values.

A model has been devised that implies that there are two categories of sites in the alignments: those that are not allowed to change (i.e., their ω value is fixed at zero) and those that are evolving according to the neutral theory of molecular evolution (i.e., their ω value is fixed at unity). A slightly more relaxed version of the preceding model is one in which there is an allowance for an additional category of sites in which the ω value is free to vary. In other words, this category of sites is assumed to exist but we would nave no *a priori* assumption concerning their ω value. The least restrictive of these kinds of discrete models is one in which there is an assumption that there are either two or three categories of sites, but in no case is the assumption being made that the values of ω for these categories are known. Each of the two or three categories within this model are estimated from the data set.

A variety of other site-specific models can be used, and usually these models assume that there are variable ω values at different sites and that the values of ω can be modeled according to either a β or a γ distribution or a combination of these distributions instead of using the continuous distribution. These models tend to use discrete approximations to these distributions.

3.4.4. Branch-Site-Specific Models

Branch-site-specific models allow ω to vary among sites and also among the branches of the input phylogenetic tree. The assumption for these models is that different evolutionary pressures on different parts of the tree for different parts of the alignment might be seen. There are two variants of this approach. One variant is to extend the neutral

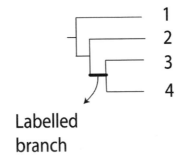

Labelled branch

Fig. 3. Graphic view of a phylogenetic tree. The labeled branch of interest is indicated in bold.

Table 4
Sample Nested Parenthesis Tree File[a]

4 3	//4 species, 3 trees
(1,2,3,4)	//tree 1
(((1,2)#1,3),4)	//tree 2 → This branch is labeled
(1,2,(3,4))	//tree 3

[a]Used as standard input for codeml, tree 2 demonstrates how branches are labeled.

model in which the ω values are fixed to either one or zero, but this can vary over the tree. This model can be compared with the neutral model using a χ^2 test.

The second branch-site model is an extension of the discrete site-specific model in which all ω values are free to vary and there are two categories of sites. The branch-site extension allows for a "background" and a "foreground" ω value. The implication is that the ω value can change in a site-specific manner from one lineage to the next. Again, the significance of adding these additional parameters can be evaluated using a χ^2 test.

3.5. Materials

The first step of this process is to download the platform-specific software bundle. Install as directed by the author. The software requires a PHYLIP sequential format sequence file in nucleotide format with the alignment being in frame, and when there are alignment gaps, they are in groups of three (representing indel codons). A PHYLIP format-nested parenthesis tree file is also required (*see* **Fig. 3**). The codeml program is executed with the assistance of a control file (*see* **Table 4**). The default name of this file is codeml.ctl.

3.6. Method

The sequence and tree files must be placed together with the codeml control file in a directory; this will be where any resulting output files will be created by the software. Edit the control file to suit your needs. The control file defines which models are applied to the data, how many site substitution categories are to be defined, and the initial start values of ω and so on. It is important to note here that a variety of ω starting values be used for any model involving estimations, because of the danger of multiple optima during the calculation. The execution run that produces the highest likelihood value should be chosen as the best estimate. Therefore, in these cases, codeml must be run multiple times for the same model and data set (we recommend at least 5, but preferably 10 sequential runs using the same data but different starting values). The program codeml is executed simply by having all the aforementioned in a directory. The software will automatically detect the presence of the control file and use the user-defined settings to carry out the analysis. Each data set should be analyzed under several different evolutionary models. These models can then be tested using an LRT.

4. Evolution of Regulatory Regions

4.1. Introduction to Eukaryotic Transcriptional Regulation

Eukaryotes employ diverse mechanisms to regulate gene expression, including chromatin condensation, transcriptional initiation, alternative splicing of RNA, mRNA stability, translational controls, and several forms of posttranslational modification. Only some of the genes in a eukaryotic cell are expressed at any given moment. The proportion and composition of transcribed genes change considerably during the life cycle, among cell types, and in response to environmental conditions. This is why transcriptional regulation is so vital to the function of a cell.

Promoters integrate multiple, diverse inputs and produce a single scalar output: the rate of transcription initiation *(33)*. There are no consistent sequence motifs that characterize the promoters of protein-coding genes. However, two functional features are always present although it can be difficult to recognize them by simply looking at the DNA sequence. The first is the basal promoter (or core promoter), the site on which the enzymatic machinery of transcription assembles. The second is a collection of transcription factor-binding sites (TFBSs). Regulatory elements, which lie upstream of a gene, are known as *cis*-elements because they are parallel with the coding sequence.

4.2. Core Promoters

Although necessary for transcription, the basal promoter is apparently not a common point of regulation, and it cannot by itself generate significant levels of mRNA *(34)*. Basal promoter sequences differ among genes. For many genes it is a TATA box, usually located about 25–30 bp 5' of the transcription start site. However, some genes lack a TATA box and instead contain an initiator element spanning the transcription start site. A key step in transcriptional initiation is attachment of TATA-binding protein (TBP) to DNA *(34)*. Transcription is carried out by the RNA polymerase II holoenzyme complex, which is composed of 10–12 proteins *(35)*. Once TBP binds, several TBP-associated factors guide the RNA polymerase II holoenzyme complex onto the DNA. After the RNA polymerase II complex assembles onto the DNA, a second point of contact is established approx 30 bp downstream. This site is the transcription start site (TSS).

4.3. Transcription Factor-Binding Sites

To produce significant levels of mRNA, the association of transcription factors with DNA sequences outside the basal promoter is necessary. These sites are known as "TFBSs." TFBSs can interact with multiple transcription factors and, conversely, each transcription factor can interact with multiple TFBSs. Binding sites typically comprise a minority of the nucleotides within a promoter region. These regions are often interspersed with regions that contain no binding sites. Nucleotides that do not affect the specificity of TFBSs are generally assumed to be nonfunctional with respect to transcription. In some cases, however, these nucleotides may influence the local conformation of the DNA, with direct consequences for protein binding *(36)*. Spacing between binding sites varies enormously, from partial overlap to tens of kilobases. Functional con-straints on binding site-spacing are often related to protein interactions that take place during DNA binding.

Clusters of nearby TFBSs sometimes operate as modules (also known as enhancers). A module is operationally defined as a cluster of binding sites that produces a discrete aspect of the total transcription profile. A single module typically contains approx 6–15 binding sites *(37)*.

4.4. Transcription Factors

Transcription factors bind to TFBSs and are known as *trans*-elements because they can regulate a gene on any chromosome. The complement of active transcription factors within the nucleus differs during the course of development in response to environmental conditions, across regions of the organism, and among cell types. This changing array of transcription factors provides nearly all of the control over when, where, at what level, and under what circumstances a particular gene is transcribed. Most transcription factors contain several functional domains. DNA-binding domains (DBDs) allow the transcription factor to bind to the TFBS. Protein–protein interaction domains allow transcription factors to engage in a variety of interactions with other proteins. Many transcription factors contain a nuclear localization signal. The activity of a transcription factor may be regulated, by controlling the ratio of cytoplasmic-to-nuclear localization of the transcription factor.

4.5. Promoter Evolution

Similar clusters of TFBSs are sometimes present in the promoters of orthologous genes of species that diverged up to 10^7–10^8 yr ago. Long-term conservation suggests constraints on promoter function. Promoter sequences can also diverge extensively among relatively closely related species, and they may include gains or losses of multiple binding sites and changes in the position of regulatory sequences relative to the TSS. Comparisons of 20 well-characterized regulatory regions in mammals revealed that approximately one-third of binding sites in humans are probably not functional in rodents *(38)*.

Analyses have revealed that one or a few binding sites are absolutely necessary for activating transcription and that others either modulate or have no impact on transcription. Regressing from this, essential binding sites should evolve relatively slowly in comparison with nonessential binding sites. In some cases, binding sites that occur several times may be functionally redundant or each may have a minor impact on the overall transcription profile. Thus, selection may tolerate more nucleotide substitutions in multiply represented sites than unique ones.

The precise affinity of a binding site for a particular transcription factor is sometimes functionally important. In cases in which high- and low-affinity variants of the binding site sequence have different phenotypic consequences, purifying selection will eliminate variants that bind protein but result in lower fitness, and, conversely, specific variants that confer a fitness advantage should be under positive selection.

The evolutionary history of transcription factor gene families includes many examples of "domain shuffling" and loss of specific domains. For example, a paralog may retain a DBD but lose a protein–protein interaction domain responsible for transcriptional activation; the resulting protein will function as a repressor if it competes for binding sites with a paralog that contains an activation domain (e.g., Sp family *[39]*). This is a plausible mode of evolution for some repressors.

Experiments often reveal that deleting a single module eliminates a specific aspect of the expression profile without disrupting the remainder, and, conversely, predictable artificial expression profiles can be built by experimentally combining modules from different promoters *(40)*. The conclusion from these results is that the modularity of promoters is a contributing factor to their evolution.

Point mutations can modulate or eliminate transcription factor binding, generate binding sites *de novo*, or result in binding by a different transcription factor. Insertions and deletions can change spacing between binding sites as well as eliminate binding sites or generate new ones *(41)*. In addition, new regulatory sequences can be inserted into promoters through transposition. For example, some Alu elements in humans contain binding sites for nuclear hormone receptors and exert influence on transcription *(42)*.

4.6. Silent Substitutions

Sequence changes might be functionally silent for several reasons. For example, they might not affect DNA–protein interactions, or perhaps because changes in spacing between distant binding sites will be neutral in many cases because interactions among proteins associated with binding sites more than approx 50 bp apart are mediated by DNA bending or looping, which may, to a large degree, be insensitive to differences in spacing. Furthermore, eliminating an entire binding site may be functionally neutral because some promoters contain multiple copies of the same binding site, raising the possibility of functional redundancy *(38)*.

4.7. Mutations in trans

The genetic basis for an observed difference in the expression of a particular gene in some cases does not reside in *cis* but within a mutation in the gene encoding a particular transcription factor. Mutations affecting the expression profile of an upstream transcription factor may result in up- or downregulation of a gene. In addition, amino acid substitutions in DBDs or protein-interaction domains of transcription factor can affect the expression of downstream genes and produce phenotypic consequences. These classes of *trans* effects are likely to have multiple phenotypic consequences because of the large number of downstream target genes that would be affected. Such changes, however, are rare because these domains are usually highly conserved.

Gene duplication must also be considered. Although analyses of gene duplication normally center on coding sequences, the associated promoters are clearly important for gene function. If the break points do not include *cis*-regulatory sequences, then the duplicated copy is likely to be transcriptionally inert in its new location and become a pseudogene even before it accumulates stop codons or frameshifts. If only part of the promoter is duplicated, the transcription profile of the new copy may differ from the original (e.g., this has been observed in nitric oxide synthase genes *[39,43]*).

4.8. Purifying Selection

Purifying selection occurs when a mutation is deleterious to the fitness of the protein and, as a result, there is a reduced chance that this mutation will become frequent in the population. Cases of long-term conservation of binding sites suggest persistent purifying selection. A comparison of human–mouse orthologs found that sequence conservation generally decayed rapidly with distance from the TSS *(44)*. This suggests that distal regions are probably evolving faster than proximal regions, which are probably under purifying selection. Furthermore, because binding sites are small and imprecise and can bind many transcription factors, binding sites will appear through random mutation at appreciable rates in large populations *(45)*. Where new binding sites interfere with transcription, purifying selection should eliminate them.

It is also suggested that purifying selection operates on the spacing between nearby binding sites. This is because protein–protein interactions associated with adjacent binding sites often rely on precise spacing and small changes in spacing can dramatically affect transcription.

There are many ways to repress transcription but relatively few ways to activate it. Furthermore, the consequences of failing to repress transcription may generally be less severe than failing to activate it. It follows that the binding sites within a promoter that activate expression may experience stronger purifying selection than those that bind repressors.

4.9. Positive Selection

There are examples of positive selection on some promoter alleles such as the cytochrome p450 allele in *Drosophila (46)*. This allele is associated with insecticide resistance in *Drosophila* and, therefore, positive selection on this allele would confer a fitness advantage to the organism. Additionally, Okuyama et al. *(47)* investigated possible positive selection acting on the subregion immediately upstream of the *Amy* coding region to diverge regulatory elements of the paralogous genes.

4.10. Compensatory Selection

There are also examples of compensatory selection. One such case in humans involves a hypomorphic allele within the coding sequence of CFTR that causes cystic fibrosis. Some haplotypes contain a second mutation within the promoter that adds a third Sp1-binding site, elevating transcription and resulting in improved prognosis *(48,49)*. The third Sp1 site never occurs in haplotypes that produce wild-type protein, suggesting that it may be under positive selection as a result of its compensatory effect.

4.11. Methods of Computational Regulatory Sequence Analysis

Empirical validation of binding sites is laborious. This has led to attempts to increase the reliability of informatic approaches to binding-site identification.

Nucleotide sequences for genomic upstream regions may be obtained from several sources, including the following:

1. Ensembl (www.ensembl.org/): This is a joint project between EMBL-EBI and the Sanger Institute to develop a software system that produces and maintains automatic annotation on eukaryotic genomes *(50)*. Ensembl presents up-to-date sequence data as well as annotation for metazoan genomes. A Web-based genome browser is provided, as well as a data-mining tool known as EnsMart. Available now are human, mouse, rat, fugu, zebrafish, mosquito, *Drosophila*, *Caenorhabditis elegans*, and *Caenorhabditis briggsae* genome sequences.

2. UCSC Genome Browser (http://genome.ucsc.edu/): This browser contains the reference sequence for the human, *C. elegans*, and *C. briggsae* genomes and working drafts for the mouse, rat, fugu, *Drosophila*, and SARS genomes. It also contains the CFTR (cystic fibrosis) region in 13 species. The Genome Browser zooms and scrolls over chromosomes showing annotations. The Family Browser shows expression, homology, and other information on groups of genes that can be related in many ways. The Table Browser provides convenient access to the underlying database. The Blat *(51)* alignment tool (similar to BLAST but structured differently), which quickly maps a sequence to the genome, is also available here.

An approach growing in popularity involves retrieving sequences from more than one species. The rationale behind it is based on the preferential conservation of functional sites over the course of evolution by selective pressure *(52)*. It is commonly known as phylogenetic footprinting.

4.12. Phylogenetic Footprinting

Phylogenetic footprinting dramatically improves the predictive reliability of bioinformatic approaches to the analysis of promoter sequences. By surveying more taxa, rather than simply one species, and incorporating functional data, it becomes possible to identify origins, losses, and turnover of binding sites. The fraction of human sequences conserved in upstream regions in mouse is estimated to be 36% *(44)*. As with all comparative analyses, dense phylogenetic sampling provides a more robust understanding of evolutionary transformations within promoters, particularly in cases of rapid sequence divergence. The effectiveness of this method is limited, however, because nucleotides can be conserved by chance and also some aspects of transcription are sequence specific. The first problem leads to false positives, whereas the second generates false negatives.

The following conserved regions in upstream sequences in human and mouse may possibly be conserved owing to their functional importance.

```
GGGGCGCAAATTTGCGAGATACAATACCAAATAGAGCGTTCTC Human
CTAGCGCAAATTCGTAGCGTATGCGGGCAAATAGAGCGAGTAC Mouse
Potential TFBS                      Potential TFBS
```

Table 5
TRANSFAC, Data Tables

Table	Description
Factor	Contains transcription factors and their interacting proteins
Gene	Contains genes which contain TFBS and genes which encode for TF
Site	DNA sequences to which binding of a TF was shown
Matrix	Nucleotide distribution matrices for the binding site of a TF.
Class	Transcription factor classes
Cell	Cellular source of the proteins that have been shown to interact with the sites.
Reference	Publications associated with TRANSFAC entries with links to PubMed.

4.13. Databases

Myriad databases are available for locating putative *cis*-regulatory elements in sequence data. TRANSFAC® and the Eukaryotic Promoter Database (EPD) are probably two of the best known databases that fall into this category.

It is important to recognize that for a variety of reasons many potential binding sites identified by these and other such programs do not bind protein in vivo and have no influence on transcription. Identifying the potential binding sites that actually bind protein requires biochemical and experimental tests. Phylogenetic footprinting can also help reduce the false-positive rate.

1. TRANSFAC *(53)* is a database on eukaryotic *cis*-acting regulatory DNA elements and *trans*-acting factors. It covers many species from yeast to human. The TRANSFAC data have been generally extracted from original literature. The user interface of TRANSFAC contains several tables of data (**Table 5**). To search TRANSFAC one must first choose the table to be searched (e.g., FACTOR). Then one must choose the search field (e.g., Species); enter the search term, e.g., "mouse" into the input field; and finish by pressing the SUBMIT button. Using this example, all transcription factor entries that belong to mouse or contain "mouse" in the species name will be retrieved.

    TRANSFAC also contains two tools into which one can submit nucleotide sequences and search for potential TFBSs in their sequence. These include MATCH, which uses a library of TRANSFAC mononucleotide weight matrices, and PATCH, which is a pattern search program based on TRANSFAC v6.0. TRANSFAC can be found at www.gene-regulation.com.

2. EPD *(54)* is an annotated, nonredundant collection of eukaryotic polymerase II promoters, for which the TSS has been determined experimentally. The main purpose of the database is to keep track of experimental data that define transcription initiation sites of eukaryotic genes. This functional information is linked to promoter sequences and positions within sequences of the EMBL nucleotide sequence database. EPD is a rigorously selected, curated, and quality-controlled database. To be included in EPD, a promoter must have its TSS mapped with accuracy and certainty, the corresponding gene must be functional, and the corresponding sequence data must be available in the public databases. At present, EPD is confined to promoters recognized by the RNA polymerase II system of higher eukaryotes. Promoter sequences, documentation, and training sets for development of promoter prediction algorithms can be downloaded from www.epd.isb-sib.ch.

Several additional methods can be applied to identify unknown binding sites. These approaches include identifying overrepresented sequence motifs *(55,56)* and examining expression data *(57)*.

4.14. Searching for Statistically Overrepresented Motifs

Two regulatory regions that have a statistically significant overrepresentation of a particular binding site may be coregulated or involved in the same pathway. Therefore, searching for genes that have similar overrepresentation of a TFBS may allow the identification of new regulatory networks.

The full range of sequences that can bind a particular transcription factor with significantly higher specificity than random DNA, under physiological conditions, is often described by a position weight matrix (PWM). The probability that each position in the binding site will be represented by a particular nucleotide is tabulated. The TRANSFAC database has a range of PWM for various TFBSs.

4.14.1. Identifying Overrepresented Motifs

First of all, it is necessary to identify functionally related proteins. Then, it is necessary to identify overrepresented motifs in the promoters of the proteins. Next, other genes with a similar promoter profile are searched. Finally, results are confirmed with expression data and a search of coregulated genes is conducted.

Elkon et al. *(55)* employed a method using PWM to identify transcription factors whose binding sites are significantly overrepresented in specific sets of promoters. They identified eight transcription factors overrepresented in promoters of genes whose expression is cell-cycle dependent. They used gene expression data to verify their results. Liu et al. *(56)* also examined overrepresentation of binding sites in immune gene promoters. They identified nine novel nuclear factor-κB-regulated immune genes in humans and confirmed their predictions with available expression data.

The use of DNA microarrays to study global gene expression profiles is emerging as a pivotal technology in functional genomics. Comparison of gene expression profiles under different biological conditions reveals the corresponding differences in the cellular transcriptional patterns. Recent studies have used microarray data and computational promoter analysis to identify novel regulatory networks. These studies have shown that genes that are coexpressed over multiple biological conditions are often regulated via common mechanisms and, hence, share common *cis*-regulatory elements in their promoters. For example, this approach has been used in *Saccharomyces cerevisiae (57)*. Using expression data to study *cis*-regulatory elements is often described as a reverse engineering approach.

Databases such as Gene Expression Omnibus (GEO) *(58)* that contain expression data for a variety of organisms are available to the public. GEO is a gene expression and hybridization array data repository, as well as a curated, online resource for gene expression data browsing, query, and retrieval. GEO was the first fully public, high-throughput gene expression data repository and can be accessed at http://www.ncbi.nlm.nih.gov/geo/.

5. Conclusion

Understanding the evolutionary mechanisms that shape DNA and protein sequences will require a thorough appreciation of informatic approaches as well as the use of comparative data from promoter sequences, biochemical assays, and functional tests. The insights into evolutionary history and mechanisms that will emerge from detailed analyses of sequence evolution are potentially enormous. This information will be essential for a complete understanding of the evolution of the genotype–phenotype relationship.

A comparative approach involving multiple species of varying degrees of divergence and polymorphism analysis may enable the identification of genomic segments that are responsible for differences in these species and differences in their reactions to the same stimuli.

References

1. Owen, R. (1843) *Lectures on the Comparative Anatomy and Physiology of the Invertebrate Animals. Delivered at the Royal College of Surgeons, in 1843.* Longman, Brown, Green, and Longmans, London.
2. Yang, Z. and Bielawski, J. P. (2000) Statistical methods for detecting molecular adaptation. *Trends in Ecol. Evol.* **15,** 496–503.
3. Zuckerkandl, E. and Pauling, L. (1965) Molecules as documents of evolutionary history. *J. Theor. Biol.* **8,** 357–366.
4. Goidts, V., Szamalek, J. M., Hameister, H., and Kehrer-Sawatzki, H. (2004) Segmental duplication associated with the human-specific inversion of chromosome 18: a further example of the impact of segmental duplications on karyotype and genome evolution in primates. *Hum. Genet.* **115,** 116–122.
5. Hughes, A. L. and Friedman, R. (2004) Differential loss of ancestral gene families as a source of genomic divergence in animals. *Proc. R. Soc. Lond. B. Biol. Sci.* **271(Suppl 3),** S107–S109.
6. Kinsella, R. J., Fitzpatrick, D. A., Creevey, C. J., and McInerney, J. O. (2003) Fatty acid biosynthesis in Mycobacterium tuberculosis: lateral gene transfer, adaptive evolution, and gene duplication. *Proc. Natl. Acad. Sci. USA* **100,** 10,320–10,325.
7. Altschul, S. F., Madden, T. L., Schaffer, A. A., et al. (1997) Gapped BLAST and PSI-BLAST: a new generation of protein database search programs. *Nucleic Acids Res.* **25,** 3389–3402.
8. Pearson, W. R. (1990) Rapid and sensitive sequence comparison with FASTP and FASTA. *Methods Enzymol.* **183,** 63–98.
9. Maddison, D. R., Swofford, D. L., and Maddison, W. P. (1997) NEXUS: an extensible file format for systematic information. *Syst. Biol.* **46,** 590–621.
10. Stewart, C. B. (1993) The powers and pitfalls of parsimony. *Nature* **361,** 603–607.
11. Swofford, D. L. (1998) *PAUP*. Phylogenetic Analysis Using Parsimony (*And Other Methods),* Sinauer Associates, Sunderland, MA.
12. Jukes, T. H. and Cantor, C. R. (1969) Evolution of protein molecules, in *Mammalian Protein Metabolism* (Munro, H. N., ed.), Academic, New York, pp. 21–23.
13. Felsenstein, J. (1981) Evolutionary trees from DNA sequences: a maximum likelihood approach. *J. Mol. Evol.* **17,** 368–376.
14. Yang, Z. (1997) PAML: a program package for phylogenetic analysis by maximum likelihood. *Comput. Appl. Biosci.* **13,** 555–556.
15. Schmidt, H. A., Strimmer, K., Vingron, M., and von Haeseler, A. (2002) TREE-PUZZLE: maximum likelihood phylogenetic analysis using quartets and parallel computing. *Bioinformatics* **18,** 502–504.

16. Rannala, B. and Yang, Z. (1996) Probability distribution of molecular evolutionary trees: a new method of phylogenetic inference. *J. Mol. Evol.* **43**, 304–311.
17. Ronquist, F. and Huelsenbeck, J. P. (2003) MrBayes 3: Bayesian phylogenetic inference under mixed models. *Bioinformatics* **19**, 1572–1574.
18. Page, R. D. (1996) TreeView: an application to display phylogenetic trees on personal computers. *Comput. Appl. Biosci.* **12**, 357–358.
19. Hughes, A. L. (1999) *Adaptive Evolution of Genes and Genomes,* Oxford University Press, New York.
20. Creevey, C. J. and McInerney, J. O. (2002) An algorithm for detecting directional and non-directional positive selection, neutrality and negative selection in protein coding DNA sequences. *Gene* **300**, 43–51.
21. Hughes, A. L., Ota, T., and Nei, M. (1990) Positive Darwinian selection promotes charge profile diversity in the antigen-binding cleft of class I major-histocompatibility-complex molecules. *Mol. Biol. Evol.* **7**, 515–524.
22. McDonald, J. H. and Kreitman, M. (1991) Adaptive protein evolution at the Adh locus in Drosophila. *Nature* **351**, 652–654.
23. Messier, W. and Stewart, C. B. (1997) Episodic adaptive evolution of primate lysozymes. *Nature* **385**, 151–154.
24. Anisimova, M., Bielawski, J. P., and Yang, Z. (2001) Accuracy and power of the likelihood ratio test in detecting adaptive molecular evolution. *Mol. Biol. Evol.* **18**, 1585–1592.
25. Creevey, C. J. and McInerney, J. O. (2003) CRANN: detecting adaptive evolution in protein-coding DNA sequences. *Bioinformatics* **19**, 1726.
26. Li, W. H. (1993) Unbiased estimation of the rates of synonymous and nonsynonymous substitution. *J. Mol. Evol.* **36**, 96–99.
27. Yang, Z. (1998) Likelihood ratio tests for detecting positive selection and application to primate lysozyme evolution. *Mol. Biol. Evol.* **15**, 568–573.
28. Yang, Z. (2000) Maximum likelihood estimation on large phylogenies and analysis of adaptive evolution in human influenza virus A. *J. Mol. Evol.* **51**, 423–432.
29. Miyata, T. and Yasunaga, T. (1980) Molecular evolution of mRNA: a method for estimating evolutionary rates of synonymous and amino acid substitutions from homologous nucleotide sequences and its application. *J. Mol. Evol.* **16**, 23–36.
30. Goldman, N. and Yang, Z. (1994) A codon-based model of nucleotide substitution for protein-coding DNA sequences. *Mol. Biol. Evol.* **11**, 725–736.
31. Yang, Z. H. (1997) Phylogenetic analysis by maximum likelihood (PAML). *CABIOS* **15**, 555–556.
32. Nielsen, R. and Yang, Z. (1998) Likelihood models for detecting positively selected amino acid sites and applications to the HIV-1 envelope gene. *Genetics* **148**, 929–936.
33. Wray, G. A., Hahn, M. W., Abouheif, E., et al. (2003) The evolution of transcriptional regulation in eukaryotes. *Mol. Biol. Evol.* **20**, 1377–1419.
34. Kuras, L. and Struhl, K. (1999) Binding of TBP to promoters in vivo is stimulated by activators and requires Pol II holoenzyme. *Nature* **399**, 609–613.
35. Orphanides, G., Lagrange, T., and Reinberg, D. (1996) The general transcription factors of RNA polymerase II. *Genes Dev.* **10**, 2657–2683.
36. Hizver, J., Rozenberg, H., Frolow, F., Rabinovich, D., and Shakked, Z. (2001) DNA bending by an adenine–thymine tract and its role in gene regulation. *Proc. Natl. Acad. Sci. USA* **98**, 8490–8495.
37. Arnone, M. I. and Davidson, E. H. (1997) The hardwiring of development: organization and function of genomic regulatory systems. *Development* **124**, 1851–1864.

38. Dermitzakis, E. T. and Clark, A. G. (2002) Evolution of transcription factor binding sites in Mammalian gene regulatory regions: conservation and turnover. *Mol. Biol. Evol.* **19,** 1114–1121.

39. Suske, G. (1999) The Sp-family of transcription factors. *Gene* **238,** 291–300.

40. Kirchhamer, C. V., Bogarad, L. D., and Davidson, E. H. (1996) Developmental expression of synthetic cis-regulatory systems composed of spatial control elements from two different genes. *Proc. Natl. Acad. Sci. USA* **93,** 13,849–13,854.

41. Ludwig, M. Z. and Kreitman, M. (1995) Evolutionary dynamics of the enhancer region of even-skipped in Drosophila. *Mol. Biol. Evol.* **12,** 1002–1011.

42. Babich, V., Aksenov, N., Alexeenko, V., Oei, S. L., Buchlow, G., and Tomilin, N. (1999) Association of some potential hormone response elements in human genes with the Alu family repeats. *Gene* **239,** 341–349.

43. Korneev, S. and O'Shea, M. (2002) Evolution of nitric oxide synthase regulatory genes by DNA inversion. *Mol. Biol. Evol.* **19,** 1228–1233.

44. Jareborg, N., Birney, E., and Durbin, R. (1999) Comparative analysis of noncoding regions of 77 orthologous mouse and human gene pairs. *Genome Res.* **9,** 815–824.

45. Stone, J. R. and Wray, G. A. (2001) Rapid evolution of cis-regulatory sequences via local point mutations. *Mol. Biol. Evol.* **18,** 1764–1770.

46. Daborn, P. J., Yen, J. L., Bogwitz, M. R., et al. (2002) A single p450 allele associated with insecticide resistance in Drosophila. *Science* **297,** 2253–2256.

47. Okuyama, E., Shibata, H., Tachida, H., and Yamazaki, T. (1996) Molecular evolution of the 5'-flanking regions of the duplicated Amy genes in Drosophila melanogaster species subgroup. *Mol. Biol. Evol.* **13,** 574–583.

48. Romey, M. C., Guittard, C., Chazalette, J. P., et al. (1999) Complex allele [-102T>A+ S549R(T>G)] is associated with milder forms of cystic fibrosis than allele S549R(T>G) alone. *Hum. Genet.* **105,** 145–150.

49. Romey, M. C., Pallares-Ruiz, N., Mange, A., et al. (2000) A naturally occurring sequence variation that creates a YY1 element is associated with increased cystic fibrosis transmembrane conductance regulator gene expression. *J. Biol. Chem.* **275,** 3561–3567.

50. Hubbard, T., Barker, D., Birney, E., et al. (2002) The Ensembl genome database project. *Nucleic Acids Res.* **30,** 38–41.

51. Kent, W. J. (2002) BLAT–the BLAST-like alignment tool. *Genome Res.* **12,** 656–664.

52. Lenhard, B., Sandelin, A., Mendoza, L., Engstrom, P., Jareborg, N., and Wasserman, W. W. (2003) Identification of conserved regulatory elements by comparative genome analysis. *J. Biol.* **2,** 13.

53. Wingender, E., Chen, X., Hehl, R., et al. (2000) TRANSFAC: an integrated system for gene expression regulation. *Nucleic Acids Res.* **28,** 316–319.

54. Praz, V., Perier, R., Bonnard, C., and Bucher, P. (2002) The Eukaryotic Promoter Database, EPD: new entry types and links to gene expression data. *Nucleic Acids Res.* **30,** 322–324.

55. Elkon, R., Linhart, C., Sharan, R., Shamir, R., and Shiloh, Y. (2003) Genome-wide in silico identification of transcriptional regulators controlling the cell cycle in human cells. *Genome Res.* **13,** 773–780.

56. Liu, R., McEachin, R. C., and States, D. J. (2003) Computationally identifying novel NF-kappa B-regulated immune genes in the human genome. *Genome Res.* **13,** 654–661.

57. Jelinsky, S. A., Estep, P., Church, G. M., and Samson, L. D. (2000) Regulatory networks revealed by transcriptional profiling of damaged Saccharomyces cerevisiae cells: Rpn4 links base excision repair with proteasomes. *Mol. Cell Biol.* **20,** 8157–8167.

58. Edgar, R., Domrachev, M., and Lash, A. E. (2002) Gene Expression Omnibus: NCBI gene expression and hybridization array data repository. *Nucleic Acids Res.* **30,** 207–210.

7

Standardization of Microarray and Pharmacogenomics Data

Casey S. Husser, Jeffrey R. Buchhalter, O. Scott Raffo,
Amnon Shabo, Steven H. Brown, Karen E. Lee, and Peter L. Elkin

Summary

This chapter provides a bottom-up perspective on bioinformatics data standards, beginning with a historical perspective on biochemical nomenclature standards. Various file format standards were soon developed to convey increasingly complex and voluminous data that nomenclature alone could not effectively organize without additional structure and annotation. As areas of biochemistry and molecular biology have become more integral to the practice of modern medicine, broader data representation models have been created, from corepresentation of genomic and clinical data as a framework for drug research and discovery to the modeling of genotyping and pharmacogenomic therapy within the broader process of the delivery of health care.

Key Words: Pharmacogenomics; clinical genomics; file format; microarray experiment; linkage disequilibrium study; genotype model; storyboard.

1. Introduction

Like the Enigma code employed by the Germans in World War II, the genomic code is proving to be a formidable cryptographic hurdle for the allied powers of modern science to clear. Although the four-base, triplet reading-frame genetic code was cracked by the mid-1960s (1–4), researchers almost immediately discovered that despite this breakthrough, unlocking the mysteries of the genome itself would be a much bigger task. The genome is multiply encrypted beyond the initial (but important) level of nucleotide sequence. Differential expression, the governance of splicing, protein folding, post-translational modification, and macromolecular interactions all play a role in conveyance of genomic information transfer, and none of these are comprehensively understood.

Information coded in biological molecules and the reactions they play a role in adeptly orchestrate the diverse yet highly ordered collection of everything that is collectively known to be *life*—and a few things that arguably are *not*. This traffic of biological information is pervasive, unrelenting, and nearly omnipresent on the surface of our planet,

From: *Methods in Molecular Biology, vol. 316: Bioinformatics and Drug Discovery*
Edited by: R. S. Larson © Humana Press Inc., Totowa, NJ

yet the key (or likely keys) to its code still escape the very finest intellectual efforts that our collective society has put forth. However, progress is slowly being made. The fruits of various genome-sequencing projects (most notably the human genome project) have previewed a better perspective on one of the genome's finest forms of obscuring its underlying message: its monolithic scale. As of this writing, the human genome alone contains some 3.2 billion bp, but just fewer than 24,000 known and speculated genes *(5)*. Now consider the fact that the presence of introns dictates that genes are not coded discretely along a given sequence of DNA. The task of finding, deciphering, and assembling the coding sequences that make up genes in the human genome amounts to a task much more intimidating than finding a needle in a haystack. It is more along the lines of finding and assembling a few handfuls of severed needles scattered across all of the haystacks of the world. The advent of microarray experiments has been a great boon to genome-sequencing projects, but their high-throughput nature adds more data to the database than knowledge to the knowledge base *(6)*. The need for mass computation has never been greater. The management of this magnitude of raw data is unprecedented in mankind's history. Likewise, the need for data standards is equally critical, so that both order and orderly commerce of information can be maintained within a pool of data that is exploding at a rate in excess of historical rates of advancement of computer processor speeds.

This chapter covers both established and emerging standards in the acquisition and storage of sequence and microarray data, as well as standards for research and clinical applications of genomic knowledge. Just as different types of information are stored at different levels of the genome and its supporting cellular machinery, different formalisms are often necessary to represent adequately each level (e.g., formalisms for collection of nucleic acid sequence information are not necessarily sufficient for representation of the three-dimensional conformational structures of the proteins for which they may [or may not] code). Unfortunately, this line of reasoning can be inappropriately overextended to justify multiple formalisms for the same area, which may often be useful for the individual(s) who create and use the formalism, but serves to stifle the free exchange of information between others in the greater scientific community conducting related research who happen to use a different—and most likely incompatible—formalism. This common problem frames the practical necessity that drives the establishment of bioinformatics standards. Although there are no current standards in the truest sense of the definition, this chapter reviews some of the more prevalent data formalisms pertaining to microarray data and pharmacogenomics.

2. Standards for Acquisition and Storage of Sequence Data

2.1. Raw or Free-Text Formats

Raw sequence data are still (and will likely remain) an accepted mode of data submission for sequence analysis applications and portals widely available on the Web. Raw data, although convenient for immediate use by an individual researcher eager to mine his or her newfound code, has its share of drawbacks and certainly cannot be considered a standard for generalized use. Without markup or annotation of any kind, raw data messages provide no information about a given sequence, be it identifiers of file source;

```
MATVPELNCEMPPFDSDENDLFFEVDGPQKMKGCFQTFDLGCPDESIQLQISQQHINKSFRQAVSLIVAVEKLWQLPVSFPWTFQDEDMSTFFSFIF
EEEPILCDSWDDDDNLLVCDVPIRQLHYRLRDEQQKSLVLSDPYELKALHLNGQNINQQVIFSMSFVQGEPSNDKIPVALGLKGKNLYLSCVMKDGT
PTLQLESVDPKQYPKKKMEKRFVFNKIEVKSKVEFESAEFPNWYISTSQAEHKPVFLGNNSGQDIIDFTMESVSS
```

Fig. 1. Amino acid sequence for mouse interleukin 1-β in raw data format, i.e., only amino acid symbols.

Table 1
JCBN Conventions for Representation of Specific and Ambiguous Nucleic Acids

Symbol	Meaning	Origin of designation	Complement
G	G	Guanine	C
A	A	Adenine	T
C	C	Cytosine	G
T	T	Thymine	A
U	U	Uracil	A
R	A or G	Purine	Y
Y	C or T	Pyrimidine	R
M	A or C	Amino	K
K	G or T	Keto	M
S	G or C	Strong interaction (3H bonds)	S
W	A or T	Weak interaction (2H bonds)	W
H	A, C, or T	not-G; **H** follows G in alphabet	D
B	G, T, or C	not-A; **B** follows A in alphabet	V
V	G, C, or A	not-T or U; **V** follows U in alphabet	B
D	G, T, or A	not-C; **D** follows C in alphabet	H
N	G, A, T, or C	Any	N

sequence identity; or, more important, clear measures of beginning, end, and quantity of data in between. Sequence formatting standards provide a measure of data integrity insurance that is important to a field in which small omissions of chemical or recorded data can lead to significant, if not fatal, changes to the original message. The raw data format provides a string of characters representing a sequence without description or annotation, as shown in **Fig. 1**.

Although raw data, by definition, is not formatted or annotated, its content must adhere to the nomenclature standards *(7–9)* set forth by the International Union of Pure and Applied Chemistry–International Union of Biochemistry and Molecular Biology (IUPAC-IUBMB, or simply JCBN, the Joint Commission on Biochemical Nomenclature) *(10)*, in order to be recognized by almost any commonly used sequence analysis software (**Tables 1** and **2**).

In a raw file format, every character is considered a sequence character, so care must be taken to avoid adding spaces, carriage returns, and other nonprintable characters to avoid errors made by applications that are instructed to read a raw file format. By contrast, the *plain* or *free-text* format only counts alphabetic characters as sequence characters; punctuation, position numbers, spaces, and other nonprintable characters are ignored.

Take care not to confuse "free-text format" with the *"free* format" used by the somewhat obscure FSAP programs (the Fristensky Sequence Analysis Package, formerly

Table 2
JCBN Conventions for Representation
of Specific and Ambiguous Amino Acids

Amino acid	Code	Symbol
Alanine	Ala	A
Arginine	Arg	R
Asparagine	Asn	N
Aspartic acid	Asp	D
Cysteine	Cys	C
Glutamic acid	Glu	E
Glutamine	Gln	Q
Glycine	Gly	G
Histidine	His	H
Isoleucine	Ile	I
Leucine	Leu	L
Lysine	Lys	K
Methionine	Met	M
Phenylalanine	Phe	F
Proline	Pro	P
Serine	Ser	S
Threonine	Thr	T
Tryptophan	Trp	W
Tyrosine	Tyr	Y
Valine	Val	V
Unspecified	Xaa	X
Asp or Asn	Asx	B
Gln, Glu, Gla[a], or Glp[b]	Glx	Z
Gap		—
Terminator		.or*

[a]4-Carboxyglutamic acid.
[b]5-Oxoproline.

known as the Cornell Sequence Analysis Package) *(11,12)*. Despite the similarity in names, the free format for FSAP is designed to be extensively annotated (to allow researchers to enter free-text laboratory notes of specific sections of sequences), and, thus, it is not at all synonymous with freetext formats. This distinction is made owing to the fact that there is still some Web presence on utilizing free format for FSAP as of this writing *(13–15)*.

2.2. FASTA File/Pearson Format

In the early 1980s, William R. Pearson and David J. Lipman began some of the earliest work on computerized nucleic and amino acid sequence analysis techniques via pairwise comparison *(16,17)*. FASTA was not the first incarnation of their designs, but it was the most successful, owing to its speed in use and its coverage of both nucleic and amino acid sequences *(18)*. These two attributes were used to coin the name FASTA (pronounced fast-aye), for its speed (FAST) and its comprehensive biopolymer cover-

Table 3
FASTA Header Conventions

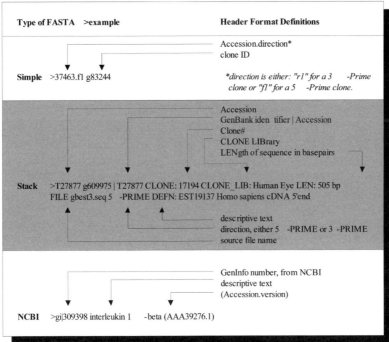

Type of FASTA	>example	Header Format Definitions
Simple	>37463.f1 g83244	Accession.direction* clone ID *direction is either: "r1" for a 3 -Prime clone or "f1" for a 5 -Prime clone.*
Stack	>T27877 g609975	T27877 CLONE: 17194 CLONE_LIB: Human Eye LEN: 505 bp FILE gbest3.seq 5 -PRIME DEFN: EST19137 Homo sapiens cDNA 5'end	Accession GenBank iden tifier	Accession Clone# CLONE LIBrary LENgth of sequence in basepairs descriptive text direction, either 5 -PRIME or 3 -PRIME source file name
NCBI	>gi|309398 interleukin 1 -beta (AAA39276.1)	GenInfo number, from NCBI descriptive text (Accession.version)

age (both amino and nucleic acids = All) *(19)*. Incidentally, FASTA has also been attributed to standing for FAST-Alignment *(20)*, but much less commonly.

FASTA has been so widely utilized over the last 20 yr, that it has become two separate but related entities. The *FASTA file format* (also referred to as the Pearson format) for sequences is a popular format for submission of sequence data to other, more sophisticated sequence analysis tools, such as gapped-BLAST, PSI-BLAST, or WU-BLAST, which, in turn, can report their results in FASTA format as well. The second entity is simply the original FASTA paired alignment tool, although numerous subtle modifications have been made since its inception *(21,22)*.

The FASTA file format, like the alignment tool that spawned it, can be used for either nucleic acid or amino acid sequences. Its minimal annotation makes it the simplest file format for sequences, adding nothing more than a header to raw sequence data. A sequence recorded in the FASTA file format begins with a one-line header that begins with a unicode "greater than" or ">" character. The header contains identifying information, usually the accession number, and a brief description of the sequence source. This information is entered by convention, but in truth, any content can be placed in this line, for it exists only for human perusal, not for any computational reference. There are several format conventions for header information, including simple FASTA, Stack FASTA *(23)*, and NCBI FASTA *(24)*; *see* **Table 3** for details on header differences for each. The sequence itself follows the header after a carriage return, and it is

```
>gi|309398 interleukin 1-beta (AAA39276.1)
MATVPELNCEMPPFDSDENDLFFEVDGPQKMKGCFQTFDLGCPDESIQLQISQQHINKSFRQAVSLIVAV
EKLWQLPVSFPWTFQDEDMSTFFSFIFEEEPILCDSWDDDDNLLVCDVPIRQLHYRLRDEQQKSLVLSDP
YELKALHLNGQNINQQVIFSMSFVQGEPSNDKIPVALGLKGKNLYLSCVMKDGTPTLQLESVDPKQYPKK
KMEKRFVFNKIEVKSKVEFESAEFPNWYISTSQAEHKPVFLGNNSGQDIIDFTMESVSS
```

Fig. 2. Same amino acid sequence as in **Fig. 1** but in FASTA file format. Note that the source of this file is NCBI's Entrez, as evidenced by its ">gi|" header.

```
>AAA1234.r1 g55
CCTCTGCGGCAGCCTTTCTTGGACTGGCAACCCACATCAAGTTGTTAAGGAAGGTATAAC
GCCAGTTTCCATGGAGAGGTTAACGCGGTAGTCATCTTTTATATGAGTTGGCATTAATCC
>AAA1235.r1 g66
ATGCTTGGCCTCTGCGGCAGCCACTGGCAACCCACATCAAGTTGTTAAGGAAGGTATAAC
CCATGGAGAGGTTAACGCGGTCATCTCCAGTTTGGTATTTATATGAGTTGGCATTAATCC
>AAA1236.r1 g25
TTTCTTGGCCTCTGCGGCAGCCACTGGCAACCCACATCAAGTTGTTAAGGAAGGTATAAC
CCATGGAGAGGTTAACGCGGTCATCTCCATATGAGTTGGCATTAATCC
```

Fig. 3. Example of concatenated simple FASTA nucleotide file containing three sequences.

formatted to have no more than 80 JCBN amino or nucleic acid characters per line, as shown in **Fig. 2**. The FASTA file format also has the capacity to store multiple sequences in a single file. This is accomplished via concatenation of FASTA sequences; that is, one sequence follows another with very little fanfare. At the end of a sequence, a carriage return is immediately followed by a ">," which designates the header for the next sequence; there are no intervening spaces or blank lines (*see* **Fig. 3**). All standard FASTA conventions apply to each sequence in the file.

2.3. Genetics Computer Group Format

Also during the early 1980s, the Genetics Computer Group (GCG) developed a sequence analysis package now commonly known as the "Wisconsin Package," owing to the group's location at the University of Wisconsin Medical Center. The more than 140 programs that make up this software package allow the user to analyze and compare protein and nucleotide sequences with those found in established databases such as EMBL, GenEMBL, PIR-Protein, Restriction Enzyme Database, and GenBank *(25)*.

In 1982, Oliver Smithies developed the initial programs for the Genetics Department at the University of Wisconsin, Madison, as a research tool. By 1985, GCG was formed in order to operate the software and develop new tools. The next decade brought GCG to a new level with the formation of a private company in 1990 and the renaming of its software to "Wisconsin Package," the release of its first graphical interface (SeqLab) in 1994, its acquisition by Oxford Molecular in 1997, the release of a Web-based package (SeqWeb) in 1998, and its acquisition by Pharmacopoeia in 2000. On June 1, 2001, Pharmacopoeia combined its software businesses, which include GCG, Oxford Molecular, Synomics, Synopsys, and MSI under the name Accelrys *(26)*.

Much like FASTA, the GCG file format is derived from its widely used sequence analysis package of the same name. It shares with the FASTA file format three other attributes: utility in representation of both peptide and nucleic acid sequences, the capacity to convey multiple sequences in a single file (GCG Multiple Sequence File, or GCG-

```
!!NA_SEQUENCE 1.0
gi|198293|gb|M15131.1|MUSIL1BA Mouse interleukin 1-beta (IL-1-beta) mRNA,
gi-198293.seq  Length: 1339  November 8, 1999 13:29  Type: N  Check: 1315  ..
        1  TGCAGGGTTC GAGGCCTAAT AGGCTCATCT GGGATCCTCT CCAGCCAAGC
       51  TTCCTTGTGC AAGTGTCTGA AGCAGCTATG GCAACTGTTC CTGAACTCAA
      101  CTGTGAAATG CCACCTTTTG ACAGTGATGA GAATGACCTG TTCTTTGAAG
      151  TTGACGGACC CCAAAAGATG AAGGGCTGCT TCCAAACCTT TGACCTGGGC
      201  TGTCCAGATG AGAGCATCCA GCTTCAAATC TCACAGCAGC ACATCAACAA
      251  GAGCTTCAGG CAGGCAGTAT CACTCATTGT GGCTGTGGAG AAGCTGTGGC
      301  AGCTACCTGT GTCTTTCCCG TGGACCTTCC AGGATGAGGA CATGAGCACC
      351  TTCTTTTCCT TCATCTTTGA AGAAGAGCCC ATCCTCTGTG ACTCATGGGA
      401  TGATGATGAT AACCTGCTGG TGTGTGACGT TCCCATTAGA CAGCTGCACT
      451  ACAGGCTCCG AGATGAACAA CAAAAAAGCC TCGTGCTGTC GGACCCATAT
      501  GAGCTGAAAG CTCTCCACCT CAATGGACAG AATATCAACC AACAAGTGAT
      551  ATTCTCCATG AGCTTTGTAC AAGGAGAACC AAGCAACGAC AAAATACCTG
      601  TGGCCTTGGG CCTCAAAGGA AAGAATCTAT ACCTGTCCTG TGTAATGAAA
      651  GACGGCACAC CCACCCTGCA GCTGGAGAGT GTGGATCCCA ...etc
```

Fig. 4. Example of nucleic acid sequence in GCG file format.

MSF), and a nonrigidly defined identification header. Header information in a GCG file does have a conventional structure, and its content offers additional functionality that FASTA does not (*see* **Fig. 4**). The simplest definition of a GCG header is any text string or stings that precede two adjacent periods (..), also known as the dividing line *(27)*. The header content is not bounded by any firm rules other than that it cannot include two adjacent periods (the dividing line can be eliminated if there is no content for a header, but this presents an undesirable condition for clear data exchange). The sequence follows the dividing line. Sequence characters are JCBN standard amino or nucleic acid letter codes, as specified by the type of sequence. Position numbers are included for ease of navigation but are ignored by applications reading GCG files for sequence data. A double slash mark (//) can denote the end of a sequence, but most applications process to the file's end without error if it is omitted *(28)*.

By convention, GCG headers begin with !!NA_SEQUENCE 1.0 for nucleic acid sequences, or !!AA_SEQUENCE 1.0 for amino acid sequences. Characters between this line and the dividing line are optional for further user specification about the sequence; they may contain accession numbers and/or text descriptions of what the sequence that follows codes for. The line ending with the dividing line typically includes: name_of_file.seq, a numeric field for length of sequence (intuitively called "Length," or "Len,"), the date and time of file creation, and the type of sequence (N = nucleic acid, P = Peptide). The final entry before the dividing line is "Check," the checksum, which is calculated from the sequence following the dividing line, and provides verification of the integrity of its sequence data (a very important feature, considering that even a tiny data omission or addition of data can lead to a frameshift "mutation" that is just as fatal to a sequence file's data as it would be to a cell's proteomic complement). See the summary in **Table 4**.

2.4. Flat-File Formats: GenBank, DDBJ, and EMBL

Flat files, by the strictest definition, are the simplest form of database, containing all of their data in a single large table or string, without metadata, application-specific

Table 4
GCG Header Conventions

		Table 4. GCG Header Conventions. Note that numbered rows in the *Sample* correspond with numbered rows in the *Example*.
Sample:	1	!!NA(nucleic acid) or AA(amino acid) _SEQUENCE 1.0
	2	optional description of sequence, no format other than cannot contain ".."
	3	GCG file name (must end in .seq) **Length of sequence in characters** Date and time of file creation Type of sequence (N = nucleotide, P = peptide) **Checksum** Dividing line (.. Marks end of header and beginning of sequence).
Example:	1	!!NA_SEQUENCE 1.0
	2	gi|198293|gb|M15131.1|MUSIL1BA Mouse interleukin 1-beta (IL-1-beta) mRNA,
	3	gi-198293.seq **Length: 1339** November 8, 1999 13:29 Type: N **Check: 1315** ..

formatting tags, or hierarchical data relationships. The advantages of working with flat files relate to their lack of formatting: they can easily be moved between different applications and databases, and working with the information they contain is quite rapid compared to relational databases. The disadvantages of working with flat files also stem from their lack of formatting: all of the logic required to relate and manipulate data within or across flat files must reside in another application. By this definition, any of the previously discussed file formats (FASTA and GCG) could qualify as flat files; however, colloquial use of the term *flat file* in the field of sequence formats is synonymous only with the much more richly documented file formats of the major genomic sequence repositories: GenBank (run by the National Center for Biotechnology Information [NCBI]), the DNA Data Bank of Japan ([DDBJ], in Mishima, Japan), and the European Molecular Biology Laboratory ([EMBL], in Heidelberg, Germany). These three repositories share sequence information freely with the public, as well as with each other under the auspices of their joint scientific effort: the International Nucleotide Sequence Database Collaboration (INSDC) *(29)*. These flat files are in fact human-friendly text reports that are automatically generated from a source database encoded in cross-platform data-interchange-friendly ASN.1 *(30)*. ASN.1, or Abstract syntax notation one, is a data specification language developed and adopted by the International Organization for Standardization (ISO Standard #8824). It was selected by NCBI for its utility in describing data types independent of particular computer structures and/or representation techniques, which allows interoperability between platforms *(31)*. By adopting ASN.1 as a standard for data specification, NCBI could accomplish two important steps in streamlining exchange of genomic data: removal of scientists from the role of creating unique file formats for their research, and by virtue of accomplishing that, and restriction of the creation of new unique file formats that are (likely) incompatible with others *(32)*.

Although the indexing of sequence information is standardized across these databases, the formatting of data differs, almost indistinguishably between GenBank and DDBJ, and more significantly between EMBL and the other two. We conducted a search of each of the three sites for files on the sequence used in several previous examples, i.e., mouse interleukin-1β (IL-1β). **Figures 5–7** illustrate the similarities and differ-

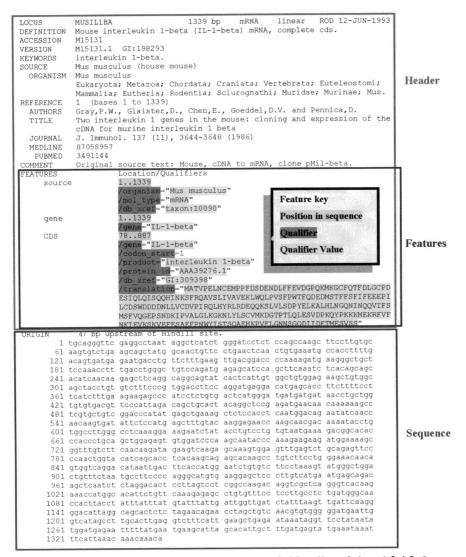

```
LOCUS       MUSIL1BA                1339 bp    mRNA     linear    ROD 12-JUN-1993
DEFINITION  Mouse interleukin 1-beta (IL-1-beta) mRNA, complete cds.
ACCESSION   M15131
VERSION     M15131.1  GI:198293
KEYWORDS    interleukin 1-beta.
SOURCE      Mus musculus (house mouse)
  ORGANISM  Mus musculus
            Eukaryota; Metazoa; Chordata; Craniata; Vertebrata; Euteleostomi;
            Mammalia; Eutheria; Rodentia; Sciurognathi; Muridae; Murinae; Mus.
REFERENCE   1  (bases 1 to 1339)
  AUTHORS   Gray,P.W., Glaister,D., Chen,E., Goeddel,D.V. and Pennica,D.
  TITLE     Two interleukin 1 genes in the mouse: cloning and expression of the
            cDNA for murine interleukin 1 beta
  JOURNAL   J. Immunol. 137 (11), 3644-3648 (1986)
  MEDLINE   87058957
   PUBMED   3491144
COMMENT     Original source text: Mouse, cDNA to mRNA, clone pMil-beta.
FEATURES             Location/Qualifiers
     source          1..1339
                     /organism="Mus musculus"
                     /mol_type="mRNA"
                     /db_xref="taxon:10090"
     gene            1..1339
                     /gene="IL-1-beta"
     CDS             78..887
                     /gene="IL-1-beta"
                     /codon_start=1
                     /product="interleukin 1-beta"
                     /protein_id="AAA39276.1"
                     /db_xref="GI:309398"
                     /translation="MATVPELNCEMPPFDSDENDLFFEVDGPQKMKGCFQTFDLGCPD
                     ESIQLQISQQHINKSFRQAVSLIVAVEKLWQLPVSFPWTFQDEDMSTFFSFIFEEEPI
                     LCDSWDDDDNLLVCDVPIRQLHYRLRDEQQKSLVLSDPYELKALHLNGQNINQQVIFS
                     MSFVQGEPSNDKIPVALGLKGKNLYLSCVMKDGTPTLQLESVDPKQYPKKKMEKRFVF
                     NKIEVKSKVEEFSAEFPNWYISTSQAEHKPVFLGNNSGQDIIDFTMESVSS"
ORIGIN      47 bp upstream of HindIII site.
        1 tgcaggggttc gaggcctaat aggctcatct gggatcctct ccagccaagc ttccttgtgc
       61 aagtgtctga agcagctatg gcaactgttc ctgaactcaa ctgtgaaatg ccacctttg
      121 acagtgatga gaatgacctg ttccttgaag ttgacggacc ccaaaagatg aagggctgct
      181 tccaaacctt tgacctgggc tgtccagatg agagcatcca gcttcaaatc tcacagcagc
      241 acatcaacaa gagcttcagg caggcagtat cactcattgt ggctgtggag aagctgtggc
      301 agctacctgt gtcttccccg tggaccttcc aggatgagga catgagcacc ttctttcct
      361 tcatctttga agaagagccc atcctctgtg actcatggga tgatgatgat aacctgctgg
      421 tgtgtgacgt tcccattaga cagctgcact acaggctccg agatgaacaa caaaaaagcc
      481 tcgtgctgtc ggacccatat gagctgaaag ctctccaacct caatggacag aatatcaacc
      541 aacaagtgat attctccatg agctttgtac aaggagaacc aagcaacgac aaaatacctg
      601 tggccttggg cctcaaagga aagaatctat acctgtcctg tgtaatgaaa gacggcacac
      661 ccaccctgca gctggagagt gtggatccca agcaatacccc aaagaagaag atggaaaagc
      721 ggtttgtctt caacaagata gaagtcaaga gcaaagtgga gtttgagtct gcagagttcc
      781 ccaactggta catcagcacc tcacaagcag agcacaagcc tgtcttcctg ggaaacaaca
      841 gtggtcagga cataattgac ttcaccatgg aatctgtgtc ttcctaaagt atgggctgga
      901 ctgtttctaa tgccttcccc agggcatgtg aaggagctcc cttgtcatga atgagcagac
      961 agctcaatct ctaggacact cctagtcct cggccaagac aggtcgctca gggtcacaag
     1021 aaaccatggc acattctgtt caaagagagc ctgtgtttcc tccttgcctc tgatgggcaa
     1081 ccacttacct atttatttat gtatttattg attggttgat ctatttaagt tgattcaagg
     1141 ggacattagg cagcactctc tagaacagaa cctcctgtc aacgtgtggg ggatgaattg
     1201 gtcatagcct tgcacttgag gtctttcatt gaagctgaga ataaataggt tcctataata
     1261 tggatgagaa tttttatgaa tgaagcatta gcacattgct ttgatgagta tgaaataaat
     1321 ttcattaaac aaacaaaca
```

Fig. 5. Outline of structure of a GenBank file. (*See* **Subheadings 2.4.** and **2.4.2.** for more information.)

ences among the file formats. Despite differences in appearance, significant efforts have been made to standardize the information across all three databases. In 1986, the INSDC set forth to adopt standards for recordable categories of sequence and sequence-related information, as well as the terminology for those categories, for the purpose of making sequence exchange seamless across GenBank and EMBL *(33)*. DDBJ joined the collaboration 1 yr later, in 1987. Their efforts have been quite successful, in that the contents of each database are synchronized and identical to within 24 h of any data submission

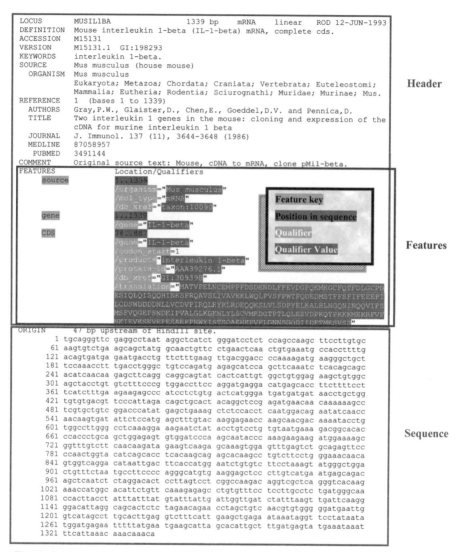

Fig. 6. Outline of structure of an EMBL file. Significant differences from GenBank/DDBJ files are highlighted. (*See* **Subheadings 2.4.** and **2.4.2.** for more information.)

(Fig. 8) *(34)*. To facilitate and maintain consistency among the three databases, the European Bioinformatics Institute (EBI) created the Feature Table (version 6.1, as of this writing), to specify an extensive set of rules on content and syntax of database entries *(35)*.

Unlike previously discussed formats for sequence information, flat files (from any of the three databases) provide context and perspective to the sequences that they record. They contain references to the research that produced them; past sequence iterations; and controlled vocabulary for taxonomy, chromosomal location, and translational infor-

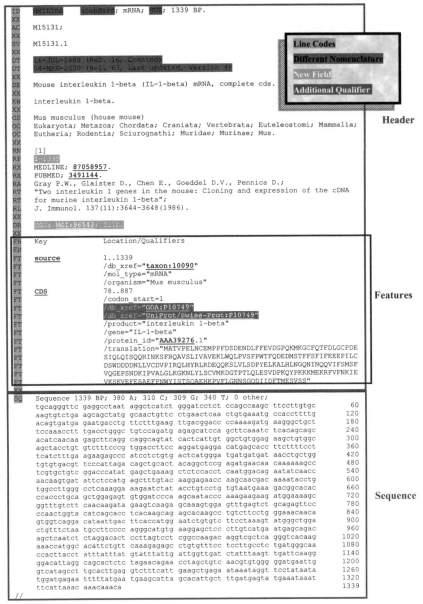

Fig. 7. Same mouse of IL-1β sequence from previous examples in AGAVE, obtained from XEMBL.

mation. The organization of GenBank files (and in almost every way DDBJ files as well) is broken down into three general sections: a header, features, and the nucleotide sequence itself (*see* **Fig. 5**).

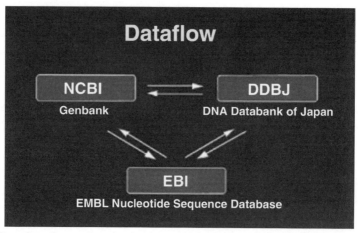

Fig. 8. Data flow for synchronization between the three regional repositories of nucleotide sequence data under INSDC.

2.4.1. Header

The header begins with the LOCUS field and terminates at the first sequence position number. GenBank/DDBJ files contain most of the information as the headers of previously discussed formats, as well as additional information for more precise identification and reference to related research and sequences. The LOCUS line defines the chromosomal sequence location, number of bases (bp) in the sequence, type of molecule (mRNA), molecule configuration (linear), GenBank division (RODent), and date that the sequence was recorded or last modified. The ACCESSION, VERSION, and GI numbers provide a precise record of the sequence and its associated information, past and present (*see* **Table 5**). The SOURCE field provides both scientific and common names for the source organism, and the ORGANISM field names the organism in context with its phylogeny via a controlled vocabulary maintained by the NCBI taxonomy project *(36)*. The REFERENCE field lists citations contributing to identification of the sequence and knowledge about the sequence (the examples in **Figs. 5** and **6** have only one reference, but multiple references are listed by repeating the REFERENCE field for each citation, oldest to most recent).

2.4.2. Features

Features are imbedded near the end of the header and are listed as indented items under the FEATURES field. The FEATURES field contains a significant amount of knowledge about sequences via sequence annotation and a controlled vocabulary. *Feature keys* define a category of knowledge about a sequence's known function. A *feature* is a specific attribute of a sequence defined by the following:

1. Its associated category (feature key).
2. Its numeric position along the sequence span.
3. Its qualifier(s), which are paired with a value to provide specific descriptive information about a given feature.

Table 5
DDBJ/EMBL/GenBank Record-Keeping Conventions

Type of record	Description
Accession	Unique identifier assigned at initial submission. This number never changes.
Version	The number to the left of the decimal is the accession number. The number of interest is the one to the right of the decimal. Each time a sequence file is updated, the number increases by one (e.g., accession.version).
GI[a]	GenInfo number. Unique identifier assigned at submission and changes to a new, unique number for every change to the sequence. This allows users to re-retrieve an exact sequence, even if it has been updated since the initial search.

[a]Currently used only in GenBank files.

There are rules on which feature keys are mandatory (e.g., source) or optional. Feature keys are well defined not only in terms of semantics, but also in terms of their hierarchical relationships to other feature keys, and contextual relationships to equally well-defined qualifiers. Some qualifiers are required for certain feature keys, and there are qualifiers that are specific to certain feature keys, required or not. For a comprehensive list of feature keys, qualifiers, and their relationships, link to the most current version of the Feature Table on any of the three data repositories. For GenBank, the current URL is www.ncbi.nlm.nih.gov/projects/collab/FT/index.html#3, under section 7.3 Appendix III: Feature keys reference.

2.4.2.1. CONVENTIONS ON FEATURE LOCATION

Locations within sequences as they pertain to features are specified by simply listing the base or base span's position number or span of position numbers, respectively. From the example in **Fig. 5**, the first listed location (from feature key "source") is 1..1339. Two numbers separated by two periods indicates that the location described is a span of sequence from the first listed base number to the last inclusive. If two numbers are separated by a single period, it indicates that the location is a single base somewhere between the two given numbered positions. If there was only a single number is listed, for example 368, the described location would simply be that specifically numbered base in the sequence. If two numbers are separated by a carat ($^\wedge$), it indicates that the specified location is between the two bases somewhere in the span (the two given numbers can be consecutive, because the location is likely to be a cleavage site, and this can only occur between, and not on, nucleotide bases). There are more sophisticated variations on describing specific sequence locations that are uncertain, spliced, found on complementary strands, and so forth in section 3 of the DDBJ/EMBL/GenBank feature table *(37)*.

2.4.3. Sequence

The sequence section begins after the ORIGIN field at the first nucleotide sequence position number and terminates at the double slash mark (//). Note that owing to the nucleic acid-centric structure of DDBJ/EMBL/GenBank flat files, the translated amino acid sequence(s) is always considered a feature and is thus included in the header, rather than in the sequence-proper section.

Table 6
Line Code Definitions for an EMBL File

Line code	Definition
ID	IDentification line
AC	ACcession
SV	Sequence Version
DT	DaTe
DE	DEcription
KW	Key Words
OS	Organism Species
OC	Organism Classification
OG	OrGanelle
RN	Reference Number
RC	Reference Comment
RP	Reference Position
RX	Reference cross-reference
RG	Reference Group
RA	Reference Author
RT	Reference Title
RL	Reference Location
DR	Database cross-Reference
AH	Assembly Header
AS	ASembly information
CO	COn(structed) or COn(tig) sequences
FH	Feature Header
FT	Feature Table
CC	Free text entry for miscellaneous info
SQ	SeQuence
XX	Spacer line
//	Sequence terminator

2.4.4. EMBL Format

EMBL files mostly contain the same information as DDBJ and GenBank files, but their formatted appearance can appear quite different at first glance (**Fig. 6**). The most obvious difference is the use of line codes in place of the fields used by GenBank and DDBJ files. Although line codes represent many of the same fields as those in GenBank and DDBJ, line codes also define blank lines, to avoid confusion with the sequence data lines *(38)* (*see* **Table 6**). Note that EMBL employs slightly different nomenclature for identifiers and dates. These differences seem trivial to the human eye, but they can be fatal to an automated parser that is expecting to see data in GenBank format. Also note that the file, albeit identical in sequence and accession to those from the other data repositories, is cross-referenced to additional databases, in both the header and the feature table. The feature table in the EMBL file is also missing a qualifier (gene) that is present in both the GenBank and DDBJ files. These differences are not in violation of the rules dictated by the INSDC feature table standards: the standards on the controlled vocabulary of feature keys, locations, qualifiers, and values remain unchanged across all three files; omissions and additions of features, however, are not as strictly governed.

2.5. Open-Source XML Schemas for Representation of Genomic Data: AGAVE and BSML

Owing to the inherent diversity, complexity, and scale of the collective biological sciences, a substantial variety of data repositories and tools for data management has been designed in support of research. Although the content and purpose of these data tools may be related or even identical, as is often the case when different data tools have different authors, these tools and repositories are incompatible in format and semantics. Because eXtensible Markup Language (XML) is designed to define and transmit data in a uniform and automatically parsed format, many in the computational biology community have looked to XML as an open-source solution for transmission, validation, and interpretation of data across different applications and formats. There are several emerging bioinformatics markup languages based on XML (e.g., AGAVE, BSML, GAME, BIOML, MGED-ML), each representing its unique data structure by means of a language-defining Document Type Definition (DTD). To properly utilize data in any XML format, one must have access to the DTD that specifies it (e.g., to parse any BSML document, one must have a browser that is XML aware and have a copy or link to the BSML DTD, because all valid BSML documents are encoded to the single set of data rules in the DTD). This section discusses AGAVE and BSML.

Despite evidence of endorsements from industry and standards bodies such as I3C and HL7, representation of BSML and AGAVE in scientific literature thus far is nearly nonexistent, as illustrated by the results of multiple literature searches specified in **Table 7**. The vast majority of publicly available information on both of these XML-based formats comes from the creator's or owner's own Web site.

2.5.1. AGAVE

AGAVE is an open-source XML format that was developed in 1999 by the now defunct DoubleTwist, for managing, visualizing, and sharing annotations of genomic sequences *(39)*. Its designer now maintains a modest site for LifeCode, to maintain the AGAVE format and schema (the latter of which is impressively documented on the site) *(40)*.

The broadly stated functional goals for AGAVE are as follows *(39)*:

- To encourage the development of tools that manipulate, visualize, and store genomic data.
- To facilitate exchange of genomic information.
- To support system and data interoperability.

AGAVE's two chief components are a Java Object Model and a corresponding XML DTD that facilitates data exchange, integration, and transformation between components. The current AGAVE DTD includes elements that represent sequence assembly, gene models, transcripts, and functional classifications *(41)*. The AGAVE DTD itself is parseable *(42)*, so that an XML parser can use the DTD to verify that data match a specification. The availability of data in AGAVE format has been quite substantial since 2001, when all INSDC nucleotide sequences became accessible through an EMBL por-

Table 7
Results of Medline Queries on July 13, 2004, Reflecting Poor Representation of AGAVE and BSML in Scientific Literature

Keyword query string	PubMed	PubMed Central	Ovid
Architecture for Genomic Annotation, Visualization, Exchange	0 hits	3 hits, none relevant	0 hits
Architecture for Genomic Annotation Visualization	2 hits, none relevant	26 hits, none relevant	0 hits
Architecture for Genomic Annotation	11 hits, none relevant	143 hits, not reviewed	0 hits
AGAVE	128 hits, not reviewed	16 hits, none relevant	100 hits, not reviewed
AGAVE NOT tequilana NOT Tequila NOT americana NOT attenuata NOT cerevisiae NOT Agavaceae NOT lecheguilla NOT sisalana NOT ferment NOT plant	18 hits, none relevant	3 hits, none relevant	19 hits, none relevant
AGAVE and XML	0 hits	0 hits	0 hits
Bioinformatic Sequence Markup Language	0 hits	3 hits, 2 relevant: 1 brief (2 sentence-long) review; 1 reference to another application that imports/exports BSML format	0 hits
Bioinformatic Sequence Markup	0 hits	3 hits, 1 relevant: 1 report of use	0 hits
Sequence Markup Language	13 hits, none relevant	30 hits, 5 relevant: all redundant	0 hits
BSML	14 hits, none relevant	11 hits, 4 relevant: 2 reports of use: 2 references to applications that import/export BSML format	16 hits, none relevant
BSML and XML	0 hits	4 hits, identical to relevant hits above	0 hits
Total nonredundant references on AGAVE	0		
Total nonredundant references on BSML	5, none of which were dedicated reports on BSML		

AGAVE, Architecture for Genomics Annotation, Visualization, and Exchange; BSML, Bioinformative Sequence Markup Language; XML, eXtensible Markup Language.

tal (XEMBL) in AGAVE format; the portal currently only supports query by INSDC accession number *(43,44)*. This free service provides the advantage of avoiding a step to initiate an automated conversion from a flat file to AGAVE on the client side.

The future of AGAVE is uncertain, given the closure of its founding company in 2002. It has never been described in peer-reviewed biomedical literature (**Table 7**), nor is it easy to find published evidence of its widespread use in general print or even on the Web (As of this writing, a Google search string, "AGAVE file" yields only four irrelevant results. Other queries meet with comparable results.) Despite the fact that visualization is part of the acronym and the mission of the schema, no viewer application is available as of this writing, and, thus, visualization of genomic data is limited to looking at the AGAVEXML file format (*see* **Fig. 7**).

2.5.2. BSML

BSML came into being in 1997, as the result of a grant from the National Human Genome Research Institute *(45)*. BSML is an open-source XML schema that was created to communicate the fruits of genomic research by encoding *(45)*

- Molecular sequence data (nucleic and protein), and its features and annotations.
- Records of research on a sequence or collection of sequences: known or novel queries, analysis, and research protocols.
- Platform-independent graphical representation of genomic data (termed *widgets*).

BSML documents possess all of the XML-bestowed attributes of cross-platform data interoperability, automatic parsing with additional software, validation of documents against rules specified in the DTD, and so on. Like AGAVE files, INSDC nucleotide sequences are also available through XEMBL in BSML format, via the same accession number query portal, an example of this is shown in **Fig. 9** *(47)*. This free service provides the advantage of avoiding a step to initiate an automated conversion from a flat file to BSML on the client side.

As of this writing, the link to download the freestanding application for viewing widgets (called the Genomic Workspace Viewer) is at www.rescentris.com, a company made up of employees from LabBook, the original creators of the BSML language specification *(46)*. The application is freely downloadable but requires a Rescentris-provided login to initiate its use. The free viewer allows the user to visualize and explore sequence information with annotation, while the commercial browser adds the ability to manipulate the data from this interface as well (**Fig. 10A,B**). Just as most computer users prefer the graphical user interface (GUI) provided by Windows™ and Mac OS™ over the traditional command-line interface of DOS, one might safely assume that this more user-friendly GUI will appeal to biological researchers who do not imagine themselves to be experienced computer professionals or hackers.

2.5.3. XML in Summary

XML's future in data representation for the biological sciences is promising, but far from predetermined. XML schemas for sequence data representation are attractive in their cross-platform integrity and conceptual extensibility, but a clear standard has yet to emerge. In fact, EBI plans to support additional types of exportable sequence formats

```xml
<?xml version="1.0" encoding="UTF-8" ?>
<?format DECIMAL="."?>
<!DOCTYPE Bsml (View Source for full doctype...)>
- <!--
   The BSML specification was created by Joseph B. Spitzner, Ph.D., LabBook, Inc. http://www.labbook.com

   -->
- <Bsml>
- <Definitions>
- <Sequences>
- <Sequence id="MMIL1BA" ic-acckey="M15131" title="MMIL1BA" comment="Mouse interleukin 1-beta (IL-1-beta) mRNA, complete cds."
      length="1339" topology="linear" molecule="rna" representation="raw">
   <Attribute name="version" content="M15131.1" />
   <Attribute name="organism-species" content="Mus musculus (mouse)" />
   <Attribute name="organism-classification" content="Eukaryota; Metazoa; Chordata; Craniata; Vertebrata; Euteleostomi; Mammalia; Eutheria;
      Rodentia; Sciurognathi; Muridae; Murinae; Mus" />
   <Attribute name="source" content="Mus musculus" />
   <Attribute name="keywords" content="interleukin 1-beta" />
   <Attribute name="date-created" content="16-JUL-1988" />
   <Attribute name="date-last-updated" content="4-MAR-2000" />
   <Attribute name="database-xref" content="MGI:MGI:96543" />
   <Attribute name="database-xref" content="UniProt/Swiss-Prot:P10749" />
   <Attribute name="database-xref" content="GOA:P10749" />
- <Feature-tables>
- <Feature-table>
- <Reference dbxref="87058957">
   <Attribute name="cross-reference" content="MEDLINE; 87058957" />
   <Attribute name="cross-reference" content="PUBMED; 3491144" />
   <RefAuthors>Gray P.W., Glaister D., Chen E., Goeddel D.V., Pennica D.</RefAuthors>
   <RefTitle>Two interleukin 1 genes in the mouse: Cloning and expression of the cDNA for murine interleukin 1-beta</RefTitle>
   <RefJournal>Journal of Immunology 137(11):3644-3648(1986)</RefJournal>
      </Reference>
- <Feature id="FTR_M15131.1_0" class="SOURCE" value-type="source" title="source" display-auto="1">
   <Qualifier value-type="organism" value="Mus musculus" />
   <Qualifier value-type="db_xref" value="TAXONOMY:10090" />
   <Interval-loc startpos="1" endpos="1339" startopen="0" endopen="0" onepos="0" complement="0" />
      </Feature>
- <Feature id="FTR_M15131.1_1" class="CDS" value-type="cds" title="IL-1-beta" display-auto="1">
   <Qualifier value-type="gene" value="IL-1-beta" />
   <Qualifier value-type="product" value="interleukin 1-beta" />
   <Qualifier value-type="codon_start" value="1" />
   <Qualifier value-type="translation"
      value="MATVPELNCEMPPFDSDENDLFFEVDGPQKMKGCFQTFDLGCPDESIQLQISQQHINKSFRQAVSLIVAVEKLWQLPVSFPWTFQDEDMSTFFSFIFEE
   EPILCDSWDDDDNLLVCDVPIRQLHYRLRDEQQKSLVLSDPYELKALHLNGQNINQQVIFSMSFVQGEPSNDKIPVALGLKGKNLYLSCVMKDGTPTLQLESVD
   PKQYPKKKMEKRFVFNKIEVKSKVEFESAEFPNWYISTSQAEHKPVFLGNNSGQDIIDFTMESVSS" />
   <Qualifier value-type="db_xref" value="GOA:P10749" />
   <Qualifier value-type="db_xref" value="UniProt/Swiss-Prot:P10749" />
   <Qualifier value-type="db_xref" value="PID:AAA39276.1" />
   <Interval-loc startpos="78" endpos="887" startopen="0" endopen="0" onepos="0" complement="0" />
      </Feature>
      </Feature-table>
      </Feature-tables>
   <Seq-data>tgcagggttcgaggcctaataggctcatctgggatcctctccagccaagc ttccttgtgcaagtgtctgaagcagctatggcaactgttcctgaactcaa
   ctgtgaaatgccaccttttgacagtgatgagaatgacctgttctttgaag ttgacggacccccaaaagatgaagggctgcttccaaacctttgacctgggc
   tgtccagatgagagcatccagcttcaaatctcacagcagcacatcaacaa gagcttcaggcaggcagtatcactcattgtggctgtggagaagctgtggc
   agctacctgtgtctttcccgtggacttccaggatgaggacatgagcacc ttcttttccttcatctttgaagaagagcccatcctctgtgactcatggga
   tgatgatgataacctgctggtgtgtgacgttcccattagacagctgcact acaggctccgagatgaacaacaaaaaaagcctcgtgctgtcggacccatat
   gagctgaaagctctccacctcaatggacagaatatcaaccaacaagtgat attctccatgagctttgtacaaggagaaccaagcaacgacaaaaataccg
   tggccttgggcctcaaaggaaagaatctatacctgtcctgtgtaatgaaa gacggcacacccaccctgcagctggagagtgtggatcccaagcaataccc
   aaagaagaagatggaaaagcggtttgtcttcaacaagataagtgcaagg gcaaagtggagtttgagtctgcagagttccccaactggtacatcagcacc
   tcacaagcagagcacaagcctgtcttcctgggaaacaacagtggtcagga cataattgacttcaccatggaatctgtgtcttcctaaagtatgggctgga
   ctgtttctaatgccttccccagggcatgtgaaggagctccttgtcatga atgacgacagctcaatcctcagtgacactccttagtcctcggccaagac
   aggtcgctcagggtcacaagaaacctggaacctcgttcaaagagagc ctgtgttttcccttcgctcttgatgggcaacacccacctaccatttatttat
   gtatttattgattggttgatctatttaagttgattcaagggggacattagg cagcactctctagaacgaacctagctgtcaacgtgtggggggatgaattg
   gtcatagccttgcacttgaggtctttcattgaagctgagaataaataggt tcctataatatgtgatgagaatttttatgaatgaagcattagcacattgct
   ttgatgagtatgaaatataatttcattaaacaaacaaaca</Seq-data>
      </Sequence>
      </Sequences>
      </Definitions>
      </Bsml>
```

Fig. 9. Same mouse of IL-1β sequence as in previous examples in BSML, obtained from XEMBL.

(GAME and BIOML) in the near future, widening the representation of easily accessed XML sequence formats, as well as the roster of future candidates for data standards *(47)*. Bioperl, a suite of open-source PERL-based bioinformatics tools, provides varying degrees of support in parsing and converting to, GAME, BSML, and AGAVE *(48)*. Ignoring supplemental GUI software, differing XML schemas are only as granular and adaptable as their respective DTDs. Because the DTDs of current schemas such as AGAVE and BSML have never been systematically compared in an unbiased environment, it is impossible to say which is more suitable to emerge as a true standard.

2.6. Format Summary

If the historical examples set by FASTA and GCG hold true, the DDBJ/EMBL/GenBank flat-file formats have an advantage over the emerging, more dynamic XML schemas,

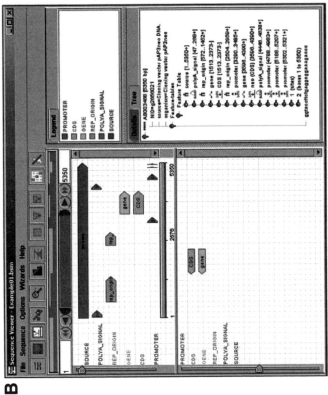

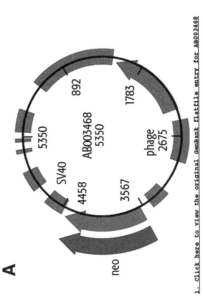

1. Click here to view the original GenBank flatfile entry for AB003468

Fig. 10. Browser visualization of (**A**) genomic XML widgets, and (**B**) exploration of sequence information from BSML source data.

Table 8
Conventions on Identifier Syntax by Database

Database name		Identifier syntax
Brookhaven Protein Data Bank	pdb	entry | chain
DDBJ, DNA Database of Japan	dbj	accession | locus
EMBL Data Library	emb	accession | locus
GenBank	gb	accession | locus
GenBank	gi	unique-identifier
General database identifier	gnl	database | identifier
GenInfo Backbone Id	bbs	number
Local Sequence identifier	lcl	identifier
NBRF PIR	pir	entry
NCBI Reference Sequence	ref	accession | locus
Patents	pat	country | number
Protein Research Foundation	prf	name
SWISS-PROT	sp	accession | entry name

because the flat files come directly from the source to which researchers submit their work. That is to say, flat files have functional value to researchers in that they need to format their work according to the standards reflected in flat files in order to share their data with the international scientific community. Additionally, because GenBank, EMBL, and DDBJ are primary databases (i.e., researchers submit the fruits of their sequence work directly), as opposed to secondary or curated databases such as SWISS-PROT and PDB (which catalog the works of researchers whose original work is based on the sequences stored in primary databases), researchers who study existing sequences must *retrieve* them in flat-file format. Of course, sequences can be (and are) converted into whatever format the researcher decides to use, but because sequence repositories adhere to ASN.1-derived flat-file formats, researchers who convert their sequence files for study must reconvert or reannotate them back to a flat-file format to submit them *(49)*. Given this paradigm of flat files in/flat files out, competing formats, such as BSML and AGAVE, must add enough functionality (including tools to make bidirectional conversion seamless, if not invisible) to make such tools appealing to researchers.

Realistically, researchers are quite far from having a single standard for genomic sequence representation, because there is currently no widely agreed on "gold standard" of file formats to impose on the scientific community. This means that readers of this chapter, and other students entering the fields of genomics, molecular biology, or bioinformatics, are almost guaranteed to encounter multiple file types in their studies and research. Deciphering an unknown file type might be vital to one's research efforts, or simply vital to one's piece of mind. Whatever the case may be, given this inevitable obstacle to productivity, **Tables 8** and **9** may be of use in identifying files by their unique data identifiers, or by their first line of text or file name extensions, respectively.

3. Microarray Experiments:
Standards for Acquisition and Storage of Genomic Data

The ability to independently replicate and, therefore, validate a reported result of an experiment is a conceptual cornerstone of modern science. This is made possible by a

Table 9
Guidelines on Identification of Unknown Files
by First Nonblank Character/Word in File, or by File Extension Type

File format	First nonblank word or character in file	File extention[a]
AGAVE	`<!DOCTYPE sciobj` (second line of file)	.xml
BSML	`<!DOCTYPE Bsml` (third line of file)	.xml
CLUSTAL	`CLUSTAL`	.aln; multiple others, as determined by user's choice of output format
DDBJ	`LOCUS`	.txt, .html, or other nonspecific
EMBL	`ID`	.txt, .html, or other nonspecific
FASTA	`>`	.fasta, .wrp
FASTA (compressed format)	Not applicable	.Z, or .gz
GCG: multiple sequence file (MSF)	`PILEUP`	.msf
GCG: single sequence file, protein	`!!AA_SEQUENCE 1.0`	.seq
GCG: single sequence file, nucleotide	`!!NA_SEQUENCE 1.0`	.seq
GDE nucleotide	`#`	.gde
GDE protein	`%`	.gde
GenBank	`LOCUS`	.txt, .html, .gbk, .gb, or other nonspecific
PHYLIP	one- or two-digit number, space three- or four-digit number	.ph, .phy, or other nonspecific
PIR	`>DL`	.pir
Plain text	JCBN character	.txt
Raw	JCBN character	.raw, .txt
SWISS	`ID`	.txt, .html, or other nonspecific

[a]Keep in mind that a file may be misnamed. It may have an incorrect file extension or no extension at all.

detailed description of the methods by which the original experiment was performed. In the biological sciences, these methods typically include the specific strain of the organism beginning tested; the type, source, and preparation of reagents; the perturbation or exposure of the system to the experimental procedure; the type, source, and implementation of instrumentation; the control procedures; and the data analyses. The same rigorous standards have been applied to the wealth of data produced by the description of the human genome beginning in the 1990; the genes have been carefully sequenced, one-by-one. To address the reality that the complexity of the biological process involved not one, but hundreds or perhaps thousands, of genes, microarray technology was developed. This powerful methodology allows the experimenter to assess gene expression in tens of thousands of genes simultaneously. The original description of the use of complementary DNA (cDNA) hybridization techniques for microarrays in 1995 *(50)* followed by the development of high-throughput technology in 1998 *(51)* has resulted in the extensive application of this technology in other laboratories. A MEDLINE database search using "microarray" as the keyword revealed 2350 publications on this technology in the year 2003 alone. This methodology has been the subject of multiple extensive reviews *(51–53)*, some with specific applications to neoplastic *(54)*, cardiac *(55)*, renal *(56)*, psychiatric *(57)*, and neurological *(58)* disorders. The fundamentals of microarray experiments are outlined next so as to provide a basis for the standards that have been suggested for this important area of research.

The primary application of this technology is in the measurement of gene expression. This is accomplished by the quantification of messenger RNA (mRNA), which is the direct product of gene transcription. The methodology involves the hybridization of labeled sample mRNA to cDNA or oligonucleotides on a microarray followed by detection of the bound label. Thus, a microarray gene expression experiment has several components: selection of tissue/specimen, extraction of mRNA, and fluorescence labeling; as well as microarray construction, reading, and data analysis.

Virtually any source of mRNA is suitable for microarray experiments including whole-tissue specimens, or RNA derived from human and animal tissues as well as cell lines. To stabilize the mRNA, it is often necessary to create its cDNA using a reverse transcriptase. Unfortunately, not all mRNAs convert easily; thus, there can be some bias, depending on which mRNAs are isolated. Quantification of message expression is achieved by adding millions of copies of mRNA to each spot on the microarray. The subsequent intensity of the signal generated by a fluorescence marker bound to the sample probe (cDNA) will be proportional to the amount of the specific mRNA in the sample. Thus, it is necessary to specify the type of tissue, amount of labeled mRNA or cDNA added to each spot, and hybridization methodology and conditions; the type, intensity, and method of exciting the fluorescence tag; the background levels of fluorescence; and the method of quantification in order to be able to reproduce this portion of the experiment.

The microarray itself is constructed by two methods. The first is the so-called spotted area in which cDNA is deposited in defined locations on a substrate (i.e., a glass slide) by robotic methods. The cDNA is selected based on the specific experiment being performed. The second technique utilizes methods derived from photolithography to synthesize the specific oligonucleotides in defined locations on the "chip." It is thus possible to detect mRNA expression from tens of thousands of genes simultaneously with this technology. In theory, the techniques by which the microarray is constructed are required to replicate the experiment. This has been limited owing to the proprietary nature of the commercially available microarray chips. In addition, the results are only as meaningful as the accuracy of the databases from which the sequences were derived. The sequences deposited in some databases are not always peer reviewed and replicated, thus allowing the possibility of error. Furthermore, random variations in the noise level owing to dust on the array, as well as variations in target placement and substrate composition, introduce errors that are difficult to control for even when appreciated.

Analysis of these extremely large data sets provides a significant challenge. A wide variety of analytical tools exists to extract meaningful conclusions from microarray data *(55,59)*. However, a multitude of potential situational errors exist regarding to differential expression of genes. Inconsistent results can be obtained from experiments on genes from different sources, from the same source but sampled at different times, and even from the same source *when sampled simultaneously*.

Additionally there is a lack of clear methods for determining what are "statistically significant" differences in expression between samples.

3.1. Minimal Information About a Microarray Experiment (MIAME)

The complexity of reporting gene expression microarray experiments and the resulting data led to the formation of the Microarray Gene Expression Data Society. The first meeting took place in 1999 and was attended by an international group of users and developers of microarray technology. The mission statement of the organization included "establishing standards for microarray data annotation and exchange, facilitating the creation of microarray databases and related software implementing these standards, and promoting the sharing of high quality, well annotated data within the life sciences community." The concept of establishing a public repository of gene microarray data was published *(60)* and five workgroups were proposed. These workgroups are described in detail on the society's Web site (www.mged.org) and include MIAME *(61)*, Microarray and Gene Expression (MAGE) *(62)*, Ontology Workgroup *(63)*, Data Transformation and Normalisation Working Group *(64)*, and the Toxicogenomics Working Group (TWG) *(65)*.

The initial draft of MIAME was made public in 2001 *(66)* and has had multiple revisions based on user input. The information that the MIAME standard would provide was to be sufficient to interpret, compare, and replicate microarray experiments and the data structure would allow efficient querying as well as automated data analysis and mining. These goals reflect the multidisciplinary nature of microarray technology as a combination of molecular biology, computer science, and informatics. The most current draft of the MIAME standards in detail and in checklist form is available on the society's Web site (www.mged.org/Workgroups/MIAME) and breaks down the standards into five sections:

1. Experimental design.
2. Samples used, extract preparation and labeling.
3. Hybridization procedures and parameters.
4. Measurement data and specifications of data processing.
5. Array design.

The experimental design standard includes basic information regarding contact information for who performed the experiment and goals of the experiment. The authors should state the type of the experiment and specimens used such as healthy vs diseased or treated vs untreated comparisons, time course, dose–response, or knockout or knock-in models.

The specific parameters of the hybridizations should be noted including the number of hybridizations, the use of a common reference, and any control measures taken.

The description of the samples used to obtain the RNA or DNA is the same as that used in any biological experiment and includes the type of organism and where it was obtained; if relevant, the age, gender, and developmental stage; alternative cell type or line; genetic variation (e.g., knock-in or knockout); and normal vs diseased. Similarly, the laboratory methodologies relating to the samples should include specific growth conditions and treatments (e.g., whole organism, cell culture), and separation techniques, if utilized, should be described. Similarly, the precise extraction method, means of amplification and type of nucleic acid extracted (e.g., DNA, mRNA) should be specified. Finally, the researchers need to describe the type and amount of labeling as well as the controls utilized.

The hybridization procedures including the preparation of reagents, blocking procedures, types of wash, quantity of labeled target, incubation parameters, and instrumentation, should be provided in enough detail to allow replication.

The measurement data and specifications of data-processing standards are in many ways the most challenging. Initially, the fluorescence is elicited by a laser scanning device and the image recorded. The instrumentation that is utilized, scan parameters, and associated software should be described. These raw data are then processed with image analysis software, the type and parameters of which should be specified. Finally, the image is normalized according to specified standards, and the data are converted into a gene expression table. Because there are no absolute units of gene expression, each step in how the values are derived needs to be precisely stated.

The array design is clearly a critical element in each experiment. One advantage of using a commercially available array is that it is available for purchase to replicate a reported experiment. However, the precise methodology of construction may be proprietary and not described in enough detail to allow independent reconstruction. Elements of the array that should be described include the substrate, means by which targets are positioned on the array, type of target (cDNA or oligonucleotide), how the target was obtained, and reference information to the gene to which it maps.

3.2. Microarray and Gene Expression (MAGE)

MAGE represents a standard data model to capture, represent, and exchange information from microarray data, specifically as outlined in MIAME *(66,67)*. The Life Science Research Committee of the Object Management Group (OMG-LSR; lsr.omg.org/) along with MGED has produced a key industry specification that addresses the representation of gene expression data and relevant annotations, as well as the mechanisms for exchanging these data. It is called MAGE-ML (MAGE Markup Language) *(68)*.

The MAGE group aims to provide a standard for the representation of microarray expression data that would facilitate the exchange of microarray information between different data systems. Currently, this is done through OMG by the establishment of a data exchange model (MAGE Object Model [MAGE-OM] and data exchange format [MAGE-ML]) for microarray expression experiments. MAGE-OM has been modeled using the Unified Modeling Language (UML) and MAGE-ML has been implemented

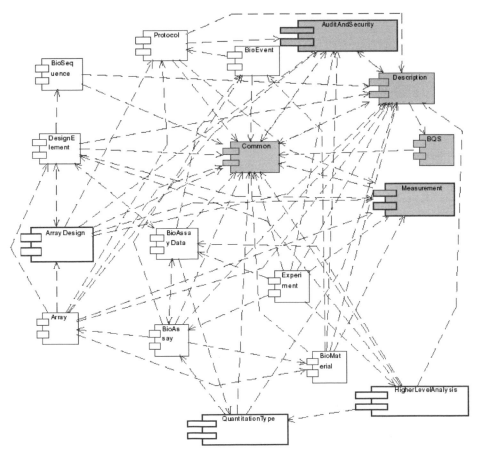

Fig. 11. Relationships among the 17 packages in MAGE-OM. (*See* color image in ebook.) (Adapted from **ref. 68a**.)

using XML. MAGE-stk (or MAGE Software Toolkit) is a collection of packages that act as converters between MAGE-OM and MAGE-ML under various programming platforms.

3.2.1. MAGE-OM

MAGE-OM, based on UML, is a graphical way of representing complex data sets such that it allows understanding by the human user. It is the primary model and the basis for MAGE-ML, which is described in the subsequent section. One major drawback of this approach is its limited ability to support data analysis.

Because of its enormous size, MAGE-OM cannot be represented usefully by a single diagram. To solve this problem data is broken up into 17 packages, including Common, BQS, Measurement, AuditAndSecurity, Description, BioSequence, ArrayDesign, Design Element, Array, BioMaterial, BioAssay, BioAssayData, Experiment, HigherLevelAnalysis, Protocol, QuantitationType (*see* **Fig. 11**). These packages are further broken down into 132 classes with 123 attributes and 223 associations among classes *(69)*. Lines represent relationships between classes. The first four packages listed (green/dark boxes in the diagram) are specific for annotation. The other twelve (yellow/ light) boxes represent the natural separation of events and objects of gene expression data. Regarding relationships and UML, further information can be gathered at http://www.uml.org/.

Based on six basic requirements, MAGE-OM allows the user to follow the natural flow of a microarray experiment. This package is not designed as a laboratory information management system, but the data are similarly organized. The six basic requirements are as follows:

1. Descriptions and protocols.
2. Array information.
3. Preparation of experimental materials, hybridizations, and scans.
4. Data model and storage.
5. Experiments.
6. Data analysis.

The work flow diagram in **Fig. 12** illustrates this concept *(69)*.

3.2.2. MAGE-ML

XML allows the definition of new vocabularies and formatting versatility. Because of this great flexibility, XML was chosen as the markup language for encoding microarray data documents, which then refers to a DTD. The DTD is specified in MAGE-ML so that XML documents designed to use MAGE-ML refer to the DTD *(69)*. As mentioned in **Subheading 3.2.1.**, MAGE-OM is the primary model and MAGE-ML is derived from it. This derivation occurs through the use of software tools such as those found in the MAGE-STK. A sample of MAGE-ML code is displayed in **Fig. 13**.

The MAGE software toolkit can be found at www.mged.org/Workgroups/MAGE/magestk.html. It is open source and available for use in an unrestricted fashion for any academic or commercial purpose *(69)*. The software toolkit not only allows the translation of MAGE-ML to and from MAGE-OM but also facilitates the development of new software by the user *(70)*. **Figure 14** visualizes the basic functionality of the MAGE-STK.

3.3. Standards for Linkage Disequilibrium Studies

Linkages between genes and clinical disorders are increasingly becoming the focus of translational research. Identification of the genetic basis for complex traits has still eluded most research efforts. The category of investigation that aims to identify these relationships is called linkage disequilibrium studies *(71)*.

3.3.1. PedHunter

Linkage analysis uses defined pedigrees for a population exhibiting a specific trait and verifies relationships within pedigrees. PedHunter (available from the NCBI), is a software package that facilitates the creation and verification of pedigrees within large genealogies *(72)*. PedHunter uses conceptual graph theory to solve two versions of the pedigree connection problem for genealogies. The pedigrees produced by PedHunter are output as files in LINKAGE format ready for linkage analysis and for drawing with PEDDRAW:

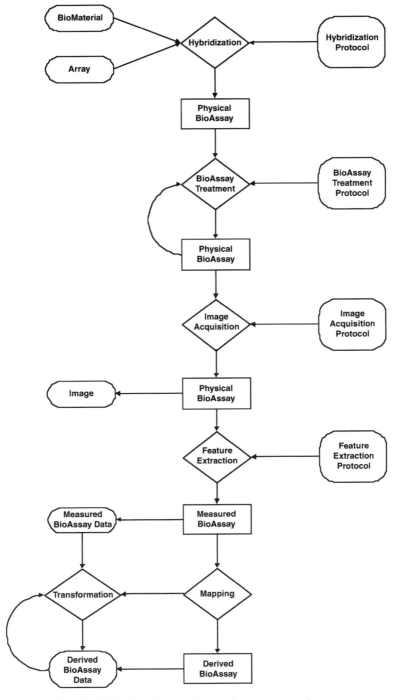

Fig. 12. Work flow diagram for a microarray experiment.

```
<?xml version="1.0" ?>
- <!--
sample MAGE-ML code snlps

-->
<MAGE-samples>
<AuditAndSecurity_package>
<Contact_assnlist>
<Person identifier="Person:John_Smith" name="John_Smith" lastName="Smith" firstName="John" phone="(800) 555 4325 x 561"
       email="jsmith@imakearrays.com" URI="http://www.imakearrays.com/~jsmith">
<Affiliation_assnref>
<Organization_ref identifier="Organization:imakearrays" />
</Affiliation_assnref>
</Person>
<Organization identifier="Organization:imakearrays" name="I Make Arrays Inc." address="1099 Pasteur Dr, San Benito, NM 79850"
       tollFreePhone="(800) 555 4325" email="orders@imakearrays.com" fax="(800) 555 4325" URI="http://www.imakearrays.com/" />
</Contact_assnlist>
<Security_assnlist>
<Security identifier="Security:Array" name="Array">
<Owner_assnref>
<Person_ref identifier="Person:Jane_N_Rogers" />
</Owner_assnref>
<ReadGroups_assnreflist>
<SecurityGroup_ref identifier="SecurityGroup:Everyone" />
</ReadGroups_assnreflist>
<WriteGroups_assnreflist>
<SecurityGroup_ref identifier="SecurityGroup:Administrators" />
</WriteGroups_assnreflist>
</Security>
</Security_assnlist>
</AuditAndSecurity_package>
<Protocol_package>
<Hardware_assnlist>
<Hardware identifier="Hardware: OligoSynthesizer1" name="Synthesizer" make="Gene Machines" />
</Hardware_assnlist>
<Software_assnlist>
<Software identifier="Software:GenePix3.0" name="GenePix" />
</Software_assnlist>
<Protocol_assnlist>
<Protocol identifier="Protocol:SepticInjury" name="Septic injury of drosophila" text="Drosophila were pricked in the abdomen with a needlet that
       had been dipped in a solution of gram positive and gram negative bacteria" />
<Protocol identifier="Protocol:OligoSynthesis" name="Oligonucleotide Synthesis" text="70mer oligos were synthesized">
<Hardware_assnreflist>
<Hardware_ref identifier="Hardware:OligoSynthesizer1" />
</Hardware_assnreflist>
</Protocol>
<Protocol identifier="Protocol:FeatureExtraction" name="Feature Extraction">
<ParameterType_assnlist>
<Parameter identifier="ParameterType:FeatureSpacing" name="Feature Spacing" />
<Parameter identifier="ParameterType:Featurepacing" name="Spot Spacing" />
<Parameter identifier="ParameterType:FeatureDiameter" name="Spot Diameter" />
</ParameterType_assnlist>
<Software_assnreflist>
<Software_ref identifier="Software:GenePix3.0" />
</Software_assnreflist>
</Protocol>
</Protocol_assnlist>
</Protocol_package>
<BioMaterial_package>
<Compound_assnlist>
<Compound identifier="Compound:Biotin" name="Biotin" isSolvent="false" />
</Compound_assnlist>
<BioMaterial_assnlist>
<BioSource identifier="BioSource:Drosophila:OregonR" name="Drosophila strain, Oregon R">
<MaterialType>
<OntologyEntry category="MGED:MaterialType" value="Organism" />
</MaterialType>
<Characteristic_assnlist>
<OntologyEntry category="MGED:Organism" value="Drosophila melanogaster" />
<OntologyEntry category="Flybase:Genotype" value="wild type" />
<OntologyEntry category="Flybase:Strain" value="Oregon R" />
<OntologyEntry category="MGED:Age:DaysPostEclosion" value="3" />
</Characteristic_assnlist>
<SourceContact>
<Person_ref identifier="Ennio_DeGregorio" />
</SourceContact>
</BioSource>
</BioMaterial_assnlist>
</BioMaterial_package>
</MAGE-samples>
```

Fig. 13. Sample code for MAGE-ML.

- Testing relationships: *is_ancestor, is_cousin, is_half_sib, is_mother, is_father, is_sibling, is_child*
- Finding people satisfying a certain relation: *mother, father, children, cousins, uncles_aunts, half_sibs, siblings, descendants, ancestors*
- Complex queries: *minimal_ancestors, inbreeding, kinship, subset, asp, all_shortest_ paths, minimal*

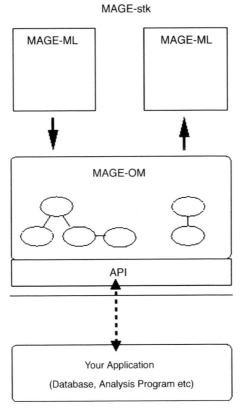

Fig. 14. Functionality of MAGE-STK.

The various types of complex queries are as follows:

- *minimal_ancestors*: given a list of people, find all persons P such that P is an ancestor of everyone in the list, but none of the children of P are ancestors of everyone in the list.
- *inbreeding*: compute the inbreeding coefficients of a list of people with respect to the entire genealogy.
- *kinship*: compute the kinship coefficients of a list of pairs of people with respect to the entire genealogy.
- *subset*: find a maximal subset of a list of people that has a common ancestor. The subset returned is "maximal" in the sense that it cannot be enlarged, but not necessarily of "maximum" size.
- *asp*: find all shortest paths pedigree for a given list of people, if any exist. The prototypical use of asp is to find a pedigree to connect several persons with the same phenotype.
- *all_shortest_paths*: print all shortest paths from an ancestor to a descendant. This function can be used to help understand the output of asp.
- *minimal*: print minimal tree connecting the given list of people who have the given 'asp' pedigree. This function can be used to find a small pedigree when the asp pedigree is too big for your purpose. Researchers have developed software for the general Steiner tree problem in conceptual graphs *(73)*.

The genealogy data to be used by PedHunter are stored as a relational database in Sybase or as column-delimited ASCII text files. PedHunter has two required tables: person information table and relationship table; it also has two optional tables: id table and generation table.

- *Person table*: this table has information specific to a person. Fields such as program identifier (required), name (optional), birth date (optional), death date (optional), address (optional), gender (required for married couples), special status (used to encode twins, adoptions; optional), and other information (optional) have been specified.
- *Relationship table*: this table encodes parent–child relationships. Fields such as program identifier of father (required), program identifier of mother (required), marriage date (optional), and delimited program identifiers for children (with these two parents, required but can be empty) have been specified.
- *Id table*: if a protocol design has a system of identifiers for its genealogy and these identifiers are not integers, then an id table with columns for program identifier and the user's identifier that expresses the 1-to-1 correspondence between them is required.
- *Generation table*: Pedhunter can generate this table automatically and is needed only if the user implements the "inbreeding" and "kinship" queries.

3.3.2. CASPAR

CASPAR is being developed by NCBI as an exploratory program designed to study the genetics of complex (polygenic) diseases. CASPAR takes as input the genetic information at multiple loci regarding families. It facilitates the exploration of hypotheses about how various genes may be involved in disease susceptibility of polygenic diseases. It semiautomatically performs an extended affected sibling pair (ASP) test for subsets of families defined by their features at one or more loci. The main advantage of CASPAR over other ASP software packages is that CASPAR allows the user to do linkage analysis at one locus, given the status of another locus. Utilizing CASPAR, one can gain insight regarding how genes in different linked regions may interact, thus leading to disease susceptibility.

CASPAR has been described for nuclear families containing at most two children and could not handle missing information *(74)*. Since that study, CASPAR has been extended the ASP test to handle pedigrees containing any number of affected sibs, multiple generations, and some missing information such as parents whose genetic information at some loci is not known.

CASPAR can handle pedigrees with any size sibships, ungenotyped parents, ungenotyped sibs, and sibs that are not genotyped at sharing locus. CASPAR handles ungenotyped parents by looping over all possible genotypes that yield compatible sibships and computing the likelihood of each choice using allele frequencies. The result is *weighted* by the probability of that genotype being the correct genotype. CASPAR should not be used if one of the regions of interest is on a sex-linked chromosome.

4. Clinical Genomics and Pharmacogenomics Standards

4.1. Pharmacogenomics Knowledge Base

The US Department of Health and Human Services National Institutes of Health is supporting a multicenter research collaborative known as the Pharmacogenetics Research

Network ([PGRN]; www.nigms.nih.gov/pharmacogenetics) to develop and disseminate knowledge about genetically determined variability of individuals' responses to medications. Such variability is manifest by broad swings in medication efficacy (or lack thereof) and/or risk of adverse reactions *(1–4)*. Genetically determined variation in an individual's response to medications may occur at any point while the drug is in the body including absorption, distribution, interaction, metabolism, or excretion. To date, most genetic variation has been detected in drug metabolism, and it has been hypothesized that virtually all paths of drug metabolism are subject to genetic variation *(2)*. Increasingly, genetic variation is being detected in drug transport and targets *(5)*. The ultimate goal of PGRN and other pharmacogenetics research efforts is to help ensure that individual patients get the correct drug at the correct dose. In the future, health care providers will increasingly include patient's genetic fingerprints in the analysis of disease states and in the choice of workup strategies and treatments. Pharmacological treatments are one important type of therapy that lends itself particularly well to individualized care. This type of understanding is essential if society is to move toward truly personalized medical care.

The primary purpose of the Pharmacogenetics and Pharmacogenomics Knowledge Base (PharmGKB; www.pharmgkb.org) is to be a central repository for data produced by PGRN members. However, PharmGKB has been designed to be more than a simple storehouse for research data. From its inception in April 2000, PharmGKB has been designed to be a collaborative work space for geographically distant laboratories by providing electronic tools that support information submission, editing, and processing *(6,7)*. Furthermore, PharmGKB has been designed to facilitate the free sharing of data among the wider scientific community while maintaining the necessary safeguards for personally identifiable health information *(8)*. Thus, although PharmGKB data are largely contributed by the members of PGRN, the resulting data are available over the Internet for use by others. PharmGKB was first online in February 2001, and the first open scientific meeting about it was held in August 2001 *(8)*.

PGRN researchers are able to submit several dozen types of data including details about gene variants (e.g., single nucleotide polymorphisms [SNPs], insertions, deletions, and repeats), gene products (i.e., proteins), and phenotypes (e.g., pharmacokinetics, enzyme kinetics, and clinical observations). The project has recently been extended to identify metabolic pathways. Submissions are not limited to experimental data. Information of potential significance that has been culled from the literature is also permitted. Information can be submitted via a Web-based form or via specifically formatted files containing XML-tagged elements *(9)*.

As of February 2004, there were 69,261 polymorphism–phenotype pairs in PharmGKB (a "pair" is defined as a single genotype, such as the identify of an SNP at a certain position, for which there is a single phenotype, such as the value of a measured parameter).

PharmGKB researchers and developers have faced and addressed a number of challenges in data standardization and knowledge representation. The core of PharmGKB's approach to knowledge representation is an ontology of pharmacogenomic concepts and their interrelationships *(10)*. Protege 2000 *(11)*, a frame-based knowledge representation system, has been used for PharmGKB ontology development. PharmGKB ontology has five top-level concepts: clinical outcomes, pharmacodynamics and drug responses, pharmacokinetics, molecular and cellular functional assays, and genotypes. Overall, the ontology includes 120 total concepts and 90 leaf-level concepts and has a maximal depth of three parent–child relationships.

Integrating heterogenous data from different independent laboratories poses significant data standardization challenges. Data models were developed and iteratively improved to provide conceptual and logical frameworks for PGRN data. Data models were necessary for pharmacokinetic and pharmacodynamic data; genomic sequence and structures; molecular, cellular, and clinical phenotype data; and other domains. PharmGKB also captures the interrelations between data objects with a rich set of hundreds of semantic relationships. For example, a particular drug may be related to a particular enzyme via the semantic relationship "is metabolized by." Extensive database and data-modeling documentation is publicly available (12,13).

Standardization of terminology is a second major challenge to PRGN data integration. PharmGKB researchers recognized this from the start and elected to reuse existing structured vocabularies when possible, and to create structured terminologies when necessary (7). The use of well-formed, high-quality terminologies is critical for the goal of data representation and integration. Terminologies with formal definitions, i.e., represented using symbolic logic, are important to support algorithmic inferencing. To date, PharmGKB researchers have adopted a number of existing terminologies including the National Library of Medicine's Medical Subject Headings (MeSH) (14) for diseases, the Hugo Gene Nomenclature Committee (HGNC) (15) for gene names and symbols, and the Department of Veterans Affairs National Drug File Reference Terminology (NDFRT™) (16). An ongoing challenge is the integration and correlation of SNP data in PharmGKB with data in other compilation databases such as HGVbase and GeneSNP (17).

PharmGKB is implemented via a multitiered architecture. The top layer is a collection of knowledge manipulation and retrieval tools. The second layer is a frame-based knowledge base implemented via protege. The third layer is a relational database. Pharm GKB researchers and implementers are involved in a number of ongoing informatics projects including integrating and cross-referencing information with other related databases (18) such as dbSNP.

4.2. Putting It All Together: HL7 Clinical Genomics Standards

The Clinical Genomics Special Interest Group (CG-SIG) of HL7 (an American National Standards Institute [ANSI]–Accredited Standards Developing Organization) addresses requirements for the interrelation of clinical and genomic data at the individual level. Many of the genomic data are still generic. The vision of "personalized medicine" is based on those correlations that make use of personal genomic data such as the SNPs that differentiate any two persons and occur about every thousand bases. Besides normal differences, health conditions such as drug sensitivities, allergies, and others could be attributed to the individual SNPs or to differences in gene expression and proteomics (such as posttranscriptional modification of proteins). The emphases in clinical genomics are personalization of the genomic data and "intelligent" linking to relevant clinical information. These links are probably the main source from which genomicists and clinicians could benefit.

Cases in which genomic data are used in health care practice vary in complexity and extent of the data used, because the current testing methods are still very expensive and not widely used. We can see simple testing such as identification of genes and mutations as well as full sequencing of alleles and use of microarrays to identify the expression of a vast number of genes in each individual. The HL7 CG-SIG group has been focusing on tests that are routinely done in health care, while preparing the information infrastructure standard for more futuristic cases.

At first sight it seems that genomic data are yet another type of observation. Although this is true, of course, there are a few characteristics that might distinguish these data from typical clinical observations such as blood pressure or potassium level:

1. Amount of data: potentially it could be the entire human genome along with associated data.
2. Personalization of the data: this is evolving as new discoveries are continually made.
3. Complexity of the data: not only the DNA sequences need to be represented, but also SNPs, annotations (automatic and manual), gene expression, protein translation, and more.
4. Emerging standard formats being used by the bioinformatics community (e.g., BSML and MAGE-ML).
5. Clinical genomic correlations are closely related to recent clinical research discoveries and its clinical reliability needs to be carefully described.

The CG-SIG develops HL7 standards to enable the communication between interested parties of the clinical and personalized genomic data. In many cases, in this domain, the exchange of genomic data is done between disparate organization (e.g., providers, laboratories, research facilities), and acceptable standards are crucial for the usefulness of the data in health care practice.

Several storyboards were explored where genomic data is actually used in health care practice, such as tissue typing for bone-marrow transplantation, cystic fibrosis genetic and BRCA testing, as well as pharmacogenomics-based clinical trials. At the same time, the group has been trying to identify the commonalities of the various storyboards resulting in the *Genotype* model intended to be a reusable standard component. This design allows every HL7 group that develops messages or documents carrying genomic data (e.g., lab order and results, clinical trials, patient care, public health) to make use of the *Genotype* model and populate its various structures. The model consists of data about a specific chromosomal locus, including alleles, variations (e.g., mutations, SNPs), sequences, gene expression levels, proteins, and determinant peptides.

The HL7 CG-SIG is taking a first principled approach to genomic knowledge representation. **Figure 15** shows some of the core knowledge classes specified by the group. These form the basis for all of the more complex knowledge structures. **Figure 16** depicts the aggregations of these types of knowledge, which are important for specifying the output or design of an experiment or some other important clinical genomics topic. **Figure 17** shows that these aggregations of concepts are useful in representing the knowledge needed for systems such as clinical trial systems or personalized medicine.

4.2.1. Genotype Model

The HL7 *Genotype* model describes a variety of genomic data types relating to a chromosomal locus, which is proposed to be the basic unit of genomic information exchange

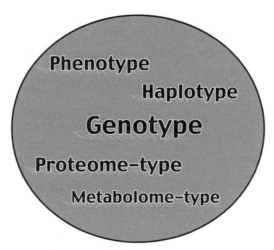

Fig. 15. This diagram depicts some of the core classes of information that need to be represented unambiguously in order to satisfy the knowledge representation needs of the clinical genomics community.

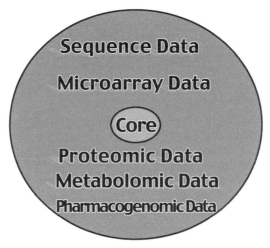

Fig. 16. Around the core one can now construct views of data that are useful data sets to define consistently and also unambiguously.

in health care. For data relating to several chromosomal loci (e.g., a clinical phenotype associated with multiple genes) there is a higher-level model named *Genetic Profile* that utilizes the *Genotype* model. The *Genotype* model is not meant to be a biological model; rather it is aimed at the needs of health care with the vision of personalized medicine in mind. In addition, it could facilitate the needs of clinical research conducted within the health care enterprises.

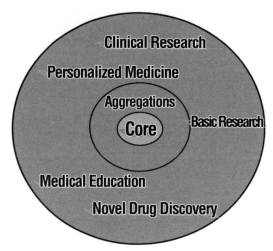

Fig. 17. Around a growing core and set of aggregations, it is now possible to define unambiguously clinical genomics application data in such a way as to support interoperability.

The *Genotype* model originally evolved from work on the bone marrow transplantation (BMT) and tissue-typing storyboard attempting to introduce modularity in this area. The first module is about the messages and documents being exchanged in the BMT use case between its major players (e.g., BMT wards, tissue-typing labs, donor banks). The second module zooms in and describes in more detail the unique observations used in tissue typing, i.e., the individual tissue-typing observation and the matching observation that indicates the level of matching between two individual tissue-typing observations (e.g., patient and donor, victim and suspect). The rationale for this modularity is that the tissue-typing observation could be used in various cases such as fatherhood testing and forensic cases. The third zoom-in is about a single human leukocyte antigen (HLA) allele, and its representation is done using the *Genotype* model. **Figure 18** describes the containment of the modules. Similarly to the use case of tissue typing in BMT, the *Genotype* model will be utilized in other use cases such as genetic testing and clinical trials.

A similar development methodology was carried out in other storyboards until it reached the level of the fine grain genomic data. As previously mentioned, the *Genotype* model is the result of these processes. **Figure 19** shows a bird's eye view of the *Genotype* model. The model itself (along with its corresponding XML schema and sample XML instances) is available from the HL7 web site (*see* www.hl7.org.)

4.2.1.1. MAIN FEATURES OF GENOTYPE MODEL

1. General notes:
   - This model can be used as an HL7 CMET (Common Message Element Type) much like *Patient, Encounter* and other CMETs that are being used in various HL7 specifications. It can be used by any message or document spec that needs to convey genomic data linked with clinical data residing either internally or externally.

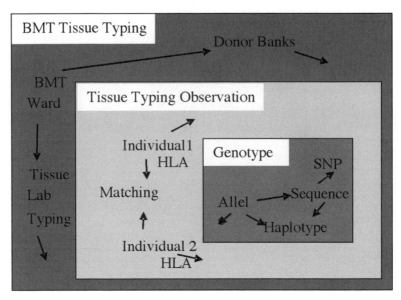

Fig. 18. Genotype model as a reusable genomic data module. HLA, human leukocyte antigen.

- The basic data framework is a chromosomal locus, typically an allele pair, one from the paternal chromosome and the other from the maternal chromosome. However, it is possible to represent a nonallelic data set, as is the typical case in gene expression, or only one allele in cases of translocations or insufficient data. More than two alleles can be also represented in cases of multiple somatic variations identified in the specimen or in the rare cases of three chromosomes as in Down syndrome.

2. Features:
   - *Starting point*: The starting point is the *GenotypeLocus* class, representing a locus or a gene, associated with any number of *IndividualAllele* classes. Note that a class in HL7 modeling refers to a refined class derived from one of the HL7 core classes, such as *Observation*, *Procedure*, or *Entity*. Refinement of a core class mainly concerns the characteristics of the class attributes, such as (a) which ones are chosen, (b) what vocabularies they are associated with, (c) what cardinalities they have, and (d) with what HL7 data types they comply.

     It is interesting to note that the result of this refinement process is sometimes called a "clone" in the HL7 RIM documentation, which obviously is not a proper name in clinical genomics and illustrates the situation where data models are developed by different communities with no common terminology.

     Instantiating the *Genotype* XML schema to represent two identified HLA alleles, for example, could result in the following XML structure:

```
<GenotypeLocus>
  <IndividualAllele>
    <value code="HLA00398" codeSystemName="IMGT/HLA Database"
    displayName="HLA B*8101"/>
  </IndividualAllele>
```

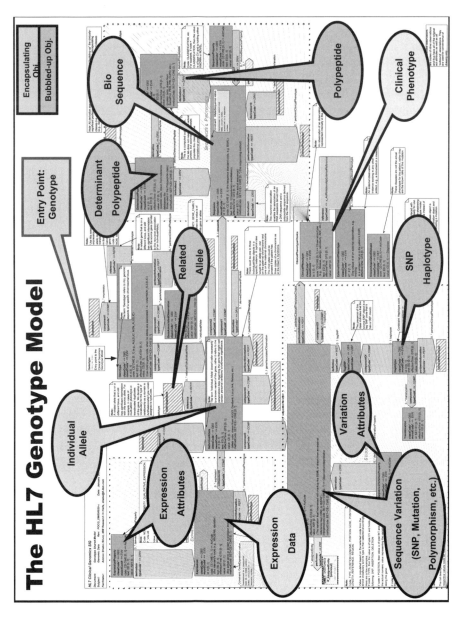

Fig. 19. Bird's eye view of HL7 Clinical-Genomics Genotype Model.

```
<IndividualAllele>
  <value code="HLA01809" codeSystemName="IMGT/HLA Database"
  displayName="HLA B*8102"/>
</IndividualAllele>
</GenotypeLocus>
```

Note that if a full sequencing procedure of the HLA genes is performed then the raw sequence data will be encapsulated in nested classes nesting within the *IndividualAllele* element.

The core genomic observations associated directly with each of the *IndividualAllele* classes are optional and include data about sequences, sequence variations and expression levels. The *Sequence* class is recursive and enables the representation of sequences of molecules, such as DNA, RNA, and protein. The *SequenceVariation* class allows the representation of any type of variation, such as SNPs, mutations, polymorphisms, and so forth. The *Expression* class allows the representation of gene expression and other expression data.

Other genomic observations associated with the core classes include classes, such as *Haplotype* and TagSNP which enable the indication of haplotype information, and *Polypeptide* and *DeterminantPeptide*, which enable the representation of proteomic data. In addition, each of the core classes is associated with a generic properties class that is populated through vocabularies that are part of the *Genotype* model. For example, it is possible to associate the zygosity of a gene with the *GenotypeLocus* class by populating the *LocusAssociatedObservation* class. The code of that object will be "zygosity" and the value could be heterozygous, homozygous, etc. The same mechanism is attached to the *Sequence*, *SequenceVariation*, and *Expression* classes. In the *Expression* class, for example, it is possible to associate properties, such as the normalized intensity of the gene expression by populating the class *ExpressionProperty*. In principle, these property classes could be populated as many times as needed to describe the data. The vocabularies are being reviewed and updated as new concepts become useful.

The essence of the model is in the linking mechanism of genomic data to clinical phenotypes, such as sensitivities, allergies, diseases, and adverse drug events. These phenotypes are best represented by HL7 classes, such as *Observations*. The phenotypes are represented by the classes *ObservedClinicalPhenotype*, *ExternalObservedClinical Phenotype*, and *KnownAssociatedPhenotype*.

The difference between the two first classes is that the former represents a phenotype that the creator of the genomic data chose to include within the genotype instance itself, whereas the latter represents a phenotype residing outside of the genotype instance, such as in the patient record's problem list. In theses cases the HL7 id attribute is being used to unambiguously identify the external phenotype. The id attribute is of type II (Instance Identifier), which includes the root and extension child elements. The root represents the OID (Object Identifier—an ISO standard) of the organization where the object resides and the extension represents the local identifier of that object within the scope of that organization. This combination allows information systems to resolve the id value and link to the "remote" object, in this case the clinical observation representing a phenotype in the context of genomic data.

As for the *KnownAssociatedPhenotype* class, it represents a potential phenotype based on the current knowledge but does not represent a phenotype actually observed in the patient.

4.2.1.2. BIOINFORMATICS FORMATS

Bioinformatics formats are utilized in the *Genotype* model to encapsulate raw genomic data such as sequencing, expression, and proteomic data. To enable the embedding of such data accepted from laboratories that work with bioinformatics formats, it is possible to assign specific XML portions into the *Sequence* and *Expression* class value attributes. Use of the XML bioinformatics markups is restricted; that is, not all tags are allowed, only a subset that relates to a specific chromosomal locus of a patient and includes the information pertinent to health care.

4.2.1.3. VALIDATION

Validation requires a receiver of an HL7 instance that carries a *Genotype* instance, a "double-validation" process: the first step is to validate the instance against the HL7 spec and the second is to validate the content of those value attributes against the respective content models. The content models of the *Sequence* and *Expression* class value attributes will be an integral part of the entire Genotype spec.

4.2.2. COEXISTENCE OF HL7 OBJECTS AND BIOINFORMATICS MARKUP

When exploring the Genotype model, one can identify the use of bioinformatics markup such as MAGE for gene expression and BSML for DNA sequencing. In addition, a few of the HL7 classes, such as the *SequenceVariation* class, overlap the elements of the bioinformatics markup. The question then arises: what are the relationships of the two and how do they coexist? The following are a few points to note about this issue:

- HL7's mission is to develop message/document specs that will be used in health care practice. The mission of the CG-SIG at HL7 is to develop message/document specs where genomic data are involved (e.g., genetic testing, clinical trials).
- Bioinformatics communities develop models/markups and are usually not ANSI-accredited Standard Developing Organizations and, thus, cannot sanction and maintain these formats. Naturally, their orientation is more toward research and the needs of information exchange among research facilities, data mining, and statistical analysis.
- HL7 CG-SIG attempts to constrain existing bioinformatics markups and embed them in the HL7 model. The bioinformatics markups are a type of raw data that might not always get into the HL7 CG-SIG actual instances; rather, they might be only referenced from the HL7 instance as supporting evidences. When they do get into an HL7 instance, then there is a blend of HL7 classes and embedded genomic markup.
- The approach taken by the HL7 CG- SIG can be described as "encapsulate and bubble-up;" that is, allowing overlaps and exploring its benefits. The HL7 classes should be seen as representing the digest of the raw genomic data that are most pertinent to the health care practice itself. There is a room here for applications that might parse the bioinformatics markup and intelligently populate the HL7 classes.
- The HL7 classes in the *Genotype* model have the advantage of being better tied with the other HL7 objects in the patient record (e.g., in a problem/allergy list) and, thus, serve better the ability to link individual genomic data to the clinical data of that individual. Note that

bioinformatics models also include clinical data, so this poses an overlapping problem in the other direction.

The integration mechanisms of bioinformatics markups could integrate various genomic sources into health care standards used for patient care, so there may not be one standard format. The issue should not be which bioinformatics model is the "best fit with HL7 Reference Information Model;" rather, it should be how mechanisms can be developed to digest data in various representations and link them to the HL7 RIM for the benefit of personalized medicine.

For example, the BSML markup is fairly simple and the HL7 CG-SIG has done some work on BSML in constraining it to be embedded in HL7 classes. For example, within the <Bsml> tags, the document is divided into three major sections, each of which is optional, but because one designs HL7 observation, it seems that there is room only for the first type:

1. Definitions—encoding of genomes and sequences, data tables, sets, and networks.
2. Research—encoding of queries, searches, analyses, and experiments.
3. Display—encoding of display widgets that represent graphical representations of biological objects.

As part of the *Genotype* specification package, XML samples are available to show how XML fragments complying with BSML are embedded in HL7-compliant instances in various uses cases, such as tissue typing observations, somatic mutations in small-cell lung cancer tissues, and genomic data in public health. The constraining process of BSML makes sure that data related to research and presentation elements are not included and that the instance includes one and only one patient's data and that this patient is uniquely identified.

4.2.3. Pharmacogenomics-Based Clinical Trial and Submission: A Sample Storyboard

Work on the pharmacogenomics storyboard is being carried out as part of the HL7 Clinical-Genomics group's ongoing activities and also as part of its participation in the Pharmacogenomics Submission Standards Initiative (joint CDISC and HL7 project coordinated by the US Food and Drug Administration [FDA] initiative on Voluntary Genomic Data Submission Guidelines).

The pharmacogenomics storyboard focuses on all clinical aspects of genomic-based clinical trials and the exchange of information needed to move from any current phase to a more advanced phase in the course of the clinical trials. It spans from patient recruitment based on genomic criteria and goes through gene selection based on haplotype information and the actual genomic testing up to the analysis of those data in conjunction with the clinical data and their reporting.

The storyboard describes a scenario that starts at clinical trial designs with Pharmacogenomics components. Institutional Review Board approval is obtained after the patient case report form and informed consent form design are prepared. Next, patient recruitment is carried out and DNA or tissue samples are received. Gene selection and a variation marker discovery process are conducted as part of the clinical trial. Clinical genotyping should be compliant with the appropriate regulation. In parallel, clinical demographics, clinical phenotype, and laboratory test results are received for each patient who participates in the trial. Haplotype or other types of markers are assigned to each patient. Statistical analysis is conducted to establish the association between the genetic markers and clinical outcomes. A validation study is then performed. Finally, reports are generated and communicated between pharmaceutical and biotechnology partners; submission materials are compiled for submission to regulatory agencies.

Following the storyboard described here, the HL7 CG-SIG groups developed an HL7 model that captures the information exchange in that storyboard. The nature of development in HL7 is that one first starts with a domain information model, called "DIM," based on the domain experts' initial input. One then derives specific message/document models from the DIM and validates them against the storyboard scenarios. In an iterative process, one refines the more specific models and updates the DIM accordingly. The DIM model is supposed to be the container of everything that matters in the domain. The more specific models are called R-MIM (refined message information models) and are derived from the DIM in such a way that the HL7 tooling can serialize them and eventually produce XML schemas for implementation purposes. **Figure 20** shows a bird's eye view of the pharmacogenomics DIM. The model itself can be obtained from HL7 (*see* www.hl7.org).

4.2.3.1. MAIN FEATURES OF PHARMACOGENOMICS MODEL

The pharmacogenomics model is focused on genomic data in the clinical trial arena. It is important to note at this point that all parts of this model that are not related to genomic data could be replaced with models developed by the HL7 Regulated Clinical Research Information Management (RCRIM) group that focuses on clinical trials. The "nongenomic" parts of this model were developed to better understand the genomic-based processes (e.g., gene selection and haplotype discovery), and for completeness of the model that might make it more convenient to read. Both HL7 groups hold joint meetings and try to harmonize their models. A dedicated mechanism in HL7 for sharing parts of models across different groups (domains) is the CMET mechanism. A CMET model is an HL7 model that can be incorporated into another model. The key for using CMETs effectively is clean modularity. The pharmacogenomics DIM model utilizes the HL7 Clinical Genomics *Genotype* model as a CMET for representing both design and selection of genes for the clinical trial, as well as for the results of the genomic testing.

4.2.3.2. PHARMACOGENOMICS MODEL WALK-THROUGH

The left side of the Pharmacogenomics model has the main participants in this model: the sponsor *(Pharma)*, the *CRO*, and the *Patient*. There are a few participants in the model, such as Collaborator and regulator, which are described below.

At the upper left corner, the patient class and its related information can be seen. Note that this model follows the HL7 V3 RIM core classes and associations. For example, there is a *Person* entity who plays the role of a *Patient* with participation of being the subject of the *PharmacogenomicsClinicalTrial* act. At the middle left, one can see the *CRO* recruiting patients—a process represented by receiving the consent form from

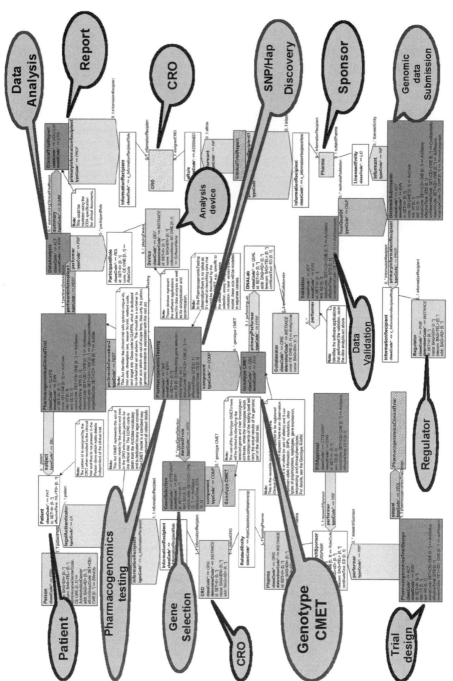

Fig. 20. Bird's eye view of Pharmacogenomics DIM.

the patient. At the lower left, the *Pharma* entity can be seen taking the role of *Clinical ResearchSponsor*, which has the participation of Performer of the *Pharmacogenomics TrialDesign* act. On the right side of the model and continuing to the bottom, the analysis and reporting process is found, starting from the pharmacogenomics trial results and its analysis on to the CRO and further to the sponsor. That is the beginning of the submission process to the regulator with validation and other necessary actions.

At the heart of the model are the genomic acts, starting from the top where one can see the main act—the *PharmacogenomicsClinicalTrial*, associated with the *PharmacogenomicsTesting* act (which is an attempt to generalize the storyboard UML class called "Genotyping"). The *PharmacogenomicsTesting* act can have any number of instances of the Genotype module (supposed to be a CMET) in two modes: downward *PharmacogenomicsTesting* is the *component* association with the Genotype module, where the actual genomic result data reside; to the left of *PharmacogenomicsTesting* is an association with the *GeneSelection* act, which is a fundamental part of a pharmacogenomics clinical trial. To represent the genes that were selected, use the *Genotype* model and populate only the gene identifiers, whereas in the use of the *Genotype* model for testing results, any part of the *Genotype* model can populate (e.g., sequencing, gene expression, SNPs, haplotypes). The *PharmacogenomicsTesting* is performed by a *DNALab*, which is a role played by the *Collaborator* entity (these classes are shown to the right of the act).

5. Conclusion

Standards for clinical genomic data were first forged by industry consortia and now by ANSI standards development organizations such as HL7. The goal is to provide mechanisms for representing, storing, and exchanging interoperable clinical genomics data. In this chapter, we have discussed formalisms for representing gene sequence data, microarray data, and pharmacogenomic data. We have described the uses of these kinds of data and the rationale for their use. Benefits stand to be gained in terms of personalized medicine, improved research into the basis for disease, and the education of current and future clinicians in this area, which, incidentally, have not been traditionally well covered by current medical education curriculums. The bioinformatics community is moving forward with standards in support of clinical genomics interoperability. This work should form a firm basis for development of clinical genomics informatics solutions of the future.

From a sequence analysis and communication standpoint, it is clear that there is a long way to go before a single standard or a set of standards is adopted by the scientific community at large. Owing to their historical and utilitarian support in the research community, raw, FASTA, and GCG file formats continue to enjoy widespread use. This is unfortunate because their "sequence(s) in isolation" paradigm is more in line with traditional genetics research than that of the much more expansive and interconnected model of genomic research. Flat-file formats represent a step toward that broader goal in the realm of data management for sequences. Not only are flat files more richly populated with biological information (both nucleotide sequence and translated reading frames, taxonomy, locus, and so on), but the detailed indexing of a sequence as a function of its discovery and its role in biology and medicine precisely positions this information within a conceptual framework of the known genome: past, present, and peer reviewed. Flat files, however, are not without failing, especially in the context of direct exchange between researchers. A measure of data integrity would provide greater confidence in working with codes that are impractical—if not impossible—to check manually, given the cryptic nature of reading a string of JCBN codes, often of overwhelming length. Options to consider are numerous, from the simple checksum utility of GCG, to more sophisticated solutions analogous to DICOM (Digital Imaging and Communications in Medicine) wrappers used in digital radiology images.

Many researchers still need to study gene and protein sequences in relative isolation, (e.g., for discovery and sequencing of SNPs, determination of posttranslational variants. For these focused areas of study, the use of simpler standards of data exchange might appear to be superior, because historical, relational, and other broader context data are less relevant to the task at hand. But does less relevant mean irrelevant? As even the simple FASTA and GCG formats demonstrate, it is very easy to instruct a computer program to *ignore* data in a file (e.g., headers, position numbers, blank spaces). Given this fact, it may be more reasonable to instruct applications of specific function (e.g., homology search) to ignore nonsequence data within flat files; however, having such data immediately available (in the same file) serves to better facilitate the grander goal of genomics, which is finding connections of information across entire genomes and proteomes. Such connections are less likely to be made when sequences are studied in isolation, as necessitated by raw, FASTA, and GCG formats (among others).

Breaking the Enigma code in WWII was a pivotal event in turning the tides for the Allies against the Axis powers. Sun Tzu recognized more than 2000 yr ago that a finely coordinated, well-communicating army was a force to be reckoned with, if not avoided altogether: "Do not engage an enemy advancing with well-ordered banners nor one whose formations are in impressive array" *(75)*. Keep in mind that all multicellular life begins as a single cell, and its organization is clearly evident in its tightly regulated network of gene expression, maintenance, and interaction with its surroundings. That level of organization is evident (to the extreme) at the tissue and organ levels, where the roaring din of 150 billion neurons finds a way to integrate into the discrete clarity of consciousness in a single human brain. The banners of the genome are "well ordered" indeed. When codes are broken, and unfettered access into vital communications is secured, be it an enemy infrastructure or a cellular genome, the battle is already won: obtaining the prize becomes a simple investment of time and labor.

References

1. Crick, F. (1966) On protein synthesis. *Symp. Soc. Exp. Biol.* **31,** 3–9.
2. Holley, R. W. (1965) Structure of a ribonucleic acid. *Science* **147,** 1462–1465.
3. Khorana, H. G. (1973) Nucleic acid synthesis in the study of the genetic code, in *Nobel Lectures: Physiology or Medicine (1963–1970)*. Elsevier, New York, pp. 341–349.
4. Nirenberg, M. W. and Leder, P. (1964) RNA codewords and protein synthesis. *Science* **145,** 1399–1407.

5. Ensembl Human Genome Browser, Sanger Institute. www.ensembl.org/Homo_sapiens/. Accessed 7/30/2004.
6. Elkin, P. L. (2003) Primer on medical genomics part V: bioinformatics. *Mayo Clin. Proc.* **78,** 57–64.
7. Nomenclature Committee of the International Union of Biochemistry (NC-IUB). (1985) Nomenclature for incompletely specified bases in nucleic acid sequences: recommendations 1984. *Biochem. J.* **229,** 281–286.
8. IUPAC-IUB Joint Commission on Biochemical Nomenclature (JCBN). (1984) Nomenclature and symbolism for amino acids and peptides: recommendations 1983. *Biochem. J.* **219,** 345–373.
9. Cornish-Bowden, A. (1985) Nomenclature for incompletely specified bases in nucleic acid sequences: recommendations 1984. *Nucleic Acids Res.* **13,** 3021–3030.
10. IUPAC-IUBMB Joint Commission on Biochemical Nomenclature (JCBN). www.chem. qmul.ac.uk/iupac/jcbn/. Accessed 8/07/2004.
11. De Banzie, J. S., Steeg, E. W., and Lis, J. T. (1984) Update for users of the Cornell sequence analysis package. *Nucleic Acids Res.* **12(1 Pt. 2),** 619–625.
12. Fristensky, B., Lis, J., and Wu, R. (1982) Portable microcomputer software for nucleotide sequence analysis. *Nucleic Acids Res.* **10,** 6451–6463.
13. Sequence File Formats. home.cc.umanitoba.ca/~psgendb/formats.html. Accessed 8/06/2004.
14. Fristensky Lab, Department of Plant Science, University of Manitoba. home.cc.umanitoba. ca/~frist/. Accessed 8/06/2004.
15. IUBio-Archive. iubio.bio.indiana.edu:7780/archive/00000252/. Accessed 8/06/2004.
16. Lipman, D. J. and Pearson, W. R. (1985) Rapid and sensitive protein similarity searches. *Science* **227,** 1435–1441.
17. Wilbur, W. J. and Lipman, D. J. (1983) Rapid similarity searches of nucleic acid and protein data banks. *Proc. Natl. Acad. Sci. USA* **80,** 726–730.
18. Pearson, W. R. and Lipman, D. J. (1988) Improved tools for biological sequence comparison. *Proc. Natl. Acad. Sci. USA* **85,** 2444–2448.
19. Pearson, W. R. (1994) Using the FASTA program to search protein and DNA sequence databases. *Meth. Mol. Biol.* **24,** 307–331.
20. Lesk, A. M. (2002). *Introduction to Bioinformatics,* Oxford University Press, New York.
21. DNA Databank of Japan. www.ddbj.nig.ac.jp/search/help/fasta-e_help.html. Accessed 7/30/ 2004.
22. European Bioinformatics Institute. www.ebi.ac.uk/Tools/homology.html. Accessed 7/30/2004.
23. Stack Pack v2.2. juju.egenetics.com/stackpack/support/format.html. Accessed 8/05/2004.
24. www.ncbi.nlm.nih.gov/BLAST/fasta.shtml. Accessed 8/05/2004.
25. Medical College of Wisconsin. www.mcw.edu/display/router.asp?docid=1717. Accessed 7/18/2004.
26. Accelrys Bioinformatics: Company, Products and Training. www.dbi.udel.edu/pdfs/Kendall. pdf. Accessed 7/18/2004.
27. Accelrys, GCG Manual. www.ccc.columbia.edu/genhelp/gcgmanual.html. Accessed 8/09/ 2004.
28. Accelrys, GCG Manual. www.ccc.columbia.edu/genhelp/reformat.html#heading. Accessed 8/09/2004.
29. International Nucleotide Sequence Database Collaboration. www.ncbi.nlm.nih.gov/projects/ collab/. Accessed 8/11/2004.
30. Felton, M. J. (2001) Bioinformatics: the child of success. *Modern Drug Des.* **4(9),** 25–28.

31. NCBI ASN.1 Summary. www.ncbi.nlm.nih.gov/Sitemap/Summary/asn1.html. Accessed 8/13/2004.

32. Ostell, J. National Center of Biotechnology Information (NCBI), National Library of Medicine, National Institutes of Health. Using ASN.1 (Abstract Syntax Notation 1): A Data Description Language. www.nal.usda.gov/pgdic/Probe/v2n2/using.html. Accessed 8/13/2004.

33. The DDBJ/EMBL/GenBank Feature Table: Definition. www.ebi.ac.uk/embl/Documentation/FT_definitions/feature_table.html. Accessed 8/11/2004.

34. 2can Bioinformatics Education Resource, Nucleotide Databases. www.ebi.ac.uk/2can/data bases/dna.html. Accessed 8/13/2004.

35. EMBL-EBI European Bioinformatics Institute Nucleotide Sequence Database Collaboration. www.ebi.ac.uk/embl/Contact/collaboration.html. Accessed 8/13/04.

36. www.ncbi.nlm.nih.gov/Taxonomy/taxonomyhome.html/. Accessed 8/13/2004.

37. www.ncbi.nlm.nih.gov/projects/collab/FT/index.html#3.5.2. Accessed 8/13/2004.

38. www.ebi.ac.uk/2can/tutorials/nucleotide/fasta5.html. Accessed 8/13/2004.

39. www.agavexml.org/. Accessed 8/13/2004.

40. www.lifecde.com/products/agave/index.html. Accessed 8/13/2004.

41. www.businesswire.com/webbox/bw.092701/212700085.htm. (BW) (CA-DOUBLETWIST) European Bioinformatics Institute Joins Initial Partners Supporting Doubletwist's AGAVE Genomic Annotation XML Format. Accessed 8/13/2004.

42. King, B. (2001) Introduction to AGAVE Genomic Annotation XML. Abstract for Bioinformatics Open Source Conference (BOSC) 2001. open-bio.org/bosc2001/abstracts/posters/king. Accessed 8/13/2004.

43. XEMBL. www.ebi.ac.uk/xembl/. Accessed 8/13/2004.

44. Wang, L., Riethoven, J. J., and Robinson, A. (2002) XEMBL: distributing EMBL data in XML format. *Bioinformatics* **18,** 1147, 1148.

45. Cibulskis, K. An Introduction to BSML. XML-Journal. http://XML-Journal.com. p1-9. Accessed 8/08/2004.

46. www.labbook.com/. Accessed 8/14/2004.

47. webservices.xml.com/lpt/a/ws/2002/05/14/biows.html. Accessed 8/13/2004.

48. bioperl.org/. Accessed 8/13/2004.

49. GenBank General Submission Information. www.ncbi.nih.gov/BankIt/help.html#gen_sub_info. Accessed 8/13/2004.

50. Schena, M., Shalon, D., Davis, R. W., and Brown, P. O. (1995) Quantitative monitoring of gene expression patterns with a complementary DNA microarray. *Science* **270,** 467–470.

51. Kononen, J., Bubendorf, L., Kallioniemi, A., et al. (1998) Tissue microarrays for high-throughput molecular profiling of tumor specimens. *Nat. Med.* **4,** 844–847.

52. Packeisen, J., Korsching, E., Herbst, H., Boecker, W., and Buerger, H. (2003) Demystified ...tissue microarray technology. *Mol. Pathol.* **56,** 198–204.

53. Leung, Y. F. and Cavalieri, D. (2003) Fundamentals of cDNA microarray data analysis. *Trends Genet.* **19,** 649–659.

54. Guo, Q. M. (2003) DNA microarray and cancer. *Curr. Opin. Oncol.* **15,** 36–43.

55. Napoli, C., Lerman, L. O., Sica, V., Lerman, A., Tajana, G., and de Nigris, F. (2003) Microarray analysis: a novel research tool for cardiovascular scientists and physicians. *Heart (Br. Cardiac. Soc.)* **89,** 597–604.

56. Kurella, M., Hsiao, L. L., Yoshida, T., et al. (2001) DNA microarray analysis of complex biologic processes. *J. Am. Soc. Nephrol.* **12,** 1072–1078.

57. Bunney, W. E., Bunney, B. G., Vawter, M. P., et al. (2003) Microarray technology: a review of new strategies to discover candidate vulnerability genes in psychiatric disorders. *Am. J. Psychiatry* **160**, 657–666.

58. Greenberg, S. A. (2001) DNA microarray gene expression analysis technology and its application to neurological disorders. *Neurology* **57**, 755–761.

59. Tefferi, A., Bolander, M. E., Ansell, S. M., Wieben, E. D., and Spelsberg, T. C. (2002) Primer on medical genomics. Part III: microarray experiments and data analysis. *Mayo Clin. Proc.* **77**, 927–940.

60. Brazma, A., Robinson, A., Cameron, G., and Ashburner, M. (2000) One-stop shop for microarray data. *Nature* **403**, 699–700.

61. Minimum Information About a Microarray Experiment—MIAME. www.mged.org/Work groups/MIAME/miame.html. Accessed 8/11/2004.

62. MicroArray and Gene Expression—MAGE. www.mged.org/Workgroups/MAGE/mage. html. Accessed 8/11/2004.

63. Ontology Working Group. mged.sourceforge.net/ontologies/index.php. Accessed 8/11/2004.

64. The MGED Data Transformation and Normalization Working Group. genome-www5. stanford.edu/mged/normalization.html. Accessed 8/11/2004.

65. Reporting Structure for Biological Investigations Working Groups (RSBI WGs) www.mged. org/Workgroups/tox/tox.html. Accessed 8/11/2004.

66. Brazma, A., Hingamp, P., Quackenbush, J., et al. (2001) Minimum information about a microarray experiment (MIAME)—toward standards for microarray data. *Nat. Genet.* **29**, 365–371.

67. Minimum Information About a Microarray Experiment—MIAME 1.1 Draft 6, Version 1.1 (Draft 6, April 1, 2002)—discussed at MGED 4. www.mged.org/Workgroups/MIAME/ miame_1.1.html. Accessed 8/11/2004.

68. Microarray Gene Expression Data Society. www.mged.org. Accessed 8/10/2004.

68a. Object Management Group, Inc. Gene Expression Specification, ver. 1.1. October 2003. http://www.omg.org/docs/formal/03-10-01.pdf_p_1-11. Accessed on 5/10/2005.

69. Spellman, P. T., Miller, M., Stewart, J., et al. (2002) Design and implementation of microarray gene expression markup language (MAGE-ML). *Genome Biol.* **3(9)**, research0046.1– 0046.9.

70. MAGE-STK: The MAGE Software Toolkit. http://mged.sourceforge.net/software/MAGE stk.php. Accessed 8/11/2004.

71. Bell, J. (1998) Medical implications of understanding complex disease traits. *Curr. Opin. Biotechnol.* **9**, 573–577.

72. Agarwala, R., Biesecker, L. G., Hopkins, K. A., Francomano, C. A., and Schaffer, A. A. (1998) Software for constructing and verifying pedigrees within large genealogies and an application to the Old Order Amish of Lancaster County. *Genome Res.* **8**, 211–221.

73. Koch, T. and Martin, A. (1998) Solving Steiner tree problems in graphs to optimality. *Networks* **32**, 207–232.

74. Buhler, J., Owerbach, D., Schaffer, A. A., Kimmel, M., and Gabbay, K. H. (1997) Linkage analyses in type I diabetes using CASPAR, a software and statistical program for conditional analysis of polygenic diseases. *Hum. Hered.* **47**, 211–222.

75. Griffith, S. B. (1971) *Sun Tzu: The Art of War.* Oxford University Press, New York.

8

Clinical Applications of Bioinformatics, Genomics, and Pharmacogenomics

Omer Iqbal and Jawed Fareed

Summary

Elucidation of the entire human genomic sequence is one of the greatest achievements of science. Understanding the functional role of 30,000 human genes and more than 2 million polymorphisms was possible through a multidisciplinary approach using microarrays and bioinformatics. Polymorphisms, variations in DNA sequences, occur in 1% of the population, and a vast majority of them are single nucleotide polymorphisms. Genotype analysis has identified genes important in thrombosis, cardiac defects, and risk of cardiac disease. Many of the genes show a significant correlation with polymorphisms and the incidence of coronary artery disease and heart failure. In this chapter, the application of current state-of-the-art genomic analysis to a variety of these disorders is reviewed.

Key Words: Single nucleotide polymorphism; bioinformatics; gene expression; microarrays; angiotensin-converting enzyme; activated protein C; coronary artery disease; glycoprotein.

1. Introduction

According to 1998 mortality rates in the United States, cardiac diseases ranked first on a list of 12 diseases, and the National Institutes of Health estimated the total cost of treatment at $183.1 billion (*1*). Environmental and genetic risk factors play an important role in the pathophysiology of most human diseases. Whereas some diseases may have a primarily environmental influence, others may be purely genetically influenced or influenced by a combination of the two. It has generally been thought that cardiovascular risk factors such as smoking, obesity, diet, and lack of exercise are environmental in nature and play a most important role in disease process. However, premature heart disease and the presence of diabetes and a definite genetic background have been identified as risk factors for coronary artery disease. Because about half of the varia-

From: *Methods in Molecular Biology, vol. 316: Bioinformatics and Drug Discovery*
Edited by: R. S. Larson © Humana Press Inc., Totowa, NJ

bility of major risk factors for cardiovascular disease is genetic, pharmacogenomics plays a major role in the diagnosis, treatment, and prevention of these disorders. Venous thromboembolism (VTE) is a common disorder worldwide. The estimated annual incidence of symptomatic thromboembolism is 117 cases per 100,000 people *(2)*, or more than 250,000 people each year in the United States. The incidence is age dependent, increasing from 0 in children to less than 1 per 10,000 in young adults and 3–5 per 10,000 in individuals over the age of 60, with further increments with each additional decade *(3)*. With a large proportion of the US population entering the older age group, VTE will become an increasingly important national health problem *(2)*. Venous thrombosis commonly develops in the deep veins of the leg (calf vein thrombosis and proximal vein involving the popliteal, femoral, or iliac veins) or the arm. Pulmonary emboli are sequelae from thrombi in the deep veins of the leg in 90% or more of patients. Deep vein thrombosis (DVT) and/or pulmonary embolism are referred to as VTE.

The emergence of pharmacogenomics-guided anticoagulant drug development has unraveled novel approaches in the management of patients and ensured individualized therapy to everyone. Gene expression profiling will be useful in the diagnosis of various diseases, in preclinical phases of drug development, and in the development of markers of adverse drug reactions, which can be avoided by withdrawing a particular drug. Through cheminformatics anticoagulant drug therapy can be tailored to the individual needs of the patient at the correct dosage and time. Now that the human genome is completely mapped, identification of gene-based single nucleotide polymorphisms (SNPs) will be valuable in the diagnosis of diseases.

Pharmaceutical industries are focusing on applying pharmacogenomics not only to develop new anticoagulant drugs but also to reduce the cost of and length of time of clinical trials. Thus, new agents could be developed and therapy individualized, i.e., tailored to treat the right patient at the correct dosage. Although genetic association studies are used to establish links between polymorphic variation in coagulation factor V gene and DVT, this approach of "susceptibility genes" directly influencing an individual's likelihood of developing the disease *(4)* has been extended to the identification of other gene variants. Variations in the drug-metabolizing enzyme gene thiopurine methyl transferase have been linked to adverse drug reactions *(5)*. Likewise, variants in drug target (5-lipoxygenase, ALOX5) have been linked to variations in drug response *(6)*. Through linkage disequilibrium or nonrandom association between SNPs in proximity to each other, tens of thousands of anonymous SNPs are identified and mapped. These anonymous genes may fall either within genes (susceptibility genes) or in noncoding DNA between genes. Through linkage disequilibrium the associations found with these anonymous SNP markers can identify a region of the genome that may harbor a particular susceptibility gene. Through positional cloning, the gene and SNP can be discovered, conferring the underlying associated condition or disease *(7)*.

The National Heart, Lung, and Blood Institute (NHLBI) has launched various programs for genomic applications (PGAs) with the goal of developing information, tools, and resources to link genes to biological function. Some of the programs include Bay Genomics (NHLBI, Bay Area Functional Genomics Consortium, http://baygenomics. ucsf.edu/), Berkeley PGA (comparative genomic analysis of cardiovascular gene regulation, http://pga.lbl.gov/), CardioGenomics (genomics of cardiovascular development, adaptation, and remodeling, www.cardiogenomics.org), and HOPGENE (applied genomics in cardiopulmonary disease, www.hopkins-genomics.org). Berkeley PGA was formed to facilitate the use of comparative genomics in the studies of heart, lung, and blood disorders. This PGA consists of bioinformatics tools for comparative sequence analysis that include VISTA server and tools (www-gsd.lbl.gov/VISTA/index.html), VISTA whole genome browser (http://pipeline.lbl.gov/), MAVID alignment tools (http://baboon.math.berkeley.edu/mavid/), and LAGAN alignment tools (http://lagan.stanford.edu/). The cross-species sequencing resources needed include BAC libraries and filters (www-gsd.lbl.gov/cheng/BAC.html, BACs containing cardiovascular genes and unprocessed sequence contigs (http://pga.lbl.gov/seq/), and a comparative genomic database for cardiovascular genes (http://pga.lbl.gov/cvcgd.html). Bioinformatics tools for comparative sequence analysis and cross-species sequencing resources are very important in facilitating the use of comparative genomics in the studies of heart, lung, and blood disorders.

2. Materials and Methods

Most of the methods described here are covered elsewhere in this book and thus are only briefly described. Detection of SNPs typically requires extraction of DNA from leukocytes of whole-blood samples and amplification of the DNA using polymerase chain reaction (PCR). From a known DNA sequence, using specific forward and reverse primers, isolation of DNA sequence containing the gene of interest is possible. The amplified DNA is then incubated with specific restriction site endonucleases to degrade the DNA into fragments. The DNA fragments are resolved using polyacrylamide gel electrophoresis and visualized with ethidium bromide. QIAamp DNA Mini and QIAamp DNA Blood Mini Kits are used for purification of total DNA. Whole blood, plasma, serum, buffy coat, bone marrow body fluids, lymphocytes, cultured cells, and tissues can be used to extract and purify the DNA. Fresh or frozen whole blood and blood treated with citrate, EDTA, or heparin can be used in the QIAamp procedure. However, prior separation of leukocytes is not a requisite. DNA is eluted in Buffer AE and phenol/chloroform extraction or alcohol precipitation is not necessary. The purified DNA free of proteins, nucleases, contaminants, and inhibitors may be stored at −20°C for later analysis.

2.1. Purification of DNA

The QIAamp procedure may be followed for purification of DNA. The QIAamp Mini and QIAamp DNA Blood Mini Kits perform rapid purification of 6 µg of total DNA from 200 µL of buffy coat.

2.2. RNA Extraction Using Trizol Reagent

1. Pipet out 250 µL of whole blood, and dilute 1:1 with diethylpyrocarbonate-treated water. Add 750 µL of Trizol reagent (lyse by pipetting several times in the tip of the pipet).
2. Incubate and mix at 15–30°C for 15 min.
3. Add 200 µL of chloroform.
4. Cap and shake vigorously for 15 s by hand, and then incubate at 15–30°C for 15 min.

5. Centrifuge at 18,659*g* for 15 min at 2–8°C. The mixture will separate into an upper color-less aqueous phase and a lower phenol-chloroform phase (interphase). The RNA remains in the upper colorless aqueous phase.

6. Transfer the aqueous phase to a clean tube and mix with 500 µL of isopropyl alcohol (do not vortex; mix by pipetting).

7. Incubate at 15–30°C for 10 min.

8. Centrifuge at 18,659*g* for 10 min at 2–8°C. The RNA precipitate with form a gel-like pellet on the sides and bottom of the tube.

9. Remove the supernatant and wash the RNA pellet for 5–10 min with 1 mL of 75% ethanol.

10. Vortex and centrifuge at 9520*g* for 5 min at 2–8°C.

11. Remove the supernatant and air-dry the RNA pellet for 5–10 min (do not let it dry com-pletely because this will decrease the solubility of the pellet and decrease the A_{260}/A_{280} ratio).

12. Dissolve the RNA in RNase-free water by passing a few times through a pipet tip, and incubate for 10 min at 55–60°C.

13. Proceed with RNA purification using a Qiagen kit.

Generally approx 6–8 µg of total RNA Smaller quantities of RNA can be amplified through different techniques, and as little as 10 ng of RNA can generate labeled cRNA in a sufficient amount to obtain reliable and reproducible microarray data. Data analysis is performed through supervised and unsupervised learning. Biological interpretation of the data is very important, and future technologies will adopt ways of minimizing over-interpretation of data. The samples are separately run in duplicates in order to validate and confirm the analysis of microarray data.

2.3. Gene Expression Analysis

There are several techniques to monitor expression of myriad genes. Some of the techniques include serial analysis of gene expression, differential display, representa-tional differential analysis, and microarrays.

2.3.1. Microarray Analysis

The DNA microarray is a very commonly used technique and can generate quantita-tive information about thousands of gene expressions in a reliable, rapid, convenient, and economical manner. There are numerous Web sites from which information on DNA microarrays can be obtained, including Stanford Genomic Resources (http://genome-www.stanford.edu), Gene Expression Omnibus database (www.ncbi.nim.nih.gov/geo), ArrayExpress database, (www.ebi.ac.uk/arrayexpress), National Human Genome Re-search Institute (http://research.nhgri.nih.gov), Broad Institute (www.broad.mit.edu/cancer), and The Jackson Laboratory (http://jax.org/staff/churchill/labsite).

Specifically designed microarrays to study angiogenesis and cell adhesion have been developed. Pathway-focused microarrays can be used to perform project-related gene expression instead of profiling the whole genome. Various available oligonucleotide arrays include angiogenesis microarrays, endothelial cell biology microarrays, and ex-tracellular matrix and adhesion microarrays. Some of the features of oligo microarrays include pathway-focused design containing 100–500 well-characterized genes belong-ing to relevant biological pathways, robust performance employing the most sensitive proprietary labeling method to achieve reproducible data, and user-friendliness and cost-effectiveness.

2.3.2. DNA Microarray Techniques

Microarrays differ with respect to the type of probe, manner in which they are arrayed on the solid support, and method of target preparation. The support on which the probes are arrayed can be made of glass slide, nylon membrane, or silicon wafer. The complement DNA or cRNA generated from sample RNA labeled with fluorescent dye is hybridized to the microarray. The scanner at the site of the probe measures fluorescence. PCR amplification of cDNA generates the cDNA fragments, which are robotically spotted onto the glass slide on which the probes are arrayed. To be consistent with the amount of each probe spotted robotically onto the glass slide, sample RNA labeled with fluorescent dye is often hybridized to the array together with a fixed amount of reference RNA labeled with a different fluorescence. Prior sequence information is not needed for DNA microarrays. Further developments in the field of DNA microarrays will lead to the development of additional oligonucleotide arrays. However, DNA microarrays are quite ideal in situations in which the genomes of the organisms are not sequenced.

2.4. Microarray Bioinformatics

Microarray bioinformatics involves microarray experimental design and data analysis involving statistical considerations and the collection, management, and analysis of microarray data. Effective data analysis involves understanding and recording information, collecting useful annotations for probes on the array, and tracking and managing data and materials in the laboratory. Data collection normalization techniques enable comparison of data on gene expression from various arrays. Data-mining algorithms help organize data and facilitate discovery of potential functional relationships. Various statistical techniques such as *t*-tests, analysis of variance, or significance analysis of microarrays may be used to identify groups of genes that distinguish different samples. Resources for microarray bioinformatics include http://jax.org/staff/churchill/labsite/index.html and http://pga.tigrr.org/PGASoftware.shtml.

3. Clinical Applications of Bioinformatics and Pharmacogenomic Analysis

Microarray analysis of different genes of interest that could be used in high-throughput sequencing in a population to detect common or uncommon genetic variants have been developed. These DNA microarrays have been accurate, high-throughput, reproducible, and low cost. So far, Food and Drug Administration-approved microarrays are on the market. Efforts should be made not only to improve the sensitivity but also to reduce the costs of identifying polymorphisms by direct sequencing.

3.1. Disorders of Thrombophilia

The functional consequences of nonsynonymous SNPs can be predicted by a structure-based assessment of amino acid variation *(8)*. The major defects associated with thrombophilia are activated protein C resistance caused by Arg 506 to Gln mutation (factor V Leiden), prothrombin polymorphism (G20210A) causing an elevated prothrombin level, hyperhomocystenemia, protein C deficiency, protein S deficiency, antithrombin deficiency, and elevated factor VIII levels. The various polymorphisms in coagulation factors are discussed next.

3.1.1. Fibrinogen Abnormalities

Various polymorphisms have been identified in all the genes located on the long arm of chromosome 4 (q23-32). However, the two dimorphisms in the β-chain gene, the *Hae*III polymorphism (a G→A substitution at position –455 in the 5' promoter region and the Bcl1 polymorphism in the 3' untranslated region, are of major importance and are in linkage disequilibrium with each other. The –455G/A substitution in different investigations was found to be a determinant of plasma fibrinogen levels *(9,10)* and linked the fibrinogen gene variation to the risk of arterial disease. Because of conflicting reports from different studies, this association between fibrinogen gene variation and arterial disease is controversial. The α-chain Thr-312 Ala polymorphism has been reported to increase clot stability *(11)*. Specific factor XIIIa inhibitors may play an important role in decreasing clot stability. Polymorphisms of the β-fibrinogen gene affect plasma fibrinogen levels *(12–15)*, the risk of peripheral arterial disease *(10,15–17)*, and the risk and extent of coronary artery disease *(18–20)*.

3.1.2. Prothrombin G20210 Polymorphism

First reported by Poort et al. *(21)* in 1996, replacement of G by A at nucleotide 20210 in the 3'-untranslated region of the prothrombin gene increases translation without altering the transcription of the gene, resulting in elevated synthesis and secretion of prothrombin by the liver. This increased synthesis and secretion of prothrombin contributes to increased thrombotic risk by causing increased thrombin generation, which can activate the thrombin activatable fibrinolytic inhibitor, resulting in fibrinolytic deficit. The A20210 allele is present in 5–7% of VTE patients and is the second most common genetic risk factor for VTE *(21–23)*. A combined mutation of factor V Leiden and prothrombin gene 20210 is associated with a higher risk of VTE *(24–30)*.

3.1.3. Activated Protein C Resistance

Factor V Leiden R506Q mutation, occurring in 8% of the population and referring to specific G→A substitution at nucleotide 1691 in the gene for factor V, is cleaved less efficiently (10%) by activated protein C. This results in DVT, recurrent miscarriages, portal vein thrombosis in patients with cirrhosis, early kidney transplant loss, and other forms of VTE *(31–34)*. A dramatic increase in the incidence of thrombosis is seen in women who are taking oral contraceptives. Both prothrombin G20210 and factor V Leiden in the presence of major risk factors may contribute to atherothrombosis. The factor V Leiden allele is common in Europe, with a population frequency of 4.4%. The mutation is very rare outside of Europe, with a frequency of 0.6% in Asia Minor *(35)*.

3.1.4. Factor VII

Polymorphisms in the factor VII gene, especially the Arg-355Gln mutation in exon 8 located in the catalytic domain of factor VII, influence plasma factor VIII levels. The Gln-353 allele caused a strong protective effect against the occurrence of myocardial infarction *(36)*. Further research in this area is warranted to understand the role of factor VII in determining arterial thrombotic risk. Because the factor VIIa/tissue factor (TF) is the initial coagulation pathway, much attention has been focused on blocking this pathway by developing factor VIIa inhibitors and tissue factor pathway inhibitors (TFPIs) *(37)*. NAPc2 and NAP-5 are two of the anticoagulant proteins isolated from the hookworm nematode *Ancylostoma caninum*. NAPc2 is currently undergoing phase II clinical trials for prevention of VTE in patients with elective knee arthroplasty. NAPc2 binds to a noncatalytic site on factor X or Xa and inhibits factor VII. NAP-5 inhibits factor Xa and factor VII/TF complex after prior binding to factor Xa.

3.1.5. Factor VIII

Increased factor VIII activity levels are associated with increased risk of arterial thrombosis. However, no specific polymorphisms in the factor VIII gene have been determined.

3.1.6. von Willebrand Factor

Although increased plasma von Willebrand factor (vWF) levels have been attributed to increased risk of arterial thrombotic events, no gene polymorphisms in the vWF gene have been identified.

3.1.7. Factor XIII

Factor XIII SNP G→T in exon 2 causes a Val/Leu change at position 34. The Val34 Leu polymorphism increases the rate of thrombin activation of factor XIII and causes increased and faster clot stabilization *(38,39)*. The Leu34 allele has been shown to play a protective role against arterial and venous thrombosis *(40,41)*. Specific factor XIIIa inhibitors, such as tridegin and others, may provide an interesting and novel approach to preventing fibrin stabilization. It is important to identify this polymorphism because the Leu34 variant associated with increased factor XIIIa activity reduces the activity of thrombolytic therapy *(38,39)*.

3.1.8. Thrombomodulin

Thrombomodulin mutations are more important in arterial diseases than in venous diseases. The thrombomodulin polymorphism G→A substitution at nucleotide position 127 in the gene has been studied regarding its relation to arterial disease. The 25Thr allele has been reported to be more prevalent in male patients with myocardial infarction than the control population *(42)*. Polymorphism in the thrombomodulin gene promoter (−33 G/A) influences plasma soluble thrombomodulin levels and causes increased risk of coronary heart disease *(43)*. Carriership of the −33A allele has also been reported to cause increased occurrence of carotid atherosclerosis in patients younger than 60 yr of age *(44)*.

3.1.9. Tissue Factor Pathway Inhibitor

Sequence variation of the TFPI gene has been reported. The four different polymorphisms reported are Pro-151Leu, Val-264Met, T384C exon 4, and C033T intron 7 *(45, 46)*. The Val-264Met mutation caused decreased TFPI levels *(46)*. It has been reported that the Pro-151Leu replacement is a risk factor for venous thrombosis *(47)*. A polymorphism in the 5' untranslated region of the TFPI gene (−287 T/C) did not alter the TFPI levels and did not influence the risk of coronary atherothrombosis *(48)*. It has recently been reported that the −33T→C polymorphism in intron 7 of the TFPI gene influences the risk of VTE independently of the factor V Leiden and prothrombin mutations, and its effect is mediated by increased total TFPI levels *(49)*.

3.1.10. Endothelial Protein C Receptor

A 23-bp insertion in exon 3 of the endothelial protein C receptor (EPCR) gene has been reported to predispose patients to the risk of coronary atherothrombosis *(50)*. Further studies are needed to relate the polymorphisms in the EPCR gene to thrombotic diseases.

3.1.11. Methylene Tetrahydrofolate Reductase

A common polymorphism, C677T, is seen in methylene tetrahydrofolate reductase (MTHFR) gene, causing hyperhomocystenemia, and is considered to be a potential risk factor for both venous and arterial diseases. Homocystenemia, most often associated with folate deficiency or deficiency of cystathione β-synthetase deficiency *(51,52)*, is found in about 10% of families in which coronary artery disease presents before the sixth decade *(53)*. It is also associated with cerebrovascular disease *(54)*. Hyperhomocystenemia appears to be a risk factor for both arterial *(55)* and venous thrombosis *(56,57)* and may cause endothelial injury. Folic acid supplementation corrects the vascular effects of homocystenemia *(58)*.

3.1.12. Platelet Surface Gene Polymorphisms

Various polymorphisms of the platelet surface proteins, such as glycoprotein (GP) Ia-Iia, GPIb-V-IX, and GPIIb/IIIa have been reported. A gene polymorphism has recently been reported in the kozac sequence of the GPIbα receptor *(59)*. The role of these polymorphisms in arterial disease warrants further studies. The GPIIb/IIIa receptors bind fibrinogen, crosslink platelets, initiate thrombus formation *(60)*, and are considered to be the final common pathway of platelet aggregation. A Leu/Pro polymorphism at position 33 occurs in about one-fourth of the population and has been linked to coronary artery stenosis *(14,61)*, myocardial infarction *(60)*, and risk of restenosis after coronary stent placement *(62)*.

3.2. Cardiac Malformations and Coronary Artery Disease

3.2.1. Congenital Cardiac Malformations

Deletions of chromosome 22q11 manifest as interrupted aortic arch in approx 50% of patients, 35% of patients with truncus arteriosus, 33% of patients with ventricular septal defect, and 16% of patients with tetralogy of Fallot, but none with transposition of great vessels *(63)*. This deletion is seen in 90% of patients with DiGeorge syndrome *(64)*. These deletions are also associated with pulmonary artery anomalies *(65,66)*. Cardiovascular malformations are frequently seen in association with various syndromes. Patients with Down syndrome (trisomy 21) also have cardiovascular malformations involving one or more loci on chromosome 21q22.2-q22.3 *(67–69)*. Microdeletions at 7q11.23 are associated with Williams syndrome, which also manifests supravalvular aortic stenosis and pulmonary artery stenosis *(70,71)*. Furthermore, Marfan syndrome manifests mitral valve prolapse and aortic root enlargement as a result of mutations in the fibrillin-1 gene *(72)*.

3.2.2. Coronary Artery Disease: GENICA Study

The GENICA Study identified novel risk factors for coronary artery disease. It has recently been reported that the C allele at the T-786C endothelial nitric oxide synthase (eNOS) polymorphism is associated with a higher risk of multivessel coronary artery disease in Caucasians *(73)*. Although an impaired endothelium-dependent vasodilation *(74)* is associated with accelerated atherosclerosis, such as arterial hypertension, cigarette smoking, diabetes mellitus, hypercholesterolemia, hyperhomocysteinemia and aging *(75,76)*, a blunted nitric oxide (NO)-mediated endothelium-dependent vasodilation was found to predict cardiovascular events independently of the common risk factors *(77)*. NO is involved in atherogenesis *(78–80)*, development of heart failure, and congenital septal defects and vascular remodeling, as shown by data from mice lacking the eNOS gene *(79,81)*. NO, by blunting the activity of the nuclear factor-κB family of transcription factors *(82,83)*, can prevent the endothelial expression of adhesion molecules and inflammatory cytokines that are responsible for atherogenesis *(84)*.

3.2.3. Polymorphisms and Coronary Atherothrombosis

The T-786 eNOS genotype has recently been reported in the GENICA Study as a novel risk factor for coronary artery disease in Caucasian patients *(73)*. NO, a major mediator of endothelium-dependent vasodilation made in the endothelium by eNOS, not only plays a key role in the regulation of vascular tone *(73,78)* and blood pressure, but is also involved in atherogenesis *(73,79,80,85)*. Although the GENICA study was limited—it was only conducted in male Caucasians—the findings in other populations from other countries and in females might be different. The T-786 and Glu298Asp polymorphisms of the endothelial NO gene affect the forearm blood flow responses of Caucasian patients with hypertension *(86)*.

3.2.3.1. Increased Low-Density Lipoprotein Cholesterol and Coronary Artery Disease

Low-density lipoprotein (LDL), the major cholesterol-carrying lipoprotein in plasma, is a causal agent in coronary heart disease. Hepatic LDL receptor (LDLR) activity normally clears the LDL from the plasma. Monogenic diseases may impair the activity of LDLR, causing elevated plasma levels of LDL. Familial hypercholesterolemia, a monogenic disorder causing elevated plasma LDL, is a result of a deficit in the LDLRs. More than 600 mutations have been identified in the LDLR gene in patients with familial hypercholesterolemia *(87)*. One in 500 patients with hypercholesterolemia are heterozygous for at least one such mutation and produce half the normal number of LDLRs, resulting in a two- to threefold increase in LDL levels. By contrast, one in a million patients is homozygous at a single locus, resulting in 6–10 times normal LDL levels, and develops severe coronary atherosclerosis and dies in childhood from acute myocardial infarction.

Other monogenic diseases that elevate plasma levels of LDL include familial ligand–defective apolipoprotein B-100, autosomal recessive hypercholesterolemia, and sitosterolemia. Mutations in the APOB-100 gene encoding apolipoprotein B-100 slow the clearance of plasma LDL by reducing the binding of apolipoprotein B-100 to LDLRs and mutation is designated familial ligand-defective apolipoprotein B-100 *(88)*. Sitosterolemia, an autosomal disorder, results from mutations in genes encoding two adenosine triphosphate (ATP)-binding-cassette (ABC) transporters, ABC G5 and ABC G8, that export cholesterol into the intestinal lumen and limit cholesterol absorption *(89, 90)*. Various mutations of APOA1-CIII-A1V gene (locus 11q23), a few mutations of cholesterol ester transfer protein (CETP) gene (locus 16q22), and mutations of lecithin cholesteryl acyltransferase (LCAT) gene (locus 16q22) cause a decrease in high-density lipoprotein levels. E2/E3/E4 polymorphism of ApoE (and C1, CII) gene (locus 19p13.3) results in increased levels of LDL and very LDL. However, KIV repeats of Apo(a) gene (locus 6q26) cause increased levels of Lipoprotein (a).

3.2.3.2. VASCULAR HOMEOSTASIS AND CORONARY ARTERY DISEASE

The A/b and Gln298Asp, I/D, C1166A, and M235T polymorphisms of ENOS, ACE, AT1, and AGT genes, respectively, have been identified. Whereas the ACE (locus 17q23) and AGT (locus 1q42) polymorphisms cause increased levels of ACE and (angiotensinogen) AGT, the functions of AT1 (locus 3q22) and ENOS (locus7q35-36) polymorphisms are unknown. Recent studies have shown an association between SNP in the promoter region of ABC transporter (ABCA1) gene and increasing severity and progression of coronary atherosclerosis *(91)*. The CYB gene is involved in maintaining a balance between oxidation and reduction in the vessel wall. CYBA gene codes for p22[phox] protein, a component of the plasma membrane–associated enzyme NADPH oxidase, a precursor to potent oxidants and an important source of superoxide anion. The P22 [phox] protein with gp91 forms a membrane-bound flavocytochrome b558 and is essential for NADPH-dependent oxygen free-radical production in the vessel wall. The Lipoprotein Coronary Atherosclerosis Study evaluated the association between the 242C/T variant of CYBA and the severity and progression of atherosclerosis and concluded that in the placebo group, subjects with mutation had more promotion and less regression of atherosclerosis and a three- to fivefold greater loss in minimum lumen diameter. Furthermore, variants of p22[phos] were involved in progression of coronary atherosclerosis *(91,92)*.

3.2.4. Genomics and Hypertension

In the United States alone, there are approx 62 million people with cardiovascular disease and 50 million with hypertension *(93)*. Hypertension, a polygenic disease, is a risk factor for cardiac morbidity and causes cardiac hypertrophy that results in sudden cardiac death. The susceptibility genes for hypertension interact with the environment and, because they are age dependent, manifest in 20–30% of the population in their elderly years. Recently, a missense mutation (leucine substituted for serine at codon 810) was identified in the mineralocorticoid receptor (MR) in a family with early onset of hypertension, decreased plasma renin activity, decreased serum aldosterone, and no other etiology of hypertension *(94)*. As a result, the receptor with the mutation activates itself without the need for 21-hydroxylase stimulation. Spironolactone instead of blocking the mineralocorticoid activity further activates it. Pregnant patients who develop hypertension may experience a serious consequence of preeclampsia or eclampsia. Normally, progesterone does not activate the MR. However, in patients with this mutation, progesterone activates the MR, resulting in increased levels of progesterone and hypertension. These patients also have decreased serum potassium and aldosterone. Spironolactone in these cases increases the hypertension-caused preeclampsia. Identification of the susceptibility genes is very important and will help in the prevention and treatment of hypertension *(94)*.

Other monogenic diseases that elevate blood pressure include glucocorticoid-remediable aldosteronism, apparent mineralocorticoid excess, hypertension exacerbated by pregnancy, and Liddle syndrome. Monogenic diseases that decrease blood pressure include aldosterone synthase deficiency; 21-hydroxylase deficiency; and pseudohypoaldosteronism type 1, both autosomal dominant and recessive forms. Monogenic diseases that cause normal or decreased blood pressure include Gitelman syndrome and Bartter syndrome *(95)*.

3.3. Familial Cardiovascular Disorders

Several of the cardiovascular disorders are familial, and for most of them, the chromosomal location has been mapped but the gene has not been identified. The broad categories of diseases in this group include the cardiomyopathies, cardiac septal defects, aortic diseases, conduction disorders, ventricular arrhythmias, and atrial arrhythmias.

3.3.1. Cardiomyopathies

3.3.1.1. FAMILIAL HYPERTROPHIC CARDIOMYOPATHY

Familial hypertrophic cardiomyopathy (FHCM) is an autosomal dominant disease characterized by an unexplained hypertrophy with minimum or no symptoms to severe heart failure and sudden cardiac death. It is the most common cause of sudden cardiac death in athletes, accounting for one-third of all sudden cardiac deaths *(96)*. The salient pathological features include myocyte hypertrophy, myocyte disarray, interstitial fibrosis, and thickening of the media of the coronary arteries *(97)*. The causal genes involved in FHCM are β-myosin heavy chain (MYH7, locus 14q12), myosin-binding protein C (MYBPC3, locus 11p11.2), cardiac troponin T (TNNT2, locus 1q32), α-tropomyosin (TPM1, locus 15q22.1), cardiac troponin I (TNN13, locus 19p13.2), essential myosin light chain (MYL3, locus 3p21.3), regulatory myosin light chain (MYL2, locus 12q23-24.3), cardiac α-actin (ACTC, locus 15q11), titin (TTN, locus 2q24.1), α-myosin heavy chain (MYH6, locus 14q1), and cardiac-troponin C (TNNC1, locus 3p21.3-3p14.3). Genetic animal models of FHCM treated with losartan or simvastatin have shown a reversal of the fibrosis, hypertrophy, and phenotype. Tissue Doppler echocardiography can diagnose FHCM in humans and in animal models before the development of cardiac hypertrophy.

3.3.1.2. DILATED CARDIOMYOPATHY

Dilated cardiomyopathy (DCM) is a primary disease of the myocardium characterized by a decreased left ventricular ejection fraction and an increased left ventricular cavity. It is clinically manifested by heart failure, syncope cardiac arrhythmias, and sudden cardiac death. The etiology of DCM is both familial (autosomal dominant) and a sporadic disease. Although in approximately half of all cases of familial DCM, the chromosomal loci have been mapped, in a significant number of families the genes have not been identified. DCM, with a diversity in causal genes and mutations, is a heterogeneous disease. The causal genes in most cases code for proteins that either are components of the mitochondrial cytoskeleton or support it. The genetic causes of DCM include genes such as cardiac α-actin (ACTC, locus 15q11-14), β-myosin heavy chain (MYH7, locus 14q11-13), cardiac troponin T (TNNT2, locus 1q32), δ-sarcoglycan (SGCD, locus 5q33-34), dystrophin (DMD, locus Xp21), Lamin A/C (LMNA, locus 1p21.2), taffazin (G4.5) (TAZ, locus Xq28), desmin (DES, locus 2q35), αβ-crystallin (CRYAB, locus 11q35), and desmoplakin (DSP, locus 6p23-25).

3.3.1.3. Arrhythmogenic Right Ventricular Dysplasia

Arrhythmogenic right ventricular dysplasia (ARVD), also known as arrhythmogenic right ventricular hypertrophy, is a primary disorder of the myocardium with progressive loss of myocytes, fatty infiltration, and fibrosis in the right ventricle. The right ventricle is arrhythmogenic and causes arrhythmias. In advanced cases, both ventricles may be involved, resulting in heart failure. Mapped loci for ARVD include 14q23-q24 (ARVD1); 1q42-q43 (ARVD2), identified as the cardiac ryanodine receptor gene (RYR2) *(98)*; 14q12-q22 (ARVD3); 2q32-q32.3 (ARVD4); 3p23 (ARVD5); and 10p14-p12 (ARVD6).

3.3.2. Cardiac Septal Defects

The genetic loci for cardiac septal defects such as Holt-Oram syndrome (12q2), DiGeorge syndrome (22q), and Noonan syndrome (12q) have been mapped.

3.3.3. Aortic Diseases

The genetic loci for aneurysms (11q23-24), supravalvular aortic disease (9q), and Marfan syndrome (15q) have been mapped.

3.3.4. Conduction Disorders

The genetic locus for familial heart block was mapped as 19q13, 1q32.

3.3.5. Ventricular Arrhythmias

The genetic loci for long QT syndrome (3p21, 4q24, 7q35, 11p15, 21q22), Brugada syndrome (3p21), and idiopathic ventricular tachycardia (3p21) have been mapped. The SCN5A gene encoding α-subunits that forms the sodium channels initiates cardiac action potentials. Familial forms of ventricular arrhythmias such as long QT syndrome, ventricular fibrillation, and cardiac-conduction disease result from mutations in SCN5A *(99–103)*. Mutations in KVLQT1, HERG, mink, and MiRP-1 result in long QT syndrome. Polymorphisms associated with long QT syndrome may increase the risk of drug-induced arrhythmias *(104)*.

3.3.6. Atrial Arrhythmias

The genetic loci for Wolf-Parkinson-White syndrome (7q3) and atrial fibrillation (9q) have been mapped.

3.3.7. Genomics and Devices

Genomics, besides having a role in therapeutics, will also impact strategies to treat patients with devices serving as endovascular therapies. Restenosis following percutaneous interventions is a major problem Identification of genetic markers of restenosis would enable effective treatment strategies. Various clinically relevant genetic polymorphisms for restenosis include insertion/deletion polymorphism of angiotensin converting enzyme (ACE) gene, apolipoprotein E gene, platelet glycoprotein receptor genes, and interleukin-1 receptor antagonist gene. Strategies involving targeting of vascular growth factors, transcription factors, cell-cycle regulators, and so on serve as experimental approaches in the treatment of restenosis and in-stent restenosis. Sirolimus-coated stents have been shown to be safe and effective in inhibiting neointimal hyperplasia in patients with stable and unstable angina *(106)*. Sirolimus binds to its cytosolic receptor, FK-binding protein-12, through an unknown pathway.

4. Conclusion

Implications of the mapping of the human genome involve identification of the genes responsible for familial cardiac disorders. Given that genetic diagnosis and management will be routinely incorporated into the cardiology practice by the end of the 2000s *(107)*, a better understanding of the etiology and pathogenesis of genetic disorders will improve the prevention, diagnosis, and management of these disorders. Molecular genetics will, therefore, provide a new paradigm in the diagnosis and management of cardiovascular diseases. With 62 million people in the United States with cardiovascular disease and 50 million people with hypertension, there were approx 946,000 deaths in the year 2000 owing to cardiovascular disease, accounting for 39% of all deaths *(93, 108)*. The NHLBI has launched 11 PGAs to advance functional genomic research in the disciplines of heart, lung, blood, and sleep disorders. The basic goal is to link genes to structure, function, dysfunction, and structural abnormalities of the cardiovascular system caused by genetic and environmental stimuli.

References

1. Department of Health and Human Services, National Institutes of Health. (2000) Disease-specific estimates of direct and indirect costs of illness and NIH support, and HHS and National Costs for 13 Diseases and Conditions (House Report 106-370), February, 2000.
2. Silverstein, M. D., Heit, J. A., Mohr, D. N., Petterson, T. M., O'Fallon, W. M., and Melton, L. J. (1998) Trends in the incidence of deep vein thrombosis and pulmonary embolism: a 25-year population-based study. *Arch. Intern. Med.* **158,** 585–593.
3. Rosendal, F. R. (1999) Venous thrombosis: a multicausal disease. *Lancet* **353,** 1167–1173.
4. McCarthy, J. J. and Hilfiger, R. (2000) The use of single nucleotide polymorphisms maps in pharmacogenomics. *Nat. Biotechnol.* **18,** 505–508.
5. Krynetski, E. Y. and Evans, W. E. (1999) Pharmacogenetics as a molecular basis of individualized drug therapy: the thiopurine-S-methyltransferase paradigm. *Pharm. Res.* **16,** 342–349.

6. Drazen, J. M., Yandava, C. N., Dube, L., et al. (1999) Pharmacogenetic association between ALOX5 promoter genotype and the response to asthma treatment. *Nat. Genet.* **22**, 168–170.
7. Collins, F. S. (1992) Positional cloning: let's not call it reverse anymore. *Nat. Genet.* **1**, 3–6.
8. Chasman, D. and Adams, R. M. (2001) Predicting the functional consequences of nonsynonymous single nucleotide polymorphisms: structure-based assessment of amino acid variation. *J. Mol. Biol.* **307**, 683–706.
9. Humphries, S. E., Ye, S., Talmud, P., Bara, L., Wilhelmsen, L., and Tiret, L. (1995) European Atherosclerosis Research Study: genotype at the fibrinogen locus (G-455-Aβ-gene) is associated with differences in plasma fibrinogen levels in young men and women from different regions in Europe: evidence for gender-genotype environment interaction. *Arterioscler. Thromb. Vasc. Biol.* **15**, 96–104.
10. Nishiuma, S., Kario, K., Yakushijin, K., et al. (1998) Genetic variation in the promoter of the β-fibrinogen gene is associated with ischemic stroke in a Japanese population. *Blood Coagulation Fibrinolysis* **9**, 373–379.
11. Muzbeck, L., Adany, R., and Mikkola, H. (1996) Novel aspects of blood coagulation Factor XIII. I. Structure, distribution, activation and function. *Crit. Rev. Clin. Lab. Sci.* **33**, 357–421.
12. De Backer, G., De Henauw, S., Sans, S., et al. (1999) A comparison of lifestyle, genetic, bioclinical and biochemical variables of offspring with and without family histories of premature coronary heart disease: the experience of the European Atherosclerosis Research Studies. *J. Cardiovasc. Risk* **6**, 183–188.
13. Carter, A. M., Mansfield, M. W., Strickland, M. H., and Grant, P. J. (1996) Beta-fibrinogen gene-455 G/A polymorphism and fibrinogen levels: risk factors for coronary artery disease in subjects with NIDDM. *Diabetes Care* **19**, 1265–1268.
14. Carter, A. M., Ossei-Gerning, N., Wilson, I. J., and Grant, P. J. (1997) Association pf the platelet P(A) polymorphism of the glycoprotein Iib/IIIa and the fibrinogen Bbeta 448 polymorphism with myocardial infarction and extent of coronary artery disease. *Circulation* **96**, 1424–1431.
15. Gensini, G. F., Comeglio, M., and Colella, A. (1998) Classical risk factors and emerging elements in the risk profile for coronary artery disease. *Eur. Heart J.* **19(Suppl. A),** A53–A61.
16. Schmidt, H., Schmidt, R., Niederkorn, K., et al. (1998) Beta-fibrinogen gene polymorphism (C148→T) is associated with carotid atherosclerosis: results of the Austrian Stroke Prevention Study. *Arterioscler. Thromb. Vasc. Biol.* **18**, 487–492.
17. Kessler, C., Spitzer, C., Strauske, D., et al. (1997) The apolipoprotein E and beta-fibrinogen G/A-455 gene polymorphism are associated with ischemic stroke involving the large vessel disease. *Arterioscler. Thromb. Vasc. Biol.* **17**, 2880–2884.
18. de Maat, M. P., Kastelein, J. J., Jukema, J. W., et al. (1998) −455G/A polymorphism of the beta-fibrinogen gene is associated with the progression of coronary atherosclerosis in symptomatic men: proposed role for an acute-phase reaction pattern of fibrinogen. REGRESS group. *Arterioscler. Thromb. Vasc. Biol.* **18**, 265–271.
19. Behague, I., Poirier, O., Nicaud, V., et al. (1996) Beta fibrinogen gene polymorphisms are associated with plasma fibrinogen and coronary artery disease in patients with myocardial infarction. The ECTIM Study: Etude Cas-Temoins sur l'Infarctus du Myocarde. *Circulation* **93**, 440–449.
20. Wang, X. L., Wang, J., McCredie, R. M., and Wilcken, D. E. (1997) Polymorphisms of factor V, factor VII, and fibrinogen genes: relevance to severity of coronary artery disease. *Arterioscler. Thromb. Vasc. Biol.* **17**, 246–251.

21. Poort, S. R., Rosendaal, F. R., Reitsma, P. H., and Bertina, R. M. (1996) A common genetic variation in the 3'-untranslated region of the prothrombin gene is associated with elevated plasma prothrombin levels and an increase in venous thrombosis. *Blood* **88,** 3698–3703.

22. Hillarp, A., Zoller, B., Svenson, P. J., and Dahlback, B. (1997) The 20210 allele of the prothrombin gene is a common risk factor among Swedish outpatients with verified venous thrombosis. *Thromb. Haemost.* **78,** 990–992.

23. Rosendaal, F. R., Siscovick, D. S., Schwartz, S. M., Psaty, B. M., Raghunathan, T. E., and Vos, H. L. (1997) A common prothrombin variant (20210 G to A) increases the risk of myocardial infarction in young women. *Blood* **90,** 1747–1750.

24. Ferraresi, P., Marchetti, G., Legnani, C., et al. (1997) The heterozygous 20210 G/A prothrombin genotype is associated with early venous thrombosis in inherited thrombophilias and is not increased in frequency in artery disease. *Arterioscler. Thromb. Vasc. Biol.* **17,** 2418–2422.

25. Zoller, B., Svensson, P. J., Dhalback, B., and Hillarp, A. (1998) The 20210 allele of prothrombin gene is frequently associated with the factor V Arg 506 to Gln mutation is not with protein S deficiency in thrombophilic families. *Blood* **91,** 2209–2211.

26. Ehrenforth, S., Ludwig, G., Klinke, S., Krause, M., Scharre, I., and Nowak-Gottl, U. (1998) The prothrombin 20210 A allele is frequently coinherited in young carriers of the factor B Arg 506 to Gln mutation with venous thrombophilia. *Blood* **91,** 2209, 2210.

27. Howard, T. E., Marusa, M., Boisza, J., et al. (1998) The prothrombin gene 3'-untranslated region mutation is frequently associated with factor V Leiden in thrombophilic patients and shows ethnic specific variation in allele frequency. *Blood* **91,** 1092.

28. Silver, D. and Vouyouka, A. (2000) The Caput medusae of hypercoagulability. *J. Vasc. Surg.* **31,** 396–405.

29. Manoussakis, M. N., Tziofas, A. G., Silis, M. P., Pange, P. J., Goudevenous, J., and Moutsopoulos, H. M. (1987) High prevalence of anti-cardiolipin and other autoantibodies in a healthy elderly population. *Clin. Exp. Immunol.* **69,** 557–565.

30. Lechner, K. and Pabinger-Fasching, I. (1985) Lupus anticoagulant and thrombosis: a study of 25 cases and review of the literature. *Haemostasis* **15,** 254–262.

31. Manucci, P. M. (2000) The molecular basis of inherited thrombophilia. *Vox. Sang.* **78 (Suppl. 2),** 39–45.

32. Foka, Z. J., Lambropoulos, A. F., Saravelos, H., et al. (2000) Factor V Leiden and prothrombin G20210 mutations but no methylenetetrahydrofolate reductase C677T are associated with recurrent miscarriages. *Hum. Reprod.* **15,** 458–462.

33. Amitrano, L., Brancaccio, V., Guardascione, M. A., et al. (2000) Inherited coagulation disorders in cirrhotic patients with portal vein thrombosis. *Hepatology* **31,** 345–348.

34. Ekberg, H., Svensson, P. J., Simanaiteis, M., and Dahlback, B. (2000) Factor V R506q mutation (activated protein C resistance) is additional risk factor for early renal graft loss associated with acute vascular rejection. *Transplantation* **69,** 1577–1581.

35. Rees, D. C., Cox, M., and Clegg, J. B. (1995) World distribution of Factor V Leiden. *Lancet* **346,** 1133–1134.

36. Iacovelli, L., Di Castelnuovo, A., de Knijiff, P., et al. (1996) Alu-repeat polymorphism in the tissue-type plasminogen activator (tPA) gene, tPA levels and risk of familial myocardial infarction (MI). *Fibrinolysis* **10,** 13–16.

37. Furie, B. and Burie, B. C. (1992) Molecular and cellular biology of blood coagulation. *N. Engl. J. Med.* **326,** 800–806.

38. Wartiovaara, U., Mikkola, H., Szoke, G., et al. (2000) Effect of Val34Leu polymorphism on the activation of the coagulation Factor XIIIa. *Thromb. Haemost.* **84,** 595–600.

39. Ariens, R. A. S., Philippou, H., Nagaswami, C., Weisel, J. W., Lane, D. A., and Grant, P. J. (2000) The Factor XIII V34L polymorphism accelerates thrombin activation of Factor XIII and affects crosslinked fibrin structure. *Blood* **96,** 988–995.

40. Kohler, H. P., Stickland, M. H., Ossei-Gernig, N., Carter, A., Mikkola, H., and Grant, P. J. (1998) Association of a common polymorphism in the Factor XIII gene with myocardial infarction. *Thromb. Haemost.* **79,** 8–13.

41. Wartiovaara, U., Perola, M., Mikkola, H., et al. (1999) Association of Factor XIII Va34Leu with decrease risk of myocardial infarction in Finnish males. *Atherosclerosis* **142,** 295–300.

42. Doggen, C. J. M., Kunz, G., Rosebdaal, F. R., et al. (1998) A mutation in the thrombomodulin gene, 127G to A coding for Ala25Thr and the risk of myocardial infarction in men. *Thromb. Haemost.* **80,** 743–748.

43. Li, Y. H., Chen, J. H., Wu, H. L., et al. (2000) G-33A mutation in the promoter region of thrombomodulin gene and its association with coronary artery disease and plasma soluble thrombomodulin levels. *Am. J. Cardiol.* **85,** 8–12.

44. Li, Y. H., Chen, C. H., Yeh, P. S., et al. (2001) Functional mutation in the promoter region of thrombomodulin gene in relation to carotid atherosclerosis. *Atherosclerosis* **154,** 713–719.

45. Kleesiek, K., Schmidt, M., Gotting, C., Brinkman, T., and Prohaska, W. (1998) A first mutation in the human tissue factor pathway inhibitor gene encoding [P151L] TFPI. *Blood* **92,** 3976–3977.

46. Moatti, D., Seknadji, P., Galand, C., et al. (1999) Polymorphisms of the tissue factor pathway inhibitor (TFPI) gene in patients with acute coronary syndromes and in healthy subjects: impact of the V264M substitution on plasma levels of TFPI. *Arterioscler. Thromb. Vasc. Biol.* **19,** 862–869.

47. Kleesiek, K., Schmidt, M., Gotting, C., et al. (1999) The 536C→T transition in the human tissue factor pathway inhibitor (TFPI) gene is statistically associated with a higher risk for venous thrombosis. *Thromb. Haemost.* **82,** 1–5.

48. Moatti, D., Haidar, B., Fumeron, F., et al. (2000) A new T-287C polymorphism in the 5' regulatory region of the tissue factor pathway inhibitor gene: association study of the T-287C and C-399T polymorphisms with coronary artery disease and plasma TFPI levels. *Thromb. Haemost.* **84,** 244–249.

49. Ameziane, N., Seguin, C., Borgel, D., et al. (2002) The –33T→C polymorphism in intron 7 of the TFPI gene influences the risk of venous thromboembolism: independently of the Factor V Leiden and prothrombin mutations. *Thromb. Haemost.* **88,** 195–199.

50. Merati, G. B., Biguzzi, F., Oganesyan, N., et al. (1999) A 23bp insertion in the endothelial protein C receptor (EPCR) gene in patients with myocardial infarction in deep vein thrombosis. *Thromb. Haemost.* **82,** 507.

51. Brattstrom, L., Isrealsson, B., Norrving, B., et al. (1990) Impaired homocysteine metabolism in early-onset cerebral and peripheral occlusive arterial disease. Effects of pyridoxine and folic acid treatment. *Atherosclerosis* **81,** 51–60.

52. Dudman, N. P., Wilcken, D. E., Wang, J., et al. (1993) Disordered methionine/homocysteine metabolism in premature vascular disease: its occurrence, cofactor therapy and enzymology. *Arterioscler. Thromb.* **13,** 1253–1260.

53. Boers, G. H. (1989) Carriership for momocystinuria in juvenile vascular disease. *Haemostasis* **19(Suppl. 1),** 29–34.

54. Brattstrom, L. E., Hardebo, J. E., and Hultberg, B. L. (1984) Moderate homocysteinemia —a possible risk factor for arteriosclerotic cerebrovascular disease. *Stroke* **15,** 1012–1016.

55. Bienvenu, T., Ankri, A., Chadefaux, B., et al. (1993) Elevated total plasma homocyteine, a risk factor for thrombosis: relation to coagulation and fibrinolytic parameters. *Thromb. Res.* **70,** 123–129.
56. Florell, S. R. and Rodgers, G. M. (1997) Inherited thrombotic disorders: an update. *Am. J. Haematol.* **54,** 53–60.
57. Simioni, P., Prandoni, P., Burlina, A., et al. (1996) Hyperhomocystinemia and deep vein thrombosis: a case-control study. *Thromb. Haemost.* **76,** 883–886.
58. Selhub, J., Jaques, P. F., Wilson, P. W., et al. (1993) Vitamin status and intake as primary determinants of homocysteinemia in an elderly population. *JAMA* **270,** 2693–2698.
59. Afshar-Kharghan, V., Khoshnevis-Als, M., and Lopez, J. (1999) A Kozak sequence polymorphism is a major determinant of the surface levels of a platelet adhesion receptor. *Blood* **94(1),** 186–191.
60. Anderson, J. L., King, G. J., Bair, T. L., et al. (1999) Associations between a polymorphism in the gene encoding of glycoprotein IIIa gene in patients with coronary artery disease. *J. Am. Coll. Cardiol.* **33,** 727–733.
61. Garcia-Ribes, M., Gonzales-Lamuno, D., Hernandez-Estefania, R., et al. (1998) Polymorphism of the platelet glycoprotein IIIa gene in patients with coronary stenosis. *Thromb. Haemost.* **79,** 1126–1129.
62. Kastrati, A., Schomig, A., Seyfarth, M., et al. (1999) PIA polymorphism of platelet glycoprotein IIIa and risk of restenosis after coronary stent placement. *Circulation* **99,** 1005–1010.
63. Goldmuntz, E., Clark, B. J., Mitchell, L. E., et al. (1998) Frequency of 22q11 deletions in patients with conotruncal defects. *J. Am. Coll. Cardiol.* **32,** 492–498.
64. Momma, K., Kondo, C., Matsuoka, R., and Tkao, A. (1996) Cardiac anomalies associated with a chromosome 22q11 deletion in patients with conotruncal anomaly face syndrome. *Am. J. Cardiol.* **78,** 591–594.
65. Seaver, L. H., Pierpont, J. W., Erickson, R. P., et al. (1994) Pulmonary atresia associated with maternal 22q11.2 deletion: possible parent of origin effect in the conotruncal anomaly face syndrome. *J. Med. Genet.* **31,** 830–834.
66. Hofbeck, M., Rauch, A., Buheitel, G., et al. (1998) Monosomy 22q11 in patients with pulmonary atresia, ventricular septal defect, and major aortopulmonary collateral arteries. *Heart* **79,** 180–185.
67. Hubert, R. S., Mitchell, S., Chen, X. N., et al. (1997) BAC and PAC contigs covering 3.5 Mb of the Down syndrome congenital heart disease region between D21S55 and MX1 on chromosome 21. *Genomics* **41,** 218–226.
68. Korenberg, J. R., Bradley, C., and Disteche, C. M. (1992) Down syndrome: molecular mapping of the congenital heart disease and duodenal stenosis. *Am. J. Hum. Genet.* **50,** 294–302.
69. Nadal, M., Mila, M., Pritchard, M., et al. (1996) YAC and cosmid FISH mapping of an unbalanced chromosomal translocation causing partial trisomy 21 and Down's syndrome. *Hum. Genet.* **98,** 460–466.
70. Del Rio, T., Urban, Z., Csiszar, K., and Boyd, C. D. (1998) A gene-dosage PCR method for the detection of elastin gene deletions in patients with Williams syndrome. *Clin. Genet.* **54,** 129–135.
71. Urban, Z., Kiss, E., Kadar, K., et al. (1997) Genetic diagnosis of Williams syndrome. *Orvi. Hetil.* **138,** 1749–1752.
72. Tynan, K., Comeau, K., Pearson, M., et al. (1993) Mutation screening of complete fibrillin-1 coding sequence: report of five new mutations, including two in 8-cysteine domains. *Hum. Mol. Genet.* **2,** 1813–1821.

73. Rossi, G. P., Cesari, M., Zanchetta, M., Colonna, S., et al. (2003) The T-786C endothelial nitric oxide synthase genotype is a novel risk factor for coronary artery disease in Caucasian patients of the Genica study. *J. Am. Coll. Cardiol.* **41,** 930–937.

74. Linder, L., Kiowski, W., Buhler, F. R., and Luscher, T. F. (1990) Indirect evidence for release of endothelium-derived relaxing factor in human forearm circulation in vivo: blunted response in essential hypertension. *Circulation* **81,** 1762–1767.

75. Celemajer, D. S., Sorensen, K. E., Spiegelhalter, D. J., et al. (1994) Aging is associated with endothelial dysfunction in healthy men years before the age-related decline in women. *J. Am. Coll. Cardiol.* **24,** 471–476.

76. Luscher, T. F., Tanner, F. C., Tschudi, M. R., et al. (1993) Endothelial dysfunction in coronary artery disease. *Annu. Rev. Med.* **44,** 395–418.

77. Al Suwaidi, J., Hamasaki, S., Higano, S. T., et al. (2000) Long-term follow-up of patients with mild coronary artery disease and endothelial dysfunction. *Circulation* **101,** 848–854.

78. Huang, P. L., Huang, Z., Mashimo, H., et al. (1995) Hypertension in mice lacking the gene for endothelial nitric oxide synthase. *Nature* **377,** 239–242.

79. Shesely, E. G., Maeda, N., Kim, H. S., et al. (1996) Elevated blood pressures in mice lacking endothelial nitric oxide synthase. *Proc. Natl. Acad. Sci. USA* **93,** 13,176–13,181.

80. Aji, W., Ravalli, S., Szabolcs, M., et al. (1997) L-Arginine prevents xanthoma development and inhibits atherosclerosis in LDL receptor knockout mice. *Circulation* **95,** 430–437.

81. Feng, Q., Song, W., Lu, X., et al. (2002) Development of heart failure and congenital septal defects in mice lacking endothelial nitric oxide synthase. *Circulation* **106,** 873–879.

82. Ishizuka, T., Takamizawa-Matsumoto, M., Suzuki, K., et al. (1999) Endothelin-1 enhances vascular cell adhesion molecule-1 expression in tumour necrosis factor alpha-stimulated vascular endothelial cells. *Eur. J. Pharmacol.* **369,** 237–245.

83. Rossi, G. P., Seccia, T. M., and Nussdorfer, G. G. (2001) Reciprocal regulation of endothelin-1 and nitric oxide: relevance in the physiology and pathology of the cardiovascular system. *Int. Rev. Cytol.* **209,** 241–272.

84. Ross, R. (1999) Atherosclerosis—an inflammatory disease. *Nature* **340,** 115–126.

85. Ohashi, Y., Kawashima, S., Hirata, K., et al. (1998) Hypertension and reduced nitric oxide–elicited vasorelaxation in transgenic mice overexpressing endothelial nitric oxide synthase. *J. Clin. Invest.* **102,** 2061–2071.

86. Rossi, G. P., Taddei, S., Virdis, A., et al. (2003) The T-786 and Glu298 Asp polymorphisms of the endothelial nitric oxide gene affect the forearm blood flow responses of the Caucasian hypertensive patients. *J. Am. Coll. Cardiol.* **41,** 838–845.

87. Goldstein, J. L., Hobbs, H. H., and Brown, M. S. (2001) Familial hypercholesterolemia, in *The Metabolic & Molecular Bases of Inherited Disease*, 8th ed., vol. 2 (Scriver, C. R., Beaudet, A. L., Sly, W. S., and Valle, D., eds.), McGraw-Hill, New York, pp. 2863–2913.

88. Kane, J. P. and Havel, R. J. (2001) Disorders of the biogenesis and secretion of lipoproteins containing the B apolipoprotein, in *The Metabolic & Molecular Bases of Inherited Diseases,* 8th ed., vol. 2. (Scriver, C. R., Beaudet, A. L., Sly, W. S., and Valle, D., eds.), McGraw-Hill, New York, pp. 2717–2752.

89. Berge, K. E., Tian, H., Graf, G. A., et al. (2001) Accumulation of dietary cholesterol in sitosterolemia caused by mutations in adjacent ABC transporters. *Science* **290,** 1771–1775.

90. Lee, M. H., Lu, K., Hazzard, S., et al. (2001) Identification of a gene, ABCG5, important in the regulation dietary cholesterol absorption. *Nat. Genet.* **27,** 79–83.

91. Cahilly, C., Ballantyne, C. M., Elghannam, H., Gotto, A. M., and Marlan, A. J. (2000) Novel polymorphisms in promoter region of ATP binding cassette transporter gene and

plasma lipids, severity, progression and regression of coronary atherosclerosis. *Circ. Res.* **86,** 391–395.

92. Marian, A. J. and Roberts, R. (2003) Molecular genetics of cardiovascular disorders, in *Evidence-Based Cardiology*, 2nd ed. (Yousef, S., Cairns, J. A., Camm, A. J., Fallen, E. L., Gersh, B. J., and Books, B. M. J., eds.), BMA House, London, UK.

93. NHLBI Morbidity and Mortality Chartbook, 2002. National Heart, Lung, and Blood Institute, Bethesda, MD, May 2002 (www.nhlbi.nih.gov/resources/cht-book.htm).

94. Geller, D. S., Farhi, A., and Pinkerton, C. A. (2000) Activating mineralocorticoid receptor mutation in hypertension exacerbated by pregnancy. *Science* **289,** 119–223.

95. Nabel, E. G. (2003) Cardiovascular disease. *N. Engl. J. Med.* **349,** 60–72.

96. Maron, B. J., Shirani, J., Poliac, L. C., Mathenge, R., Roberts, W. C., and Mueller, F. O. (1996) Sudden death in young competitive athletes. Clinical, demographic and pathological profiles. *JAMA* **276,** 199–204.

97. Maron, B. J., Anan, T. J., and Roberts, W. C. (1981) Quantitative analysis of the distribution of cardiac muscle cell disorganization in the left ventricular wall of patients with hypertrophic cardiomyopathy. *Circulation* **63,** 882–894.

98. Tiso, N., Stephan, D. A., Nava, A., et al. (2001) Identification of mutations in the cardiac ryanodine receptor gene in families affected with arrhythmogenic right ventricular cardiomyopathy type 2 (ARVD2). *Hum. Mol. Genet.* **10,** 189–194.

99. Bennett, P. B., Yazawa, K., Makita, N., and George, A. L. Jr. (1995) Molecular mechanism for an inherited cardiac arrhythmia. *Nature* **376,** 683–685.

100. Wang, Q., Shen, J., Splawski, I., et al. (1995) SCN5A mutations associated with an inherited cardiac arrhythmia, long QT syndrome. *Cell* **80,** 805–811.

101. Chen, Q., Kirsch, G. E., Zhang, D., et al. (1998) Genetic basis and molecular mechanism for idiopathic ventricular fibrillation. *Nature* **392,** 293–296.

102. Schott, J. J., Alshinawi, C., Kyndt, F., et al. (1999) Cardiac conduction defects associate with mutations in SCN5A. *Nat. Genet.* **23,** 20–21.

103. Tan, H. L., Bink-Boelkens, M. T., Bezzina, C. R., et al. (2001) A sodium channel mutation causes isolated cardiac conduction disease. *Nature* **409,** 1043–1047.

104. Splawski, I., Shen, J., Timothy, K. W., et al. (2000) Spectrum of mutations in long QT syndrome genes: KVLQT1, HERG, SCN5A, KCNE1 and KCNE2. *Circulation* **102,** 1178–1185.

105. Fiala, M., Popik, W., Roos, K., Cashman, J., and Arthos, J. (2003) Molecular pathogenesis of HIV cardiomyopathy and drug-induced heart disease, in *From Genome to Disease: A Symposium of High Throughput Biology*.

106. Sousa, J. E., Costa, M. A., Abizaid, A., et al. (2001) Lack of neointimal proliferation after implantation of sirolimus-coated stents in human coronary arteries: a quantitative angiography and three dimensional intravascular ultrasound study. *Circulation* **103,** 192–195.

107. Roberts, R. (2000) A perspective: the new millennium dawns on a new paradigm for cardiology—molecular genetics. *J. Am. Coll. Cardiol.* **36,** 661–667.

108. NHLBI Factbook, Fiscal Year 2002. National Heart, Lung and Blood Institute, Bethesda, MD, February 2003 (www.nhlbi.nih.gov/about/factpdf.htm.).

9

Protein Interactions Probed With Mass Spectrometry

Suma Kaveti and John R. Engen

Summary

Understanding the interactions of proteins with other proteins and/or with drug molecules is essential for understanding the progression of diseases. In this chapter, we present several methods utilizing mass spectrometry (MS) for the analysis of protein–protein, protein–drug, and protein–metal interactions. We describe the analysis of protein interactions with hydrogen exchange MS methods. Hydrogen exchange methods can be used to analyze conformational changes on binding, to estimate dissociation constants, and to locate the sites of interaction/binding between binding partners. We also discuss more direct MS methods, including the analysis of metal ion complexation with proteins.

Key Words: Hydrogen exchange; dissociation constant; conformational changes; mass spectrometry; deuterium.

1. Introduction

Mass spectrometry (MS) is a powerful technique for studying protein interactions. Only within the last 10 yr has its utility for this purpose been realized. Conventionally, analytical techniques such as nuclear magnetic resonance (NMR), X-ray crystallography, ultracentrifugation, and various spectroscopic techniques (fluorescence, circular dichroism, light scattering, surface plasmon resonance) have been used to study such interactions. Despite their specific advantages, most of these techniques require significant amounts of sample (greater than or equal to a few micromoles), which are generally difficult to obtain from real-life samples. MS, however, requires only small amounts of sample (less than or equal to nanomoles), is highly selective, and can be faster than other techniques. In this chapter, we provide examples of using MS for studying protein interactions.

Cellular functions are often a result of protein interactions with target molecules. Targets may be substrates, antibodies, other proteins, or drug molecules. For example, many cellular machines and signaling events in vivo often involve significant protein-protein interactions *(1–3)*. It is essential to know not only what the individual components

From: *Methods in Molecular Biology, vol. 316: Bioinformatics and Drug Discovery*
Edited by: R. S. Larson © Humana Press Inc., Totowa, NJ

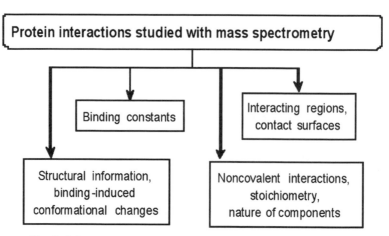

Fig. 1. Selected uses of MS for investigating protein interactions.

of protein complexes are but also their stoichiometry. It may also be necessary to determine the nature of interactions, the kinetics, and any resulting conformational changes during complex formation. MS can be used to investigate all of these areas of protein interactions (**Fig. 1**).

Many protein interactions are noncovalent interactions and can be investigated with MS if the experimental conditions favor retention of noncovalent association (*see* **Note 1**). Mass spectral peaks characteristic of the individual constituents may be observed along with those that represent complexes (**Fig. 2A,B**). The ligand in these cases may either be another protein(s) or a small molecule such as a drug compound (*see* **Subheading 3.3.**). A number of noncovalent interactions *(4–10)* have been studied with electrospray MS. The effects of pH, heat, and salt concentrations on these noncovalent complexes have also been probed *(11,12)*, as well as the stoichiometry of noncovalent macromolecular assemblies *(12)*. Matrix-assisted laser desorption ionization (MALDI) MS has been used to study noncovalent complexes as well *(13)*.

Proteolysis by specific enzymes (*see* **Note 2**) when combined with MS can provide information about interactions. The rationale behind this technique is that when a protein is bound to a ligand (**Fig. 2**, center), some of the sites or domains of the protein that were accessible to protease may be blocked in the ligand-bound form. A chemical crosslinking approach may also be used to link the interacting partners irreversibly and covalently *(14–16)*. After enzymatic digestion, peptides containing the crosslink may be observed in mass spectra (**Fig. 2E**). Using an isotope-coded affinity tag as the crosslinker, peptides can be purified selectively by biotin/avidin technology and analyzed to locate the binding surfaces directly *(17)*. A certain degree of luck is required in any crosslinking experiment because if functional groups that react with the crosslinker are not present in the interface between the protein and ligand, no meaningful crosslinking will occur.

Binding between a protein and a ligand such as a drug molecule may alter the activity of the protein such that it induces or prevents some disease condition. In addition, many

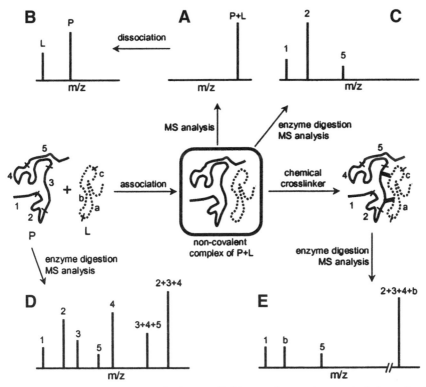

Fig. 2. Noncovalent complex analysis, crosslinking studies, and proteolysis investigations with MS. Two proteins (P and L) may associate and form a noncovalent complex (center). Direct analysis of this noncovalent complex can be accomplished with electrospray methods (*see* **Subheading 3.1.**). (**A**) Peaks corresponding to the combined mass (P + L) indicate formation of the complex. (**B**) Subsequent dissociation into the individual components verifies that the peak of P + L was indeed composed solely of P and L. In more complicated complexes involving multiple partners, dissociation can help sort out the stoichiometry. (**C, D**) Binding may alter the enzymatic digestion pattern. P can be digested into peptides 1–5 and L into peptides a, b, and c (enzyme cutting sites indicated by short, perpendicular lines). Analysis of P peptides after complex formation (**C**) is compared with the peptides produced when P was alone before complex formation (**D**). Changes to the digestion pattern can indicate which enzyme sites are occluded by complex formation. After complex formation, a chemical crosslinker may also be utilized to link covalently the two proteins together. The resulting mass spectrum (**E**) will contain peptides with m/z values of the combination of peptide(s) from P that were crosslinked to peptide(s) from L. In this example, the diagnostic peak is 2 + 3 + 4 + b. With spectra of the peptides from each protein without crosslinking, simple addition calculations of peptide masses indicates which peptides have been linked together.

protein–protein interactions that take part in cellular processes have interfaces that can be potential sites of docking for novel drug molecules that interfere with complex formation (*18*). Determining the details of protein–protein and protein–drug interactions is important. With combinatorial chemical libraries for drug molecules being generated instead of individual drug target molecules, rapid methods such as MS are necessary to identify the potential compounds for further testing *(19)*. Both electrospray and MALDI MS have been used to study protein–drug interactions *(20–23)*. MS can be used to probe noncovalent interactions between a protein and a drug molecule, the stoichiometry of such interactions, and the stability of the complex. Drug binding may interfere with proteolysis as detected by MS. Drug molecules may be crosslinked to proteins, just as a proteinaceous ligand would, and the regions of interaction identified with MS.

Drug binding to proteins may alter the structural dynamics of the protein or cause conformational changes that inactivate regular protein function. Hydrogen exchange (HX) when combined with MS (*see* **Subheading 3.2**). can provide information about structural changes occurring in proteins on drug binding. Such information is difficult to obtain with other methods. HX MS can also be used to investigate other aspects of protein–protein interactions, including multimeric states that cannot be analyzed with the previously described noncovalent methods.

A final area of protein interactions in which MS is important involves metal ion binding. Metal ions not only play many important roles in cellular processes but as part of metalloenzymes are essential for catalytic activity. There are three important aspects of studying protein interactions with metal ions, all of which can be accomplished with MS: (1) the specificity of a protein for a given metal, (2) the protein:metal stoichiometry, and (3) conformational changes of the protein on metal ion binding. Electrospray MS has been used for studying the stoichiometry of protein-metal binding for a number of proteins *(24–27)*. Conformational changes on complexation have been probed in combination with HX MS *(28,29)*, and cooperative binding has been studied *(30)*.

2. Materials

2.1. Proteins

Proteins are usually overexpressed in *Escherichia coli* and purified with classic affinity chromatography. They may also be obtained from overexpression in mammalian cells (i.e., Sf 9-baculovirus) (*see* **Note 3**).

2.2. Proteases

1. Pepsin (cat. no. P6887; Sigma-Aldrich, St. Louis, MO) immobilized on POROS-20AL beads (cat. no. 1-602906; Perseptive) (*see* **Note 4** and **Subheading 2.5., item 3**).
2. Trypsin, sequencing grade (from Sigma-Aldrich, Promega, or Roche).

2.3. Chromatography

1. Acetonitrile and water (high-performance liquid chromatography [HPLC] grade).
2. Trifluoroacetic acid (99+ purity) (Sigma-Aldrich).
3. Formic acid (ACS reagent grade) (Sigma-Aldrich).

2.4. HX MS Buffers

1. Phosphate buffers (50:50 mixture of K_2HPO_4 and KH_2PO_4): these are recommended for HX experiments because they offer good buffering capacity at the key pHs (7.0, 2.5). Citrate buffers can also be used for quenching because they provide efficient buffering at pH 2.5.

2. Deuterium chloride (DCl) and sodium deuteroxide (NaOD), obtained from Sigma-Aldrich and MDS Isotopes (Montreal, Canada), respectively. These are used for moderating the pD of labeling buffers (*see* **Note 5**).

2.5. Columns, Packing Materials, and Other Materials for Chromatography

1. Stainless steel transfer lines: These are recommended over PEEK transfer lines for efficient cooling and minimal deuterium loss in HX MS experiments (*see* **Note 6**).
2. POROS 10-R2 packing material (Perseptive Biosystems) packed into empty 254 μm id × 10 cm steel columns (Alltech, Deerfield, IL) for perfusion chromatography; MAGIC C18 (5 μ 200 Å; 1.0 × 50 mm) microbore columns or similar for conventional reverse-phase HPLC.
3. Empty stainless steel column (no. 65175; Alltech), to prepare immobilized pepsin digestion columns (*see* **Note 4**).
4. Protein (no. 004/25108/03) or peptide (no. 004/25109/02) trap columns (Michrom, Auburn, CA).

2.6. Matrices for MALDI

1. α-Hydroxy-4-cyano cinnamic acid (4HCCA), 2,5-dihydroxy benzoic acid from Sigma-Aldrich, or HP-Agilent (*see* **Note 7**).

2.7. Software for Data Processing

The data-processing software provided with each mass spectrometer is used to determine the m/z values and deconvolute charged spectra from electrospray. To determine the centroid m/z values in HX MS analyses, MagTran *(31)* can be used to calculate the center of mass of any selected isotopic distribution.

3. Methods

3.1. Direct MS Methods

An outline for studying protein interactions with other molecules by direct MS methods is given next. This outline is not meant as an exact protocol but, rather, as a guide for establishing a working method. Because each protein may behave differently, the conditions often must be determined empirically.

1. Estimate the concentrations of individual protein(s) and ligand(s) (*see* **Note 8**).
2. Incubate stoichiometric ratios of protein and the target molecules first independently and then together for 30 min at appropriate pH and in a buffer that retains protein–ligand complexation (*see* **Note 9**).
3. Analyze protein–ligand complex with either electrospray or MALDI MS. For electrospray, conditions that favor noncovalent complexes may be used. The complex may or may not hold together under the more typical acidic electrospray conditions or during MADLI crystallization *(13)*, so complex retention should be checked.
4. Establish the effect of pH, temperature, and concentration of the various constituents on the mass spectra.
5. Measure peak abundances and peak areas (particularly if an internal standard was added) for quantification.

3.2. Hydrogen Exchange Mass Spectrometry

3.2.1. General Protocol for Continuous Labeling HX

1. Estimate the concentration of the purified protein(s) (*see* **Note 8**).
2. Mix various molar ratios of protein A and protein B (or other ligands) for a final concentration of ≥150 pmol/sample after dilutions (depends on instrument sensitivity). Allow the mixture to stand for at least 10–15 min for stabilization (*see* **Note 10**).
3. Start HX by diluting the protein–protein mixture 15-fold or more with labeling buffer (i.e., 10 mM phosphate buffer, 99% D$_2$O, pD 6.60).
4. Quench HX by transferring an aliquot of labeling mixture to a vial containing quench buffer (i.e., 100 mM phosphate buffer, H$_2$O, pH 2.6) and reduce the temperature (*see* **Note 11**).
5. As unbound controls, induce HX reactions following **steps 1–4** for the protein (or proteins if the complex involves multiple proteins) alone (*see* **Note 12**).

3.2.2. Intact Protein Analysis

1. Inject quenched sample (*see* **Subheading 3.2.1.**) onto a perfusion column (10 cm × 0.254 mm id, packed with POROS 10-R2 material) or conventional reverse-phase microbore HPLC column and desalt for at least 2 to 3 min (*see* **Note 6**).
2. Run a rapid gradient of acetonitrile (30–70% of acetonitrile over 3 min) to elute the protein directly into an electrospray mass spectrometer.
3. Measure the relative deuterium uptake from the deconvoluted mass spectrum using MagTran *(31)* or the software provided with the mass spectrometer. Where necessary, only gently smooth raw data using a Savitkzy-Golay algorithm. Mass accuracy should be, in general, ±1 Dalton.

3.2.3. Peptide Analysis

1. For an on-line proteolytic digestion, allow the protein from **step 4** or **5** in **Subheading 3.2.1.** to pass through an immobilized pepsin column (*see* **Note 6**). Collect the resulting peptides on an in-line peptide trap and wash for 2 to 3 min (*see* **Note 13**).
2. For an off-line digestion with pepsin, incubate quenched protein from **step 4** or **5** in **Subheading 3.2.1.** with pepsin (usually 1:1 [w/w] ratio) for a maximum of 5 min, and inject the resulting peptides directly onto the separation column of the HPLC (*see* **Note 14**).
3. Separate the peptic peptides with a 4 to 5-min gradient of 5–60% acetonitrile. The peptides are eluted directly into the mass spectrometer (*see* **Note 15**).
4. Analyze the deuterium uptake of each peptide with a method similar to that used for intact protein in **Subheading 3.2.2.**, **step 3**. Mass accuracy should be ±0.25 Daltons for peptides.

3.2.4. HX MS for Titrations

1. Follow **steps 1–5** in **Subheading 3.2.1.** to prepare proteins.
2. Analyze as in section **Subheading 3.2.2.** or **3.2.3.**
3. Plot the relative deuterium uptake vs time.
4. Choose a time point at which the HX is maximally affected (*see* **Subheading 3.4.2.** and **Fig. 5A**).
5. Using the time determined in **step 4** as the labeling time, change the ratio of protein:ligand and repeat **steps 1–3**. It is easiest to hold one protein concentration constant while changing the other.

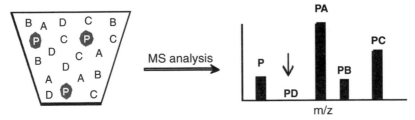

Fig. 3. Measuring binding of a protein to various ligands. The protein (P) is mixed with four ligands (A, B, C, D). The ligands may be drug molecules, metal ions, peptides, or other proteins. The affinities follow the order A > C > B >> D. The ligands may be either drug molecules or metal ions. After mass spectrometric analysis, the peak intensity is a reflection of which ligand has bound to the protein. In this example, the protein (P) showed highest affinity for ligand A, followed by C and B, with no affinity for D. The peak corresponding to protein–ligand D complex (PD) is negligible, and the arrow indicates where it is expected.

6. Observe the effect of changing the relative protein concentration(s) on the deuterium uptake, and prepare a plot of the relative concentration vs deuterium level for the whole protein, or for a diagnostic peptide.

3.3. Protein–Drug Interactions

Studying protein–drug interactions using mass spectral techniques involves finding lead drug molecules from a mixture of analogs or combinatorial libraries that bind to the target protein, determining the affinity of the protein–drug complex, and analyzing the conformational changes of the protein on drug binding. This information may provide a better understanding of the interaction, leading to more efficient drug development.

3.3.1. Determination of Drug Binding to Target Proteins

A generalized approach of determining whether or not a small-molecule drug will bind to a protein of interest includes a procedure similar to that in **Subheading 3.1.** wherein the ligand is replaced with a drug molecule(s). The mass spectrometer can differentiate components of mixtures by mass and, thus, is used to identify protein–drug complexes simultaneously in both bound and unbound forms. The presence or absence of peaks corresponding to protein–drug complexes under native conditions reflects the affinity of drug molecule(s) for the given protein. As illustrated by the example in **Fig. 3**, protein P has the highest affinity for drug A and no affinity at all for drug D. MALDI, with its high sensitivity and fast analysis time, can be used for quick screening of proteins against combinatorial libraries containing thousands of potential drug molecules. Such studies have been reported for affinity ranking of drug ligands for proteins *(22)*. A number of groups have also used separation and preconcentration of bound and unbound protein–drug molecules based on size; affinity; or ion mobility chromatographic techniques such as size exclusion, gel filtration, and electrophoresis followed by mass spectral analysis *(22,23,32)*.

3.3.2. Determination of Binding Affinity

In principle, binding constants for protein–drug (or any other ligand, including another protein) complexes are measures of the strength of the complex and are generally expressed in terms of the molar concentration of drug/ligand with respect to the protein ($K_d = [P][L]/[C]$, in which P = is the protein concentration, L is the free ligand concentration, and C is the concentration of the complex). Mass spectral peak areas of P, L, and C give a rough estimate of the concentrations in solution. There are, however, pitfalls associated with using these values to determine the K_d that should be considered when making such a measurement. One important aspect is mutual ion suppression effects in mixtures, especially in the case of electrospray *(33,34)*. To combat this, it may be necessary to screen each potential compound individually in addition to screening mixtures of potential compounds. In addition, highly accurate mass spectral quantification requires an internal standard. This point is usually minor because the interesting information is the relative affinity of several compounds and not the absolute affinity of one compound. Finally, concentration information alone does not provide any information about the nature of interactions taking place, which is critical to improving the binding ability of the molecule.

The affinity of a protein–ligand complex can also be estimated with HX methods. HX MS can provide simultaneous information about where the interaction occurs on the protein and reveal any conformational changes taking place within the protein on binding. Detailed aspects of these types of experiments are discussed further in the next section for protein–protein complexes but are equally applicable to protein–drug interactions.

In summary, as applied to protein–drug interactions, the drug/ligand is titrated against a constant amount of protein. For concentrations at which there is a change in the HX behavior of the protein, the approximate K_d value can be extracted *(35)*.

3.4. Protein Interactions Probed With HX MS

HX when used in combination with MS provides many details about the structural changes of individual proteins as well as proteins in complex. As already mentioned, it can be used to locate sites of drug–protein interaction and to investigate structural changes on drug binding. The number of hydrogens, particularly the backbone amide hydrogens, that can be exchanged with hydrogens from the solvent is related to the structure of the protein. Two main parameters that alter the rate of the exchange reaction are hydrogen bonding and solvent accessibility. If either of these are altered during protein–protein interactions or drug binding, the HX rate(s) will be changed.

Katta and Chait *(36)* showed that MS can be used to measure HX rates if the regular H_2O solvent is replaced with D_2O (where deuterium is the first isotope of hydrogen with a mass of two rather than a mass of one). The details of HX MS have been recently reviewed *(37–39)*. HX MS can be used to probe conformational changes, analyze protein–drug binding, and identify/characterize intermediates in protein folding and unfolding *(40–43)*. Although HX MS is dominated by electrospray methodology, MALDI has also been used to measure HX. Mandell et al. *(44)* showed that MALDI can be used for HX MS studies of protein–ligand interactions and for analysis of proteolytic digests without separation.

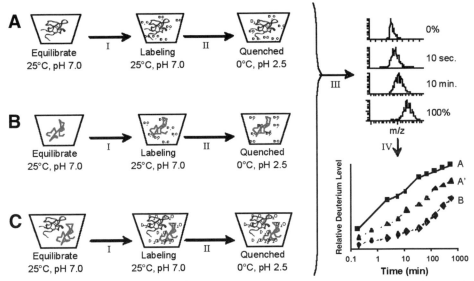

Fig. 4. General hydrogen exchange (HX) mass spectrometry (MS) methodology for protein interaction studies. Two proteins are analyzed separately (**A,B**) to provide baseline information and then together as a complex (**C**). In each case, the protein or protein mixture is incubated in an equilibrium buffer at 25°C, pH 7.0 in H$_2$O. D$_2$O is then added (I) to initiate the HX reaction. At various times after the introduction of D$_2$O HX of an aliquot of the labeling sample is quenched (II) by adjusting the pH to 2.5 and the temperature to 0°C. The quenched samples are then analyzed individually by MS (III) either as whole proteins or after pepsin digestion (not shown). The resulting mass spectra indicate the amount of deuterium incorporation at each exchange time point. These results are plotted (IV) as deuterium level vs time. In this example, the deuterium uptake of protein A when by itself and protein B when by itself were plotted. When protein A was in the presence of protein B (indicated as A'), its deuterium uptake was less than when it was alone. The deuterium level of protein B in the presence of protein A is not shown. *See* **Subheadings 3.2.** and **3.4.** for more details.

The use of HX MS to investigate the interaction(s) of two proteins, referred to as A and B, respectively, is illustrated schematically in **Fig. 4**. These techniques can be applied to any proteins or other ligands. HX into the intact protein or into short peptides created after HX can be investigated. Deuterium incorporation into each of the proteins independently (for the time course of 10 s to 8 h) is usually established first, followed by HX MS for the two proteins mixed together. **Figure 5A** shows example data of deuterium uptake reduction when two proteins bind to each other *(35)*. These results can be attributed to conformational changes and occlusion of some exchangeable hydrogens in protein A on interaction with protein B. However, the average mass of each protein after HX provides an overview of only the extent of change, not the location of the changes. Localization of the regions of change can be achieved after proteolytic digestion of deuterium-labeled proteins, as discussed in the following section.

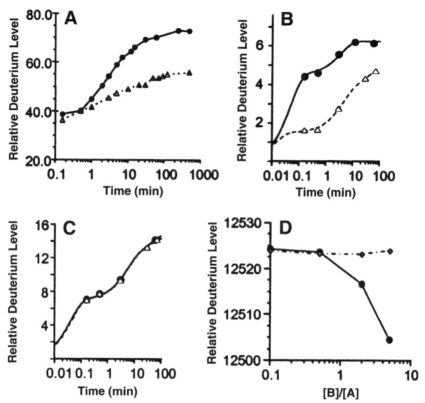

Fig. 5. Protein–protein interactions by hydrogen exchange (HX) and determination of K_d. Plots of deuterium incorporation with time (as in **Fig. 4**, lower right) were prepared for a protein when incubated with a binding partner. (**A**) Relative deuterium uptake of protein A alone (●) and in presence of protein B (△). Although not shown, HX into protein B was unaffected by the presence of protein A. (**B**) Representative deuterium uptake of region of protein A where deuterium exchange was altered on binding (symbols same as in [A]). (**C**) Peptic fragment from protein B that showed no difference in deuterium uptake as a result of interaction with protein A (protein B alone [●] and in presence of protein A [△]). (**D**) Relative deuterium uptake of protein A plotted against different mixtures of proteins A and B ([B]/[A]): (—●—) wild-type protein A and (—○—) mutant form a protein A *(35)* that cannot bind to protein B.

3.4.1. Location Information Provided by HX MS

A combination of enzymatic digestion and HX MS *(45)* allows HX information to be localized to short peptide segments, thereby increasing the spatial resolution. A number of groups have effectively used similar methodology in experiments to probe protein–ligand and protein–protein interactions *(46–52)*. A general protocol is presented **Subheading 3.2.3.**

For the example proteins illustrated here (**Fig. 5**), pepsin digestion of the HX-quenched samples was performed to understand which regions of the proteins underwent interaction. It is important to note that pepsin digestion is carried out after HX is completed and quenched. Hence, the structural information captured by deuterium incorporation is present in the peptides. Some regions (or peptides) from protein A or B may have altered exchange rates in a complex either because the domain or the region is blocked by the other protein, or as a result of changes that led to a tighter or looser conformation. In fact, in the present example, a peptide that showed reduced deuterium uptake (**Fig. 5B**) comes from a region of protein A identified by NMR *(53)* as located in the interface region between proteins A and B. According to the HX MS results, protein B structure was not affected by the presence of protein A because there was no evidence for differences in deuterium uptake in protein B when incubated with protein A. To illustrate this, HX MS data for a representative peptic fragment from protein B that is located at the interface region between protein A and protein B is shown in **Fig. 5C**. Proteolytic digestion in combination with HX MS gives a much more detailed picture of protein-protein interactions. A similar approach can be used for studying protein interactions with other molecules such as drugs and peptides.

3.4.2. Using HX MS to Estimate K_d Values

HX MS can be used to determine the dissociation constant (K_d) for complexes. The concentration of one of the proteins is varied such that various amounts of binding occur (between 0 and 100% bound). If deuterium uptake in one of the proteins is sensitive to the percentage of protein molecules bound, a binding curve can be generated. The deuterium uptake of the example protein A was determined when various amounts of proteins B were incubated with it. Measuring HX into protein A was chosen because its HX was sensitive to the presence of protein B, as indicated by the decreased amount of deuterium that was incorporated into protein A at a 1:5 ratio of A:B (**Fig. 5A**). For the titration illustrated here, an HX labeling time of 30 min was used because after 30 min in deuterium, a maximal difference between free and complexed protein A deuterium levels was observed. The experimental protocol remained the same (*see* **Subheading 3.2.4.**) except for varying the ratio of proteins. The mass of the full protein (or any given charge state of the protein) was plotted against the relative concentration (**Fig. 5D**). The concentrations of A and B at the halfway point in the titration curve were used to estimate the K_d (*see* **Note 16**). Hence, the point of maximum slope corresponded to B:A = 5:1, or approx 60–100 µ*M* protein B. The K_d is, therefore, also in the same range. To investigate the role of specific amino acids at the identified interface, mutants were made that abolished binding. The absence of binding of one of the mutants, as determined by HX MS, is illustrated in **Fig. 5D**.

3.5. Using HX MS to Determine
Binding-Induced Conformational Changes

The conformation of proteins may be altered by the presence of other proteins or other molecules. Conformational changes in proteins may cause alterations in the HX within the protein. Using methods similar to those discussed for the analysis of protein–protein complexes (*see* **Subheading 3.2.**), proteins can be analyzed individually. Conformational changes occurring in the order of seconds to hours can be monitored by regular manual sample preparation. Using automated techniques such as quench flow techniques, the exchange times can be reduced to milliseconds. These methods have been applied to study various aspects of protein biophysics *(54,55)*. The populations of different conformers or intermediates, if they exist at equilibrium, can be studied by pulse-labeling experiments in combination with HX MS.

3.6. Protein–Metal Ion Interactions

Protein–metal ion interactions are highly specific to both the metal ion and the protein. Interaction depends on the selectivity of protein for a given metal ion, its topological orientation, and also the nature of the metal ion. For example, a protein (P) with affinity toward various metal ions (A, B, C, D) forms complexes with an order of affinity of A > C > B >> D, the latter having almost negligible affinity for the protein (*see* **Fig. 3**). Under such conditions, the ion abundances of mass spectra peaks of protein and metal ions, when analyzed by MS using the general protocol discussed in **Subheading 3.1.**, provide information about stoichiometry and the relative binding affinity. It is important to maintain the physiological pH because acid-induced dissociation of metal ions from substrate may occur *(56)*. Using these kinds of methods, various MS studies have determined the relative binding affinities and stoichiometry of protein-metal complexes, mostly by electrospray *(24–27,29,57–59)*. HX has also been used in conjunction with MS to study metal ion-induced conformational changes. The procedure for studying these changes is practically the same as that described for drugs and protein-protein (*see* **Subheading 3.2.**), but the ligand is replaced with a metal ion.

MS has been shown to be a very useful tool for detecting minor to moderate changes in protein conformation on metal ion complexation *(60)* and also for identifying the site(s) of metal ion binding *(61)*. Because electrospray is sensitive to conformational differences in solution (e.g., *see* **refs.** *47, 62,* and *63*), it can be used to assess metal ion binding to proteins. A tightly folded protein conformer will have relatively fewer charges in electrospray spectra compared with an unfolded or denatured form. Distinctly different charge-state envelopes are therefore apparent in electrospray mass spectra (**Fig. 6**). A change in conformation on the addition of metal ion (or other ligand) may lead to a more tightly folded, metal-coordinated complex. The result of such complexation is a shift in the bimodal distribution to the envelope with fewer charges (**Fig. 6B**). Metal-bound ternary complexes can also be analyzed in the same fashion *(29)*.

3.7. Conclusion

As illustrated with these few examples, MS is a very powerful tool for probing protein interactions with other molecules. The interacting molecules vary in size, nature, and complexity. HX methods when combined with MS provide finer details in all of these interactions as well as information difficult to obtain with other techniques. With the development of more and more drugs targeted at proteins, MS should continue to contribute extensive information, ultimately increasing the speed of drug discovery.

4. Notes

1. Instrumental parameters can have a drastic effect on the analysis of noncovalent interactions with MS. Particularly important is tuning the pressure inside the mass spectrometer. If there are large pressure changes at each pumping stage, the noncovalent complexes will not

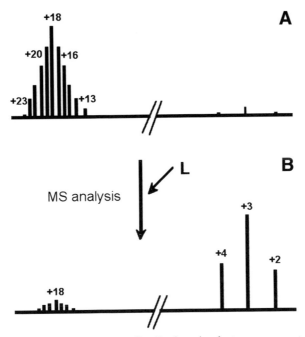

Fig. 6. Complexation and charge-state distributions in electrospray spectra. (**A**) A protein exhibits a bimodal distribution of charge states, indicating the presence of two distinct conformational forms in solution. The unfolded or higher charge-state distribution centered around +18 is the predominant form in the absence of "L" (where "L" is a ligand that could be a metal ion/ drug molecule/peptide or another protein), and so on. (**B**) Ligand complexation causes a conformational change in the protein leading to a more compact conformation that accommodates relatively fewer charge states (+2 to +4) compared to uncomplexed form.

hold together during transit inside the mass spectrometer. Collisional cooling of the ions by a gradual pressure gradient helps retain noncovalent interactions. Other variables that need to be considered are the capillary and cone voltages; source temperature; pH; salt/buffer concentration; and amount, if any, of organic solvent. In general, it is essential to retain what are referred to as "native conditions" (mildly acidic conditions with pH 5.0–6.0, very low or absence of organic solvent, low source temperature [≤20°C]) during electrospray.

2. Trypsin, normally active in the poststomach gut, is active at pH 7.5–8.5. It cleaves protein C terminally to lysine and arginine. Other proteases have different specificities (e.g., V8 cleaves at acidic sites such as aspartic acid and glutamic acid). Choice of the protease is key to producing partial digestion because different sites will be accessible for different proteases owing to their unique specificities. Often, digestion with a battery of proteases (trypsin, Asp-N, Glu-C, V8, carboxypeptidases) may be necessary.

3. Proteins A and B discussed here are both 6xHis-tagged proteins. Their overexpression and purification using Ni-NTA agarose affinity column chromatography are discussed elsewhere (*48*), but, generally, the directions provided by the supplier of the Ni-agarose beads work well.

4. Immobilized pepsin columns may be easily packed in-house. Pepsin is first, immobilized on POROS-20AL beads from Perseptive according to the directions supplied with the POROS beads. Then the beads are slurry packed with a normal HPLC into an empty stain-less steel column (*see* **Subheading 2.5., item 3**). No special packing equipment is required. Pepsin columns made in this fashion typically can be reused many times without significant loss in enzyme efficiency. It is important, however, never to introduce samples or buffers above pH 6.0 into the pepsin column because pepsin is irreversibly inactivated above this pH. Detailed directions for pepsin-column packing have been published elsewhere (*64*).

5. pH Adjustment of deuterated solvents using DCl or NaOD is measured directly with a hydrogen electrode rather than a deuterium electrode. As such, the pH reading (pH_{read}) must be corrected according to the equation $pD = pH_{read} + 0.4$ (*65*). The pD should never be adjusted with HCl or NaOH for labeling buffers in which the deuterium level is to remain 99% or greater.

6. PEEK tubing does not allow efficient cooling, especially when the mobile phase is flowing. A premixer coil (placed before the A/B mobile phase mixing tee) of approx 40–50 cm of stainless steel tubing is employed to ensure efficient mobile phase cooling before the mobile phase reaches the injector and column. The cooling loop, all transfer lines, injector, traps, and column are all immersed in an ice bath.

7. It is advisable to recrystallize 4HCCA and to use freshly prepared matrix solution for analyzing samples on MALDI (*66*).

8. A Bradford assay (*67*) is normally used to determine the protein concentration. This assay is an estimate and may provide a concentration value significantly different from the true protein concentration. However, if samples are prepared relative to each other based on a Bradford estimate, it is in most cases not necessary to have an exact concentration value. Alternatively, concentration may be determined more accurately using extinction coefficients.

9. Incubation time, concentration of protein and ligand, stoichiometry, pH, and so forth need to be optimized for every protein–ligand combination. The conditions referred to in the text are general recommendations. Good starting conditions are pH 5.0–7.0 in weak (10–25 m*M*) ammonium acetate or ammonium bicarbonate buffer. Spraying directly from water has also been successful for some complexes.

10. It is not advisable to reconstitute proteins directly into D_2O buffer for HX because resolvation may alter deuterium exchange rates at early time points. The proteins should be as near to their native state as possible before the introduction of deuterium.

11. Quenching to a lower pH reduces the HX reaction by approx 10^4, and lowering the temperature to 0°C further reduces exchange rates by another order of magnitude. Quenched samples may be immediately frozen on dry ice and stored at −80°C until analysis. Because deuterium losses may still occur at −80°C, our experience dictates that the time between sample preparation and mass spectral analysis should be minimized as much as possible.

12. A potential problem with these studies is protein self-association or aggregation, particularly at higher concentrations necessary for titration experiments. Control experiments should be performed for each protein to determine whether concentration alters the HX properties for that protein.

13. Pepsin is a nonspecific protease, meaning that its digestion products cannot be predicted based on sequence. It is, however, very reproducible under identical conditions. Therefore, each peptide observed in the mass spectra must be identified/sequenced with MS/MS experiments before HX MS results can be fully interpreted.

14. Pepsin solutions are made in pure water (pH < 5.0) and placed at 0°C. Usually a small volume of pepsin solution is added to a much larger volume of protein solution. Therefore,

the sample solution must be acidic (have been quenched) for digestion to proceed. Pepsin is ideal for digestion in HX MS experiments because it is active at a quench pH of 2.5.

15. The time required for peptide separation should be reduced in order to minimize deuterium back-exchange. Poor chromatographic resolution is not problematic because the mass spectrometer can provide additional resolution by mass.

16. Ion suppression, as was the case in this example, may prevent creation of the typical sigmoidally shaped titration curve. At very high concentrations of protein B, all the signal from protein A is suppressed by the overwhelming amount of protein B. Improvements in chromatography can overcome this problem by separating signals from the binding partners.

Acknowledgments

We wish to acknowledge funding from the NIH-BRIN program of the National Center for Research Resources (P20-RR16480), the National Cancer Institute (R24-CA88339), and the University of New Mexico.

References

1. von Mering, C., Krause, R., Snel, B., et al. (2002) Comparative assessment of large-scale data sets of protein-protein interactions. *Nature* **417**, 399–403.
2. Scott, J. D. and Pawson, T. (2000) Cell communication: the inside story. *Sci. Am.* **282**, 72–79.
3. Rout, M. P., Aitchison, J. D., Suprapto, A., Hjertaas, K., Zhao, Y., and Chait, B. T. (2000) The yeast nuclear pore complex: composition, architecture, and transport mechanism. *J. Cell Biol.* **148**, 635–651.
4. van Berkel, W. J., van den Heuvel, R. H., Versluis, C., and Heck, A. J. (2000) Detection of intact megaDalton protein assemblies of vanillyl-alcohol oxidase by mass spectrometry. *Protein Sci.* **9**, 435–439.
5. Sanglier, S., Leize, E., Van Dorsselaer, A., and Zal, F. (2003) Comparative ESI-MS study of approximately 2.2 MDa native hemocyanins from deep-sea and shore crabs: from protein oligomeric state to biotope. *J. Am. Soc. Mass Spectrom.* **14**, 419–429.
6. Rostom, A. A. and Robinson, C. V. (1999) Detection of the intact GroEL chaperonin assembly by mass spectrometry. *J. Am. Chem. Soc.* **121**, 4718–4719.
7. Sobott, F. and Robinson, C. V. (2002) Protein complexes gain momentum. *Curr. Opin. Struct. Biol.* **12**, 729–734.
8. Sobott, F., Benesch, J. L., Vierling, E., and Robinson, C. V. (2002) Subunit exchange of multimeric protein complexes: real-time monitoring of subunit exchange between small heat shock proteins by using electrospray mass spectrometry. *J. Biol. Chem.* **277**, 38,921–38,929.
9. Hanson, C. L., Fucini, P., Ilag, L. L., Nierhaus, K. H., and Robinson, C. V. (2003) Dissociation of intact *Escherichia coli* ribosomes in a mass spectrometer: evidence for conformational change in a ribosome elongation factor G complex. *J. Biol. Chem.* **278**, 1259–1267.
10. Hernandez, H. and Robinson, C. V. (2001) Dynamic protein complexes: insights from mass spectrometry. *J. Biol. Chem.* **276**, 46,685–46,688.
11. Benesch, J. L., Sobott, F., and Robinson, C. V. (2003) Thermal dissociation of multimeric protein complexes by using nanoelectrospray mass spectrometry. *Anal. Chem.* **75**, 2208–2214.
12. Fandrich, M., Tito, M. A., Leroux, M. R., et al. (2000) Observation of the noncovalent assembly and disassembly pathways of the chaperone complex MtGimC by mass spectrometry. *Proc. Natl. Acad. Sci. USA* **97**, 14,151–14,155.

13. Farmer, T. B. and Caprioli, R. M. (1998) Determination of protein-protein interactions by matrix-assisted laser desorption/ionization mass spectrometry. *J. Mass. Spectrom.* **33,** 697–704.

14. Bennett, K. L., Matthiesen, T., and Roepstorff, P. (2000) Probing protein surface topology by chemical surface labeling, crosslinking, and mass spectrometry. *Methods Mol. Biol.* **146,** 113–131.

15. Farmer, T. B. and Caprioli, R. M. (1991) Assessing the multimeric states of proteins: studies using laser desorption mass spectrometry. *Biol. Mass Spectrom.* **20,** 796–800.

16. Alley, S. C., Ishmael, F. T., Jones, A. D., and Benkovic, S. J. (2000) Mapping protein-protein interactions in the bacteriophage T4 DNA polymerase holoenzyme using a novel trifunctional photo-cross-linking and affinity reagent. *J. Am. Chem. Soc.* **122,** 6126–6127.

17. Lee, W. C. and Lee, K. H. (2004) Applications of affinity chromatography in proteomics. *Anal. Biochem.* **324,** 1–10.

18. Archakov, A. I., Govorun, V. M., Dubanov, A. V., et al. (2003) Protein-protein interactions as a target for drugs in proteomics. *Proteomics* **3,** 380–391.

19. Blom, K. F., Larsen, B. S., and McEwen, C. N. (1999) Determining affinity-selected ligands and estimating binding affinities by online size exclusion chromatography/liquid chromatography-mass spectrometry. *J. Comb. Chem.* **1,** 82–90.

20. Henion, J., Li, Y. T., Hsieh, Y. L., and Ganem, B. (1993) Mass spectrometric investigations of drug-receptor interactions. *Ther. Drug Monit.* **15,** 563–569.

21. Lewis, J. K., Chiang, J., and Siuzdak, G. (1999) Monitoring protein-drug interactions with mass spectrometry and proteolysis protein mass mapping as a drug assay. *J. Assoc. Lab. Automation* **4,** 46–48.

22. Wabnitz, P. A. and Loo, J. A. (2002) Drug screening of pharmaceutical discovery compounds by micro-size exclusion chromatography/mass spectrometry. *Rapid Commun. Mass Spectrom.* **16,** 85–91.

23. Dunayevskiy, Y. M., Lyubarskaya, Y. V., Chu, Y. H., Vouros, P., and Karger, B. L. (1998) Simultaneous measurement of nineteen binding constants of peptides to vancomycin using affinity capillary electrophoresis-mass spectrometry. *J. Med. Chem.* **41,** 1201–1204.

24. Loo, J. A. (1997) Studying noncovalent protein complexes by electrospray ionization mass spectrometry. *Mass Spectrom. Rev.* **16,** 1–23.

25. Salmain, M., Caro, B., Le Guen-Robin, F., Blais, J. C., and Jaouen, G. (2004) Solution- and crystal-phase covalent modification of lysozyme by a purpose-designed organoruthenium complex: a MALDI-TOF MS study of its metal binding sites. *Chembiochem.* **5,** 99–109.

26. Chitta, R. K. and Gross, M. L. (2004) Electrospray ionization-mass spectrometry and tandem mass spectrometry reveal self-association and metal-ion binding of hydrophobic peptides: a study of the gramicidin dimer. *Biophys. J.* **86,** 473–479.

27. She, Y. M., Narindrasorasak, S., Yang, S., Spitale, N., Roberts, E. A., and Sarkar, B. (2003) Identification of metal-binding proteins in human hepatoma lines by immobilized metal affinity chromatography and mass spectrometry. *Mol. Cell Proteomics* **2,** 1306–1318.

28. Zhu, M. M., Rempel, D. L., Zhao, J., Giblin, D. E., and Gross, M. L. (2003) Probing Ca(2+)-induced conformational changes in porcine calmodulin by H/D exchange and ESI-MS: effect of cations and ionic strength. *Biochemistry* **42,** 15,388–15,397.

29. van den Bremer, E. T., Jiskoot, W., James, R., et al. (2002) Probing metal ion binding and conformational properties of the colicin E9 endonuclease by electrospray ionization time-of-flight mass spectrometry. *Protein Sci.* **11,** 1738–1752.

30. Gehrig, P. M., You, C., Dallinger, R., et al. (2000) Electrospray ionization mass spectrometry of zinc, cadmium, and copper metallothioneins: evidence for metal-binding cooperativity. *Protein Sci.* **9,** 395–402.

31. Zhang, Z. and Marshall, A. G. (1998) A universal algorithm for fast and automated charge state deconvolution of electrospray mass-to-charge ratio spectra. *J. Am. Soc. Mass Spectrom.* **9,** 225–233.

32. Nikolic, D., Habibi-Goudarzi, S., Corley, D. G., Gafner, S., Pezzuto, J. M., and van Breemen, R. B. (2000) Evaluation of cyclooxygenase-2 inhibitors using pulsed ultrafiltration mass spectrometry. *Anal. Chem.* **72,** 3853–3859.

33. Wang, G. and Cole, R. B. (1994) Effect of solution ionic strength on analyte charge state distributions in positive and negative ion electrospray mass spectrometry. *Anal. Chem.* **66,** 3702–3708.

34. Buhrman, D. L., Price, P. I., and Rudewicz, P. J. (1996) Quantitation of SR 27417 in human plasma using electrospray liquid chromatography-tandem mass spectrometry: a study of ion suppression. *J. Am. Soc. Mass Spectrom.* **7,** 1099–1105.

35. Engen, J. R. (2003) Analysis of protein complexes with hydrogen exchange and mass spectrometry. *Analyst* **128,** 623–628.

36. Katta, V. and Chait, B. T. (1991) Conformational changes in proteins probed by hydrogen-exchange electrospray-ionization mass spectrometry. *Rapid Commun. Mass Spectrom.* **5,** 214–217.

37. Engen, J. R. and Smith, D. L. (2001) Investigating protein structure and dynamics by hydrogen exchange MS. *Anal. Chem.* **73,** 256A–265A.

38. Kaltashov, I. A. and Eyles, S. J. (2002) Studies of biomolecular conformations and conformational dynamics by mass spectrometry. *Mass Spectrom. Rev.* **21,** 37–71.

39. Hoofnagle, A. N., Resing, K. A., and Ahn, N. G. (2003) Protein analysis by hydrogen exchange mass spectrometry. *Annu. Rev. Biophys. Biomol. Struct.* **32,** 1–25.

40. Miranker, A., Robinson, C. V., Radford, S. E., Aplin, R. T., and Dobson, C. M. (1993) Detection of transient protein folding populations by mass spectrometry. *Science* **262,** 896–900.

41. Engen, J. R., Smithgall, T. E., Gmeiner, W. H., and Smith, D. L. (1997) Identification and localization of slow, natural, cooperative unfolding in the hematopoietic cell kinase SH3 domain by amide hydrogen exchange and mass spectrometry. *Biochemistry* **36,** 14,384–14,391.

42. Wang, F. and Tang, X. (1996) Conformational heterogeneity of stability of apomyoglobin studied by hydrogen/deuterium exchange and electrospray ionization mass spectrometry. *Biochemistry* **35,** 4069–4078.

43. Ramanathan, R., Gross, M. L., Zielinski, W. L., and Layloff, T. P. (1997) Monitoring recombinant protein drugs: a study of insulin by H/D exchange and electrospray ionization mass spectrometry. *Anal. Chem.* **69,** 5142–5145.

44. Mandell, J. G., Falick, A. M., and Komives, E. A. (1998) Measurement of amide hydrogen exchange by MALDI-TOF mass spectrometry. *Anal. Chem.* **70,** 3987–3995.

45. Zhang, Z. and Smith, D. L. (1993) Determination of amide hydrogen exchange by mass spectrometry: a new tool for protein structure elucidation. *Protein Sci.* **2,** 522–531.

46. Mandell, J. G., Baerga-Ortiz, A., Akashi, S., Takio, K., and Komives, E. A. (2001) Solvent accessibility of the thrombin-thrombomodulin interface. *J. Mol. Biol.* **306,** 575–589.

47. Maier, C. S., Schimerlik, M. I., and Deinzer, M. L. (1999) Thermal denaturation of Escherichia coli thioredoxin studied by hydrogen/deuterium exchange and electrospray ioniza-

tion mass spectrometry: monitoring a two-state protein unfolding transition. *Biochemistry* **38,** 1136–1143.

48. Engen, J. R., Bradbury, E. M., and Chen, X. (2002) Using stable-isotope-labeled proteins for hydrogen exchange studies in complex mixtures. *Anal. Chem.* **74,** 1680–1686.

49. Chen, J. and Smith, D. L. (2000) Unfolding and disassembly of the chaperonin GroEL occurs via a tetradecameric intermediate with a folded equatorial domain. *Biochemistry* **39,** 4250–4258.

50. Resing, K. A. and Ahn, N. G. (1998) Deuterium exchange mass spectrometry as a probe of protein kinase activation: analysis of wild-type and constitutively active mutants of MAP kinase kinase-1. *Biochemistry* **37,** 463–475.

51. Wang, F., Scapin, G., Blanchard, J. S., and Angeletti, R. H. (1998) Substrate binding and conformational changes of Clostridium glutamicum diaminopimelate dehydrogenase revealed by hydrogen/deuterium exchange and electrospray mass spectrometry. *Protein Sci.* **7,** 293–299.

52. Zhang, Y. H., Yan, X., Maier, C. S., Schimerlik, M. I., and Deinzer, M. L. (2002) Conformational analysis of intermediates involved in the in vitro folding pathways of recombinant human macrophage colony stimulating factor beta by sulfhydryl group trapping and hydrogen/deuterium pulsed labeling. *Biochemistry* **41,** 15,495–15,504.

53. Liu, Q., Jin, C., Liao, X., Shen, Z., Chen, D. J., and Chen, Y. (1999) The binding interface between an E2 (UBC9) and a ubiquitin homologue (UBL1). *J. Biol. Chem.* **274,** 16,979–16,987.

54. Tsui, V., Garcia, C., Cavagnero, S., Siuzdak, G., Dyson, H. J., and Wright, P. E. (1999) Quench-flow experiments combined with mass spectrometry show apomyoglobin folds through and obligatory intermediate. *Protein Sci.* **8,** 45–49.

55. Deng, Y. and Smith, D. L. (1999) Rate and equilibrium constants for protein unfolding and refolding determined by hydrogen exchange-mass spectrometry. *Anal. Biochem.* **276,** 150–160.

56. Liang, Y., Du, F., Sanglier, S., et al. (2003) Unfolding of rabbit muscle creatine kinase induced by acid: a study using electrospray ionization mass spectrometry, isothermal titration calorimetry, and fluorescence spectroscopy. *J. Biol. Chem.* **278,** 30,098–30,105.

57. Hu, P., Ye, Q. Z., and Loo, J. A. (1994) Calcium stoichiometry determination for calcium binding proteins by electrospray ionization mass spectrometry. *Anal. Chem.* **66,** 4190–4194.

58. Veenstra, T. D., Johnson, K. L., Tomlinson, A. J., Naylor, S., and Kumar, R. (1997) Determination of calcium-binding sites in rat brain calbindin D28K by electrospray ionization mass spectrometry. *Biochemistry* **36,** 3535–3542.

59. Lafitte, D., Capony, J. P., Grassy, G., Haiech, J., and Calas, B. (1995) Analysis of the ion binding sites of calmodulin by electrospray ionization mass spectrometry. *Biochemistry* **34,** 13,825–13,832.

60. Nemirovskiy, O., Giblin, D. E., and Gross, M. L. (1999) Electrospray ionization mass spectrometry and hydrogen/deuterium exchange for probing the interaction of calmodulin with calcium. *J. Am. Soc. Mass Spectrom.* **10,** 711–718.

61. Wang, F., Li, W., Emmett, M. R., Marshall, A. G., Corson, D., and Sykes, B. D. (1999) Fourier transform ion cyclotron resonance mass spectrometric detection of small Ca(2+)-induced conformational changes in the regulatory domain of human cardiac troponin C. *J. Am. Soc. Mass Spectrom.* **10,** 703–710.

62. Konermann, L. and Douglas, D. J. (1998) Equilibrium unfolding of proteins monitored by electrospray ionization mass spectrometry: distinguishing two-state from multi-state transitions. *Rapid Commun. Mass Spectrom.* **12,** 435–442.

63. Chowdhury, S. K., Katta, V., and Chait, B. T. (1990) Probing conformational changes in proteins by mass spectrometry. *J. Am. Chem. Soc.* **112,** 9012–9013.

64. Wang, L., Pan, H., and Smith, D. L. (2002) Hydrogen exchange-mass spectrometry: optimization of digestion conditions. *Mol. Cell Proteomics* **1,** 132–138.

65. Glasoe, P. K. and Long, F. A. (1960) Use of glass electrodes to measure acidities in deuterium oxide. *Anal. Chem.* **64,** 188–191.

66. Uljon, S. N., Mazzarelli, L., Chait, B. T., and Wang, R. (2000) Analysis of proteins and peptides directly from biological fluids by immunoprecipitation/mass spectrometry. *Methods Mol. Biol.* **146,** 439–452.

67. Bradford, M. M. (1976) A rapid and sensitive method for the quantitation of microgram quantities of protein utilizing the principle of protein-dye binding. *Anal. Biochem.* **72,** 248–254.

10

Discovering New Drug-Targeting Sites on Flexible Multidomain Protein Kinases

Combining Segmental Isotopic and Site-Directed Spin Labeling for Nuclear Magnetic Resonance Detection of Interfacial Clefts

Thomas K. Harris

Summary

A novel structure-based approach to study the structure and dynamics of flexible multidomain monomeric protein kinases, which otherwise do not yield diffraction quality crystals, is described. A combination of segmental ^{15}N-isotopic labeling of a regulatory domain with site-directed paramagnetic nitroxide spin labeling of the kinase domain is employed. Nuclear magnetic resonance studies of the enhancement of amide proton relaxation rates of the ^{15}N-isotopically labeled regulatory domain caused by insertion of the paramagnetic nitroxide spin label on the kinase domain provide long-range distance restraints for determination of both the average positional structure and the relative flexibility exhibited between the two contiguous domains. Clefts and crevices detected around the dynamic domain–domain interface provide new targeting sites for tethered-based extension of current small-molecule lead compounds to produce more potent and selective pharmaceutical agents.

Key Words: Structure-based drug discovery; fragment-based drug discovery; tethering; protein engineering; segmental isotopic labeling; site-directed spin labeling; nuclear magnetic resonance; nuclear spin relaxation; paramagnetic enhancement effect; protein dynamics.

1. Introduction

Protein kinases are already the second largest group of drug targets after G protein-coupled receptors, and they account for 20–30% of the drug discovery programs of many companies (1). There is clearly no shortage of potential targets; protein kinases comprise the largest enzyme family, with approx 500 being encoded by the human genome.

From: *Methods in Molecular Biology, vol. 316: Bioinformatics and Drug Discovery*
Edited by: R. S. Larson © Humana Press Inc., Totowa, NJ

In addition, the availability of more cell-permeant protein kinase inhibitors would be extremely useful in helping to delineate the physiological roles of these enzymes. Despite the large amount of effort that has been directed toward the development of inhibitors of protein kinases *(2)*, only two compounds have been approved by the Food and Drug Administration for clinical use: rapamycin (Wyeth-Ayerst) and Gleevec (Novartis). Rapamycin has been shown to inhibit the mammalian serine–threonine protein kinase target of rapamycin (mTOR). It is the primary drug of choice for use as an immunosuppressant for organ transplantation, because it effectively and specifically inhibits the proliferation of T-cells *(3)*. Similarly, Gleevec has been shown to effectively inhibit the Abelson tyrosine kinase oncogene (ABL), found in nearly all patients with chronic myelogenous leukemia *(4)*. The success of these compounds has led to the development of numerous other relatively selective inhibitors of protein kinases, which are now in human clinical trials involving the treatment of a variety of other cancer-related illnesses, in addition to several inflammatory and degenerative diseases *(1,2)*.

The primary reason that so few protein kinase inhibitors have been approved for clinical use is that the overwhelming majority of compounds that inhibit a targeted protein kinase mimic adenosine triphosphate (ATP) and bind in the ATP-binding pocket, causing inhibition of numerous other kinases and adenosine triphosphatases *(5,6)*. Although SB203580 and Gleevec have been shown to be competitive with ATP, X-ray diffraction studies indicate that the relatively high affinity and specificity observed for these compounds is owing to an additional hydrophobic moiety, which extends into a hydrophobic pocket near the ATP-binding site of only the inactive form of the kinase *(7)*. The extended hydrophobic moiety exemplifies the additive nature of binding free energies of chemically linked molecular fragments *(8)*. Thus, additive binding can facilitate the search for drugs in fragments, which offers a tremendous combinatorial advantage over discovery of drugs intact. However, the primary challenge of detecting weak interactions of small molecular fragments with proteins continues to hinder fragment-based drug design and development.

One of the most recent and promising methods of fragment-based drug discovery entails Tethering™ *(9)*. The basic method of Tethering is to engineer a single-site surface-exposed cysteine residue within 5–10 Å of a potential binding pocket of interest. Then, the protein is reacted with a library of disulfide-containing fragments under partially reducing conditions. If one of the fragments has inherent affinity to a site near the cysteine, the thioldisulfide equilibrium will be shifted in favor of the disulfide for this fragment. Owing to the change in mass by the amount of the particular disulfide-linked fragment, the predominant chemically modified protein species can be identified by mass spectrometry (MS). Then selected fragments can be elaborated, combined with other molecules, or combined with one another to provide high-affinity drug leads. The primary advantage of Tethering is that it provides a site-directed basis for fragment-based drug discovery based on low to moderate binding activities in contrast to selection based on high-affinity inhibition of enzyme activity by intact drugs required of high-throughput screening assays. One major limitation of the Tethering approach, as well as of other structure-based drug discovery methods such as X-ray crystallography and nuclear magnetic resonance (NMR), is the feasibility of obtaining three-dimensional

(3D) models of all target proteins and detecting additional small-molecule binding sites in flexible loop regions that may exist some distance from the active site.

Structure-based approaches represent the newest and most promising areas of focus for drug discovery programs *(10)*. Numerous companies have begun to automate the structural biology process to rapidly crystallize gene products on a massive scale (e.g., Astex, Structural Genomix, and Syrrx). However, it is becoming evident that X-ray diffraction quality crystals are difficult to obtain for many of the most important protein targets, because they behave as flexible multidomain proteins *(11)*. In such cases, X-ray or NMR structures can be solved only for individual functional domains. For example, **Fig. 1** shows domain organizations of a number of well-characterized serine–threonine protein kinases of pharmaceutical interest. Of these members, X-ray structures have been reported only for isolated kinase domain constructs of phosphoinositide-dependent protein kinase-1 (PDK1), protein kinase B/AKT (PKB), protein kinase A (PKA), c-JUN NH_2-terminal protein and 38-kDA protein kinases (JNK/p38), extracellular signal-regulated protein kinases (ERK1,2) cyclin-dependent protein kinases (CDK), and checkpoint kinases (CHK); and X-ray or NMR structures have been reported only for the corresponding isolated regulatory domain constructs of the pleckstrin homology (PH) domain of PKB, the diacyclglycerol (DAG) and Ca^{2+} domains of PKC, the cyclic adenosine monophosphate (cAMP)-regulatory subunit of PKA, the cyclin-regulatory subunit of CDK, the conserved region 1 (CR1) domain of the first identified downstream effector kinases (RAF1,A,B), and the forkhead-associated (FHA) domain of CHK. Fragment-based drug discovery methods such as Tethering™ could be better exploited if structures of the full-length multidomain protein kinases could be determined. Then, chemically linked compounds could be developed that could simultaneously interact with either known binding pockets of proximal domains or unknown potential binding pockets that may exist within clefts or crevices near the interface between contiguous domains.

In this chapter, a novel structure-based approach to study the structure and dynamics of flexible multidomain monomeric protein kinase drug targets in which high-quality 3D models have been determined for the isolated domains but cannot be determined for the full-length kinase is presented. **Figure 2** illustrates site-directed spin labeling of the N-terminal kinase domain and isotopic labeling of the C-terminal regulatory PH domain of PDK1, and **Fig. 3** illustrates isotopic labeling of the N-terminal regulatory PH domain and site-directed spin labeling of the C-terminal kinase domain of PKB2. By using intein-mediated protein ligation, the isotopic labeled regulatory domain is chemically joined to the site-directed, spin-labeled kinase domain to generate the full-length native protein with a native peptide bond. First, NMR is used to determine the chemical shift assignments of the isotopic-labeled backbone amides of the regulatory domain while in its intact position of the native kinase. Second, NMR relaxation studies are performed to determine long-range distance restraints between the site-directed spin label on the kinase domain and backbone amide protons of the regulatory domain.

Unpaired electrons of spin labels, such as the nitroxide spin label, produce local fluctuating magnetic fields, which can influence the relaxation times of magnetic nuclei in a distance-dependent manner. In general terms, the magnetic interaction between the

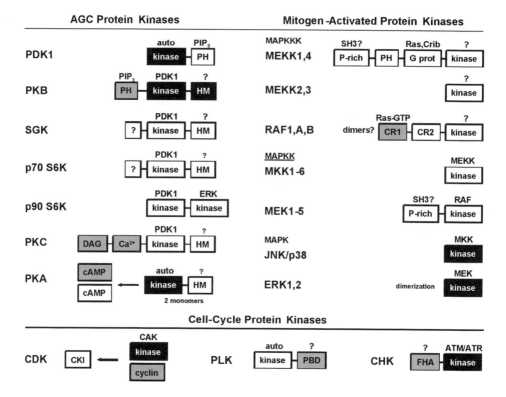

Fig. 1. Domain organization of well-characterized serine–threonine protein kinases of pharmaceutical interest. The isolated kinase domain constructs for which X-ray 3D structures have been reported are indicated in black: phosphoinositide-dependent protein kinase-1 (PDK1); protein kinase B/Akt (PKB); cyclic adenosine monophosphate (cAMP)-dependent protein kinases (PKA); c-JUN NH$_2$-terminal protein and 38-kDa protein kinases (JNK/p38); extracellular signal-regulated protein kinases (ERK1,2); cyclin-dependent protein kinases (CDK); and checkpoint kinases (CHK). The active kinase domains of each family member must be phosphorylated, and the upstream protein kinase activator is indicated above each domain. Interestingly, PDK1 serves as the upstream activator of serum- and glucocorticoid-induced protein kinase (SGK), 40- and 90-kDa 40S ribosomal protein S6 kinase (p70 and p90 S6K), and Ca^{2+}-activated protein kinase (PKC). No upstream activator has been clearly identified for phosphorylation of the C-terminal hydrophobic motif (HM) domains of PKB, SGK, p70 S6K, PKC, and PKA. The regulatory domain constructs for which X-ray or NMR structures have been reported are indicated in gray: pleckstrin homology (PH) domain of PKB; diacylglycerol (DAG) and Ca^{2+} domains of PKC; cAMP-regulatory subunit of PKA; cyclin-regulatory subunit of CDK; the conserved region 1 (CR1) domain of the first identified downstream effector kinases (RAF1,A,B) of the mitogen-activated G protein (RAS); the polo box domain (PBD) of polo-like kinase (PLK) and the forkhead-associated (FHA) domain of CHK. Regulatory domains that bind either small-molecule sec-ond messengers or regulatory proteins are indicated. PIP$_3$, phosphatidylinositol 3,4,5-triphosphate; CAK, CDK-activating kinase; MEK, MAPK/ERK kinase; SH3, Src-homology 3 domain; ATM/ATR, ataxia telangiectasia mutated kinase/ataxia- and Rad-related kinase; MAPK, mitogen-activated protein kinase.

unpaired electron of a site-directed spin label and a proton *in the same molecule* is similar to the nuclear Overhauser effect (NOE) between pairs of protons. Unlike an NOE, whose measurable effect is limited to distances ≤5.5 Å, the electron–proton interaction extends over approx 20–35 Å, depending on the particular spin label. Finally, distance geometry/simulated annealing protocols in CNS(XPLOR) are used to calculate the average position of the known structure of the regulatory domain relative to the known X-ray structure of the larger kinase domain.

The combined use of X-ray crystallography, segmental isotopic and site-directed spin labeling, and NMR structural studies may prove to become a powerful method to study other flexible multidomain proteins, which otherwise do not yield diffraction quality crystals. The effects of ligand binding on the position of one domain with respect to the other domain would provide firsthand accounts of how binding events regulate domain organization and dynamics. Knowledge of the position of a ligand-binding site on one domain with respect to the binding site on another proximal domain will be highly useful toward the rational or structure-based design of bivalent inhibitors. If the ligand-binding sites are reasonably close, then the free energies of binding of these two sites could be chemically "linked." Not only will this produce high-affinity inhibitors, but specific linkage geometries will provide for highly selective binding. In addition, new-found clefts and crevices leading to the interface between two contiguous protein domains will provide tactical sites of interest to which small molecular fragments can be targeted for binding interactions.

2. Materials

2.1. Molecular Biology

1. Human tissue Marathon-Ready™ cDNA library and Advantage 2 Polymerase Mix, for polymerase chain reaction (PCR) amplification of protein kinase genes from human cDNA library (Clontech, Palo Alto, CA).
2. Oligonucleotide primers for all PCR reactions (Operon, Alameda, CA).
3. KOD proofreading polymerase for high-fidelity PCR reactions except PCR from human cDNA library (Novagen, Madison, WI).
4. pCR®-Blunt II-TOPO® vector and One Shot® TOP10 Chemically Competent *Escherichia coli* for initial cloning purposes (Invitrogen, Carlsbad, CA).
5. QIAquick® Gel Extraction Kit and QIAprep® Spin Miniprep Kit for DNA preparative procedures (Qiagen, Valencia, CA).
6. QuikChange® Single and Multi Site-Directed Mutagenesis kits (Stratagene, La Jolla, CA).
7. Restriction enzymes and DNA polymerization mix (deoxynucleotide 5'-triphosphates) (Boehringer Mannheim, Indianapolis, IN)
8. All other chemicals, salts, and buffers (Sigma, St. Louis, MO).

2.2. Protein Expression and Purification

1. Bac-to-Bac® Baculovirus Expression System, pFastBac™1 cloning plasmid, DH10Bac™ competent cells of *E. coli*, S.N.A.P.™ MidiPrep Kit, *Taq* DNA polymerase High Fidelity, M13 forward (−40) and M13 reverse primers, Cellfectin® Reagent, unsupplemented Grace's Medium, and Sf9 insect cells for expression of human protein kinases and their catalytic kinase domain constructs (Invitrogen).

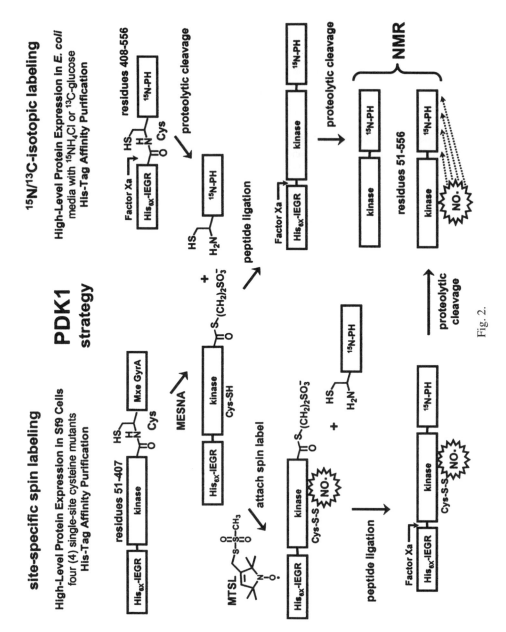

Fig. 2.

204

2. BL21(DE3) competent cells of *E. coli* and pET protein expression vectors for bacterial expression of ^{15}N- and ^{13}C-isotopic-labeled regulatory domains (Novagen).
3. Factor Xa protease and benzamidine column for His$_6$ tag removal and generation of an NT-Cys (Novagen).
4. ÄKTAbasic fast performance liquid chromatography (FPLC), Ni Sepharose High Performance Resin, and Prepacked HisTrap HP columns for affinity tag purification and removal of His$_6$ tag (Amersham, Piscataway, NJ).

2.3. Segmental Isotopic and Paramagnetic Spin Labeling

1. Ammonium-^{15}N chloride and D-Glucose-^{13}C$_6$, for isotopic labeling of regulatory domains (Isotec, Miamisburg, OH).
2. MTSL, for site-directed paramagnetic spin labeling of kinase domains (Toronto Research Chemicals, Canada).
3. MESNA, for generation of C-terminal thioester; ninhydrin (indane 1,2,3-trione), for NT-Cys protection; and Ellman's reagent (5,5'-dithio-*bis*[2-nitrobenzoic acid], or DTNB), for thiol titration (Sigma).
4. 7-Diethylamino-3-(4'-maleimidylphenyl)-4-methylcoumarin (CPM), for thiol titration of spin-labeled proteins (Molecular Probes, Eugene, OR).
5. BioGel 501 organomercurial thiol affinity column (Bio-Rad, Hercules, CA).

2.4. Determination of Structure

2.4.1. Hardware

1. High-field NMR instrumentation (≥500 MHz) with cryoprobe, for high-sensitivity protein structural and dynamic studies.
2. Standard EPR instrumentation with capability of containing a small-diameter capillary for data collection on protein samples in aqueous solution.

Fig. 2. *(Opposite page)* Overall strategy utilized to combine site-directed nitroxide spin labeling of N-terminal kinase domain with uniform ^{15}N-isotopic labeling of C-terminal regulatory pleckstrin homology (PH) domain of phosphoinositide-dependent protein kinase-1 (PDK1). A His$_6$-tagged single-site cysteine mutant of the N-terminal kinase domain fused with a C-terminal Mxe GyrA intein is expressed and affinity purified from Sf9 insect cells. Thiolytic cleavage of the C-terminal Mxe GyrA intein with 2-mercaptoethanesulfonate (MESNA) generates a C-terminal thioester on the N-terminal kinase domain. The C-terminal regulatory PH domain is expressed as a fusion protein containing an N-terminal His$_6$ tag with a factor Xa protease cleavage site and affinity purified from *Escherichia coli* grown in minimal media supplemented with the desired nuclear magnetic resonance (NMR) active isotopic label. Cleavage with factor Xa generates an N-terminal cysteine (NT-Cys). As a result of the chemical reactivity between the C-terminal thioester and the NT-Cys, native peptide bond formation occurs on mixing the N-terminal kinase domain with the C-terminal regulatory PH domain. Full-length PDK1 is affinity purified, and the His$_6$ tag is cleaved to form segmental isotopic-labeled PDK1 for NMR structural and dynamic studies. To provide for site-directed spin labeling, the thioester derivative of the N-terminal kinase is first reacted with (1-oxyl-2,2,5,5-tetramethyl-3-pyrroline-3-methyl)methanesulfonate (MTSL), which modifies the single-site cysteine with the nitroxide (NO) spin label through disulfide bond formation. NMR relaxation studies of the paramagnetic enhancement effect caused by insertion of the spin label yield distances between the unpaired electron of the spin label and the ^{15}N-isotopic-labeled backbone amide protons of the regulatory PH domain.

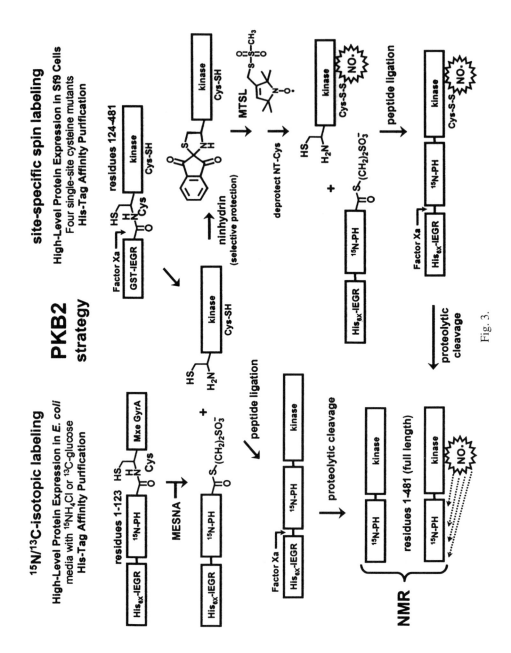

Fig. 3.

3. Either an Apple computer with Mac OS X operating system, any personal computer (PC) with a Linux operating system, or a Unix-based computer (e.g., Silicon Graphics and Sun), to perform the required NMR data processing and structural analysis. The Apple PowerBook laptop computer with Mac OS X operating system is portable and requires little modification for installing all necessary software. Although several PC laptops (e.g., Dell, IBM, and Gateway) with Linux operating systems are available, some degree of modification is required.

2.4.2. Software

1. NMRPipe, NMRDraw, and NMRView for NMR data processing compatible with either Mac OS X, Unix, or Linux operating systems (http://spin.niddk.nih.gov/bax/software/NMR Pipe/info.html).
2. CNS for structure calculations (http://cns.csb.yale.edu/v1.1/).

3. Methods

To perform NMR structural studies of flexible multidomain protein kinases, two different arrangements of the kinase and regulatory domains must be considered: (1) site-directed spin labeling of an N-terminal kinase domain and isotopic labeling of a C-terminal regulatory domain (*see* **Fig. 2**), and (2) isotopic labeling of an N-terminal regulatory domain and site-directed spin labeling of a C-terminal kinase domain (*see* **Fig. 3**). **Subheading 3.1.** describes protein engineering strategies for generating protein kinases with isotopic labeling of the regulatory domain present at either the N- or C-terminus. **Subheading 3.2.** describes protein engineering strategies for generating protein kinases with site-directed spin labeling of the kinase domain present at either the N- or C-terminus. Finally, **Subheading 3.3.** describes the NMR experiments and structural calculations

---

Fig. 3. *(Opposite page)* Overall strategy utilized to combine uniform ^{15}N-isotopic labeling of N-terminal regulatory pleckstrin homology (PH) domain with site-directed nitroxide spin labeling of C-terminal kinase domain of PKB2. The N-terminal regulatory PH domain is expressed as a fusion protein containing an N-terminal His$_6$ tag and a C-terminal Mxe GyrA intein and affinity purified from *Escherichia coli* grown in minimal media supplemented with the desired nuclear magnetic resonance (NMR) active isotopic label. Thiolytic cleavage of the C-terminal Mxe GyrA intein with 2-mercaptoethanesulfonate (MESNA) generates a C-terminal thioester on the N-terminal regulatory PH domain. The C-terminal kinase domain is expressed as a fusion protein containing an N-terminal His$_6$ tag with a factor Xa protease cleavage site and affinity purified from Sf9 insect cells. Cleavage with factor Xa generates an N-terminal cysteine (NT-Cys). As a result of the chemical reactivity between the C-terminal thioester and the NT-Cys, native peptide bond formation occurs on mixing the two protein fragments. Full-length phosphoinositide-dependent protein kinase-2 (PKB2) is affinity purified, and the His^6 tag is cleaved to form segmental isotopic-labeled PKB2 for NMR structural and dynamic studies. To provide for site-directed spin labeled of the C-terminal kinase domain, the NT-Cys is first protected with ninhydrin before chemical modification of the internal single-site cysteine with the MTSL nitroxide (NO) spin label. On deprotection of NT-Cys, the spin-labeled kinase domain is ligated to the thioester derivative of the N-terminal isotopic-labeled regulatory PH domain. NMR relaxation studies of the paramagnetic enhancement effect caused by insertion of the spin label yield distances between the unpaired electron of the spin label and the ^{15}N-isotopic-labeled backbone amide protons of the regulatory PH domain.

required for determining the overall structural dynamics of flexible multidomain protein kinase drug targets, which otherwise do not yield diffraction quality crystals.

3.1. Segmental Isotopic Labeling of Either an N-Terminal or a C-Terminal Regulatory Domain

Because many protein kinases are already established drug targets *(1,2)*, the procedures for cloning, expression, and purification of numerous soluble and functional kinase constructs are provided in the literature. To facilitate structural and dynamic studies of yet-uncharacterized protein kinases, all general procedures necessary for generating the required soluble and functional domain constructs from the full-length kinases are described herein. It is first essential to identify soluble and functional "full-length" kinase constructs that contain both the intact contiguous catalytic and regulatory domains of interest. The "full-length" protein kinase should be tested for soluble expression in a number of different organisms (e.g., bacteria, yeast, or insect cells). If no soluble expression is observed, then amino acid sequence alignments should be performed with sequences of related kinase and regulatory domains from other enzymes and proteins for which 3D structures have been determined. Often, a slightly modified construct may be identified in which a small fragment of the N- and/or C-terminal regions are deleted. Then, sets of primers covering differing ranges of residues are used to generate different constructs to test for soluble expression in the organism of choice. If a construct that contains the contiguous domains of interest is identified, then soluble and functional constructs of the two individual domains can be more easily identified by limited proteolysis, which ultimately facilitates combined segmental isotopic and site-directed spin labeling for NMR studies.

Subheadings 3.1.1.–3.1.6. describe protein engineering strategies for generating segmental isotopic labeling of a C-terminal regulatory domain (e.g., the PH domain of PDK1, as depicted in **Fig. 2**) and segmental isotopic labeling of an N-terminal regulatory domain (e.g., the PH domain of PKB2, as depicted in **Fig. 3**). This includes descriptions for PCR amplification of full-length protein kinase genes from a human cDNA library, expression and purification of soluble and functional human protein kinases from Sf9 insect cells, identification of soluble and functional catalytic and regulatory domain constructs for intein-mediated protein ligation, generation of an NT-Cys on a C-terminal kinase domain or an isotopic-labeled C-terminal regulatory domain, generation of C-terminal thioesters on an N-terminal kinase domain or an isotopic labeled N-terminal regulatory domain, and chemical ligation of the isotopic-labeled regulatory domain to the kinase domain.

3.1.1. Molecular Cloning of Full-Length Protein Kinase Genes From a Human cDNA Library

The most efficient method for obtaining the cDNA encoding a target protein kinase, whether previously described or computer identified through bioinformatic analysis, is by PCR amplification of the full-length gene from a cDNA library and subsequent efficient ligation into a cloning vector as described in **Subheadings 3.1.1.1. and 3.1.1.2.**, respectively. Alternatively, PCR-based gene synthesis provides a robust alternative approach for generating cDNA sequences for predicted genes/cDNA that either are difficult to clone or for which the corresponding mRNA sources are difficult to obtain. Detailed protocols for PCR-based gene synthesis have been evaluated *(12)*.

3.1.1.1. TOUCHDOWN PCR AMPLIFICATION FROM A cDNA LIBRARY

The cDNA coding sequence is obtained for the full-length target protein kinase (e.g., PDK1, accession no. NM002613; and PKB2, accession no. NM005163). PCR is used to generate full-length copies of the human cDNA coding sequence. Human tissue Marathon-Ready cDNA libraries (Clontech) serve as convenient templates. Advantage 2 Polymerase Mix (Clontech), which includes TaqStart Antibody for automatic hot-start PCR, is found to be more effective than other polymerase mixes. To increase further the efficiency of gene-specific PCR amplification from the cDNA library, it is best that the forward and reverse primers complement the 5' and 3' termini of the coding sequence and contain no flanking restriction sites. Each primer should have a GC content of 50–70% and a $T_m \geq 70°C$. To increase the specificity of gene amplification, the following optimized protocol for "touchdown" PCR may be employed: incubation at 94°C for 30 s, 5 cycles of 94°C for 30 s and 72°C for 3 min, 5 cycles of 94°C for 30 s and 70°C for 3 min, and 25 cycles of 94°C for 30 s and 68°C for 3 min. The resulting DNA products are efficiently isolated by gel purification (1% agarose) using a QIAquick Gel Extraction Kit (Qiagen).

3.1.1.2. EFFICIENT LIGATION AND CORRECTIVE MUTAGENESIS

The 3'-dA nucleotide overhangs generated by the Advantage 2 Polymerase Mix (Clontech) must be removed by incubation with a blunt-ended pfu-type high-fidelity polymerase mix (e.g., KOD proofreading polymerase; Novagen). The blunt-ended cDNA PCR products can be efficiently cloned into pCR-Blunt II-TOPO plasmid vector (Invitrogen), which is supplied linearized with *Vaccinia* virus DNA topoisomerase I covalently bound to the 3' end of each DNA strand (*see* **Note 1**). The products of the ligation reactions are transformed into any number of strains of competent cells of *E. coli* (e.g., One Shot TOP10 Chemically Competent *E. coli*; Invitrogen), and selected colonies are grown in 10 mL of enriched media (e.g., Luria Broth) containing an appropriate antibiotic (e.g., ampicillin for the pCR-Blunt II-TOPO plasmid vector). High-quality plasmid preparations can be obtained using a QIAprep Spin Miniprep Kit (Qiagen) for sequence verification. Plasmids shown to contain the fewest alterations in the cDNA sequence are saved for further corrective mutagenesis using either QuikChange Single or Multi Site-Directed Mutagenesis kits (Stratagene) to obtain the native full-length sequences for the target proteins (*see* **Note 2**). The newly generated plasmid PCR products are transformed back into competent cells of *E. coli*, and the plasmids are isolated and sequenced to verify the corrective mutations.

3.1.2. Expression and Purification of Human Protein Kinases

To date, baculovirus-mediated protein expression in either Sf9 or Sf21 insect cells is the most effective method for generating high levels of soluble and active human protein kinases for structural and drug-screening studies. It has been underreported but overestablished that a majority of human protein kinases are poorly expressed and purified as inclusion bodies from both bacterial and yeast protein expression strains under a wide variety of growth and induction conditions. **Subheadings 3.1.2.1.–3.1.2.5.** describe procedures for high-level protein expression in Sf9 insect cells, affinity tag purification, and PDK1 (residues 51–556) and PKB2 (full length, residues 1–481). Removal of the first 50 amino acid residues of PDK1 significantly increases its stability in solution and does not alter its catalytic and regulatory activities.

3.1.2.1. PCR Subcloning Into pFastbac 1 and Generation of Recombinant Bacmid for Producing Recombinant Baculovirus

PCR is used to generate cDNA encoding for an N-terminal His_6-tagged fusion protein of the "full-length" kinase (e.g., residues 51–556 of PDK1 and residues 1–481 of PKB2) containing a PreScission protease recognition sequence for removal of the His_6 tag and flanking restriction enzyme recognition sequences for directional ligation into the pFastbac 1 vector (*see* **Note 3**). A sequence-verified restriction fragment is ligated into the pFastBac 1 vector (Invitrogen), which is used to generate recombinant bacmid for producing recombinant baculovirus using a Bac-to-Bac Baculovirus Expression System (Invitrogen). The recombinant FastBac 1 plasmid is transformed into DH10Bac competent cells of *E. coli*. When transformed DH10Bac cells are grown on Luria-Bertani (LB) agar plates containing kanamycin (50 μg/mL), gentamicin (7 μg/mL), tetracycline (10 μg/mL), Bluo-gal (100 μg/mL), and isopropyl-β-D-thiogalactoside (IPTG) (40 μg/mL), colonies containing recombinant bacmid are white, whereas colonies containing unaltered bacmid are blue (*see* **Note 4**). After selected white colonies are restreaked, a single isolated large white colony is used to inoculate LB media containing kanamycin (50 μg/mL), gentamicin (7 μg/mL), and tetracycline (10 μg/mL), and the high molecular weight recombinant bacmid DNA is isolated using a S.N.A.P. MidiPrep Kit (Invitrogen). Because the recombinant bacmid DNA is greater than 135 kb in size, PCR analysis must be used to verify the presence of the kinase construct using *Taq* DNA polymerase High Fidelity, the M13 Forward (−40) and M13 Reverse primers, and the protocol provided by Invitrogen.

3.1.2.2. Production of Recombinant Baculovirus in Sf9 Insect Cells

1. As suggested in the manufacturer's protocol, dilute 1 μg of recombinant bacmid and 6 μL of Cellfectin Reagent in 200 μL of unsupplemented Grace's Medium, incubate for 45 min at room temperature, and then further dilute with 0.8 mL of unsupplemented Grace's Medium (i.e., no antibiotics). Then add this mixture to individual wells of a 35-mm tissue culture plate containing 9×10^5 attached Sf9 cells/well (>97% viability), and incubate the cells at 27°C for 5 h.
2. Replace the bacmid solution with 2 mL of complete growth media (i.e., Sf-900 II serum-free media with antibiotics), and incubate the cells at 27°C for 72 h.
3. Collect the recombinant P1 viral stock as the clarified supernatant after centrifuging the media containing the cells from which viral budding has been confirmed using an inverted phase microscope at ×250–400.
4. Amplify the recombinant P1 viral stock by infection of a 10-mL suspension culture at 2×10^6 cells/mL, and incubate the cells at 27°C for 48 h.

5. After centrifugation, collect the recombinant P2 stock as the clarified supernatant; a titer of $\geq 1 \times 10^7$ plaque-forming units/mL should be obtained. Store aliquots of the recombinant P2 viral stock at either −80°C (long-term storage) or 4°C (immediate use).

3.1.2.3. HIGH-LEVEL PROTEIN KINASE EXPRESSION IN SF9 INSECT CELLS

1. Use recombinant P2 viral stocks to infect 500-mL spinner flask cultures of Sf9 cells in the midlogarithmic phase of growth (1.5×10^6 cells/mL) at a multiplicity of infection of 1, yielding 1.5×10^6/mL.
2. Incubate the infected cells at 27°C for 72 h, harvest by centrifuging at 200–400g for 10 min at 4°C in a Sorvall centrifuge with a GS-3 rotor, and store the whole cell pellets at −80°C.
3. Allow the frozen pellets to thaw on ice before resuspending in 20 mL of lysis buffer (per 500-mL spinner flask) containing 50 mM Tris-HCl, pH 7.5; 300 mM NaCl; 5 mM ethylenediaminetetraacetic acid (EDTA); 1 mM dithiothreitol (DTT); 1 mM sodium orthovanadate; 5 mM sodium fluoride; 1% (v/v) glycerol; 0.2% (v/v) Triton X-100; and complete protease inhibitor cocktail (one tablet/50 mL). Lyse the cells by incubating for 20 min, followed by freezing and thawing, and pellet the cell debris by centrifuging at $\geq 1600g$ for 30 min at 4°C in a Sorvall centrifuge with an SS-34 rotor. Collect the supernatants containing the soluble components of the cell lysate.

3.1.2.4. NICKEL SEPHAROSE HISTRAP HP AFFINITY PURIFICATION OF N-TERMINAL HIS$_6$-TAGGED PROTEIN KINASE

1. Directly load the soluble lysate by FPLC (1 mL/min) onto a 5-mL bed volume of Ni Sepharose HisTrap HP affinity column (Amersham) equilibrated at 4°C in 50 mM Tris-HCl, pH 7.5; 300 mM NaCl; 50 mM imidazole; 5 mM EDTA; 1 mM DTT; and 1% (v/v) glycerol. Subsequently wash the column until the absorbances at 260 and 280 nm return to baseline.
2. Elute the recombinant His$_6$ affinity–tagged enzyme by increasing the imidazole concentration from 50 to 500 mM. Analyze fractions by sodium dodecyl sulfate polyacrylamide gel electrophoresis (SDS-PAGE), and pool and concentrate fractions containing >85% pure recombinant protein. If no soluble protein expression is obtained, then expression of alternative "full-length" constructs should be attempted.

3.1.2.5. CHARACTERIZATION OF PURIFIED RECOMBINANT PROTEIN KINASES

When adequate amounts of soluble full-length kinase are obtained (e.g., ≥ 20 mg of enzyme/L of culture), the basic structural and enzymatic properties should be characterized.

1. Confirm the identity of the purified enzyme by N-terminal Edman sequencing and also by Western blotting if an antibody is available.
2. Determine the overall molecular weight of the purified kinase by electrospray ionization mass spectrometry (ES-MS) on enzyme preparations that have been either treated or not treated with a variety of protein phosphatases. A reduction in the apparent molecular weight on treatment with phosphatase indicates that the purified kinase underwent phosphorylation during protein expression and/or purification. Conduct phosphopeptide mapping studies to identify the precise sites of phosphorylation and those sites that are dephosphorylated by treatment with specific phosphatases.
3. Evaluate the activity of the protein kinase before and after treatment with specific phosphatases toward model synthetic peptide substrates.
4. Evaluate the stability of the purified enzyme regarding ionic strength, temperature, pH, and freeze/thaw cycling. Whereas the enzymatic activity of most human protein kinases,

which have been expressed and purified from Sf9 insect cells, is prolonged at lower temperatures (4°C) in buffers of physiological ionic strength (≥0.15 *M*) and mild pH, NMR protein structural studies are optimally performed at higher temperatures (≥20°C) in buffers of lower ionic strength (≥0.15 *M*) and slightly acidic pH.

3.1.3. Identification of Soluble and Functional Catalytic and Regulatory Domain Constructs for Intein-Mediated Protein Ligation

The "full-length" kinase target construct (20–50 μg) is cleaved at 37°C with trypsin (0.2–0.5 μg) in 50 m*M* Tris-HCl, pH 8.0, with 100 m*M* NaCl. Aliquots are taken every min over 20 min, supplemented with 10 m*M* benzamidine, and analyzed by SDS-PAGE. The protein fragments are purified from the gel and subjected to N-terminal Edman sequencing and matrix-assisted laser desorption ionization analysis. From knowledge of the N-terminal sequence, the molecular mass, and the trypsin cleavage sites, soluble domain constructs can be identified. After identifying soluble domain constructs, the first approach toward selection of a suitable ligation site is to identify an X-Cys pair between the boundaries of the N- and C-terminal domains to be ligated. X will be the C-terminal residue of the N-terminal domain, and Cys will be the N-terminal residue of the C-terminal domain (*see* **Note 5**) *(13,14)*. If no X-Cys pair (in which X is preferably His, Cys, or Gly and preferably not Asp, Pro, Ile, or Val) exists between the boundaries, then an X-Ser pair is chosen, because a Ser→Cys mutation is both isosteric and isoelectronic and often causes very little effects in protein activity and stability. If an X-Ser pair does not exist, care must be taken to identify a pair of residues for which mutagenesis to form an X-Cys pair is least likely to induce structural perturbations and lower the stability of the enzyme.

3.1.4. Generation of NT-Cys on C-Terminal Kinase or Regulatory Domains

Proteolytic cleavage of an N-terminal affinity tag using the factor Xa protease is the most convenient method for generating an NT-Cys, because factor Xa cleaves at the C-terminus of arginine in the recognition sequence IEGR *(13,14)*. Although the procedure described next is for removal of an N-terminal His$_6$ tag, any N-terminal affinity tag may be substituted.

1. Because a C-terminal larger-sized kinase domain does not require isotopic label, high-level and soluble protein expression is best achieved in Sf9 insect cells. Generate a fusion protein construct containing an N-terminal His$_6$ tag with a factor Xa protease cleavage site prior to an NT-Cys of the kinase domain construct in FastBac 1 vector (Invitrogen). Use recombinant pFastBac 1 vector to generate recombinant baculovirus using the Bacto-Bac Baculovirus Expression System (Invitrogen), and express and purify the His$_6$-tagged kinase domain from Sf9 insect cells (*see* **Subheading 3.1.2.**).

2. To facilitate uniform ^{15}N and/or ^{13}C-isotopic labeling, a C-terminal regulatory domain must be expressed in either bacterial or yeast cells. Generate a protein expression vector containing an N-terminal His$_6$ tag with a factor Xa protease cleavage site prior to an NT-Cys of the regulatory domain construct by PCR and transform into protein expression strains of either *E. coli* bacteria or *Pichia pastoris* yeast. Optimize the temperature, time, and chemical inducer (e.g., IPTG) concentration for high-level expression of a soluble His$_6$-tagged fusion regulatory domain construct. If no soluble protein can be generated, then

consider alternative ligation sites. If high-level expression of soluble protein is achieved, then carry out uniform ^{15}N- and/or ^{13}C-isotopic labeling by growing the cells in minimal media containing ^{15}NH$_4$Cl as the sole source of nitrogen, either ^{13}C- or ^{12}C-glucose as the sole source of carbon, and the appropriate selective antibiotic before His$_6$ tag affinity purification.

3. Optimal conditions for factor Xa proteolytic cleavage of individual affinity tagged fusion proteins must be established. Add varying amounts of factor Xa protease to the purified His$_6$-tagged C-terminal domain, and carry out digestion at varying temperatures for varying times. The extent of cleavage may be followed by high-performance liquid chromatography (HPLC), ES-MS, or SDS-PAGE.

4. After the reaction is carried out under optimized conditions, remove factor Xa by passage over a benzamidine column. Remove simultaneously the cleaved His$_6$ tag and any remaining uncleaved protein containing the His$_6$ tag by incubating with nickel Sepharose HisTrap HP (200 µL) resin (Amersham). After incubation for 15 min, centrifuge the mixture, and concentrate ($\geq$0.05 mM) the supernatant containing the cleaved enzyme and store at −80°C.

3.1.5. Generation of C-Terminal Thioester on N-Terminal Kinase and Regulatory Domains

A C-terminal thioester on either an N-terminal kinase domain or an N-terminal regulatory domain is generated by designing a construct in which a cleavable N-terminal His$_6$ tag preceding the domain construct is fused to a C-terminal Mxe GyrA intein *(13, 14)*. Depending on whether the N-terminal construct is expressed in bacteria, yeast, or insect cells, such fusion protein constructs are generated by PCR and subsequent ligation into any number of protein expression vectors. Addition of the thiol reagent MESNA to the purified fusion protein causes cleavage of the C-terminal Mxe GyrA intein and formation of a C-terminal thioester derivative of MESNA with the N-terminal domain. MESNA is particularly advantageous over other thiolytic reagents (e.g., ethanethiol or thiophenol), because it is significantly more soluble and is completely odorless.

1. Since an N-terminal kinase domain requires expression in Sf9 insect cells, generate an N-terminal His$_6$ tag with a PreScission protease cleavage site preceding the kinase domain construct fused to the C-terminal Mxe GyrA intein in FastBac 1 vector (*see* **Note 6**). Use recombinant pFastBac 1 vector to generate recombinant baculovirus using the Bac-to-Bac Baculovirus Expression System (Invitrogen), and express the Mxe GyrA fusion construct of the kinase domain is expressed in Sf9 insect cells and His$_6$ tag affinity purify (*see* **Subheading 3.1.2.**). If no soluble fusion construct can be obtained, then it is necessary to select a new ligation site, and new domain constructs must be engineered.

2. Since an N-terminal regulatory domain requires uniform ^{15}N- and/or ^{13}C-isotopic labeling by *E. coli* expression in minimal media, generate a fusion protein construct containing a cleavable N-terminal His$_6$ tag preceding the regulatory domain construct fused to a C-terminal Mxe GyrA intein in a chosen bacterial protein expression vector (*see* **Note 7**). Even if high levels of insoluble protein are produced, we find it often possible to obtain the regulatory domain in soluble form after thiolytic cleavage with MESNA of the Mxe GyrA intein under partially denaturing conditions ($\leq$4 M guanidine HCl or urea). Smaller regulatory domains can often be refolded to be soluble and functional. Once it has been established that thiolytic cleavage can yield a soluble domain construct (*see* **step 3**), express the His$_6$-tagged regulatory domain–Mxe GyrA construct in minimal media for isotopic labeling and His$_6$ tag affinity purify (*see* **Subheading 3.1.2.4.**).

3. Subject the N-terminal His$_6$-tagged kinase–Mxe GyrA or isotopic-labeled regulatory domain–Mxe GyrA construct to thiolytic cleavage in mild aqueous buffer (pH 6.0–8.0) by adding MESNA in a fourfold excess molar ratio to the protein. The extent of the cleavage reaction may be followed by subjecting small aliquots of the reaction mixture to HPLC, ES-MS, or SDS-PAGE analysis. The reaction rate and extent of cleavage is increased under slightly acidic conditions (pH 6.0–7.0). The MESNA thioester derivative of the N-terminal domain may be stored under normal protein domain storage conditions until native chemical ligation with the C-terminal domain is to be performed.

3.1.6. Native Chemical Ligation of Kinase and Regulatory Domains

Native chemical ligation between the N-terminal domain containing the C-terminal thioester derivative of MESNA and the C-terminal domain containing an NT-Cys is typically carried out in mild aqueous buffers (pH 6.0–8.0) at temperatures between 4 and 40°C, depending on the stability requirements of the protein components *(13,14)*. The reaction is further catalyzed by including 2% (w/v) MESNA as a "cofactor" in the ligation buffer in the presence of the protein components at the highest possible concentration (≥0.05 mM). The rates of native chemical ligation vary, depending on the temperature, protein concentration, and the amino acid residues near the termini being joined. The extent of the ligation reaction may be monitored by either HPLC, ES-MS, or SDS-PAGE. Once it has been established that the reaction has proceeded to near completion, the ligated full-length kinase is His$_6$ tag affinity purified, and the affinity tag is proteolytically removed (*see* **Subheading 3.1.4.**). The enzymatic properties (e.g., activity, regulation, and stability) of the segmentally labeled full-length protein kinase must be evaluated and compared with those determined for the native full-length protein kinase (*see* **Subheading 3.1.2.5.**). In addition, protein NMR spectra should be obtained for the segmentally labeled full-length protein kinase and compared with spectra of the isolated regulatory domain construct (*see* **Subheading 3.3.1.**).

3.2. Site-Directed Paramagnetic Spin Labeling of Either an N-Terminal or a C-Terminal Kinase Domain

Once it has been established that a soluble isotopic-labeled regulatory domain may be successfully ligated to a soluble kinase domain and that high-quality ^{1}H–^{15}N HSQC NMR spectra (*see* **Subheading 3.3.1.**) can be obtained for the segmentally-labeled construct, the final protein engineering step involves site-directed, paramagnetic nitroxide spin labeling of the individual kinase domain. The site-directed, spin-labeled kinase domain is ligated to the isotopic-labeled regulatory domain for ultimate determination of long-range distance restraints between the two domains. **Subheading 3.2.1.** describes methods for selecting and generating single-site cysteines in the kinase domain. **Subheading 3.2.2.** describes a basic procedure for chemical modification with the nitroxide spin label of a single cysteine residue in the case of an N-terminal kinase domain (e.g., PDK1, as depicted in **Fig. 2**). **Subheading 3.2.3.** describes additional procedures for chemical protection and deprotection of the NT-Cys of a C-terminal kinase domain (e.g., PKB2, as depicted in **Fig. 3**) in order to provide site-directed spin labeling of a single internal cysteine.

3.2.1. Generation of Single-Site Cysteine Mutants of Kinase Domains

Alkylation of the thiolate of cysteine residues provides a highly site-specific method for the introduction of spin labels on proteins *(15)*. However, many of the kinase domains contain numerous cysteine residues. If the number of cysteine residues in the kinase domain construct is less than five, then it is practical to use the QuikChange Single or Multi Site-Directed Mutagenesis kits (Stratagene) in order to mutate all of the cysteine residues to serine residues (*see* **Note 2**). If the kinase domain contains more than five cysteine residues, then it is preferable to generate a cysteine-free mutant by PCR-based gene synthesis of an engineered kinase domain in which all of the cysteines have been mutated to serines *(12)*. With a cysteine-free kinase domain, site-directed mutagenesis can be further used to substitute any amino acid residue with a single cysteine, allowing a spin label to be introduced at any position in the kinase domain.

Using the known X-ray structure of a given kinase domain, four to six residues for cysteine substitution should be chosen. Single-site cysteine mutant constructs should be generated so that spin label modifications are obtained on both the N- and C-lobes at positions both near and far from the kinase active site. Residues with highly solvent-accessible side chains should be given preference, particularly the native cysteine and serine residues. However, substitution of any charged residue will likely yield a stable mutant.

3.2.2. Chemical Modification of Single Cysteine With Nitroxide Spin Label

1. Directly modify an N-terminal kinase domain (e.g., PDK1, as depicted in **Fig. 2**) with a C-terminal thioester derivative of MESNA with the spin label reagent MTSL (Toronto Research Chemicals) (*see* **Note 8**) *(15)*. Dissolve the protein in the preferred buffer (pH 8.0), and remove oxygen by flushing the solution with argon gas. Add a threefold molar excess of MTSL from a 40 mM stock in acetonitrile to the protein (0.05–0.5 mM), and incubate the reaction mixture in the dark at room temperature overnight. The reaction rate may be increased by incubating with higher concentrations of MTSL (≤10-fold molar excess).
2. Remove excess MTSL reagent by gel filtration on a P4 column.
3. To remove any unlabeled protein with a free sulfhydryl group, pass the reaction product over an organomercurial thiol-affinity column (Bio-Gel 501; Bio-Rad).
4. A sensitive method for determining the extent of modification is titration of an aliquot of the reaction product with the thiol-specific fluorophore CPM (Molecular Probes) (*see* **Note 9**). The nitroxide must be reduced prior to fluorescence measurements to prevent paramagnetic quenching of the CPM fluorophore. Collect fluoresence emission spectra using the ratio of corrected emission intensities at $\lambda_{max} = 480$ nm on excitation at 340 nm.
5. Evaluate the efficiency of spin labeling by direct electron paramagnetic resonance (EPR) measurements of the spin-labeled protein (*see* **Subheading 3.3.3.**).
6. Chemically ligate the N-terminal kinase domain containing both a C-terminal thioester and a site-directed nitroxide spin label to the C-terminal isotopic-labeled regulatory domain (*see* **Subheading 3.1.6.**).

3.2.3. Chemical Protection and Deprotection
of NT-Cys of a C-Terminal Kinase Domain

In the case in which a C-terminal kinase domain (e.g., PKB2, as depicted in **Fig. 3**) requires a single-site cysteine to attach the spin label but also requires an N-terminal cysteine for intein-mediated ligation, the N-terminal cysteine must be chemically protected before chemical modification with the nitroxide spin label. NT-Cys residues are distinguished from internal cysteine residues by the presence of *two* vicinal nucleophiles, β-thiol and α-amine, which confer unique chemical reactivity with ninhydrin (indane-1,2,3-trione). It is known that ninhydrin reacts with uncharged primary amines ($-NH_2$) under mild aqueous conditions to form the chromophore Ruhman's purple, which has been greatly utilized for quantitative amino acid analysis. However, the β-thiol of free cysteine or an NT-Cys further reacts with the Schiff's base intermediate of ninhydrin bonded to the N-terminal amino group to form a cyclic five-membered spiro-thiazolidine (Thz) ring *(16)*. The Thz structure effectively protects the NT-Cys so that the internal single-site Cys can be chemically modified with the nitroxide spin label (*see* **Note 10**). Following attachment of the nitroxide spin label, ninhydrin is removed to facilitate native chemical ligation of the C-terminal site-directed, spin-labeled kinase domain to the N-terminal regulatory domain.

1. Cleave the N-terminal His_6 tag with factor Xa protease to generate the C-terminal kinase domain with an NT-Cys and a single internal Cys (*see* **Subheading 3.1.4.**).
2. Add a 10-fold molar excess of ninhydrin (≤10 m*M*) from a concentrated stock solution to the purified C-terminal kinase domain, and incubate in buffer (pH 5.0–7.0) at room temperature for 2 h.
3. Remove excess ninhydrin by gel filtration on a P4 column, and evaluate the extent and specificity of the ninhydrin reaction.
4. Assess the extent of possible lysine modification by observing of Ruhman's purple color formation. Ninhydrin can be prevented from reacting with lysine by lowering the pH of the protection reaction.
5. Assess the extent of NT-Cys and internal cysteine modification by Ellman's reaction. Dilute 100-μL aliquots of the test reaction with 850 μL of phosphate buffer (pH 7.5) and 50 μL of 3 m*M* (DTNB or Ellman's reagent) and measure the absorbance at 412 nm. Under these conditions, the test reaction should show approximately half the titratable sulfhydryl groups of an identical protein sample that did not undergo reaction with ninhydrin (corrected for protein concentration). If more than half of the sites are obtained, the ninhydrin can be further removed from the internal cysteine by repassaging over the P4 gel filtration column. If less than half of the sites are obtained, the ninhydrin reaction should be carried out for longer times.
6. React the ninhydrin-protected NT-Cys kinase domain with MTSL, and evaluate the extent of modification by CPM titration and EPR (*see* **Subheading 3.2.2.**).
7. Remove ninhydrin from the NT-Cys of the spin-labeled domain by treating with a 10-fold molar excess of free cysteine at pH 7.5–8.0 for 30 min at room temperature (*see* **Note 11**).
8. Remove free cysteine and the ninhydrin–cysteine compounds by gel filtration, and evaluate the extent of the deprotection reaction by thiol titration with CPM.
9. Chemically ligate the C-terminal kinase domain containing both an NT-Cys and a site-directed nitroxide spin label to the N-terminal isotopic-labeled regulatory domain (*see* **Subheading 3.1.6.**).

3.3. NMR Structural Studies

Once it has been established that a soluble, isotopic-labeled regulatory domain can be successfully ligated to a soluble kinase domain, which contains a single nitroxide spin label, NMR experiments and structural calculations may be performed in order to determine the overall structural dynamics of a target multidomain protein kinase. **Subheading 3.3.1.** describes the standard NMR approaches for determining the NMR solution structure of the regulatory domain, either in its isolated form or while ligated to its kinase domain. **Subheading 3.3.2.** describes the NMR relaxation experiments for determining the effects that placing the paramagnetic nitroxide spin label on the kinase domain has on the relaxation rates of the backbone amide protons of the regulatory domain, and how these effects can be converted into distance restraints between the site-directed spin label and each of the backbone amide protons. **Subheading 3.3.3.** describes methods for calculating the effective rotational correlation times, τ_c, required for distance calculations. **Subheading 3.3.4.** describes methods for calculating the relative structures from distance restraints derived from the paramagnetic relaxation enhancement effects and assessing the relative degree of domain–domain flexibility.

3.3.1. NMR Structural Studies of Regulatory Domain

The solution structure of the isotopic-labeled regulatory domain while spliced and intact with its kinase domain is determined by standard heteronuclear multidimensional NMR methods *(17)*. However, the overall rotational correlation times, τ_c, of segmental isotopic-labeled full-length kinases will be greater than those of the equivalent isotopic-labeled individual regulatory domains, which will cause broadening of the NMR peaks and loss of resolution. By collecting NMR spectra at higher temperatures (e.g., 37°C), effective rotational correlation times of larger proteins can be reduced, thus enhancing the spectral resolution. If the target full-length protein kinase is not stable at higher temperatures for prolonged data collection times, then NMR peak broadening can be reduced by selective incorporation of amino acids with aliphatic side chains containing carbon-bound deuterium instead of hydrogen (e.g., Ala, Val, Leu, and Ile) into the ^{15}N- and ^{13}C-isotopic-labeled domain *(18)*. If deuterium labeling is necessary to obtain NMR spectra, then advanced TROSY-modified forms of the NMR experiments described in the following paragraphs will yield quality data on higher-field NMR instruments (e.g., ≥600 MHz) *(19)*. Although this approach provides enhanced ability to perform heteronuclear multidimensional NMR experiments for assignment of backbone resonances and determination of backbone secondary structure, tertiary structural information is compromised owing to the loss of NOE signals that would otherwise indicate hydrophobic packing between side-chain methyls from residues distant in residue sequence. In such cases, the structure of the isolated domain construct should be determined and used with the X-ray structure of the kinase domain for overall model calculations.

If the isolated regulatory domain construct or the segmentally labeled full-length protein kinase is sufficiently stable in low-salt (≤0.15 *M*) buffer solutions for up to 3 d, then sequential backbone assignments are initially obtained from ^{15}N-edited NOESY and TOCSY spectra and confirmed and completed by ^{15}N- and ^{13}C-edited HNCACB and CBCA(CO)NH triple resonance spectra. Side-chain assignments are primarily obtained from ^{15}N- and ^{13}C-edited HCCH-TOCSY, CC(CO)NH, and HC(CO)NH experiments. Intramolecular distance constraints between protons of the regulatory domain are obtained from ^{15}N- and ^{13}C-edited NOESY spectra. NOE signals to specific residues of the ^{13}C-isotopically labeled regulatory domain from protons of the unlabeled kinase domain are distinguished by performing a ^{12}C/^{13}C-isotope-edited NOESY experiment, which detects NOEs to methyl protons on ^{13}C-labeled residues only from ^{12}C-bound protons. Dihedral angle restraints are determined from $^3J_{NH\alpha}$ values calculated from HNCA-J and HNHA experiments. If an adequate number of NOE signals between amino acid residues distant in primary sequence (long-range NOE) are determined, structures of the isolated or segmentally labeled regulatory domain can be calculated from randomized initial structures using the hybrid distance geometry-simulated annealing and protocol in the program CNS(XPLOR) *(20)*. A set of substructures is selected to undergo a simulated annealing refinement to select for a final ensemble of energy-minimized structures that satisfy the criteria of no NOE violations of more than 0.5° and no dihedral violations of more than 5° to be used to define the tertiary structures of the regulatory domain construct.

To determine the position of the regulatory domain with respect to the kinase domain, it is necessary to confirm or redetermine as many chemical shift assignments as possible for regulatory domain backbone amide cross peaks in two-dimensional (2D) ^{1}H–^{15}N HSQC spectra of the full-length kinase. Backbone amide chemical shift assignments of the intact regulatory domain ultimately facilitate the NMR relaxation experiments combining segmental isotopic and site-directed spin labeling (*see* **Subheadings 3.3.2.–3.3.4.**).

3.3.2. Distance Restraints Between Backbone Amides of Regulatory Domain and Site-Directed Spin Label of Kinase Domain

Distances between the unpaired electron of the nitroxide spin label on the kinase domain and each of the backbone amide protons of the ^{15}N-labeled regulatory domain can be calculated from the amount that either the longitudinal ($\Delta R1$; **Eq. 1**) or transverse ($\Delta R2$; **Eq. 2**) relaxation rates of the amide protons is increased in the presence of the spin label according to a modified form of the Solomon-Bloembergen equation *(15,21)*:

$$r = 6 \sqrt{\frac{2K}{\Delta R1} \times \frac{3\tau_c}{1 + \omega_H^2\tau_c^2}} \qquad (1)$$

$$r = 6 \sqrt{\frac{K}{\Delta R2} \times 4\tau_c + \frac{3\tau_c}{1 + \omega_H^2\tau_c^2}} \qquad (2)$$

in which K is a constant (1.23×10^{-32} cm^6 s^{-2}) for paramagnetic nitroxide, ω_H is the Larmor frequency of the amide proton (s^{-1}), τ_c is the correlation time for the electron-amide proton vector (s), and r is the vector distance between the electron and the proton (cm). The paramagnetic enhancement of the longitudinal ($\Delta R1$) and transverse ($\Delta R2$) relaxation rates is calculated from **Eqs. 3** and **4**:

$$1/T1_p = \Delta R1 = R1_{para} - R1_{dia} \qquad (3)$$

$$1/T1_p = \Delta R2 = R2_{para} - R2_{dia} \qquad (4)$$

in which $R1_{para}$ and $R2_{para}$ are, respectively, the longitudinal and transverse relaxation rates of the amide proton in the presence of oxidized *para*magnetic nitroxide, and

$R1_{dia}$ and $R2_{dia}$ are, respectively, the longitudinal and transverse relaxation rates of the amide proton in the presence of reduced *dia*magnetic nitroxide or no spin label at all.

With good approximations of τ_c and paramagnetic relaxation enhancement values for either $\Delta R1$ or $\Delta R2$, long-range distance restraints for electron-amide proton vectors are obtained from **Eqs. 1** and **2**, which can be used to evaluate the overall structural dynamics of the contiguous regulatory and kinase domains. Although the distance restraints obtained from only one site-directed spin label will give a good indication of the overall arrangement between the regulatory and kinase domains, additional distance restraints obtained from NMR studies of other engineered constructs in which the spin label is positioned at different locations on the kinase domain will give a better indication of the overall structural dynamics of the full-length protein kinase.

3.3.2.1. Distance Restraints Derived From Either $\Delta R1$ or $\Delta R2$

Longitudinal $R1$ and transverse $R2$ relaxation rates of the backbone amide protons of a ^{15}N-labeled regulatory domain are measured using standard ^1H–^{15}N HSQC pulse sequences, which have been modified to include either an inversion recovery sequence ($R1$) or a CPMG phase-cycled spin echo ($R2$) *(22,23)*. Inversion recovery HSQC spectra are collected with varying recovery delay times (e.g., 0, 25, 75, 150, 300, 500, 700, 1000, 1500, 2000, 2500, and 3000 ms), and CPMG HSQC spectra are collected with a constant spin echo delay of 0.5 ms and with varying echo trains (e.g., 0, 5, 10, 20, 30, 50, 75, 100, and 150 echos).

Integrated peak volumes (V) are measured for each amide cross peak in the 2D spectra and plotted as a function of either the inversion recovery delay time for $R1$ measurements or the time in the transverse plane (number of echo trains × constant echo delay of 0.5 ms) for $R2$ measurements. To account for the small decrease in peak volume that occurs during the HSQC pulse sequence (*see* **Note 12**), it is preferable that the peak volumes be fitted to **Eq. 5** *(24)*:

$$V(\tau) = V_D[1 - B(1 - \exp(-\kappa R)) \times \exp(-\tau R)] \qquad (5)$$

in which V_D is the initial peak volume, κ is the sum of acquisition and preparation times during the ^1H–^{15}N HSQC experimental pulse sequence, B is an adjustment parameter for incomplete magnetization inversion, and R can be either the longitudinal ($R1$) or transverse ($R2$) relaxation rate constant.

Longitudinal $R1$ or transverse $R2$ relaxation rates are determined for the amide proton relaxation rates under both diamagnetic and paramagnetic conditions, and the paramagnetic enhancements ($\Delta R1$ or $\Delta R2$) are calculated by either **Eq. 3** or **4**, respectively (*see* **Note 13**).

3.3.2.2. Rapid Determination of $\Delta R2$ for Unstable Protein Kinases

The primary drawback of determining values of $\Delta R1$ and $\Delta R2$ is that successive HSQC experiments must be carried out with varying inversion recovery or CPMG periods. As these periods become longer, the data collection times of the experiments become longer. With minimal sample concentrations (~0.3 mM), many transients must be collected, and a complete $R1$ or $R2$ data set may require days to obtain good signal-to-noise ratios ($S/N \geq 10$), which ultimately reduces propagated errors in distance calculations. This can become a hindrance when extensive NMR time is not readily available or when the stability of the engineered protein kinase construct is in question. In such cases, it is possible to simply collect a standard HSQC spectrum of the protein kinase in the presence (paramagnetic conditions) and absence (diamagnetic conditions) of the spin label. Values of the paramagnetic relaxation enhancement effect on the transverse relaxation rate ($\Delta R2$) for each amide proton are determined from the ratio of the intensity (height) of the HSQC cross peak in the paramagnetic sample (I_{para}) to the intensity of HSQC cross peak in the diamagnetic sample (I_{dia}) according to **Eq. 6** *(25,26)*:

$$\frac{I_{para}}{I_{dia}} = \frac{R2_{dia}\,\exp(-\Delta R2t)}{R2_{dia} + \Delta R2} \tag{6}$$

in which t is the duration of the INEPT delays (~9 to 10 ms) in the HSQC pulse sequence and $R2_{dia}$ is calculated from the line width at half height ($R2_{dia} = \pi \times LW$) of the amide cross peak in the proton dimension. Values of $\Delta R2$ are obtained by computer fitting of I_{para}/I_{dia} to **Eq. 6** with substitution of known values of $R2_{dia}$ and t. These $\Delta R2$ values are substituted into **Eq. 2** to obtain distances. Since intensity ratios (I_{para}/I_{dia}) are used to calculate $\Delta R2$, it is required that the two HSQC spectra be collected and processed with identical parameters and that the sample conditions also be identical, especially protein concentration.

3.3.3. Calculation of Electron-Amide Proton Vector Correlation Times, τ_c

The correlation time, τ_c, required for calculating distances in **Eqs. 1** and **2** is described by the sum of contributions from the relaxation of the electron plus motions of the electron–proton vector according to **Eq. 7** *(15)*:

$$\frac{1}{\tau_c} = \frac{1}{\tau_S} + \frac{1}{\tau_R} \tag{7}$$

in which τ_S is the longitudinal relaxation time of the nitroxide free radical (≥ 100 ns) and τ_R is the effective rotational correlation time of the vector (~1–30 ns). Since the effective rotational correlation times of the electron-amide proton vectors (τ_R) in protein kinase constructs containing a single catalytic kinase domain (~35–50 kDa) and a small regulatory domain (~10–20 kDa) will always be significantly shorter than the longitudinal relaxation time of the nitroxide free radical (τ_S), the value of τ_c can be approximated from measurements of τ_R. Since the distance r depends on the sixth root of τ_c, distance calculations will be relatively insensitive to errors in estimate values of τ_c. Thus, typical errors of ±10% in ΔR and ±50% in τ_c measurements result in an error of only ±8% in the distance. **Subheadings 3.3.3.1.–3.3.3.3.** describe three different methods for measuring τ_c values, which can be used as estimates for τ_c in **Eq. 1** or **2**.

3.3.3.1. ESTIMATE OF τ_c: NMR MEASUREMENTS OF $\Delta R1$ AT TWO FIELD STRENGTHS

The correlation times, τ_c, for each of the individual electron-amide proton vectors may be obtained by measuring $\Delta R1$ at two different magnetic field strengths. For example, τ_c for each of the electron-amide proton vectors is calculated from the frequency dependence of the paramagnetic effects at 500 and 700 MHz according to **Eq. 8** *(21)*:

$$\tau_c = \sqrt{\frac{T1_{p700} - T1_{p500}}{T1_{p500}\,\omega^2_{500} - T1_{p500}\,\omega^2_{700}}} \tag{8}$$

in which ω is the Larmor frequency of the proton and $T1_p = 1/\Delta R1$ at either 500 or 700 MHz.

3.3.3.2. ESTIMATE OF τ_c: NMR MEASUREMENTS OF $\Delta R1$ AND $\Delta R2$ AT ONE FIELD STRENGTH

The correlation times, τ_c, for each of the individual electron-amide proton vectors may also be obtained by measuring both $\Delta R1$ and $\Delta R2$ at one magnetic field strength. For example, τ_c for each of the electron-amide proton vectors is calculated from the ratio of $\Delta R2$ to $\Delta R1$ using **Eq. 9 (15)**:

$$\tau_c = \sqrt{\frac{6(\Delta R2/\Delta R1) - 7}{4\omega^2_H}} \tag{9}$$

in which ω is the Larmor frequency of the proton.

3.3.3.3. ESTIMATE OF τ_c: EPR MEASUREMENT AND SPECTRAL SIMULATION

The electronic rotational correlation time of the nitroxide unpaired electron can be measured by generating simulated EPR spectral lines that reproduce the spectral lines observed from direct EPR studies of the spin-labeled protein *(21)*. Spectral simulations can be performed with the available software provided by the EPR manufacturer, and this τ_c can be used to calculate the distance for each individual electron-amide proton vector. Although distances calculated in this manner have a larger uncertainty than those calculated using individual correlation times, it can save considerable time and provide reliable overall structures.

3.3.4. STRUCTURAL CALCULATIONS

Changes in the position of the isotopically labeled domain relative to the site-directed spin-labeled domain can be calculated using distance geometry/simulated annealing protocols in CNS(XPLOR) *(21,26,27)*. First, the NMR solution structure of the isotopically labeled domain construct is chemically connected to the known X-ray structure of the site-directed spin-labeled domain, and only the peptide bonds located in the loop region of the junction between the two domains are allowed to sample different conformations. Distances between the site-specific spin label and the amide protons of the ^{15}N-labeled domain are given the energy function normally used for NOE restraints in CNS(XPLOR). This is possible because both NOE and paramagnetic distance restraints have an r^{-6} distance dependence. For each construct, lower and upper bounds for distance restraints are initially derived by propagation of errors for taking the mathematical difference between relaxation rate constants measured under paramagnetic (R_{para}) and diamagnetic (R_{dia}) conditions, as well as the estimated error in τ_c. The most accurate protocol is to generate an annealing process using distance restraints from the backbone amides to the site-directed spin label. In such a case, the amino acid site in the X-ray structure must be replaced with the disulfide-linked nitroxide molecule, and this modification must be parameterized for computer-simulated annealing calculations. Owing to considerable error in distance calculations, much time can be saved if the terminal heteroatom of the native amino acid is used for distance geometry location point of the nitroxide ion while simply increasing the upper bound of the distance restraints.

The observation that no suitable crystals have been obtained for X-ray diffraction studies of any full-length serine–threonine protein kinase with a regulatory domain strongly suggests that multiple tertiary arrangements may exist between the two domains. Therefore, it is unreasonable to quantify a degree of resolution for such dynamic structures. For example, the sixth-power relationship between r and ΔR will cause the calculated distances to be heavily biased in favor of the shortest distances attained by the regulatory domain amides to the spin label. Although this is not a concern for a well-defined rigid domain–domain interaction, it can be misleading for highly flexible domains that sample a wide variety of relative positioning. Nevertheless, the dynamic range of relative orientations between two domains can best be observed by performing distance restraint calculations for numerous additional individual constructs containing the nitroxide spin label on four opposite faces of the kinase. By comparing structures derived for each of the individual constructs, the relative degree of domain–domain flexibility will be determined. If the relative positions of the two domains are very similar for all of the spin-labeled constructs, then structure calculations can be carried out using all of the distance restraints.

4. Notes

1. The TOPO enzyme catalyzes ligation of the 3' ends of each vector strand to the 5' ends of the PCR product, while releasing itself in an energy-conserved reaction. In addition, pCR-Blunt II-TOPO allows direct selection of recombinants via disruption of the lethal *E. coli* gene *ccd*B, permitting growth of only positive recombinants on transformation.

2. QuikChange Single or Multi Site-Directed Mutagenesis kits (Stratagene) use corrective primers to generate full-length corrected copies of the entire plasmid containing the mutated gene. The plasmid template containing the mutation is then digested away using *Dpn*I endonuclease.

3. The full-length protein kinase gene in the pCR-Blunt II-TOPO plasmid vector is used as the template to generate the desired coding region. The nucleotide coding region must not contain the restriction enzyme recognition sequences selected for directional ligation, and the amino acid sequence must be checked for recognition sites for the protease selected for removal of the His_6 or other affinity tag. The reverse or downstream primer (kinase-R) is designed complementary to the 3'-terminal coding region and extended to include the desired restriction enzyme recognition sequence. Two forward or upstream 5' primers can be used to extend the cDNA protein-coding region to include a His_6 tag with a PreScission protease cleavage site and a flanking restriction enzyme recognition sequence. The PreScission-kinase-F1 primer is designed complementary to the kinase-coding region and extended in the 5' direction to include nucleotides coding for the PreScission protease peptide recognition sequence (LEVLFQGP). The His_6-PreScission-F2 primer is designed complementary to the protease peptide recognition sequence (LEVLFQGP) and extended in the 5' direction to include the N-terminal His_6 tag and the restriction enzyme recognition sequence. The T_m values for all of the overlapping regions should be temperature optimized for the high-fidelity PCR polymerase mix. Standard PCR reaction conditions using 100 ng

of plasmid template, 500 nM kinase-R reverse primer, 200 nM PreScission-kinase-F1 primer, and 300 nM His$_6$-PreScission-F2 primer will yield the full-length cDNA with flanking restriction enzyme cloning sites.

4. DH10Bac cells contain a baculovirus shuttle vector (bacmid) with a mini-*att*Tn7 target site and a helper plasmid. On transformation, transposition occurs between the mini-Tn7 element on the recombinant pFastBac 1 vector and the mini-*att*Tn7 target site on the bacmid to generate a recombinant bacmid. The transposition reaction is catalyzed by transposition proteins supplied by the helper plasmid. Insertion of the mini-Tn7 into the mini-*att* Tn7 attachment site on the bacmid disrupts expression of the LacZa peptide.

5. All 20 naturally occurring amino acids have been shown to support native chemical ligation when placed at the C-terminus of a thioester peptide, but the kinetics of ligation can be significantly different *(13,14)*. For example, rapid ligation reactions are observed when X is either His, Cys, or Gly and extremely slow ligation reactions are observed with Ile, Val, and Pro. The nature of X also appears to influence the thiolytic cleavage of the intein to yield the C-terminal thioester derivative of the N-terminal protein fragment. For example, high levels of premature in vivo cleavage of the intein fusion protein may occur when X is an Asp residue, and in vitro thiol-mediated cleavage of the intein is inhibited when X is a Pro residue.

6. First, the cDNA encoding for the kinase domain construct with an N-terminal restriction enzyme recognition sequence, His$_6$ tag, and protease recognition sequence is obtained by PCR using the recombinant pFastBac 1 vector containing the full-length kinase gene as the template. Second, the cDNA encoding for the Mxe GyrA intein is obtained by PCR using the pTWIN1 vector (New England Biolabs) as the template. The Mxe GyrA forward primer is complementary to the N-terminus of the Mxe GyrA intein and extended in the 5' direction to generate an overlapping region with the C-terminal residues of the kinase domain construct. The Mxe GyrA reverse primer is complementary to the C-terminus of the Mxe GyrA intein and extended in the 5' direction to include a stop codon and a restriction enzyme recognition sequence. Finally, the cDNA PCR products encoding for the N-terminal kinase domain and the Mxe GyrA intein are joined by further PCR, since both fragments share the nucleotide-coding region coding for the C-terminus of the kinase domain construct. Then, a sequence-verified restriction fragment of the His$_6$-tagged kinase domain fused at the C-terminus to the Mxe GyrA intein is ligated into the pFastBac 1 vector (Invitrogen).

7. First, the cDNA encoding for the regulatory domain with an N-terminal cloning recognition sequence is obtained by PCR. Second, the cDNA encoding for the MxeGyrA intein is obtained by PCR and extended in the 5' direction to generate an overlapping region with the C-terminal residues of the regulatory domain. The cDNA PCR products encoding for the regulatory domain and the Mxe GyrA constructs are joined by further PCR, ligated to a bacterial protein expression vector, and optimized for high-level bacterial expression.

8. The electrophilic thiosulfonate group of MTSL will not react favorably with the electrophilic C-terminal thioester group. Rather, the MTSL reagent is very susceptible to nucleophilic attack by the sulfhydryl group of the single cysteine, resulting in disulfide bond formation to the nitroxide spin label.

9. CPM has been found to be more sensitive than DTNB for quantifying residual amounts of thiol in a large backgound of nitroxide-labeled protein *(25)*.

10. The reaction of ninhydrin with NT-Cys is highly specific under slightly acidic conditions (pH < 5.0), which eliminates the reaction of ninhydrin with the side-chain ε-amino group of lysine residues more prevalent at pH > 7.0. While ninhydrin does react with the side-

chain sulfhydryl group of the internal cysteine, the presumed hemithioketal is fascile and decomposes on removal of free ninhydrin by gel filtration *(16)*.

11. The exchange reaction of ninhydrin from NT-Cys to free cysteine is driven under mass action and is much more rapid than the exchange of the nitroxide spin label from the internal cysteine to free cysteine.

12. Prior to signal acquisition, the coherence transfer pathway in the conventional HSQC pulse sequence involves a total of ~9 to 10 ms of fixed delays during which the ^{15}NH proton magnetization resides in the transverse plane. During these delays the peak volume in the HSQC spectrum decreases owing to transverse relaxation of the proton.

13. Traditionally, relaxation spectra are first collected with the spin label in its paramagnetic or oxidized form; identical data are then collected on the same sample in which the spin label has been reduced to its diamagnetic form. To reduce the nitroxide free radical to its secondary amine, a threefold molar excess of ascorbate is added and the sample is allowed to incubate at pH 5.3 and room temperature overnight *(15)*. The pH must be readjusted before collecting the HSQC on the reduced sample. If the protein sample is unstable toward treatment with ascorbate, it is possible to determine the $R1_{dia}$ or $R2_{dia}$ values on a segmentally labeled protein kinase that has not been chemically modified with the spin label under identical solution conditions (e.g., buffer, temperature, and protein concentration) to the samples that contain a spin label. Then, the $R1_{dia}$ and/or $R2_{dia}$ values can be subtracted from $R1_{para}$ and/or $R2_{para}$ values determined for all of the different single-cysteine, site-directed spin-labeled constructs, and values of $\Delta R1$ and/or $\Delta R2$ may be used to calculate distances for each of the electron-amide proton vectors according to **Eqs. 2** and/or **3**, respectively.

References

1. Cohen, P. (2002) Protein kinases—the major drug targets of the twenty-first century? *Nat. Rev. Drug Discov.* **1,** 309–315.
2. Noble, M. E., Endicott, J. A., and Johnson, L. N. (2004) Protein kinase inhibitors: insights into drug design from structure. *Science* **303,** 1800–1805.
3. Kahan, B. D. (2002) The limitations of calcineurin and mTOR inhibitors: new directions for immunosuppressive strategies. *Transplant. Proc.* **34,** 130–133.
4. Druker, B. J. (2002) STI571 (Gleevec) as a paradigm for cancer therapy. *Trends Mol. Med.* **8,** S14–S18.
5. Cohen, P. (1999) The development and therapeutic potential of protein kinase inhibitors. *Curr. Opin. Chem. Biol.* **3,** 459–465.
6. Davies, S. P., Reddy, H., Caivano, M., and Cohen, P. (2000) Specificity and mechanism of action of some commonly used protein kinase inhibitors. *Biochem. J.* **351,** 95–105.
7. Tong, L., Pav, S., White, D. M., et al. (1997) A highly specific inhibitor of human p38 MAP kinase binds in the ATP pocket. *Nat. Struct. Biol.* **4,** 311–316.
8. Jencks, W. P. (1981) On the attribution and additivity of binding energies. *Proc. Natl. Acad. Sci USA* **78,** 4046–4050.
9. Erlanson, D. A., Wells, J. A., and Braisted, A. C. (2004) Tethering: fragment-based drug discovery. *Annu. Rev. Biomol. Struct.* **33,** 199–223.
10. Mountain, V. (2003) Astex, Structural Genomix, and Syrrx, I can see clearly now: structural biology and drug discovery. *Chem. Biol.* **10,** 95–98.
11. Harris, T. K. (2003) PDK1 and PKB/Akt: ideal targets for developing new strategies to structure-based drug design. *IUBMB Life* **55,** 117–126.

12. Gao, X., Yo, P., Keith, A., Ragan, T. J., and Harris, T. K. (2003) Thermodynamically balanced inside-out (TBIO) PCR-based gene synthesis: a novel method of primer design for high-fidelity assembly of longer gene sequences. *Nucleic Acids Res.* **31,** e143.
13. Blaschke, U. K., Silberstein, J., and Muir, T. W. (2000) Protein engineering by expressed protein ligation. *Methods Enzymol.* **328,** 478–496.
14. Cowburn, D. and Muir, T. W. (2001) Segmental isotopic labeling using expressed protein ligation. *Methods Enzymol.* **339,** 41–54.
15. Kosen, P. A. (1989) Spin labeling of proteins. *Methods Enzymol.* **177,** 86–121.
16. Pool, C. T., Boyd, J. G., and Tam, J. P. (2004) Ninhydrin as a reversible protecting group of amino-terminal cysteine. *J. Pept. Res.* **63,** 223–234.
17. Cavanaugh, J., Fairbrother, W. J., Palmer, A. G., and Skelton, N. J. (1996) *Protein NMR Spectroscopy: Principles and Practice,* Academic, San Diego.
18. Goto, N. K. and Kay, L. E. (2000) New developments in isotope labeling strategies for protein solution NMR spectroscopy. *Curr. Opin. Struct. Biol.* **10,** 585–592.
19. Fernandez, C. and Wider, G. (2003) TROSY in NMR studies of the structure and function of large biological molecules. *Curr. Opin. Struct. Biol.* **13,** 570–580.
20. Brünger, A. T. (1992) *X-PLOR (Version 3.1), A System for X-Ray Crystallography and NMR,* Yale University Press, New Haven, CT.
21. Gaponenko, V., Howarth, J. W., Columbus, L., et al. (2000) Protein global fold determination using site-directed spin and isotope labeling. *Protein Sci.* **9,** 302–309.
22. Carr, H. Y. and Purcell, E. M. (1954) Effects of diffusion on free precession in nuclear magnetic resonance experiments. *Phys. Rev.* **94,** 630–641.
23. Meiboom, S. and Gill, D. (1958) Modified spin-echo method for measuring nuclear relaxation times. *Rev. Sci. Instrum.* **91,** 688–691.
24. Ferretti, J. A. and Weiss, G. H. (1989) One dimensional Overhauser effects and peak intensity measurements. *Methods Enzymol.* **176,** 3–11.
25. Gillespie, J. R. and Shortle, D. (1997) Characterization of long-range structure in the denatured state of Staphylococcal nuclease. I. Paramagnetic relaxation enhancement by nitroxide spin labels. *J. Mol. Biol.* **268,** 158–169.
26. Battiste, J. L. and Wagner, G. (2000) Utilization of site-directed spin labeling and high resolution heteronuclear nuclear magnetic resonance for global fold determination of large proteins with limited nuclear Overhauser effect data. *Biochemistry* **39,** 5355–5365.
27. Gillespie, J. R. and Shortle, D. (1997) Characterization of long-range structure in the denatured state of Staphylococcal nuclease. II. Distant restraints from paramagnetic relaxation and calculation of an ensemble of structures. *J. Mol. Biol.* **268,** 170–184.

11

Nuclear Magnetic Resonance-Based Screening Methods for Drug Discovery

Laurel O. Sillerud and Richard S. Larson

Summary

Nuclear magnetic resonance (NMR) techniques are widely used in the drug discovery process. The primary feature exploited in these investigations is the large difference in mass between drugs and receptors (usually proteins) and the effect that this has on the rotational or translational correlation times for drugs bound to their targets. Many NMR parameters, such as the diffusion coefficient, spin diffusion, nuclear Overhauser enhancement, and transverse and longitudinal relaxation times, are strong functions of either the overall tumbling or translation of molecules in solution. This has led to the development of a wide variety of NMR techniques applicable to the elucidation of protein and nucleic acid structure in solution, the screening of drug candidates for binding to a target of choice, and the study of the conformational changes that occur in a target on drug binding. High-throughput screening by NMR methods has recently received a boost from the introduction of sophisticated computational techniques for reducing the time needed for the acquistion of the primary NMR data for multidimensional studies.

Key Words: Nuclear magnetic resonance; diffusion; nuclear Overhauser enhancement; chemical shift; nuclear spin; drug candidate; transferred nuclear Overhauser effect spectroscopy; saturation transfer difference; structure-activity relationships; residual dipolar couplings.

1. Introduction to Nuclear Magnetic Resonance Methods Used for Identification and Screening of Lead

Nuclear magnetic resonance (NMR) methods have such general applicability that there is hardly a branch of modern science that has not been favorably impacted by this technology. The basis for this broad scope of applications lies in the existence of a magnetic isotope for almost every nucleus in the periodic table. Nuclear resonances are exquisite magnetometers, revealing, through their frequencies, the local molecular magnetic fields in great detail. The local molecular magnetic fields arise from the density, within the nucleus, of the very magnetic electrons whose role in covalent bonding puts them right at the heart of molecular and chemical physics. For this reason, nuclear

From: *Methods in Molecular Biology, vol. 316: Bioinformatics and Drug Discovery*
Edited by: R. S. Larson © Humana Press Inc., Totowa, NJ

resonance frequencies reveal molecular structures and interactions, from both a static and a dynamic point of view, from molecules in the gaseous, liquid, and solid state. The dependence of nuclear resonance properties on the masses of the molecules enables one to differentiate between large receptor proteins and small drug molecules. When suitable external field gradients are applied to the sample, anatomical structures in living systems can also be observed. It is no surprise, then, that NMR methods continue to have a great impact on drug discovery, and this chapter seeks to review the most important applications of current interest.

The properties of NMR signals are modulated by the dynamics of the chemical structure containing the nucleus of interest. Foremost among these dynamic effects is the coupling between the nuclear spin and the surrounding radiation bath, which is manifest in the rates of transverse (R_1) and longitudinal (R_2) nuclear magnetic relaxation. This coupling is a very strong function of the rotational correlation time for the chemical framework. Because chemical exchange processes influence the lifetimes of the excited nuclear states, exchange processes also modulate the observed properties of nuclear resonances. In addition to tumbling and exchanging among differing environments, nuclei diffuse in solution locked to their chemical structures with a diffusion coefficient that varies according to molecular mass. Each of these physical effects is a rich source of spectroscopic information about a chemical species by itself, but for our purposes, the emphasis is placed on the applications of these effects to the screening of molecules for interactions with a given drug target. A spectral editing scheme has been developed for each of these dynamic interactions, including relaxation, chemical shift perturbations, translational diffusion, and magnetization transfer. NMR methods can even reveal the metabolism of drugs in living systems and provide metabolite identification. Advances in solvent suppression, coherent and incoherent magnetization transfer pathway selection, isotope editing and filtering, and diffusion filtering have made it possible to examine the interactions between small molecules and proteins or nucleic acids in great detail *(1)*.

The main feature that is exploited in the use of NMR methods in screening for drug candidates is the large difference in molecular masses between drugs (~500 Daltons) and their targets ($M_r > 25$ kDa). This large mass difference leads to large disparities in either the rotational correlation or diffusion times for these two classes of molecules, which can then be used to filter the spectra. For example, the strength of the nuclear Overhauser effect (NOE) depends on the rotational correlation time. The transferred nuclear Overhauser effect (trNOE) has been employed to determine the bound conformations of carbohydrates and other bioactive molecules in complex with protein receptors. The corresponding experiments in the rotating frame and selective editing experiments (e.g., QUIET-NOESY [NOE spectroscopy]) are used to eliminate indirect cross-relaxation pathways (spin diffusion), to minimize errors in the data used for calculation of conformations. Saturation transfer difference NMR experiments reveal detailed information about intermolecular contacts between ligand and protein *(2)*. An additional advantage of these techniques is that low-affinity ligands, which might be missed by high-throughput screening (HTS), can be detected and could serve as synthetic precursors for higher-affinity ligands *(3)*.

In addition to editing schemes based on mass differences, another powerful filtration technique involves the replacement of the nuclei in either the drug or the target with isotopes that are either magnetic or nonmagnetic. The most common isotopes used are ^{2}H, ^{13}C, and ^{15}N, which can replace ^{1}H, ^{12}C, and ^{14}N, respectively, in biomolecules. Because the NMR frequencies for the nuclei in a biomolecule are sensitive to molecular structure, isotopic labeling and NMR methods are used extensively to determine macromolecular structure. Approximately 25% of the structures in the Protein Data Bank (www.rcsb.org/pdb/) have been developed using NMR methods. Of particular interest is the fact that these NMR structures were determined in solution, so no time-consuming crystallization was necessary.

NMR methods also fit perfectly into the modern, structure-based drug design program. The biological target is a macromolecule that is crucial for the biological activity or process that is to be inhibited. For example, human immunodeficiency virus (HIV-1) is expressed as a single polypeptide within an infected host cell. This polypeptide is then processed by a virally encoded protease; the processed proteins are packaged and the virus erupts from within the infected cell. The HIV protease was critical for virus maturation and was an important biological target for drug discovery and development. This has led to several highly effective therapeutics for HIV *(4)* based on the structure of the binding site for proteins on the HIV protease.

A structure-based drug design program will have the following components. The gene of the target of interest is cloned and the protein or macromolecule is expressed and purified. The initial lead compound is then discovered by a variety of techniques such as HTS, in which hundreds of thousands of compounds are examined en masse for binding to the purified target. In a concurrent effort, the three-dimensional (3D) structure of the target macromolecule is determined using NMR or X-ray crystallography, or the structure can be modeled using molecular modeling techniques. Once the structure of the target macromolecule has been determined or modeled, and a lead compound has been isolated, the structure of the target-compound complex can be determined using the same techniques. These target-compound structures can then be examined using computational chemistry techniques and possible modifications to the compound can be determined. Finally, all of the data are collated and used in designing the next series of compounds, which are then synthesized. This cycle is repeated until a compound is sufficiently potent (able to inhibit the biological target at extremely low, typically picomolar, concentrations), at which point it is sent to preclinical (animal testing) and clinical (human) testing. In the current discovery cycle, an average time to reach preclinical investigation is 3 yr. We present here a brief review and introduction to the role that NMR techniques play in each of these components.

2. Materials

2.1. NMR Supplies

NMR tubes are available in all of the necessary shapes and sizes for the study of proteins, drugs, and nucleic acids from the following sources:

1. Aldrich (www.sigmaaldrich.com).
2. Wilmad (www.wilmad.com/index.html): maker of some of the very best NMR tubes, standards, and other NMR-related items.
3. Chemglass (www.nmrtubes.com): NMR tubes, caps, valves, and NMR tube cleaners.
4. RototecSpintec (www.rototec-spintec.com/): a distributor for Wilmad consumables in Europe.
5. New Era Enterprises (http://newera-spectro.com/): NMR 5-mm sample tubes.
6. Shigemi (www.geocities.com/~shigemi/): makes magnetic-susceptibility matched plugs for all types of solvents, as well as NMR tubes and other diposables.
7. Norell (www.nmrtubes.com): a supplier of NMR sample tubes, NMR solvents, Teflon tubing, books, and a discussion forum for NMR professionals.
8. NMR pages from Kontes (www.kontes.com/html/NMR.html): Kontes has several useful NMR consumables.
9. Deutero GmbH (http://home.t-online.de/home/deutero/): isotopes, solvents and consumables for NMR in Europe.
10. AmpolNMR.com/Europe (http://ampolnmr.com/): a supplier of NMR sample tubes and accessories.
11. Worldwide Glass Resource Ltd. (www.wwglassresource.co.uk): UK suppliers of NMR consumables.

2.2. Stable Isotopes for Labeling Drugs and Receptors, and for NMR Solvents

1. Cambridge Isotope Laboratories (www.isotope.com/cil/index.html): a manufacturer of stable isotope-labeled compounds, stable isotope separations, and some fine deuterated solvents.
2. Silantes GmbH (www.silantes.com/): stable isotope-labeled biopolymers (^2H, ^{13}C, ^{15}N).
3. Isotec (www.sigmaaldrich.com): a member of the Sigma-Aldrich family, manufacturer of stable isotope-labeled compounds. It makes some of the most unique and novel labeled compounds.
4. C/D/N ISOTOPES (www.cdniso.com/): a large listing of deuterated compounds and carbon 13- and nitrogen 15-labeled compounds; in English, German, or French.
5. Medical Isotopes (www.medicalisotopes.com/): nearly a complete line of enriched biochemicals; nice selection of fatty acids enriched with C13.
6. NMR Shift Reagents (www.rareearthproducts.com/Prodnmr%20Shift%20Reagents.htm): a supplier of NMR shift reagents.
7. Novachem Pty Ltd. (www.novachem.com.au/): stable isotopes in Australia.
8. U.S. Department of Energy (DOE) Isotope Programs (http://nuclear.gov/isotopes/default-mine.asp): information about US DOE production of isotopes programs.
9. Spectra Gases (www.spectra-gases.com/): isotopic enrichment of gases for research.
10. International Isotope Society (www.intl-isotope-soc.org/): provides a forum for all chemists involved in radiochemical synthesis and analysis to obtain and share information outside of their immediate area of employment and expertise.
11. Martek Biosciences (www.martekbio.com/): isotopically enriched biochemicals and media for the growth of microorganisms.
12. U.S. DOE Isotope Production & Distribution (www.ornl.gov/sci/isotopes/catalog.htm): US DOE isotopes catalog.
13. Isoflex (www.isoflex.com/): stable isotopes for use in science, medicine, and industry from Russian producers.

14. Moravek Radiochemicals (www.moravek.com/): a manufacturer of tritium- and carbon 14-labeled radiochemicals for acquired immunodeficiency syndrome and cancer research.

15. The National Stable Isotope Resource at Los Alamos (http://sir.lanl.gov): advances biomedical applications of compounds labeled with the stable isotopes ^{13}C, ^{15}N, ^{17}O, ^{18}O, ^{33}S, ^{34}S, and ^{77}Se.

16. STB Isotope Germany Gmbh (www.stb-isotope.com/): stable isotopes for science, medicine, and industry, including some rare and unusual stable isotopes.

17. RITVERC GmbH (www.ritverc.com/): a producer and worldwide supplier of radioisotope products for science, industry, and medicine. The product list includes radiation sources, labeled compounds, stable isotopes, and radiopreparations.

18. Techsnabexport (www.tenex.ru/): a supplier of Russian-produced radioisotopes and labeled compounds.

19. Advanced Materials Technologies Ltd. (www.isotope-amt.com): a supplier of stable isotopes, deuterated solvents, and high-purity materials for medical and chemical research.

20. PicoTrace (www.picotrace.de/): equipment for trace element and isotope analysis.

21. Chemgas (www.chemgas.com/): a supplier of high-purity rare gases and isotopically enriched gases.

22. Omicron Biochemicals (www.omicronbio.com/): a supplier of single, multiple, and uniform stable isotope-labeled saccharides and nucleosides (^{13}C, ^{2}H, ^{15}N, ^{18}O).

23. Wellington Laboratories (www.well-labs.com/): a producer of ^{12}C and ^{13}C halogenated reference standards of environmental concern, including chlorinated and brominated dioxins, furans, biphenyls, and diphenyl ethers.

24. IsoSciences (www.isosciences.com/pages/1/index.htm): custom stable isotope labeling and small-scale organic synthesis including the preparation of metabolites and positron emission tomography precursors and standards.

25. Gas-Oil JSC (www.c13.ru): a manufacturer of [^{13}C]-CO_2 using lasers.

26. CNL Scientific Resources (www.cnlscientific.com/main.html): a supplier of isotopes, metals, crystals, and other engineered materials to manufacturers of pharmaceuticals and instruments.

2.3. NMR Acquistion and Processing Software

1. Bruker Biospin (www.bruker-biospin.com/nmr/products/software.html): XWIN-NMR^{TM} is the main software package for Bruker spectrometer control, data acquisition, and processing, and XWIN Plot^{TM} is an interactive graphical plot editor, which facilitates the manipulation of plot layouts directly on the display so that the user can quickly tailor the results. This software can be purchased for off-line processing on Silicon Graphics Incorporated and PC-based computers.

2. Acorn NMR (www.acornnmr.com/): offers desktop NMR data-processing software and operates a high-resolution NMR spectroscopy service in Fremont, CA.

3. VNMR (www.varianinc.com/cgi-bin/nav?products/nmr/software/vnmr&cid=OPOILPK FP): Varian's X Window packages (VNMRX for the Sun, VNMRSGI for Silicon Graphics computers, and VNMRI for IBM RS/6000 workstations) provide full functionality in that environment.

4. GoNMR (www.gonmr.com/): is a software package for data acquisition and processing. It is supposed to make VNMR (Varian software) much easier to use for the beginner and the expert, for routine day-to-day uses. GoNMR provides fully automated software for obtaining NMR spectra.

5. NMRPipe (http://spin.niddk.nih.gov/bax/software/NMRPipe/): is a multidimensional spectral processing system based on UNIX pipes.

6. TRIAD (www.tripos.com/sciTech/inSilicoDisc/nmrAnalysis/triad.html): Spectra, spread-sheets, and structure all in one time-saving program.
7. MestReC (www.mestrec.com/): is an advanced NMR data-processing package for Windows. MestReC is a software package for WinNT/2K/XP systems that offers state-of-the-art facilities for data processing, visualization, and analysis of high-resolution NMR data, combined with a robust, user-friendly graphical interface.
8. MRUI (www.mrui.uab.es): is a graphical user interface that allows MR spectroscopists to perform easily time-domain analysis of in vivo MR data.
9. FELIX (www.accelrys.com/pharma/target/nmr/dataproc.html): is an industry standard for off-line data-processing software for all types of high-resolution, one- to four-dimensional homonuclear and heteronuclear NMR data.
10. NUTS (www.acornnmr.com/nuts_price.htm): is a complete NMR data-processing package that runs on PCs under Windows (95, 98, NT, 2K, ME, and XP) and on PowerMacs.
11. Other specialized software can be found on the often-updated NMR Information Server at www.spincore.com/nmrinfo/.

3. Methods

The theoretical basis for the use of various filters on the NMR spectra from drug candidates and protein targets rests on fundamental classical and quantum physics. We examine here each of the filter techniques with the goal of providing an understanding of the underlying physical phenomena, including a summary equation of the process and often a graphical illustration of the strength of the effect as a function of the relevant parameters.

3.1. Diffusion Filtering

Self-diffusion of a solute in a solvent can easily be measured using now-classic, pulsed-gradient, spin-echo NMR techniques first proposed by Stejskal and Tanner *(5)* in 1965, in which the nuclear signal, S, decays owing to the diffusion coefficient, D, during the time, B, between two gradient pulses of amplitude, G, and duration, A, according to

$$S(2\tau) = S(0)\exp(-\gamma^2 b^2 D G^2)$$

in which γ is the nuclear gyromagnetic ratio (~4.23 kHz/G for protons); $2\tau = t_1 + t_2 + A + B$ is the total time from the $\pi/2$ pulse to the center of the echo in the acquisition window; and $b^2 = A^2 B$. Here, t_1 is the time from the first $\pi/2$ pulse to the first gradient pulse, and t_2 is the time from the π pulse to the center of the acquisition window. This exponential dependence of the NMR signal amplitude on the diffusion coefficient provides an efficient filter to discriminate the nuclear resonances from small molecules free in solution from those bound to macromolecules. For example, the diffusion coefficient for a small molecule in water at 25°C is about 10^{-5} cm²/s, whereas that for a 30,000-Dalton protein is approx 6×10^{-8} cm²/s. This large disparity leads to a 10- to 20-fold relative difference in the NMR signals of the two species (**Fig. 1**).

Use of diffusion filters in drug screening involves mixing a putative drug with its receptor and examining the resulting NMR spectra taken in the presence and absence

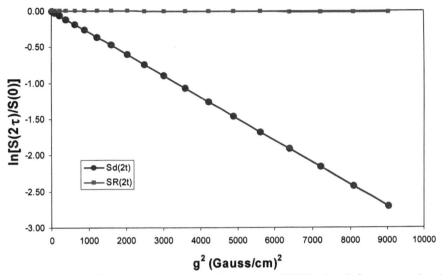

Fig. 1. Example of decay of nuclear magnetic resonance (NMR) signals from two molecules with differing molecular masses of 113 (solid circles = drug) and 30,000 Daltons (solid squares = receptor) in a pulsed-field gradient of strength up to 95 G/cm. Note that at the highest gradient strength, the NMR signal from the smaller molecule has decayed by a factor of 15 with respect to the macromolecule.

of a pulsed magnetic field gradient (*6*). If the drug binds to the protein, then it will adopt the diffusion coefficient of the larger molecule and the NMR signals will survive diffusion editing with gradients that would otherwise remove the signals from a drug free in solution (*7*). Often diffusion editing is applied through digital difference spectroscopy on mixtures of small candidate molecules with their receptor. The resulting difference spectra will contain only signals from those (if any) small molecules that bind to the macromolecule and can be readily identified from the mixture by their unique chemical shifts. This editing scheme depends on exchange between the bound and free forms of the drugs, so that if the association constants are too large, the bound form of the drug(s) will not be observable owing to T_2 relaxation from the macromolecule. Diffusion coefficients can be miscalculated, however, owing to magnetization transfer between the receptor and ligand. This trNOE disrupts the observed signal decay owing to diffusion as a function of the experimental diffusion time (*8*).

3.2. Relaxation Editing

Much like a spinning gyroscope, which, owing to the conservation of classical angular momentum, resists realignment of its spin axis, a spinning nucleus prefers to remain with its quantum-mechanical angular momentum (spin) aligned parallel to the applied magnetic field in an NMR spectrometer magnet. And, just as a gyroscope requires a large impulsive force to tip its spin vector away from its initial axis, a spinning nucleus in a magnetic field requires a large, impulsive orthogonal field to tip its magnetization vector away from the static field direction. Once perturbed, both a spinning gyroscope and a spinning nucleus tend to return to their original positions. The rate of return for a nucleus is on the order of seconds for small molecules in aqueous solution because nuclei are extremely weakly coupled to their environments. This return to equilibrium, or relaxation, of the polarized nuclear spin is often dominated by dipolar interactions with neighboring nuclei that have components of molecular motion at frequencies either near zero (transverse relaxation) or at the Larmor (NMR) frequency (longitudinal relaxation). The longitudinal relaxation time (rate) is termed T_1 ($R_1 = 1/T_1$), and the transverse relaxation time (rate) is T_2 ($R_2 = 1/T_2$). For rotational motion of a nucleus characterized by a correlation time, τ, in a fluid of low viscosity, such as water, the dipolar relaxation rates are given by

$$R_1 = \frac{2\gamma^4 h^2 I(I + 1)}{5\pi^2 r^6} \left(\frac{\tau}{1 + \omega^2 \tau^2} + \frac{4\tau}{1 + 4\omega^2 \tau^2} \right)$$

and

$$R_2 = \frac{\gamma^4 h^2 I(I + 1)}{5\pi^2 r^6} \left(3\tau + \frac{5\tau}{1 + \omega^2 \tau^2} + \frac{2\tau}{1 + 4\omega^2 \tau^2} \right)$$

in which γ is, again, the nuclear gyromagnetic ratio; h is Planck's constant; I is the nuclear spin quantum number (1/2 for protons); r is the internuclear distance; and ω is the Larmor frequency (these are shown in **Fig. 2** for two different NMR frequencies). In the extreme narrowing limit, in which $\omega\tau \ll 1$ is satisfied, both R_1 and R_2 become equal to

$$R_1 = R_2 = \frac{2\gamma^4 h^2 I(I + 1)}{\pi^2 r^6} \tau$$

Now, since the rotational correlation time is proportional to the mass through Stoke's Law;

$$\tau = \frac{\eta M}{\rho k T}$$

in which η is the viscosity, M is the molecular mass, and ρ is the density, the relaxation rates for molecules in solution are a strong function of their masses. To illustrate this, we have calculated the dipolar relaxation rates for the same two molecular masses (113 Daltons and 30 kDa) used in the diffusion example shown in **Fig. 1** (**Table 1**), including the nuclear Overhauser enhancement, η (τ), as if an observed proton were relaxed by an adjacent proton 1.75 Å away. The large difference in mass results in an equally large difference in rotational correlation times and relaxation rates between the drug and the receptor.

It is clear from the relaxation curves shown in **Fig. 2** that the most efficient agent that leads to transverse relaxation (R_1) for a given proton is another proton nearby with Fourier components of motion at the Larmor frequency; the relaxation rates peak at correlation times approximately equal to the reciprocal of the Larmor frequency. The physical basis for this results from Einstein's work on the matrix elements for stimulated emission of radiation in which a photon of the proper frequency can stimulate the decay of an excited quantum state. Since adjacent protons can cause the relax-

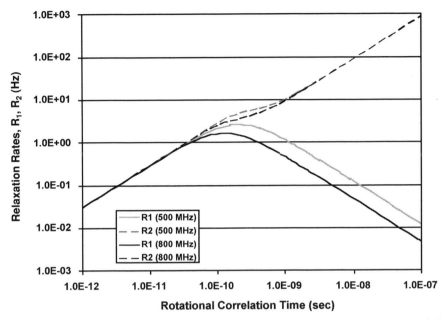

Fig. 2. Relationship between the proton relaxation rates R_1 and R_2 and rotational correlation time for two different nuclear magnetic resonance frequencies, 500 and 800 MHz.

Table 1
Comparison of NMR Relaxation Properties for a Drug and a Receptor

M_r (Daltons)	ν (MHz)	τ (s)	R_1 (Hz)	R_2 (Hz)	η (τ)	D (cm²/s)
113	500	1.2×10^{-12}	3.7×10^{-4}	3.7×10^{-4}	0.50	1×10^{-5}
113	800	1.2×10^{-12}	3.7×10^{-4}	3.7×10^{-4}	0.50	1×10^{-5}
30,000	500	2.1×10^{-9}	5.0×10^{-3}	2.2×10^{3}	−1.00	6×10^{-8}
30,000	800	2.1×10^{-9}	2.1×10^{-1}	2.0×10^{1}	−0.95	6×10^{-8}

ation of an observed polarized proton, it is then logical to suppose that nearby protons can also influence the populations of excited states. This is indeed true and forms the basis for another very important physical property of nuclear spins, the nuclear form of the Overhauser effect (NOE).

3.3. Nuclear Overhauser Effect

Although most modern NOE experiments are performed as two-dimensional (2D) acquisitions (NOESY), the theory of the NOE is most easily understood with reference to the simplest one-dimensional (1D) experiment. For a pair of nuclei (e.g., protons)

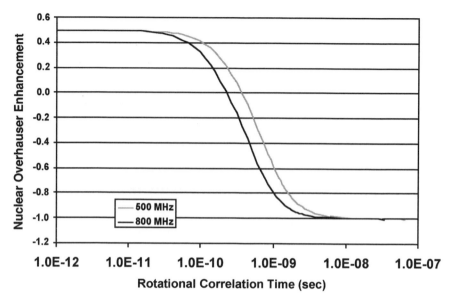

Fig. 3. Relationship between rotational correlation time of a molecule and maximum nuclear Overhauser enhancement (NOE) for a proton relaxed by a neighboring proton for two different proton resonance frequencies, 500 and 800 MHz. Note that there is also a $1/r^6$ distance dependence of the NOE that attenuates this maximal interaction.

with distinct chemical shifts, irradiation of one nuclear resonance will result in changes in the intensity of the other, as long as the second nucleus is within range (<6 Å) so that dipolar coupling between the two will result in spin-lattice (T_1) relaxation. The NOE arises from the changes in populations of the nuclear spin states owing to enhanced relaxation of the observed state as a result of irradiation of the dipolar-coupled state. There is a strong dependence of the NOE on the rotational correlation time (**Fig. 3**). The fractional enhancement for the resonance integral of one proton on saturation of the resonance of a second, nearby proton is given by

$$\eta\,(\tau) = \frac{5 + \omega^2\tau^2 - 4\omega^4\tau^4}{10 + 23\omega^2\tau^2 + 4\omega^4\tau^4}$$

The maximum enhancement for protons is 0.5 for the small correlation times appropriate for drugs in water, and for macromolecules with longer correlation times, the NOE becomes negative (**Fig. 3**) with a limiting magnitude of −1.0. This serves as another means by which drug interactions with receptors can be studied and used for screening.

A drug in solution will acquire the NOE of the receptor if it binds, and this forms the basis for the transferred-NOESY (trNOESY) method, which can be used to reveal the structure of the bound ligand in solution. The other main use of the NOE is to derive internuclear distances and, hence, molecular structures in solution. Because the NOE is a dipole–dipole interaction, its amplitude decreases as the inverse sixth power of the distance between the nuclei. Therefore, by measuring the NOEs for several nuclei in a molecule, and by referring these to an internal, known calibration distance (e.g., a methylene with nondegenerate resonances), one can generate accurate solution structures; this is the basis for the thousands of protein structures determined by NMR and deposited in the Protein Data Bank (www.rcsb.org/pdb/).

3.4. Transferred NOE Spectroscopy

The binding of molecules to receptors is an equilibrium process in which there is chemical exchange between the free and bound forms of the ligand. Exchange results in the drug adopting the different physical properties of the receptor with attendent alterations in the correlation times and effective masses of the drugs. During the drug's residence in its receptor-binding site, it will adopt the bound configuration, which may bring remote groups into proximity. The resulting intramolecular NOEs in the NMR spectrum will give useful information about the distances between these groups in the bound state. Chemical exchange with drug molecules free in solution will transfer the bound NOE from the bound drug to the free drug, resulting in a trNOE. Protein-drug interactions cause significant relaxation enhancement even when the drug concentration is in excess by 10- to 100-fold over that of the receptor. In this way, the trNOE is amplified and visible in the narrow resonances of the drug in solution. trNOE methods work particularly well for the very large receptor molecules traditionally thought to be too massive for direct, conventional NMR methods.

The theoretical basis for the analysis of structures by trNOE methods is the subject of an excellent review by Ni *(9)*. In brief, a trNOE can be observed if the drug-receptor dissociation is fast enough, which in NMR terms means that the drug must move on and off the receptor a few times during the NOE mixing time ($\tau_m \sim$ 100–200 ms, or K_d ~5–10 s^{-1}). For a drug interacting with a receptor, R, there are at least four separate mechanisms by which magnetization can be transferred from one proton, A, on a drug to another, nearby proton on the drug, B, or on the receptor. These can be summarized by

$$A_{\text{free}} \xrightarrow{k} A_{\text{bound}} \xrightarrow{\sigma} B_{\text{bound}} \tag{1}$$

$$A_{\text{free}} \xrightarrow{k} A_{\text{bound}} \xrightarrow{\sigma} B_{\text{bound}} \xrightarrow{k} B \tag{2}$$

$$A_{\text{free}} \xrightarrow{k} A_{\text{bound}} \xrightarrow{\sigma} R \tag{3}$$

$$A_{\text{free}} \xrightarrow{k} A_{\text{bound}} \xrightarrow{\sigma} R \xrightarrow{\sigma} B_{\text{bound}} \xrightarrow{k} B_{\text{free}} \tag{4}$$

in which k and σ are the rate constants for chemical exchange and cross relaxation, respectively. The cross-relaxation rate involves zero and double quantum transitions for the A and B protons, which is the basis for the use of the NOE to determine internuclear distances by NMR, and is given by **Eq. 5** for a pair of protons separated by a distance r. Note that the cross-relaxation rate is a dipole–dipole interaction and, hence, decreases as the inverse sixth power of the distance:

$$\sigma = \frac{h^2\gamma^4}{40\pi^2 r^6}\tau\left(\frac{6}{1 + 4\omega^2\tau^2}\right) - 1 \qquad (5)$$

In the motional narrowing limit, in which $\omega^2\tau^2 \ll 1$, σ is proportional to the correlation time. For typical drugs and receptors, with correlation times of about 0.4 and 20 ns, respectively, the process outlined in **Eq. 2** is the dominant mode of magnetization transfer, in which cross relaxation occurs for the bound form of the drug, which is then transferred, by chemical exchange, to the free form of the drug.

3.5. Saturation-Transfer Difference NMR

The foregoing discussion of NOE methods brought to light the concept of cross relaxation in which a given polarized nucleus can transfer its magnetization to a nearby nucleus, if the resonance frequencies for the two nuclei are similar. This leads to the concept of spin diffusion in which magnetization of a given site in, say, a protein receptor, would diffuse away from the initial site onto other adjacent protons. Spin diffusion is a highly efficient mechanism for magnetization transfer in proteins because there are large numbers of coresonant, nearby protons. Although this process must be taken into account in any quantitative analysis of internuclear distances based on NOE measurements, like many physical phenomena, it can also be exploited to provide useful information in other contexts.

Because spin diffusion is so efficient, it is easy to saturate most (if not all) of the protons in a protein simply by irradiating the aliphatic resonance envelope. Saturation then diffuses from the aliphatic protons onto the other classes of protons. If a drug is bound to the protein, while the protein spins are magnetized, a portion of the magnetization is transferred onto the drug as well. This can be used as a powerful screening method in which mixtures of drugs are added to a protein solution and the protein proton resonances are then irradiated. A control spectrum is also obtained in which the saturation is moved off resonance for the protein. The difference between the on- and off-resonance spectra will contain signals from any drug molecules that have bound to the protein and received magnetization from it. This has the added advantage that interpretation of the resulting spectra is very simple and contains data only on those drugs that have interacted with the protein so that identifying these molecules is straightforward in mixtures. One can also determine the drug functional groups involved in recognizing the receptor because these will be closest to the protein and will receive the largest magnetization transfer, whereas more remote groups will receive less or none, owing to the fact that spin diffusion is much less efficient for small molecules.

3.6. Heteronuclear Single Quantum Coherence

We have so far discussed drug-screening methods based on NMR observations of the drug resonances in solution. The advantages of this approach reflect the fact that small molecules tumble rapidly in solution, giving rise to narrow NMR signals that are easy to detect. Of course, one can also take the other approach and monitor the NMR signals from the receptor as well. Tremendous progress has been made along these lines, leading to the development of robust methods for resonance assignment and structural determination of proteins with molecular masses up to approx 50 kDa. Direct observation of the receptor gives valuable information about the nature of the drug-binding site residues, and this can be compared with other structural information to develop modifications of drugs to enhance binding. One of the most popular methods for protein structural studies is to label the protein with ^{15}N, a low natural abundance, spin half of the nucleus present in the amides, and some side chains of amino acids. ^{15}N is not particularly expensive and can be incorporated into cloned proteins grown in microorganisms using ^{15}N-enriched nitrogen sources, such as ammonium nitrate, or sulfate. The resulting ^{15}N-labeled protein will have a single ^{15}N at each amide, which can then be detected at proton sensitivity using the ^{15}N-^1H J-coupling via 2D heteronuclear single quantum coherence (HSQC) spectroscopy.

When a drug binds to a ^{15}N-labeled protein, the resulting conformational change in the protein, coupled with the juxtaposition of the drug, causes chemical shift changes in those residues involved in drug binding and, sometimes, in remote residues that are sensitive to the conformational changes but are not directly involved in binding. Interpretation of these spectral changes requires knowledge of the resonance assignments for the protein, which is not a trivial undertaking, but as long as one is confident that the spectral changes are directly related to drug binding, one can use the magnitude of these changes to assess the relative affinities of different drugs to the receptor and to determine relative differences in binding modes, or for the involvement of different residues in the binding of alternative drugs.

HSQC has, in this context, been given the misnomer structure-activity relationship (SAR) by NMR in the literature. This is not an actual SAR method, unless one can confidently use the chemical shift changes as a surrogate for affinities for different drug molecules and then correlate the structures with other measures of their binding affinities. However, the approach that has been taken is to bind drug fragments to two adjacent sites on ^{15}N-labeled proteins and then to link chemically those most active fragments to produce a more potent drug lead.

3.7. Transverse Relaxation Optimized Spectroscopy

The direct observation of protein resonances has been traditionally limited to molecules with masses less than 50 kDa because the resonance line widths become too large owing to T_2 relaxation. The advent of higher-field (~21 T) superconducting magnets has increased the sensitivity and spectral resolution of NMR, and the applications to protein structure have followed in like fashion. Superconducting probes and preamplifiers have also been responsible for an additional increase in sensitivity. However, neither of these welcome developments has solved the basic problem of line width for large molecules.

The discussion in **Subheading 3.2.** has shown that the transverse relaxation rate of a proton in a large protein is dominated, at moderate magnetic fields, by direct dipolar interactions with adjacent protons. One method for lowering R_2 for amide protons is to deuterate all of the other hydrogen sites. The lower γ of deuterium will then markedly lower R_2 for the amide proton, and the resulting narrower resonances will allow NMR structural studies of larger proteins. This will not address another problem that crops up

at the higher magnetic field strengths useful for higher-sensitivity and spectral disper-
sion, that of the frequency dependence of chemical shift anisotropy (CSA).

Because the bonds in molecules are not spherically symmetric, the chemical shift
of a nucleus depends on the angle between the molecular principal axes and the applied
magnetic field. For protons, this CSA is measured by the difference between the chemical shifts of a nucleus when the principal axis is parallel and perpendicular to the field;
the CSA assumes a value of approx 5–10 ppm, or a few kilohertz, at modest magnetic
fields. If molecules were static, the NMR signals would be this wide, and difficult to
detect, but rotation in solution at 10^9–10^{12} Hz effectively averages the CSA so that one
observes very narrow lines (<1 Hz) for small molecules. This rotation, however, also
modulates the chemical shifts of the nuclei and acts as a source of relaxation enhancement. The contribution of CSA relaxation to R_2 is given by

$$R_2\,(CSA) = \frac{h^2\gamma^4}{90\pi^2 r^6} \left(\frac{6\tau}{1 + 4\omega^2\tau^2} + 8\tau \right) \omega^2 \Delta s^2$$

in which $\Delta s^2 = s_{\parallel} - s_{\perp}$ is the difference between the parallel and perpendicular components of the chemical shift tensor. The fact that the CSA contribution to R_2 is proportional to the square of the Larmor frequency means that it becomes more important as
a relaxation mechanism at higher fields, such as 800 and 900 MHz.

The work of Wüthrich on transverse relaxation optimized spectroscopy (TROSY)
was therefore greeted with great enthusiasm because it demonstrated how to circumvent this basic limitation on direct NMR studies of larger proteins. For a system of two
protons in a protein, the relaxation matrix *(10)* can be written as

$$\frac{d}{dt}\,[M] = -\begin{bmatrix} f(\omega, R, T_2, T_1) & 3\,(p^2 - \delta^2)J(\omega) - g(T_1) \\ 3\,(p^2 - \delta^2)J(\omega) - g(T_1) & f'(\omega, R, T_2, T_1) \end{bmatrix}[M]$$

in which M is the magnetization matrix, and f is a function of the Larmor frequency,
ω; the relaxation times; and R, the transverse relaxation rates for the members of the
spin- coupled doublet, but not of the CSA. $J(\omega)$ is the now-familiar spectral density

$$J(\omega) = \frac{2\tau}{5(1 + \tau^2\omega^2)}$$

and $g(T_1) = 1/2T_1$. The main feature of interest here is that the dipolar contribution to
relaxation, p, and the CSA contribution, δ, enter as their difference, so if these two
terms are comparable ($p \sim \delta$; $p \sim \gamma I\,\gamma s\,/\,r_{Is}^3$, and $\delta_I \sim \gamma I\,B_o\Delta s_I$), then their contribution
vanishes and one may have slow transverse relaxation even for large molecules. The
result is that in combination with various isotope-labeling techniques, TROSY allows
one to observe narrow lines even for very large proteins, up to 1 million Daltons by
solution NMR, particularly at the highest fields now available (900 MHz).

Important recent applications of TROSY include the structure determination of membrane proteins in detergent micelles, structural and functional studies of large proteins
in both monomeric form and macromolecular complexes, and investigations of intermolecular interactions in large complexes *(11)*. TROSY improves the measurement of

residual dipolar couplings and the detection of scalar couplings across hydrogen bonds —techniques that promise to enhance further the determination of solution structures of large proteins and oligonucleotides.

3.8. Solvent-Exposed Amide—TROSY

Solvent-exposed amide (SEA) TROSY *(12)* is an advanced NMR technique for spectral simplification in very large molecules. It is based on the assumption that for drug binding to a receptor, only the surface amino acid residues are of importance, because the buried residues do not directly participate in binding. The technique uses a double ^{15}N filter, which does not affect the water signal, to transfer magnetization only from solvent H_2O molecules to the surface amide protons in ^{15}N-labeled, perdeuterated proteins. Amides exposed to the water protons take up magnetization by hydrogen-deuterium exchange with water during the mixing time, and these amides can then be observed in a TROSY experiment. The strength of the SEA-TROSY signal, I, from an amide proton in the ^{15}N, ^1H correlation spectra depends on the exchange rate, k, and the mixing time, τ_m, according to $I(k, \tau_m) = I_0(1 - e^{-k\tau_m})$. Backbone amides vary markedly in their exchange rates, depending on their position in the secondary structure of the protein, with amides in surface loops exchanging rapidly and buried amides exchanging much more slowly. Amide protons in direct contact with bound water molecules and in the neighborhood of Thr, Ser, and Tyr hydroxyl groups may also exchange magnetization with water. The spectral simplification associated with SEA-TROSY is evident in **Fig. 4**, where filtering of the surface amides reduced the spectral complexity of this 71-kDa protein fragment by at least threefold. The SEA-TROSY method has now been modified *(13)* to eliminate the need for deuteration of the observed proteins. SEA-TROSY spectra may be contaminated with exchange-relayed NOE contributions from fast exchanging protons on hydroxyl or amine groups, and T_1 relaxation contributions. Furthermore, for nondeuterated proteins or protein–ligand complexes, SEA-TROSY spectra may contain NOE contributions from aliphatic protons. A modified version of the SEA element, a Clean SEA element, has been introduced to eliminate these artifacts *(13)*.

3.9. HTS by NMR

Companies and research institutes often generate thousands of compounds using combinatorial chemistry, in hopes of finding one lead compound. Whether the compounds are just off the shelf, purchased, or produced by synthetic means, all of these potential candidates must be screened. The development of HTS assays gave scientists the ability to test large numbers of molecules for a desired biochemical activity, including binding and enzymatic catalysis. Designing such a specific assay is not always trivial; the assays can be complicated and may require several components that can interfere with the interaction of the drug candidate and the target protein. These assays also lend themselves to other problems such as low sensitivity, in the case of a weak signal or high background, and false positives.

Several recent developments support the development of NMR as a high- throughput sampling technique so that the breadth and sophistication of the technique can be

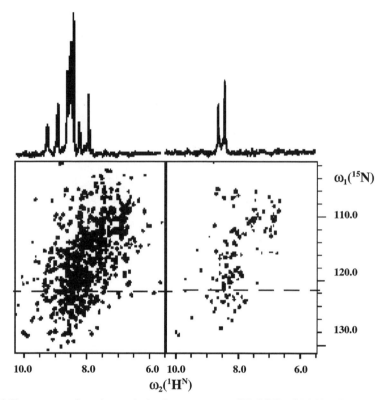

Fig. 4. Transverse relaxation optimized spectroscopy (TROSY) of P450 reductase (*see* **Note 1**) from rat liver (**left**) compared with solvent-exposed amide (SEA)-TROSY (**right**). The SEA-TROSY spectrum is much simpler than the TROSY spectrum because the SEA element only picks up resonances from amides exposed to the solvent water protons. (Adapted from **ref. *12*.**)

brought to bear as a key component of the drug discovery process. These include the production of automated sample changers that read bar-coded samples; acquire spectra automatically; and, with the addition of suitable software, can measure spectra and produce reports from hundreds of proton samples per day.

The small value of the nuclear magnetic moments and the relatively weak polarizing fields available combine to make NMR a rather insensitive method, compared with, e.g., mass spectrometry. At room temperature, the NMR signal, S, is proportional to the negative exponential of the ratio of the NMR transition energy, $\Delta\nu$ (which is on the order of a few Hertz) to that of the thermal background, given by kT (which is a few megaHertz), in which k is Boltzmann's constant:

$$S \approx \exp\left(-\Delta\nu/kT\right)$$

For most situations, S is on the order of 10^{-6}, which means that only one spin in a million will give rise to an NMR signal. Clearly, cooling the sample to very low temperatures would allow the fixed NMR transition energy to dominate over kT and improve the sensitivity, but for biological samples involved in drug discovery, this is impractical owing to the high freezing point of water. One possibility for sensitivity enhancement that has been recently exploited, however, is to cool the NMR detector and preamplifier to liquid helium temperatures to diminish their contribution to the electrical noise inherent in any electronic system. This has the effect of improving the signal-to-noise ratio for a given sample by about a factor of four, so that the acquisition time can be reduced by 16-fold. These cryoprobes are now in use at several hundred sites worldwide.

Another facet of the push to speed up the NMR data collection is particularly useful for the multidimensional experiments so important in drug discovery. Here, the data in the directly detected dimension, typically protons, can be acquired in a few seconds to minutes, but the indirectly detected dimension must be built up from large numbers (256–1024) of phase-shifted directly detected signals, resulting in data acquisition times that can be days or even weeks. There are two methods for speeding up data acquisition in multidimensional experiments, using G-matrices *(14)* and imaging-style gradients *(15)*, but only the former is suitable for use in drug discovery. In G-matrix Fourier transform (GFT) NMR, the data are obtained from several 1D scans simultaneously in an experiment that generates multiplets instead of the traditional single peaks at a given chemical shift. The multiplets occur as linear combinations of chemical shifts that require a collection of linear equations (or G-matrices) and Fourier transforms to resolve the spectrum into component frequencies. Here, the method results in significant data compression as well, so the computational tasks are markedly reduced. The GFT method can reduce the data acquistion time from weeks to hours for a five-dimensional spectrum.

Data analysis can also be a bottleneck for the use of NMR in drug discovery. One way to ease this problem is to preprocess the samples so that the resulting spectra are simpler than those for the entire complex mixture. This was the approach taken by Nicholson's group at Imperial College (London), where they used liquid chromatography (LC) to separate and assign the 1D NMR spectra from a randomly synthesized mixture of 27 tripeptides containing Ala, Tyr, and Met in a single 30-min LC run *(16)*. Along these lines, the cost of producing hundreds or thousands of NMR samples can be prohibitive if standard precision tubes (~$10 each) and deuterated solvents (~$0.50 each) are required, but the development of flow probes and robust water suppression NMR pulse sequences means that the cost of high-throughput NMR can still be reasonable.

NMR-based screening has become an important tool in the pharmaceutical industry. Methods that provide information on the location of small-molecule-binding sites on the surface of a drug target (e.g., SAR by NMR and related techniques) are of particular interest. To extend the applicability of such techniques to drug targets of higher molecular weight, selective labeling strategies may be employed *(16)*. Dual amino acid selective labeling and site-directed nonnative amino acid replacement allow the selective detection of NMR signals of a specific amino acid residue. This results in significantly reduced spectral complexity, which not only enables application to higher molecular weight systems, but also eliminates the need for sequential resonance assignments in order to identify the binding site. Regioselective (or segmental) labeling of an entire protein domain of a multidomain protein may also be achieved. Labeling only a selected part of a multidomain protein (e.g., a catalytic or ligand-binding domain) is an attractive way to simplify spectral interpretation without disturbing the system under study.

3.10. Multiquantum NMR

The spin coupling among nuclei leads to the possibility of concerted transitions involving two or more nuclear quantum states simultaneously, in addition to the classical transitions involving only two states. These concerted transitions have been called multiquantum resonances in analogy with similar phenomena that occur in optical spectroscopy. It may seem strange that essentially any order of transition is allowed, as long as there are enough states to provide the requisite number of transitions, including zero quantum transitions. A zero quantum transition is not one in which zero quanta are absorbed, but one in which a simultaneous two-spin transition is made between a pair of identical states distinguished only by the labels on spins. For example, in a two-spin system of spin 1/2 particles, the states can be numbered according to the projections of each spin as $|\alpha\alpha\rangle$, $|\alpha\beta\rangle$, $|\beta\alpha\rangle$, and $|\beta\beta\rangle$, in which β is spin up and α is spin down. A zero quantum transition involves the change $|\alpha\beta\rangle \rightarrow |\beta\alpha\rangle$, in which both spins flip simultaneously. A double quantum transition is $|\alpha\alpha\rangle \rightarrow |\beta\beta\rangle$, and there are two single quantum transitions, $|\alpha\alpha\rangle \rightarrow |\alpha\beta\rangle$ and $|\alpha\alpha\rangle \rightarrow |\beta\alpha\rangle$, in this manifold. It should also be noted that the two spins do not necessarily need to be from a single nuclide; for example, the first could be a proton, and the second could be from ^{15}N. Multiple quantum transitions are also possible for spins greater than ½.

Of particular interest for drug development is the use of multiquantum techniques for the filtering of spectra to remove signals from unwanted transitions, or to edit the spectra for a specific order of multiquantum coherence. This has led to the widely used HSQC experiments, which rely on the transfer of single quantum coherence between ^{13}C or ^{15}N and ^1H for spectral editing of, e.g., the amide nitrogens in a protein, and for sensitivity enhancement through the detection of proton signals instead of the signals from the lower-sensitivity heteronuclei. The problem of spectral overlap and poor resolution for large macromolecules has partially been solved by exploiting multiquantum techniques in a multidimensional NMR approach.

3.11. Residual Dipolar Couplings

The first robust method for determination of protein structure, X-ray diffraction, required crystallization of the macromolecule under consideration. This was often the rate-limiting step in structural studies. NOE-based NMR methods were introduced in the early 1980s to enable solution structures to be determined, but the accuracy of these methods is limited by the small number of constraints observable owing to NOEs from nuclei within about 5 Å of an observed proton, and particularly from long-range, intrasubunit NOEs, which are valuable for establishing the overall folding pattern of the protein. What has become clear in the past few years is that there exist other NMR parameters that are sensitive to structure that can be used to develop the solution structures of macromolecules. These methods include the use of chemical shifts in concert with refined models of the electromagnetic fields generated in the neighborhood of amino acids to solve for the distances and orientations of chemical groups in proteins.

The use of chemical shift data as the sole NMR data used for structural analysis is currently a topic of interest and has seen limited use, but the chemical shift index is a robust method for parsing assigned resonance shifts into basic structural features (α-helix or β-sheet). Further information is available from the spin–spin coupling constants, which reveal restraints on the bond angles for certain portions of the protein, mainly the backbone ϕ angle. Many schemes have been introduced to measure these coupling constants, both in natural-abundance molecules, where proton–proton splittings are the only parameters possible to determine, and in isotopically labeled molecules, where a much broader range of couplings is measureable. Because the proton–proton coupling constants are on the order of 5–10 Hz, one only observes them in spectra from smaller proteins whose motion is characterized by correlation times of 10–30 ns, or molecular masses of 30–70 kDa. These coupling constants are independent of molecular motion, so they are visible for rapidly tumbling molecules in solution and were the first couplings exploited for structural studies.

Other couplings are present in molecular NMR spectra but were not exploited because they are averaged out by the predominantly isotropic molecular motion in solution. From elementary chemical exchange NMR theory, it is known that two states differing in frequency by 10 Hz will only be visible if the molecular motion is slower than approx 30 Hz; otherwise, only an average line is observed centered on the average frequency. However, a 30-kDa protein, with a 2.1-ns correlation time, will have motions in solution with frequencies on the order of 500 MHz! In 1995, Tolman et al. *(17)* pointed out that one could observe small residual dipolar couplings of this magnitude (~10 Hz) if a molecule is partially oriented by, e.g., the intrinsic anisotropic magnetic susceptibility of the heme group in a heme-containing protein, or through the use of an anisotropic solvent, such as a liquid crystal or bicelle.

The dipolar coupling between two spin 1/2 nuclei I and K arising from partial alignment in an anisotropic environment is given by

$$D_{IK} = D_o A_a S \left\{ [3 (\cos \theta)^2 - 1] + \frac{3}{2} R [(\sin \theta)^2 \cos 2\phi] \right\}$$

in which $D_o = -(1/2\pi)(\mu_o/8\pi^2)h\gamma_I\gamma_K r_{IK}^{-3}$ is the dipolar interaction constant; S is the order parameter, which reflects the isotropic averaging owing to rapid local motions; A_a is the axial component of the molecular alignment tensor; R is its rhombicity; and θ and ϕ are the polar angles of the IK internuclear vector in the molecular alignment coordinate system *(18)*. The Euler angles $\{\alpha,\beta,\gamma\}$ specify the orientation of the alignment frame with respect to a fixed molecular frame, e.g., the X-ray coordinate frame. The equation for D_{IK} shows that the residual dipolar couplings specify a position-independent vector orientation and that they may be considered structural parameters in a global sense. Because two parallel N-H vectors produce the same D_{NH} values independent of their position in the backbone of the protein, these residual dipolar couplings are particularly useful for the determination of large-scale properties such as the relationship between domains in solution. Measurement of the residual dipolar couplings is accomplished by examination of the splittings between, e.g., ^{15}N-^{1}H signals in an HSQC experiment on a ^{15}N-labeled protein partially oriented in solution; the nominal amide $^1J_{NH}$ is 94 ± 1 Hz and residual dipolar couplings will lower or raise this value by 5–10 Hz.

There are also practical advantages in measuring couplings from the ^{15}N, ^1H correlation spectra. Several dipolar couplings measured conveniently from 2D ^{15}N-^1H correlation spectra can give insight into conformational changes induced by ligand binding, in a manner similar to that of the SAR by NMR studies in which binding epitopes can be localized from changes in chemical shifts (19,20). Amide nitrogen and proton chemical shifts are extremely sensitive to changes in chemical environment and conformation. It is therefore conceivable that changes in residual dipolar couplings induced by ligand binding could also be observed concomitantly with chemical shift changes to delineate conformational changes.

4. Applications of NMR Techniques

Given the previous introduction to the basic physics used in the various schemes for filtering NMR spectra from drug–receptor interactions, we now turn to an examination of applications of these techniques in specific examples applied to different classes of drug discovery. We begin with diffusion, as we did in **Heading 3.**, and follow in the same order of presentation.

4.1. Applications of Diffusion Filtering

Combinatorial chemistry has been widely used for the synthesis of mixtures of large numbers of compounds in the search for active drug leads. The resulting mixtures can be separated and the compounds screened one at a time, but this is a difficult and time-consuming step. Of more interest would be a method for screening the entire mixture in a single NMR experiment. One way of studying such mixtures is with diffusion-weighted total correlation spectroscopy (TOCSY) in which the superior resolution of 2D methods is combined with selection on the basis of diffusion coefficient (22). Differences in molecular mass of only 14 Daltons from a single $-CH_2-$ were shown to produce measureable changes (5% decrease) in the diffusion coefficient in a series of low molecular mass (102–172 Daltons) esters.

Larger changes in the diffusion coefficient are produced by the binding of small molecules to proteins. This has served as the basis for a screening technique in which mixtures of putative ligands are added to a protein solution and the resulting spectra are diffusion filtered. Hajduk et al. (20,23) used this approach to isolate single, stromelysin-binding compounds from a mixture of nine molecules. Their results (**Fig. 5**) showed that the 1D NMR spectrum of this mixture of compounds (**Fig. 5A**), even in the absence of protein, produced severe spectral overlap. The use of field gradients in the presence of protein (**Fig. 5B**) still produced a complex spectrum. However, the difference spectrum (**Fig. 5C**) showed only the signals from the molecule, 2-phenylimidazole (**Fig. 5D**), that bound to stromelysin. The absence of 2-phenylimidazole in the mixture produced no positive signals (**Fig. 5E**).

Many compounds of interest in drug development bind weakly to target proteins but are nevertheless useful as leads on which to build additional substituents. Diffusion NMR methods are useful for measuring the affinities of such weak binders to proteins.

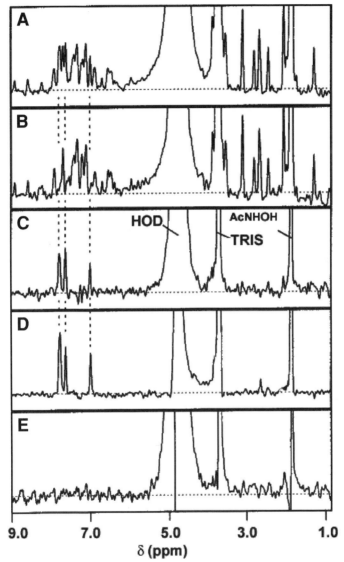

Fig. 5. Diffusion editing of a mixture of molecules to discover compounds that bind to stromelysin. (**A**) Nuclear magnetic resonance (NMR) spectrum of mix without protein; (**B**) spectrum of mix in presence of stromelysin taken with gradients; (**C**) difference spectrum ([A] – [B]) showing signals from single binding molecule, 2-phenylimidazole; (**D**) NMR spectrum of only 2-phenylimidazole; (**E**) control difference spectrum like in (C) but without 2-phenylimidazole. (Adapted from **ref. 20**.)

For example, one potential method for the sequestration of the Alzheimer's amyloid β-peptide (Aβ) is to bind it to cyclodextrins to prevent self-aggregation. Danielsson et al. *(24)* used the changes in the diffusion coefficients of Aβ to determine the dissocia-

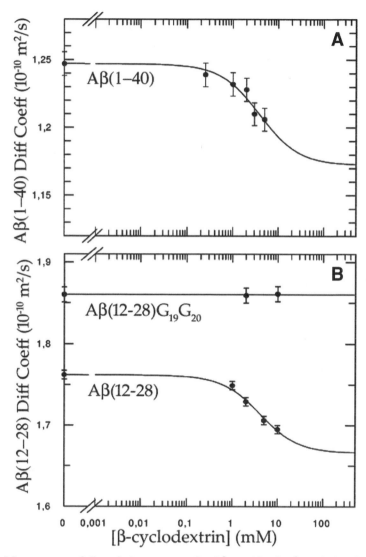

Fig. 6. Measurement of dissociation constant for Aβ peptides for β-cyclodextrin by diffusion-filtered nuclear magnetic resonance: (**A**) Aβ(1–40) and (**B**) Aβ(12–28) and Aβ(12–28) $Gly_{19}Gly_{20}$. (Adapted from **ref. 24.**)

tion constants for the full-length Aβ (1–40) peptide, and for truncated Aβ (12–28) and sequence-variant Aβ (12–28) $Gly_{19}Gly_{20}$ versions (**Fig. 6**). Aβ(1–40) and Aβ(12–28) both bound to β-cyclodextrin with a K_d of 3.8 mM, whereas replacement of the hydrophobic phenylalanines at positions 19 and 20 with glycines to form Aβ(12–28)Gly_{19} Gly_{20} abolished binding (**Fig. 6B**). The phenylalanines at postions 19 and 20 are partially responsible for self-aggregation of Aβ(1–40).

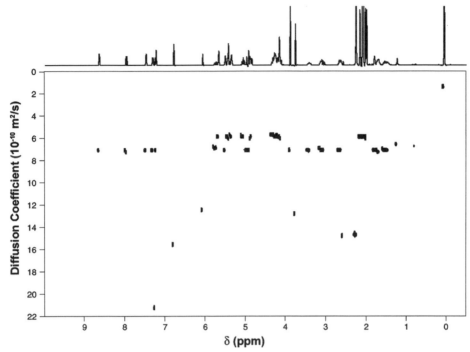

Fig. 7. Diffusion-ordered spectrum of a mixture of polydimethylsiloxane, mesitylene, tri-methoxybenzene, sucrose octaacetate, and quinine. Sixteen transients were acquired for each of 20 gradient values ranging from 5 to 25 G/cm in a total time of 32 min. (Adapted from **ref. 25.**)

The power of diffusion filtering is elegantly revealed in the diffusion ordered spectroscopy (DOSY) experiment. In this 2D scheme, the normal chemical shift dimension is acquired at varying gradient strengths; these spectra form the basis for the second dimension. The 2D data set consists of the spectra of molecules in a mixture ordered according to their diffusion coefficients. Newer pulse sequences *(25)* allow the rapid measurement of DOSY spectra using one-shot methods in a few minutes. These techniques are well suited to the screening of mixtures and avoid the difference methods used earlier. Results of DOSY on a mixture of polydimethylsiloxane, mesitylene, tri-methoxybenzene, sucrose octaacetate, and quinine in $CDCl_3$ (**Fig. 7**) show excellent separation of the spectra on the basis of the constituents' diffusion coefficients. Clearly, the addition of a protein with a binding site for one of these molecules would dramatically alter the diffusion coefficient for one of the small molecules and shift its position along the diffusion coefficient axis. The analytical dynamic range for the method then is determined by the difference between the free and bound diffusion coefficients. Derrick et al. *(26)* calculated this difference for tryptophan bound to human serum albumin (**Fig. 8**). Their calculation assumed an albumin concentration of 0.1 m*M* with a dif-fusion coefficient of 0.63×10^{-10} m^2/s, and a free tryptophan diffusion coefficient

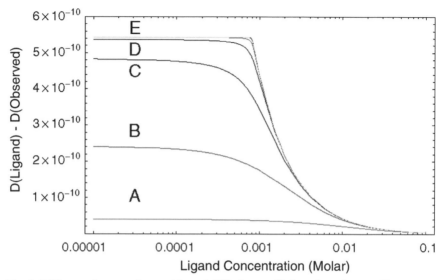

Fig. 8. Difference between free and bound diffusion coefficients for mixture of human serum albumin and tryptophan (see text for parameters) for various dissociation constants, K_d, as function of ligand concentration. $K_d = 0.01\ M$, $0.001\ M$, $0.1\ \text{mM}$, $10\ \mu M$, and $10\ \text{nM}$, for curves A, B, C, D, and E, respectively.

of $6.1 \times 10^{-10}\ \text{m}^2/\text{s}$. For the experiment to produce useful data, the ligand must be in fast exchange with the protein, and the ligand should be in excess. Curve E in **Fig. 8** shows that the maximum change in curve D occurs if the ligand is completely bound to the protein at a high-affinity site, but under these conditions the relaxation properties (R_2) of the ligand are unfavorable for NMR detection, so one should raise the ligand concentration to provide a free ligand signal for detection. 1D NMR measurements of this type are not too useful because the protein background present at the optimal low ligand-to-protein ratios skews measurements of the ligand diffusion coefficient. The 2D DOSY experiment avoids these problems altogether. These techniques are also useful for studying the interactions of small molecules with other small molecules *(27)*.

Diffusion filters are profitably combined with other filters to provide even greater control over the selectivity. One popular combination is to use a T_2 filter to attenuate protein resonances in combination with a diffusion filter to select resonances from small molecules. In this way, NOEs could be observed between lysozyme and very weakly binding solvent molecules, such as N,N-dimethyl-formamide *(28)*. Isotope filtration has also been used in combination with a diffusion filter. Many proteins are labeled with either ^{13}C or ^{15}N, or both, in order to perform HSQC studies on the protein structure in response to ligand binding. These proteins can also be used for binding studies in which the protein proton signals are filtered out with the use of a heteronuclear filter *(29,30)*.

4.2. Applications of Relaxation Editing

The large differences in T_1 and T_2 relaxation times between small molecules and proteins naturally leads one to suppose that relaxation editing can be an effective means for filtering drug-binding spectra. The side chains involved in drug binding change motional characteristics from the unliganded state *(31)*. Relaxation editing has been used to determine which component of a mixture bound to the FK506 binding protein *(20)*. The proton T_2 for the protein was 40 ms, whereas those for the ligands in a mixture were approx 2 s. This difference resulted in a 99% attenuation of the protein signals in a spin-echo spectrum with a 400-ms echo time. An application of transverse relaxation editing is shown in **Fig. 9**. This technique can identify a molecule that binds to a protein directly, without deconvolution of the mixture. For example, 2-phenylimidazole binds to the FK506 binding protein with an affinity of 200 μ*M*. The NMR spectrum of this molecule (**Fig. 9D**) is identical to that of the spectrum of the compound selected by transverse relaxation editing (**Fig. 9C**) and no other signals arise from this mixture of nine compounds (**Fig. 9C**).

4.3. Applications of NOE and trNOE Editing

While diffusion and relaxation editing of NMR spectra are relatively straightforward techniques for the screening of drug candidates in the presence of macromolecules, more subtle NMR effects have also received attention. One of these is the trNOE (*see* **Subheading 3.4.**) *(9,32,33)*. This is useful for drug screening because the proton NOE is a function of the rotational correlation time of a small molecule, and binding to a macromolecule lengthens this time markedly. The NOE changes sign on binding from positive for small values of τ_c to negative for larger values of τ_c when bound (**Fig. 3**).

Mixtures of compounds can be screened for binding by examining the NOEs for the mixture in the presence of the macromolecule. Transferred NOEs owing to binding have the opposite sign from those owing to rapid rotation in solution, build up faster than for the unbound molecules, and are larger than from unbound molecules. Meyer et al. *(34)* used these facts to monitor the binding of α-L-Fuc(1 → 6)-β-D-GlcNAc-OMe to the agglutinin from *Aleuria aurantia*. A comparison of the NOEs for the free and bound disaccharide (**Fig. 10**) showed that the transferred NOEs were negative, built up faster, and were larger for the bound sugar.

The compound(s) that bind to a macromolecule can even be ascertained from mixtures of 6–15 separate compounds. Under favorable conditions, the structure of the bound form of the ligand can also be deduced from the transferred NOEs. In attempting to use transferred NOEs to monitor binding, the NOE spectrum of the mixture must first be obtained, and often weakly negative NOEs may be observed for a few resonances at lower temperatures. These may be converted into positive NOEs at slightly higher temperatures. The molar ratio of ligand to macromolecule will need to be adjusted for the maximum trNOE, but often this ratio is in the range of 15–20:1 for ligands with dissociation constants between 10^{-3} and 10^{-7} *M*. Thus, only small amounts of macromolecules are required (one-twentieth of the number of moles of the ligands), and these can be recovered by dialysis after the NMR experiments.

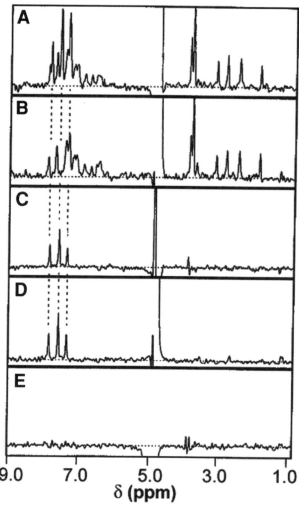

Fig. 9. Transverse relaxation editing of ligand binding to FK506 binding protein: (**A**) T_2-edited ^{1}H spectrum of a mix of nine compounds, one of which was the FKBP ligand, 2-phenyl-imidazole; (**B**) T_2-edited spectrum of same mix in presence of FKBP; (**C**) difference spectrum (A – B); (**D**) reference spectrum of 2-phenylimidazole alone; (**E**) difference spectrum as in (C) but without 2-phenylimidazole. (Adapted from **ref. 21**.)

Because the interproton NOE changes sign for NMR frequencies and rotational correlation times on the order of $\omega\tau \sim 1$ (**Fig. 3**), potential drug molecules with a mass of approx 1000 Daltons (where $\tau \sim 1/\omega$) will only give weak NOEs by themselves. These molecules in a mixture can readily be distinguished from genuine binders whose NOEs become strongly negative. The NOE spectrum can also give significant clues as

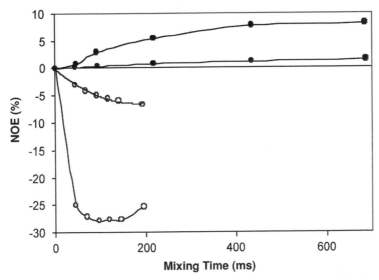

Fig. 10. Nuclear Overhauser effect (NOEs) for two proton pairs of α-L-Fuc(1 → 6)-β-D-GlcNAc-OMe in absence (closed symbols) and presence (open symbols) of *Aleuria aurantia* agglutinin. The transferred NOEs (open symbols) are larger, build up faster, and are negative with respect to the NOEs for the disaccharide free in solution (closed symbols). (Based on data from **ref. 34**.)

to the structure of the binders in a mixture without deconvolution because the unique chemical shifts reflect the functional groups on a binder.

Spin diffusion is often an aid in the determination of the structure of the binder in a mixture (*35*). If the spectrum of the mixture suffers from signal overlap even after the trNOE filter step, additional dimensions of NMR space can be exploited to reveal the structure of the binder. The addition of a TOCSY dimension to a trNOESY (*36*) can often provide the extra information needed to identify unambiguously the binder from a mixture.

Since peptides derived from interface peptides or from phage display are often used as starting molecules in the drug discovery process, it is useful to consider how one uses trNOESY data to derive the conformation of the bound drug by examining the applications to the interactions between peptides and macromolecules. There also exist a variety of native peptide hormones of interest that are potent physiological activators of G protein-coupled receptors (GPCRs). To utilize trNOESY the ligand must be in fast exchange with the receptor; the exchange rate must be significantly larger than the cross-relaxation rate so that the ligand residence time is small compared to the T_1 for the free ligand. The molar ratio of ligand to receptor is often on the order of 10–20:1 and can range as high as 5000:1 for macromolecular assemblies, such as ribosomes (*37*). This ratio depends on the binding affinity and on the mass of the receptor, with larger receptors serving as more efficient sources of cross relaxation to be transferred to the ligand.

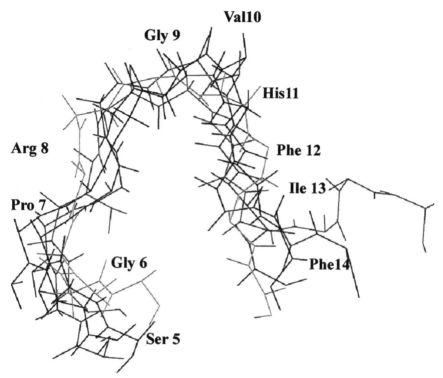

Fig. 11. Structure of SGPRGVHFIF region of gp91*phox* C-terminal peptide bound to p47*phox*. Shown are the five lowest energy structures having the best agreement with the transferred nuclear Overhauser effect spectroscopy data (Adapted from **ref. 38.**)

The C-terminal peptide from neutrophil gp91*phox* (SNSESGPRGVHFIFNKEN) has been found by trNOESY to bind to cytosolic p47*phox* in an extended conformation with immobilization of all of the residue side chains in the RGVHFIF region except the histidine *(38)*. At a molar ratio of 10:1 (peptide:p47) 126 trNOESY cross peaks were found, which led to the elucidation of the structure shown in **Fig. 11**. Immobilization of side chains deduced from the NMR data was found to agree closely with biological data from alanine replacement studies by Kleinberg et al. *(39)*.

trNOESY effects are largest for the largest receptors, in contrast to those of most other NMR experiments, in which increases in size are a hindrance. This fact has been exploited to study the interactions of peptides with very large receptors, such as antibodies. Myasthenia gravis is a disease caused by the production of autoantibodies against the acetylcholine receptor. trNOESY methods are ideal for the study of the interaction of the main immunogenic region peptide (WNPDDYGGVK) derived from the α-subunit of the acetylcholine receptor with antiacetylcholine receptor autoantibodies (Fv198). trNOESY data from a 50:1 molar ratio of peptide to Fv198 yielded 73 distance restraints *(40)* and showed that the N-terminal loop of the peptide adopted a β-turn, imposed by

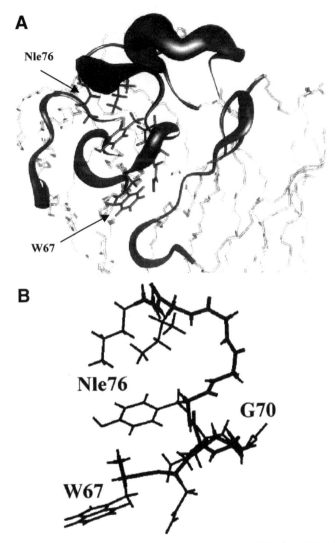

Fig. 12. (**A**) Fit of peptide into recognition site of antibody Fv198; the width of the backbone drawing is proportional to the root mean square deviation. (**B**) Conformation of main immunogenic region peptide (WNPDDYGGVK) from α-subunit of acetylcholine receptor with antiacetylcholine receptor autoantibodies (Fv198). (Adapted from **ref. 40**.)

the proline residue, and contained bulky hydrophobic groups (W67, Y72) that made numerous contacts with the antibody (**Fig. 12A,B**).

Membrane proteins are the subject of intense interest owing to their role as transducers of extra- and intracellular signals, and they represent a difficult, but potentially very rewarding, target for drug development. However, they are also difficult to work with. Crystallography cannot be used to study their structures because the proteins often

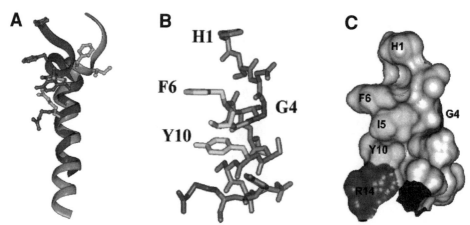

Fig. 13. (**A**) Comparison of N-terminal β-coil conformation of 21-residue fragment of pitu-itary adenylate cyclase-activating peptide (HSDGIFTDSYSRYRKQMAVKK) bound to G pro-tein-coupled receptor (light gray) and full-length, 27-residue peptide (dary gray) bound to dodecyl-phosphocholine micelles. (**B**) N-terminal β-coil structure and (**C**) its solvent-accessible surface. (Adapted from **ref. *41*.**)

are insoluble when taken out of the membrane, so the only fruitful course has been to attempt to crystallize them in the presence of detergents. This has met with limited suc-cess, at best. Solid-state NMR techniques are making significant inroads for the direct structural elucidation of membrane proteins.

trNOESY studies are very favorable because one can prepare the proteins in deter-gent or phospholipid micelles and study them in solution without crystallization. trNOESY methods have therefore been applied to the elucidation of the structures of peptide hormones bound to integral membrane receptors. The pituitary adenylate cyclase-activat-ing peptide functions through a GPCR that is present in the membranes of target cells. Inooka et al. *(41)* used the trNOESY approach to determine the conformation of a trun-cated, 21-residue form of the pituitary adenylate cyclase-activating peptide (H_1SDGI FTDSYSRYRKQMAVKK_{21}YLAAVL_{27}) bound to the GPCR at a molar ratio of 42.5:1. Binding to the receptor induced a unique β-coil structure (**Fig. 13**) in the N-terminus (residues 3–7), which was not observed in the full-length, 27-residue peptide bound to dodecylphosphocholine micelles. Several N-terminal residues (His-1, Phe-6, and Thr-7) are conserved among a number of physiological peptide ligands for this GPCR, and ala-nine replacement studies have shown the critical importance of Phe-6, Tyr-10, and Arg-14 for binding activity. The α-helical C-terminal tail binds the peptide to the membrane, from which subsequent lateral diffusion brings the peptide to the receptor. Although the receptor–peptide complex could likely have been crystallized, it is difficult to imagine the crystallization of the peptide–micelle complex; here, NMR methods in solution pro-vided unique biophysical information.

Integrins are an important class of cell-adhesion molecules *(42)* that have been the target for many drug design efforts *(43)*. The crystal structure of the integrin heterodimer

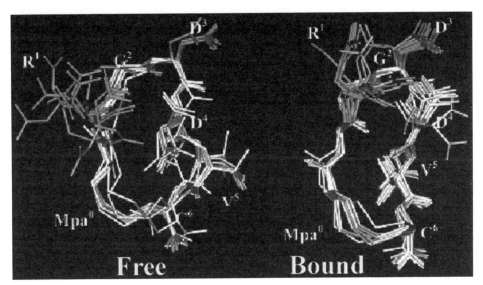

Fig. 14. Conformations of free (**left**) and bound (**right**) forms of integrin $\alpha_1\beta_5$ inhibitor c[Mpa RGDDVC]-NH$_2$ determined by means of ^{15}N-edited QUIET-nuclear Overhauser effect spectroscopy (Adapted from **ref. 54**.)

$\alpha_v\beta_3$ has recently been solved in complex with an Arg-Gly-Asp ligand *(44)*. There are many other important integrins whose structures have not been solved; among these is $\alpha_1\beta_5$, an integrin found on the surfaces of endothelial cells that binds to fibrinogen, and is important in cancer metastasis. The integrins are very large integral membrane proteins, with heterodimeric masses more than 200 kDa, making them prime candidates for trNOESY studies of peptide-binding sites that mimic the binding to the extracellular matrix.

One of the pitfalls of any cross-relaxation NMR experiment (NOESY, trNOESY, and so on) is that spin diffusion can bleed magnetization away from the polarized nucleus and give rise to NOE-style cross peaks that are less intense than would be expected solely on the basis of nearest-neighbor distances, and give internuclear distances larger than actually exist. The earliest methods for dealing with spin diffusion used several mixing times and extrapolated the NOE-derived distances to zero mixing time. Zwahlen et al. *(45)* pioneered an even better approach in which doubly selective inversion pulses were used to cancel spin diffusion effects to first order. This technique, called QUIET-NOESY, was used, along with ^{15}N labeling, to suppress spin diffusion and to determine the conformation of an ArgGlyAsp (RGD) peptide (cyclo-[MpaRGDDVC]-NH$_2$) bound to the integrin $\alpha_1\beta_5$ (**Fig. 14**). The RGD peptide changed conformation on binding. The distance between the Arg-1(C$_\beta$) and Asp-3(C$_\beta$) decreased from 7.5 Å in the free form to 5.6 Å in the bound conformation, indicating that the binding pocket for $\alpha_5\beta_1$ is narrower than found for the related integrin $\alpha_{IIb}\beta_3$ *(46)*.

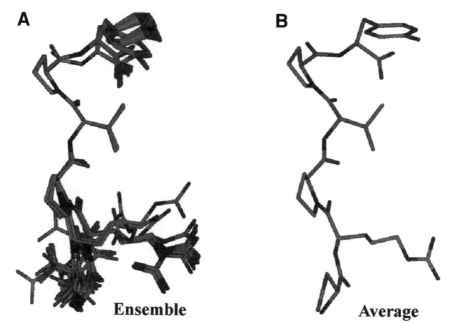

Fig. 15. QUIET-trNOESY of DRPVPY hexapeptide mimic of trisaccharide repeating unit, L-rhamnose-α-(1 → 2)-(D-*N*-acetylglucosamine-β-(1 → 3))-α-L-rhamnose, of *Streptococcus* group A cell-wall polysaccharide bound to SA-3 monoclonal antibody: (**A**) ensemble of 27 lowest-energy structures; (**B**) average of structures shown in (A). (Adapted from **ref. *47*.**)

Peptides can mimic carbohydrates because peptides can recognize polysaccharide-binding sites on antibodies. With masses on the order of 140 kDa, antibodies are too large for the traditional NMR structural analyses but are excellent candidates for study with trNOESY. Antibodies against carbohydrates have been used to isolate peptides from phage display libraries to find peptide mimics of carbohydrate structures. The hexapeptide DRPVPY is a functional molecular mimic of the *Streptococcus* group A cell-wall-branched trisaccharide repeating unit, L-rhamnose-α-(1 → 2)-(D-*N*-acetylglu-cosamine-β-(1 → 3))-α-L-rhamnose. QUIET-trNOESY NMR data show that this pep-tide, at a molar ratio of 20:1, adopted a tight turn conformation (**Fig. 15**) with close contacts observed between the side chains of Val and Tyr when bound to to the SA-3 monoclonal antibody *(47)*. Even though this peptide contained only six residues, its bound stucture was well defined by the extensive trNOEs, and QUIET-trNOESY showed that spin diffusion effects could be ruled out.

As a final example of the application of trNOESY to extremely large macromolec-ular ensembles, we show that these methods are applicable to studies of the binding of antibiotic-resistance peptides to the bacterial ribosome, a topic of great importance for the development of drugs to defeat the resistance that bacteria have evolved against

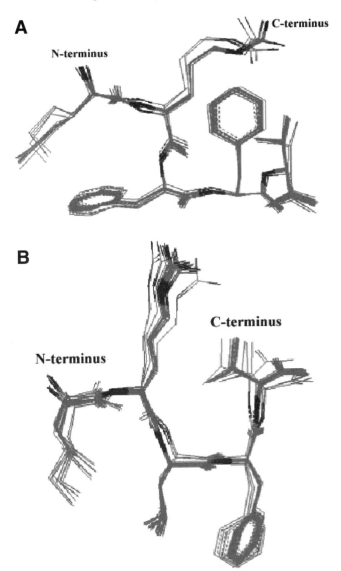

Fig. 16. Structures of ribosome-bound (**A**) K-peptide and (**B**) E-peptide, determined by means of transferred NOESY data. These are superpositions of the 20 lowest energy structures determined by simulated annealing. (Adapted from **ref. *37*.**)

many antibiotics. Two antibiotic-resistance peptides, the E-peptide (MRLFV) and the K-peptide (MRFFV) from *Staphylococcus aureus*, were found to bind to bacterial ribosomes in a way similar to that found for macrolide and ketolide antibiotics (*37*). No trNOEs were observed for these peptides free in solution, but at a molar ratio of 5000:1, peptide:ribosomes, 52 trNOEs were measured, particularly between L3 H_δ and H_β, and between F4 $H_{\delta 1, \delta 2}$ and $H_{\epsilon 1, \epsilon 2}$ for the E-peptide, and 87 NOEs were measured for the K-peptide, including important interactions between the proton pairs: V5 $H_\gamma \rightarrow$ F3,4 $H_{\delta, \epsilon}$; R2 $H_\beta \rightarrow$ F4 $H_{\delta, \epsilon}$; and M1 $H_\beta \rightarrow$ F3 $H_{\delta, \epsilon}$. These NOEs defined ribosome-bound conformations of the peptides that mimicked those of the previously determined macrolide and ketolide antibiotics, erythromycin and telitromycin (**Fig. 16**).

4.4. Applications of Water-LOGSY

A related magnetization transfer technique for monitoring the binding of small molecules to macromolecules is that of water-ligand observation with gradient spectroscopy (water-LOGSY), which involves magnetization transfer from the protons in solvent water to those of the ligand. In reality, this method is a trNOE-type experiment in which water molecules bound with the ligand to the macromolecule have long residence times, ranging from a few nanoseconds to hundreds of microseconds. At these residence times, the water-protein NOEs change sign (**Fig. 3**), and a bound molecule picks up magnetization of the same sign as the protein. This technique has been used to discover which molecules in a mixture of drugs interact with a given protein; the interacting molecules give rise to positive NMR signals, and those that do not interact produce negative signals. For a water molecule tightly buried at a protein–ligand interface, the intermolecular NOE cross-relaxation rate, σ_{wp}, from the protein to water is given by (**48**)

$$\sigma_{wp} = \frac{\gamma^4 h^2 \mu_o^2}{640\pi^4 r_{wp}^6} \left(\frac{\tau_r \tau_p}{\tau_r + \tau_p}\right) \left\{ \left[1 + \frac{6}{\frac{4\omega_o^2 \tau_r^2 \tau_p^2}{(\tau_r + \tau_p)^2}} \right] \right\}^{-1}$$

in which τ_r and τ_p are the residence times for the water within the protein-binding site and the rotational correlation time of the protein, respectively; r_{wp} is the separation of the protein and water protons; and ω_o is the Larmor frequency. For a field of 14.1 T (600 MHz) and a proton separation of 2.5 Å, we have calculated the intermolecular NOE for various residence times (**Fig. 17**). It is seen that the NOEs change sign at 0.3 ns and that the magnetization transfer is more efficient for longer protein correlation times.

4.5. Saturation Transfer

Application of the saturation transfer method to mixtures of compounds in the presence of a putative binding protein shows that one can discriminate between binders and nonbinders. For example, Dalvit et al. (**48**) used this technique to monitor the binding of a mixture of 10 putative cyclin-dependent kinase 2 inhibitors to their target at a molar ratio of 20:1 (**Fig. 18**). Their results showed that binders displayed positive magnetization transfer from water, whereas nonbinders gave rise to negative signals. One can also use this method to measure binding constants and to perform competition experiments (**49**) allowing high-affinity ligands to be identified. This has been a drawback of all the NMR screening methods developed to date in that only weak ligands could be identified.

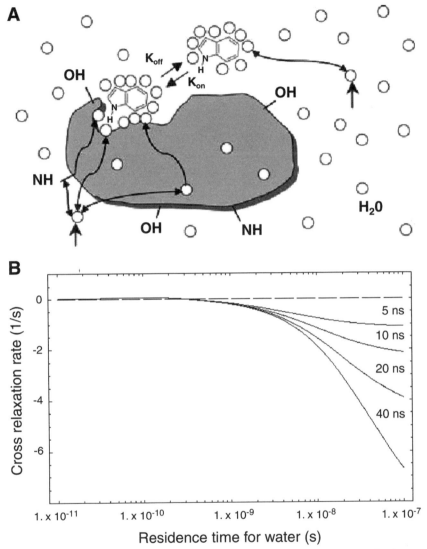

Fig. 17. **(A)** Mechanisms for nuclear Overhauser effect magnetization transfer from water (circles) bound with ligand at binding site of a macromolecule. Spin diffusion and exchange with bulk water brings magnetization into the binding cavity. **(B)** Cross-relaxation rate for water molecules at 600 MHz, 2.5 Å from protein proton as function of water residence time in binding site and for values of protein correlation time. (Adapted from **ref. *48*.**)

4.6. Applications of Saturation Transfer Difference Spectroscopy

Along the lines of trNOESY and water-LOGSY is a method in which magnetization is transferred, not from water or from cross relaxation in the bound state, but directly from the protein spin reservoir to the ligand. This is known as saturation transfer dif-

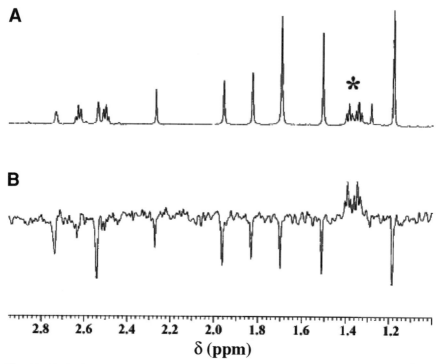

Fig. 18. **(A)** Reference proton nuclear magnetic resonance spectrum of mixture of 10 compounds in presence of 10 mM cdk2; **(B)** spectrum showing magnetization transfer from water to the drugs. The methyl group resonances from the cdk2 binder ethyl-α-(ethoxycarbonyl)-3-indoleacrylate are denoted by an asterisk. (Adapted from **ref. 48**.)

ference (STD) spectroscopy, because one needs to subtract a spectrum in which the protein resonances have been saturated from one where the saturating field is applied far off resonance from the protein protons. The method works because the protein contains protons that absorb radiofrequency radiation over a broad range of frequencies, essentially a continuous envelope of absorption. Then, because spin diffusion is so efficient in proteins, in a relatively small amount of time, the saturation spreads over the entire protein molecule, eventually arriving at the ligand-binding site where this saturation is transferred to the bound ligand. Exchange between the free and bound states for the ligand then results in the appearance of magnetization in the free ligand resonances, much like trNOESY and water-LOGSY. STD spectroscopy has the distinct advantage that one can directly determine from a simple, 1D NMR spectrum those protons on the ligand that directly interact with the protein, something of great interest for structure-based drug design. This method also appears to work for higher-affinity ligands and in cases in which trNOESY methods are no longer applicable. STD spectroscopy works best for fast exchange. The saturation transfer difference method is applicable to mixtures. For large numbers of putative drugs, multidimensional methods are needed, but the STD technique can be incorporated into many standard 2D and 3D sequences, so the binding components can readily be identified.

These techniques have been applied to examine the binding epitopes of the Lewis-B hexasaccharide (lacto-*N*-difucosylhexaose; **1** in **Fig. 19**) for the fucose-binding lectin, *A. aurantia* agglutinin *(50)*. STD TOCSY results (**Fig. 19**) indicate that only the fucosyl-V and -VI residues are in contact with the lectin and thereby obtained saturation directly. Saturation progressed down the hexasaccharide chain, so the more remote Gal-IV, GlcNAc-III, and Gal-II residues showed only 60% of the saturation of the fucosyl residues, and Glc-I showed even less (30%) saturation. STD NMR can even be applied to proteins attached to controlled pore glass beads using magic angle spinning *(51)*. Membrane receptors can also be studied using this technique.

Cyclo(RGDfV) is a potent integrin antagonist, with an IC_{50} against fibrinogen binding to activated platelets of approx 20 μM *(52)*, and a dissociation constant about the same value *(53)*. The epitopes for the binding of cyclo(RGDfV) to liposome-incorporated integrin $\alpha_{IIb}\beta_3$ have been determined (**Fig. 20**) to be the D-phe, the Val methyl groups, the Arg α, β, and γ protons, one H_β of Asp and one H_α of Gly *(53)*. The structure of the complex of cyclo(RGDfV) with the integrin $\alpha_v\beta_3$ was determined by X-ray crystallography *(44)*, and the complex of $\alpha_5\beta_1$ with the closely related peptide cyclo[Mpa RGDDVC]-NH$_2$ was determined by ^{15}N-edited trNOESY experiments (**ref. 54** and **Fig. 14**). Data from the STD NMR determination of the binding epitopes for cyclo(RGDfV) in its interaction with $\alpha_{IIb}\beta_3$ were in complete agreement with this related work (**Fig. 20**), and it is likely that the STD NMR data required only a fraction of the time and expense of the other two methods. Other applications of the STD NMR method have been made to determine the antibody-bound conformation of a carbohydrate-mimetic peptide *(47)*, to screen a collection of small molecules for binding to the active site of human factor Xa protein *(55)* and for epitope mapping of the *O*-chain polysaccharide of *Legionella pneumophila* serogroup 1 lipopolysaccharide *(56)*. Finally, Wang et al. *(57)* have recently shown how to use STD NMR spectroscopy to detect high-affinity ligands, a problematic task for other NMR-based screening methods. They detected the presence of a competing high-affinity ligand by monitoring the reduction or disappearance of the STD signals from a lower-affinity indicator ligand.

A note of caution with respect to the use of STD NMR for epitope mapping was raised by Yan et al. *(58)*, who pointed out that T_1 relaxation of the protons from the ligand can interfere with the epitope map, particularly if there is a marked difference in T_1s for the different ligand protons. They suggest that measurement of the ligand T_1s is essential prior to designing the STD NMR study and that saturation times less than T_1 are to be used to improve epitope mapping.

Because the STD NMR method is one that relies on the transfer of cross relaxation, the theoretical methods that have been developed for the analysis of cross relaxation can be applied. A complete relaxation and conformational exchange matrix analysis (CORCEMA) has shown *(59)* that changes in the intensity of ligand resonance integrals depended on a number of factors, including the spin saturation time, distance between the saturated receptor protons and the ligand protons, structure of the ligand-binding

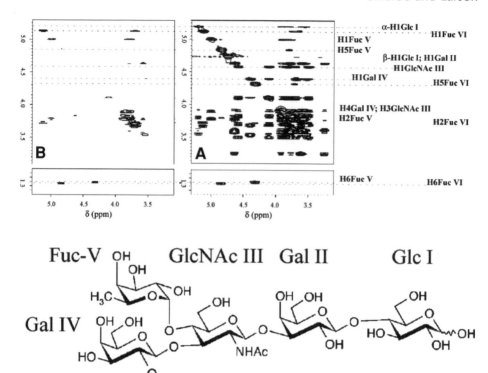

Fig. 19. Saturation transfer TOCSY nuclear magnetic resonance spectra of Lewis-B hexasaccharide (**1**) in (**A**) absence and (**B**) presence of agglutinin from *A. aurantia*. In (B) only the fucosyl residues of **1** are seen to acquire saturation from the protein. The on-resonance ($\delta = 10$ ppm) and off-resonance ($\delta = 30$ ppm) TOCSY spectra were taken at 300 K from 1 mmol of hexasaccharide and 10 nmol of protein. (Adapted from **ref. 50**.)

Fig. 20. *(Opposite page)* (**A**) Structure of cyclo(RGDfV) peptide antagonist of $\alpha_{IIb}\beta_3$. (**B**) Conventional nuclear magnetic resonance spectrum (a) of cyclo(RGDfV) and RGD peptides in presence of $\alpha_{IIb}\beta_3$ and saturation transfer difference (STD) NMR spectrum (b) of cyclo(RGDfV) and RGD peptides in presence of $\alpha_{IIb}\beta_3$ showing only signals from high-affinity peptide. The inset shows an expanded region of the spectra from (a) and (b) and displays only the resonances from the better binder, cyclo(RGDfV), and not from RGD. (**C**) Relative STD responses for distinct protons of cyclo(RGDfV) peptide. Note the strong response of the phe δ, ϵ, ζ protons. (**D**) Stereo view of a CPK model of cyclo(RGDfV) peptide with asterisks indicating medium and strong STD responses of individual protons revealing the fact that these protons directly interact with integrin. (Adapted from **ref. 53**.)

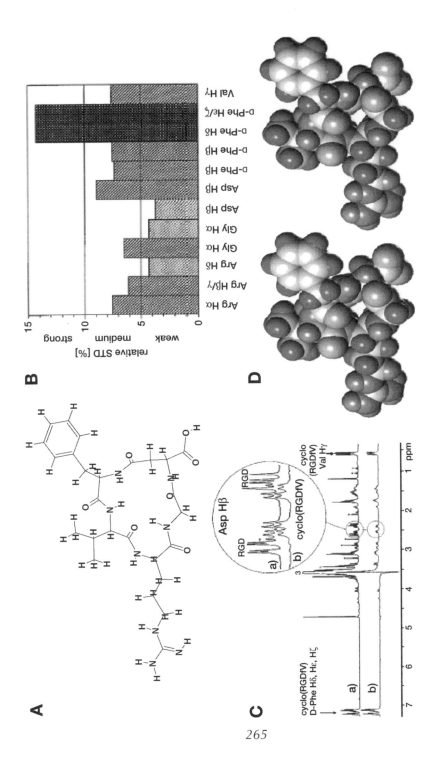

Fig. 20

265

pocket, molecular rotational correlation times, exhange kinetics, and ratio of ligand to receptor. A new method for refining approximate structures of ligands bound to proteins has been developed *(60)* based on the use of STD NMR data on weak binding complexes. The minimum energy bound conformation of the ligand is found by CORCEMA calculation of intensities, with simulated annealing optimization of torsion angles of the bound ligand, using STD-NMR intensities as experimental constraints and the NOE R-factor as the pseudoenergy function to be minimized.

4.7. Applications of HSQC, Chemical Shift Mapping, and Multiguantam NMR with Isotopic Labeling

One of the early methods that stimulated interest in NMR applications to drug discovery was the development of ^{15}N HSQC spectroscopy of ^{15}N-labeled proteins in the absence and presence of weakly binding potential ligand fragments. High-affinity ligands were built up by linking together these weaker-binding fragments *(19)*. The ^{15}N chemical shifts of the backbone amides in a protein are sensitive to the global conformation and folding characteristics of the protein, including the presence of nearby aromatic rings, or charged residues, and to local perturbations arising from the binding of ligands. Changes in the chemical shifts for specific assigned residues then can reveal the approximate nature of the ligand-binding site. Because chemical shift changes arise at both local and remote sites in a protein on substrate binding, interpretation of these effects is not simple or straightforward *(61)*. More precise information on the nature of the binding site can be obtained if one compares the ^{1}H ^{13}C and ^{15}N chemical shift changes induced in a protein by a series of closely related compounds *(62)*. For example, most of the FK506 binding protein resonances shift on binding of the FK506 analog ascomycin, making it difficult to locate the binding pocket, and more difficult to orient the analog (**Fig. 21**). However, when differential chemical shift changes are mapped onto the protein structures, it is easy to pick out those residues involved in interactions with specific modifications to the ligands.

A fragment-based approach was successfully applied to the development of nanomolar ligands for the FK506-binding protein *(19)*. Chemical shift changes of the protein on ligand binding were observed in HSQC spectra of ^{15}N-labeled proteins (**Fig. 22**). By examining these changes for the FK506-binding protein *(63)* in complex with small molecules, a putative binding site for compound **2** (**Fig. 23**) could be determined. An additional, nearby site for another compound (**9**; **Figs. 23** and **24**) was found by map-

Fig. 21. *(Opposite page)* Differential proton, carbon, and nitrogen chemical shifts of FK506-binding protein in presence of ascomycin with respect to (**A**) free FK506-binding protein, (**B**) 31-keto-32-desoxy-ascomycin, (**C**) 24-desoxy-ascomycin, and (**D**) FK506. Similar data are shown for the Bcl-X$_L$ complex with a Bak 16mer peptide compared with (**E**) free Bcl-X$_L$, (**F**) a V307A Bak mutant, (**G**) an R320A Bak mutant, and (**H**) a G315A Bak mutant. In each panel the nuclei showing significant chemical shift changes ($\Delta\delta$, ppm) are represented as spheres, with the size of the sphere representing the magnitude of the changes ($0.03 < \Delta\delta^1$H, ^{15}N < 0.13; $0.15 < \Delta\delta^{13}$C < 0.65). Note that in (**A**) and (**E**) the $\Delta\delta$ values are large for most of the nuclei, and in (**B**)–(**D**) and (**F**)–(**H**) the only significant changes occur for nuclei at the site of the ligand modifications (circled). (From **ref. 62** with permission.)

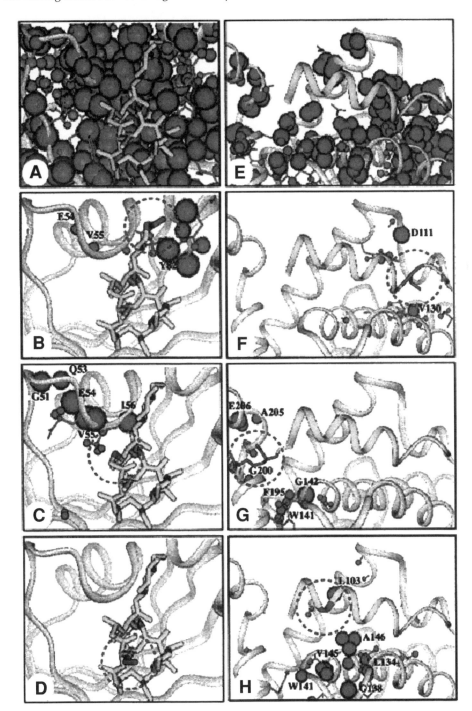

Fig. 21

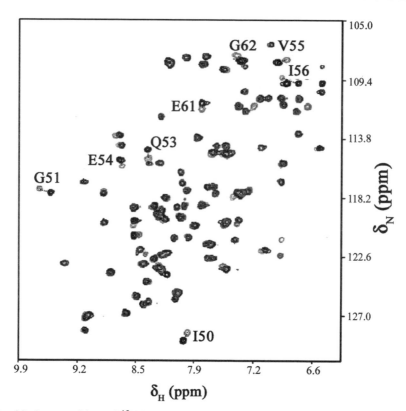

Fig. 22. Superposition of ^{15}N heteronuclear single quantum conerence nuclear magnetic resonance spectra of FK506-binding protein without (gray) and with (black) compound **3** (**Fig. 23**). The labeled amide signals display significant chemical shift changes on binding **3**. Each spectrum was taken in the presence of saturating amounts of compound **2**, which bound to a site on the protein adjacent to that occupied by **3**. (Adapted from **ref. *19*.**)

ping the chemical shift changes for the protein when **9** was added in the presence of **2**. Linkage of **2** and **9** to form compounds **10–13** (**Fig. 23**) and the synthesis of a related compound **14** led to the attainment of compounds with nanomolar affinities for the FK506-binding protein, which bind to the same site as the fragments (**Fig. 25**). In a similar fashion, inhibitors that block DNA binding by the human papillomavirus E2 protein were produced *(22)*. Here, biphenyl compounds were found to bind to a site close to the DNA-binding site, and compounds with a benzophenone group were found to bind to the β-barrel at the E2 dimer interface. These two separate fragments were then combined to produce [5-(3'(3'',5''-dichlorophenoxy)-phenyl)-2,4-pentadienoic acid], which had an IC_{50} of 10 μ*M*.

Matrix metalloproteases (MMPs) are a group of zinc-requiring enzymes of importance in tissue remodeling and tumor metastases. Fragment-based screens of compounds using ^{15}N HSQC of the MMP stromelysin *(64)* produced two molecules that bound to

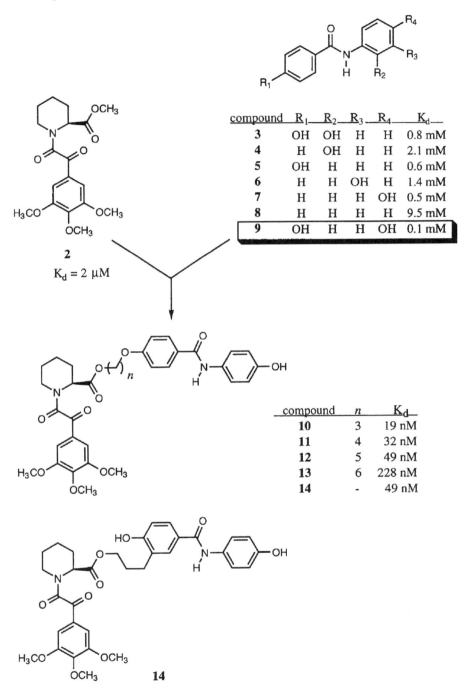

compound	R₁	R₂	R₃	R₄	Kd
3	OH	OH	H	H	0.8 mM
4	H	OH	H	H	2.1 mM
5	OH	H	H	H	0.6 mM
6	H	H	OH	H	1.4 mM
7	H	H	H	OH	0.5 mM
8	H	H	H	H	9.5 mM
9	OH	H	H	OH	0.1 mM

2

$K_d = 2\ \mu M$

compound	n	Kd
10	3	19 nM
11	4	32 nM
12	5	49 nM
13	6	228 nM
14	-	49 nM

14

Fig. 23. Structures of fragments used in assembly of a nanomolar inhibitor of FK506-binding protein. (From **ref. *19*** with permission.)

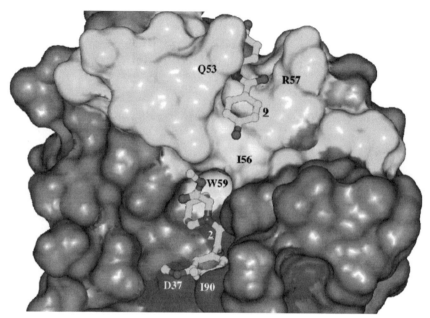

Fig. 24. Surface of FK506-binding protein showing binding sites of compounds **2** and **9** (**Fig. 23**), as determined from ^{15}N-^{13}C-filtered nuclear Overhauser effect data (*see* **Note 2**). Residues that exhibited the largest chemical shift changes on the binding of **2**, **9**, or both **2** and **9** are D37, I90, Q53, R57, W59, I56, respectively. Chemical shift changes for **9** are those observed on the addition of **9** to FKBP in the presence of saturating amounts of **2** (2.0 m*M*). Weighted averaged chemical shifts were used ($\Delta(^1\text{H}, ^{15}\text{N}) = |\Delta(^1\text{H})| + 0.2*|\Delta(^{15}\text{N})|$), and indicated residues are those for which $\Delta(^1\text{H}, ^{15}\text{N})$ exceeded 0.15 and 0.05 ppm for **2** and **9**, respectively. (From **ref. 19** with permission.)

stromelysin (MMP-3) at distinct but adjacent sites, acetohydroxamate (site 1, $K_D = 17$ m*M*) and 1-hydroxy,4'-cyano-biphenyl (site 2, $K_D = 0.02$ m*M*). Linkage of these two molecules produced a biarylhydroxamate with a K_D of 57 n*M*, again illustrating the power of fragment-based NMR screening and linkage to produce high-affinity ligands from lower-affinity fragments. Compounds binding at site 1 interact with the active-site zinc atom. Replacement of the hydroxamate with 1-naphthylhydroxamate gave a compound which bound to site 1 ($K_D = 0.05$ m*M*) with higher affinity than hydroxamate itself and allowed the binding of other molecules at site 2. An NOE-based structure of the complex between stromelysin and 1-naphthylhydroxamate using ^{13}C-edited and ^{12}C-filtered NOESY data sets (**Fig. 26**) showed that the naphthyl group of 1-naphthylhydroxamate engaged in hydrophobic interactions with Tyr-155, Tyr-168, Phe- 86, His-205, and Val-163 of stromelysin, and that there was still room for a biaryl compound to bind at site 2. Linkage of 1-naphthylhydroxamate with 1-*O*-mesitylated-4'-cyano-biphenyl produced 2-[2-[(4'-cyano[1,1'-biphenyl]-4-yl)oxy]ethoxy]-*N*-hydroxy-1- naphthalene-carboxamide ($K_D = 340$ n*M*), which bound to stromelysin and showed NOEs between the biaryl moiety and Val-163, Leu-197, Val-198, and Leu-218, which were the same as

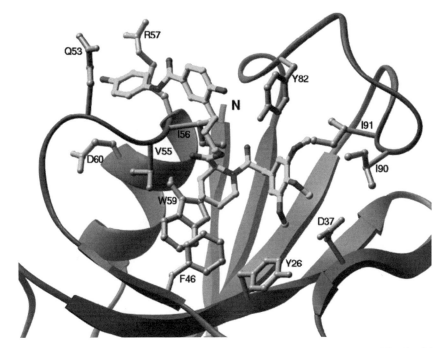

Fig. 25. Ribbon depiction of structure of FKBP (gray) when complexed to **14** (**Fig. 23**; unlabeled carbon atoms). Labeled FKBP residues are those residues that have nuclear Overhauser effects to the ligand. (From **ref. *19*** with permission.)

observed for 1-hydroxy-4'-cyano-biphenyl at site 2, and the naphthyl moiety-induced chemical shift changes at Tyr-155, Val-163, Ala-165, Ala-167, Tyr-168, and Ala-169 of stromelysin at or near site 1. Finally, this compound was modified to pruduce *N*-hydroxy-2-[2-[[3'-(cyanomethyl)[1,1'-biphenyl]-4-yl]sulfonyl]ethoxy]-1- naphthalenecarboxamide (K_D = 62 n*M*), which had the same K_D (57 n*M*) as the original biarylhydroxamate, but had superior oral availability, showing the robustness of the fragment-based screening and linkage approach using HSQC to monitor the protein–ligand interaction sites. This approach works well for proteins that bind two substrate molecules.

A final example of the use of HSQC is the fragment-based design of an inhibitor of protein tyrosine phosphatase 1B, a molecule involved in insulin and leptin signal transduction (*65*). *N*-Phenyloxamic acid is a nonphosphorus-containing phosphotyrosine analog. Mimics of this oxamate structure could serve as ligands for site 1 on the phosphatase. One molecule synthesized was 5-(4-bromophenyl)-3-carboxy-5*H*-isoxazol-1-ium (**Fig. 27**), which had a K_D of 0.8 m*M*. The second site (*66*) bound salicylic acid (K_D = 1.2 m*M*). Linkage of these produced 3-carboxy-5-{5-[(1*E*)-3-(2-carboxy-3-hydroxyphenoxy)prop-1-enyl]-2-fluorophenyl}-5*H*-isoxazol-1-ium (**Fig. 27**). The X-ray crystal structure of protein tyrosine phosphatase 1B complexed to 3-carboxy-5-{5-[(1*E*)-3-(2-carboxy-3-hydroxy-phenoxy)prop-1-enyl]-2-fluorophenyl}-5*H*-isoxazol-1-ium (**Fig. 27**) showed

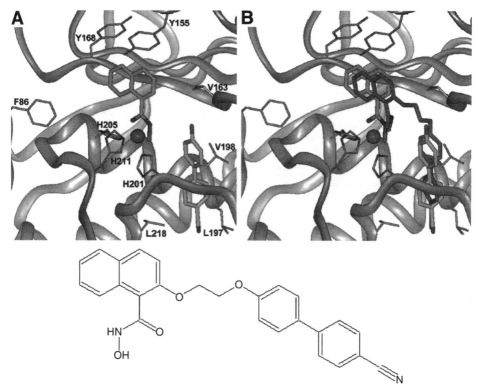

2-[2-[(4'-Cyano[1,1'-biphenyl]-4-yl)oxy]-ethoxy]-N-hydroxy-1-naphthalenecarboxamide

Fig. 26. (**Top**) Structure of inhibitors bound to active site of stromelysin. (**A**) 1-naphthylhydroxamate. (**B**) 2-[2-[(4'-cyano[1,1'-biphenyl]-4-yl)oxy]ethoxy]-*N*-hydroxy-1-naphthalenecarboxamide. In both panels is the biaryl compound 1-hydroxy-4'-cyano-biphenyl. The labeled residues engage in nuclear Overhauser effect magnetization exchange with the bound molecules, and the ball represents the zinc atom. (**Bottom**) Structure of 2-[2-[(4'-cyano[1,1'-biphenyl]-4-yl)oxy] ethoxy]-*N*-hydroxy-1-naphthalenecarboxamide. (Adapted from **ref. *64*.)

that this molecule now spanned both sites with the isoxazole and phenyl rings occupying the hydrophobic pocket otherwise occupied by the phosphotyrosine ring. The use of fragment-based HSQC NMR screening allowed the generation of a potent phosphatase inhibitor without the need to screen blindly thousands of compounds because weak binders for both sites could be identified based on simple ligands already known.

4.8. Applications of Residual Dipolar Couplings

One of the potential shortcomings of NMR-based determination of macromolecular structure is that methods that rely on the observation of NOEs only give short-range (<6 Å) constraints on distances between nuclei. This is fine for determining local structure, but often longer-range information on overall molecular folding and relative domain

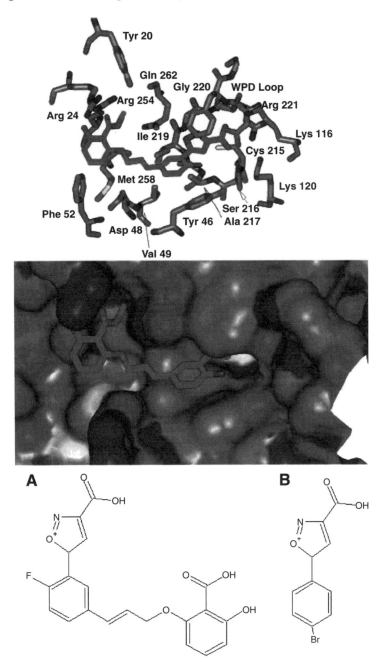

Fig. 27. (**Top**) Stick drawing and X-ray structure of protein tyrosine phosphatase 1B complexed with 3-carboxy-5-{5-[(1*E*)-3-(2-carboxy-3-hydroxyphenoxy)prop-1-enyl]-2-fluorophenyl}-5*H*-isoxazol-1-ium (**A**). (**B**) Structure of 5-(4-bromophenyl)-3-carboxy-5*H*-isoxazol-1-ium, a weak binder to site 2 of protein tyrosine phosphatase 1B ($K_D = 0.8$ m*M*). (Adapted from **ref. 65**.)

orientation is both necessary and important for an understanding of the functions of new proteins obtained from genetics or molecular biological investigations. The measurement of residual dipolar couplings (RDCs) provides data that nicely complement those from NOE experiments *(67)* in that RDCs show the relative orientations of backbone vectors *(17,68)*. For example, an extensive set of RDC measurements *(18)* showed that packing of the maltodextrin-binding protein into a crystal lattice appeared to change the relative orientation of its two domains by 11° from that found in solution. Several algorithms now exist that can give the structure of a protein from RDC measurements combined with sparse NOE and hydrogen bond restraints *(69–71)*.

Our principal interest in RDC measurements is not only in the ability to use these as additional data for the determination of macromolecular structure in solution, but in the potential utility of the data for elucidating the structures of ligands in solution, bound to receptors, and for determining conformational changes in proteins. In a study of the structure of the catalytic fragment of human fibroblast collagenase (MMP-1), Huang et al. *(72)* found that superposition of the active-site backbone atoms from both a high-quality MMP-1 structure and a minimal-restraint MMP-1 structure yielded an RMSD of 0.68 Å. The size and shape of the S1' catalytic pocket were found to be nearly identical in both structures. Additionally, the structure of an MMP-1-CGS-27023A complex based on RDCs and a minimal set of NOE-based restraints reliably reproduced the structure of the complex and established the usefulness of the structures for drug design.

Direct analysis of ligand binding using RDC data is beginning to appear in the literature. The ligand-binding properties of the 53-kDa mannose-binding protein (MBP) have been investigated using RDCs. The determined geometry of the bound trimannoside ligand and orientational constraints allowed docking of the ligand in the binding site of MBP and gave a structural model for MBP-oligosaccharide interactions *(73)*. The conformational and motional properties of flexible trisaccharides, such as methyl-3,6-di-*O*-(α-D-mannopyranosyl)-α-D-mannopyranoside, have been determined in solution using RDCs *(74)*. The conformation of the carbohydrate recognition domain of the galactose-binding lectin Galectin-3 was studied in the presence and absence of the ligand *N*-acetyllactosamine using residual dipolar couplings from NMR spectra *(75)* to determine the backbone structure of the protein and the binding geometry of the ligand, with the result that the ligand-binding geometry was consistent with that found in a crystal structure of the complexed state. As more research groups become familiar with the orientational requirements of RDC measurements, an expansion of the use of this technique in structure-based drug design will be seen.

4.9. Applications of TROSY

The discovery of the cancellation between transverse relaxation time (T_2) and CSA-induced line broadening by Pervushin et al. *(10)* has opened the way for the study of very large proteins, and, in particular, protein complexes, which were previously believed to be too large for NMR study. The inhibition of protein–protein interactions constitutes a new and important area of development in drug discovery *(76)*, so knowledge of the interaction sites for proteins with other proteins is now of critical importance. Many bacteria infect their hosts by means of adhesive interactions between pili or fimbriae,

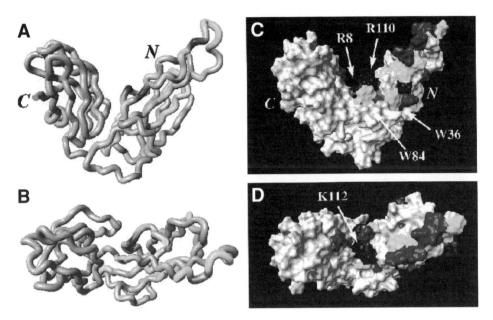

Fig. 28. (**A**) Mapping of ^{15}N and ^{1}H chemical shift differences for FimC–FimH complex onto 3D structure of FimC. Part (**B**) is the same as (**A**) after rotation by 90° about a horizontal axis so that the two wings of the structure point toward the viewer. (From **ref. 77**. Copyright by Nature Publishing Group. Used with permission.) Molecular surface of nuclear magnetic resonance structure of FimC 3 showing binding surface for FimH. The residues with $\delta\Delta > 0.1$ ppm are dark. Part (**D**) is the same as (**C**) after a 90° rotation of the molecule.

which also act as virulence factors, and cell-surface proteins on host cells. Drugs that interfere with either the assembly of the pili or their attachment to the host cell would then be useful as alternative antibiotics different from the classic protein synthesis inhibitors, to which bacteria are evolving resistance. Type 1 pili from *Escherichia coli* are filamentous oligomers of the 28-kDa mannose-binding FimH monomer. The assembly of the pilus involves the chaperone-mediated assembly of FimH monomers by the 23-kDa, two-domain periplasmic chaperone, FimC. TROSY-assisted chemical shift mapping of the interaction sites between [^{15}N, ^{2}H]-FimC and FimH in the 51-kDa complex *(77)* showed that the FimH-binding surface of FimC is formed almost entirely by the N-terminal domain, and its extent and shape indicate that FimC binds a folded form of the pilus subunits. Chemical shift changes were found to be large for the solvent-exposed residues Trp-36 and Trp-84, and for Arg-8 and Arg-110 at a basic site near Lys-112 (**Fig. 28**) when FimC bound to FimH. It is well known that Trp and Arg residues function as critical residues at the sites of protein-protein interactions *(76)* and that these residues can likely be incorporated into peptide mimics to form inhibitors of pilus assembly.

TROSY methods are also of great interest for the study of membrane proteins. Genes for these proteins make up approx 30% of the human genome. Membrane proteins are great potential drug targets because these proteins are involoved in cell signaling and cell–cell interactions. Studies of membrane proteins have lagged because most membrane proteins are insoluble in water. To circumvent their insolubility, they are often studied as large aggregates, with masses larger than 50 kDa, of mixed micelles with detergents; therefore, they are not candidates for classic solution NMR techniques. Larger proteins also give rise to severe spectral crowding, even in multidimensional NMR experiments. The use of intein technology (78,79) can reduce the complexity of the resulting NMR data sets by offering the means to label selectively only single domains, or specific sequence regions. Nevertheless, labeling of membrane proteins with ^{15}N, ^{2}H, and ^{13}C enables NMR studies to progress even in the presence of detergents or phospholipid micelles because only the labeled molecules are detected, and the micellar background protons are filtered out of the spectrum.

Initial TROSY NMR studies of membrane proteins examined the well-characterized outer-membrane proteins, OmpA (325 residues; 36.2 kDa) and OmpX (148 residues; 16.5 kDa) from E. coli (80,81) as approx 60-kDa aggregates with dihexanoylphosphatidylcholine micelles. For OmpX, complete sequence-specific NMR assignments were obtained for the protein backbone. ^{13}C chemical shifts and NOE data allowed the identification of regular secondary structure elements of OmpX/dihexanoylphosphatidylcholine in solution and gave sufficient conformational constraints for the computation of the global fold of the protein. For OmpA, the NMR assignments were limited to about 80% of the polypeptide chain, perhaps owing to different motional characteristics of the reconstituted OmpA β-barrel from those of OmpX. Both of the intramembranous portions of these proteins formed a β-barrel structure of high regularity within the lipid bilayer (**Fig. 29**). NMR data sets obtained by means of 3D [^{15}N, ^{1}H]-TROSY-HNCA and [^{13}C]-ct-[^{15}N, ^{1}H]-TROSY-HNCA experiments provided ^{13}C chemical shifts that enabled sequential backbone assignments to be made for C_α and C_β carbons for the first 171 of 176 residues. These assignments were used to generate an unambiguous map of the eight membrane-spanning β strands (**Fig. 29**). The development of additional techniques will be required before the side-chain assignments necessary for a complete structural analysis will be possible, but this study of the Omp proteins was a significant beginning.

The applications of NMR to the study of large macromolecular systems are illustrated by the successful use of TROSY techniques to examine the control of tryptophan biosynthesis genes in bacteria (82). Tryptophan synthesis is regulated by tryptophan-dependent binding of the Trp RNA-binding attenuation protein (TRAP) to the leader region of the Trp operon mRNA. TRAP is a 90.6-kDa protein composed of 11 identical subunits, clearly too large for study by classic solution NMR techniques. However, triple-resonance TROSY-based NMR spectra recorded at 55°C provided backbone resonance assignments for uniformly ^{2}H,^{13}C,^{15}N-labeled TRAP from Bacillus stearothermophilus in the absence and presence of tryptophan (82). Trp binding to TRAP is temperature dependent in this thermophile. Ligand-dependent differential line-broadening, chemical shift perturbations (**Fig. 30**) and biochemical measurements suggested that

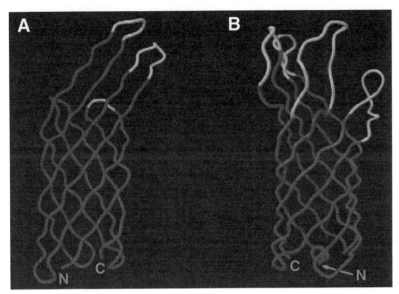

Fig. 29. Transferse relaxation optimized spectroscopy nuclear magnetic resonance-derived backbone structure of the intramembranous portion of *E. coli* outer membrane proteins (**A**) OmpX (residues 1–148) and (**B**) OmpA (residues 1–176) determined in micelles of dihexanoylphosphatidylcholine. The gray loops in (A) and (B) contain flexible residues not observed in prior X-ray structures *(80,81)*. The molecules are oriented with their peri-plasmic ends (containing the N- and C-termini) down and the extracellular portions up. (Reproduced from **ref.** *80* with permission.)

tryptophan-modulated protein flexibility played a central role in the allosteric control of TRAP function by altering its RNA-binding affinity.

TROSY techniques are now being applied to transient protein-protein interactions between components of the respiratory chain. Wienk et al. *(83)* used chemical shift mapping to investigate the molecular interaction between two components of the electron-transfer chain from *Paracoccus denitrificans*: a fragment of cytochrome-c_{552} and the Cu_A domain from cytochrome-*c* oxidase. Comparison of [^{15}N, ^{1}H]-TROSY spectra of the ^{15}N-labeled cytochrome-c_{552} fragment in the absence and presence of the Cu_A fragment led to the finding of chemical shift changes for the backbone amide groups of several uncharged residues around the exposed heme edge in cytochrome-c_{552}. The contact areas on the cytochrome-c_{552} surface were found to be similar under both reduced and oxidized conditions, implying that these chemical shift changes represented biologically relevant protein–protein interactions.

The development of effective anticancer drugs constitutes one of the great current drug design challenges. TROSY NMR techniques have now been applied to the study of interactions of drugs with targets and for the solution structures of oncoproteins (e.g., gankyrin; *[84]*). Polyphenols found widely in nature are derived from plant structural lignins. Certain of these molecules have received wide attention because they have

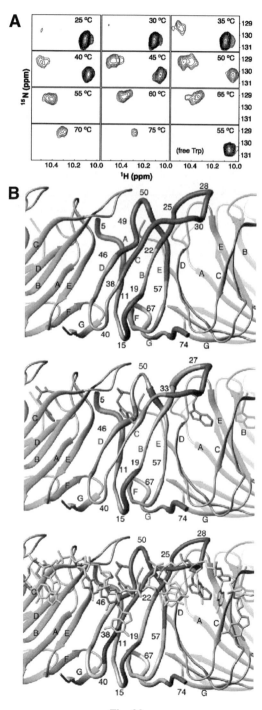

Fig. 30

demonstrated antitumor activity through the inhibition of protein-protein interactions involved in the intrinsic apoptosis pathway. Two such molecules, gossypol and pur-purogallin, have been found, by using TROSY NMR techniques, to bind to the hydro-phobic crevice on Bcl-x$_L$, which controls heterodimerization with BH3-containing proteins *(85)*, providing a mechanism to explain their ability to induce apoptosis even in Bcl-2- or Bcl-x$_L$-overexpressing cells. A pharmacophore model was developed that gave an important foundation from which to design even more potent and selective anticancer drugs targeting Bcl-2 family proteins.

The development of vaccines has also been aided by TROSY NMR. MSP1[19], the C-terminal fragment of merozoite surface protein 1 from *Plasmodium falciparum*, is a leading candidate antigen for development of a vaccine against the blood stages of the malaria parasite. Morgan et al. *(86)* used TROSY NMR spectroscopy to produce high-quality spectra of Fab complexes that allow the mapping of epitopes by the chemical shift perturbation technique on a complete, folded protein antigen MSP1[19]. NMR chemical shift changes were measured in the complexes of *P. falciparum* MSP1[19] with Fab fragments from three MAbs, two of which had parasite-inhibitory activity in vitro, and a third antibody that was noninhibitory. A close spatial relationship was found between the binding sites for the two inhibitory antibodies, but the noninhibitory antibody bound at a different location. The results revealed a surface on MSP1[19] where inhibitory antibodies bound, information that will be valuable for optimizing the MSP1[1] antigen by rational vaccine design.

4.10. Applications of HTS with NMR

It is clear that the enormous amount of information available from an NMR- spectroscopic approach to drug screening makes it a method of choice for all aspects of the discovery process. However, NMR is an intrinsically low-sensitivity method that is also slow and requires large amounts of difficult-to-produce materials. What can be done to improve these shortcomings?

Sensitivity can be increased in several ways. The HSQC experiment uses the higher-sensitivity proton for detection of spin-coupled ^{13}C or ^{15}N. The highest field magnets can be used, currently 19 T, although these are the most expensive, costing in excess

---

Fig. 30. *(Opposite page)* Application of transverse relaxation optimized spectroscopy nuclear magnetic resonance (NMR) spectroscopy to study the interaction of tryptophan with Trp RNA-binding attenuation protein (TRAP) from the thermophilic bacterium *Bacillus stearothermophilus*. (**A**) The binding of Trp to TRAP is temperature dependent. ^{1}H, ^{15}N heteronuclear single quantum coherence spectra of TRAP in the presence of Trp from 25 to 75°C show free Trp at low temperature (signal at δ_H = 10.3 ppm, δ_N = 130.5 ppm, and lower right panel) changing to bound Trp (signal at δ_H = 10.5 ppm, δ_N = 129 ppm) at 35°C. (**B**) Trp-induced NMR spectral changes mapped onto the backbone of TRAP derived from the crystal structure (protein databank code 1CS9): (**top**) Proton line widths in absence of Trp. Darker gray residues indicate significant line broadening. (**Middle**) Proton line widths in presence of Trp. The backbone is drawn with a ribbon whose width is proportional to the line width. (**Bottom**) Trp-induced proton, carbon, and nitrogen chemical shift changes are largest (darker gray) for strand C, indicating transmittal of the Trp-binding information to the RNA-binding surface. (From **ref.** *82* with permission.)

of \$5 million. A less expensive approach is the retrofitting of existing spectrometers with cryoprobe technology, which costs around \$200,000, and gives a factor of 2–4 increase in signal-to-noise ratio for a given sample. This cuts the time needed per spectrum by up to an order of magnitude, so a 2D ^{15}N/^{1}H correlation spectrum on 50 μM protein samples using cryogenic NMR probe technology can be obtained in less than 10 min *(87,88)* and up to 200,000 compounds can be screened in less than 1 mo. Cryoprobe technology coupled with the automated analysis of HSQC data, could dramatically improve the throughput of NMR-based drug screenings.

An outgrowth of the development of TROSY methods is an increase in sensitivity produced through line narrowing because the signal-to-noise ratio is defined in terms of signal heights, rather than integrals. It is easier to detect narrow lines than broad ones. Most of the HSQC NMR studies have used ^{15}N labeling of the backbone amides of the protein, but ^{13}C-labeled methyl groups have more potential because they contain three protons instead of the single proton in the amides *(64)*, so they produce three times the NMR signal for a given protein concentration *(64)*. In addition, TROSY methods have now been introduced for the observation of these labeled methyls in proteins *(89)* as large as 810 kDa (lysine decarboxylase). Often the target protein is uniformly labeled with isotopes, and for very large molecules, the resulting NMR spectra are extremely complex. Studies of protein interaction sites have shown that only a few residues actually contribute the bulk of Gibb's free energy of interaction; these residues include Tyr, Trp, and Arg *(76,90)*. Therefore, specific labeling of Trp can greatly simplfy the spectra while preserving information about specific binding sites *(91)*.

Another method for increasing the effectiveness of NMR arises from the unique aspects of the technique. HSQC of a protein target in the presence of drugs indicates where a drug binds to a protein and therefore gives clues to the functions of unknown proteins derived from expression of new sequences from the human genome. Instead of screening 200,000 compounds against an expressed protein of unknown function, it is more efficient to use a mixture of a smaller number of compounds, but to include in this mix examples of the broad spectrum of known protein ligands, such as kinase inhibitors, saccharides, protease inhibitors, or nucleosides. *(64)*. In this way the NMR data not only reveal binders but give clues as to the protein's function, with less time expended on the data production phase. The mixture of compounds could also consist of molecular fragments, which can then be optimized by linkage *(19)*. A prescreen, such as MS, can narrow the list of potential binders so that NMR can be applied where it has its greatest strength and impact—in the identification of true ligands and their interaction sites.

HTS NMR methods that focus on the ligands have also been proposed. Dalvit et al. *(92)* used the high relative sensitivity of ^{19}F NMR spectroscopy (83% of the proton) and the lack of background fluorine nuclei to perform enzyme assays using substrates containing –CF_3 groups. Enzyme inhibitors can then be detected at high sensitivity using ^{19}F cryoprobes. Applications of this technique to the screening of inhibitors of the Ser/Thr kinase AKT1 and the protease trypsin were examined.

The DNA sequences generated through the Human Genome Project give rise to many proteins of unknown function. NMR methods can greatly assist in functional genomic studies of the nature of these molecules. To have a high-throughput impact, automated methods for the production of isotopically labeled cloned, expressed proteins must be available. Major bottlenecks in high-throughput recombinant protein production with the *E. coli* expression systems include low expression levels and the insolubility of eukaryotic gene products. One way around these problems could be to focus on separate protein domains. A fast, microtiter plate-based expression and solubility screening procedure has been developed that is capable of purifying 24 protein samples/wk for the production of protein samples for NMR *(93)*. Starting with 81 cloned human protein domains, in vivo expression was detected in 54 cases, and from 28 of those, milligram quantities of protein could be purified. An informative HSQC spectrum was recorded for 18 proteins (22%), half of which were indicative of a folded protein. Similar work by Scheich et al. *(94)* analyzed 88 different *E. coli* expression constructs for 17 human protein domains using high-throughput cloning, purification, and folding analysis to obtain candidates suitable for structural analysis. Six constructs (representing two domains) were quickly identified as well folded and suitable for structural analysis. This procedure was found to be especially effective as a rapid and inexpensive screen for high-copy-number proteins from structural genomics. It is clear from these results that NMR methods have a significant role to play in HTS.

4.11. Applications of Computational Methods

Just as NMR methods have impacted many areas of drug discovery, so have computational techniques impacted NMR spectroscopy. The very conduct of NMR experiments is impossible today without the use of control software and computers. NMR data analyses also depend on computers and software for storage, processing, and display of multidimensional spectra. The construction of restrained molecular models is integrated into NMR software, such as Felix (Accelrys, San Diego, CA) and its associated modules, and the software produced by Tripos (St. Louis, MO). Numerous useful NMR software is available free of charge on the Internet, or through contact with software developers (*see* **Subheading 2.3.**). Good Web sites containing many links to NMR software are www.spincore.com/nmrinfo/software_s.html and www.organik.uni-erlangen.de/research/NMR/software.html.

Among several interesting new computational developments, the radical G-matrix approach to data acquisition, GFT *(95)*, ranks highly. Multidimensional Fourier transform NMR spectroscopy suffers from the need to measure N-1 indirect dimensions in an N- dimensional data set. These indirect dimensions require the accumulation of many (e.g., 256–1024) separate spectra at differing time delays to build up adequate digital resolution in the indirect dimensions. This makes the measurements time-consuming and a constant compromise between digital resolution and measuring time. GFT NMR uses phase-sensitive joint sampling of the indirect dimensions to produce chemical shift multiplet subspectra, which are then linearly combined using a G-matrix prior to Fourier transformation. The chemical shifts, which are multiply encoded in the multiplets, give statistically indendent multiple measurements from which the shifts can be obtained with high precision *(14)*. The dramatic reduction in time (4- to 18-fold) needed to build up the indirect dimensions means that determination of macromolecular structure can achieve the high-throughput speed necessary for modern drug discovery schemes *(96)*.

After the NMR data sets are measured, new computational methods are required to deal with the massive amounts of spectral information produced. Even a simple HSQC screen of a ^{15}N-labeled protein in the presence of a mixture of compounds can easily produce 500 data sets, which must be assigned and measured, and the relevant chemical shift changes must be sorted from irrelevant structural changes. Processing schemes based on multivariate methods such as linear discriminant analysis, support vector machines, or three-way decomposition have been developed to deal with the increased data flow. One of these methods (three-way decomposition) has been incorporated into the software MUNIN (multidimensional NMR spectral interpretation; *[97–100]*), which can automatically process large groups of HSQC data sets and extract signals that change chemical shifts owing to compound binding to a target molecule *(101)*. Because this technique is based on the extraction of orthogonal feature vectors (called "shapes" in MUNIN) in three dimensions, it does not require full experimental sampling of all of the indirect dimensions and can therefore reduce data acquisiton times by up to a factor of 4. Application of MUNIN to drug discovery treats a set of 2D HSQC spectra as a 3D object in which the third dimension is the spectrum number. The output appears to distinguish clearly binding from nonbinding ligands in an automatic fashion.

Another method for compressing the large amounts of 3D structural information found in protein–ligand complexes generated either with X-ray diffraction, NMR, or computer-aided docking studies, is to generate 1D feature vectors (bit strings) based on the interaction sites between ligands and macromolecules. These vectors can be clustered and compared quickly, revealing common binding modes and interactions *(102)*, and can be used for data mining.

So far, we have concentrated on the use of experimental NMR data for the elucidation of binding features of drug candidates, but computational methods can take this one step further and use calculated molecular NMR properties in cases in which the molecules may be difficult or expensive to synthesize or time factors preclude actual synthesis. Such a scheme involves developing quantitative spectral activity relationships based on empirical data for a class of related compounds binding to a given target, and then using chemical shift prediction algorithms to provide input data for unsynthesized molecules. This approach has been successfully used to model steroid inhibitor activity *(103, 104)* in relation to the aromatase enzyme, a cytochrome P450 complex that converts androgens to estrogens, which is therapeutically significant with respect to control of breast cancer. Further studies of ^{13}C NMR spectral features were used to develop accurate models of steroid binding to the corticosteroid-binding globulin *(105)* and of polychlorinated dibenzodioxins, dibenzofurans, and biphenyls binding to the aryl hydrocarbon receptor *(106)*.

4.12. Conclusion

NMR methods have had an impact on all aspects of the drug discovery process. We have not mentioned several other areas because they are outside the scope of this chapter, but NMR is also an important player in metabolomics *(107)*, which can reveal the response of organisms to the presence of drugs, or to specific genetic manipulations.

NMR imaging is also very useful in the discovery process but has been well covered elsewhere. Other aspects of the use of NMR in drug discovery are provided in reviews by Homans *(108)* and Pellecchia et al. *(109)*, particularly the techniques of NMR-DOC and NMR-SOLVE, two fragment-based methods *(110)* similar to HSQC (SAR by NMR; *[87,88]*). Further applications of NMR in this area will only be limited by investigator's insights.

5. Notes

1. ^{15}N, ^1H correlation spectra of 0.5 mM ^2H, ^{15}N-labeled P450 reductase from rat liver obtained in 95% H_2O, 5% D_2O; $T = 303$ K, pH 7.5.
2. The NMR samples of the ternary complex were composed of uniformly ^{15}N-, ^{13}C-labeled FKBP (2.0 mM), 2 (2.0 mM), and 9 (5.0 mM) in a D_2O or a mixture of H_2O and D_2O (9 to 1) phosphate-buffered solution (50 mM, pH 6.5) containing 100 mM NaCl and 0.05% sodium azide. The ^1H, ^{13}C, and ^{15}N backbone and side-chain resonances of FKBP in the complex were assigned from an analysis of several 3D ^5N- and ^{13}C-edited NMR experiments *(111)*. A total of 17 intermolecular restraints were used to dock 9 to the known structure of FKBP *(112–114)*. Compound 2 was placed in a location similar to that observed in the ascomycin complex, which was consistent with the chemical shift changes observed on binding of 2 (**Fig. 22**) *(19)*.

References

1. Pochapsky, S. S. and Pochapsky, T. C. (2001) Nuclear magnetic resonance as a tool in drug discovery, metabolism and disposition. *Curr. Top. Med. Chem.* **1,** 427–441.
2. Johnson, M. A. and Pinto, B. M. (2004) NMR spectroscopic and molecular modeling studies of protein-carbohydrate and protein-peptide interactions. *Carbohydr. Res.* **339,** 907–928.
3. Chen, A. and Shapiro, M. J. (1999) Affinity NMR. *Anal. Chem.* **71,** 669A–675A.
4. De Clercq, E. (2002) Strategies in the design of antiviral drugs. *Nat. Rev. Drug Discov.* **1,** 13–25.
5. Stejskal, E. O. and Tanner, J. E. (1965) Spin diffusion measurements: spin echoes in the presence of a time-dependent field gradient. *J. Chem. Phys.* **42,** 288–292.
6. Luo, R. S., Liu, M. L., and Mao, X. A. (1999) NMR diffusion and relaxation study of drug-protein interaction. *Spectrochim. Acta A Mol. Biomol. Spectrosc.* **55A,** 1897–1901.
7. Utsumi, H., Seki, H., Yamaguchi, K., and Tashiro, M. (2003) Segment identification of a ligand binding with a protein receptor using multidimensional T1rho-, diffusion-filtered and diffusion-ordered NOESY experiments. *Anal. Sci.* **19,** 1441–1443.
8. Lucas, L. H., Yan, J., Larive, C. K., Zartler, E. R., and Shapiro, M. J. (2003) Transferred nuclear overhauser effect in nuclear magnetic resonance diffusion measurements of ligand-protein binding. *Anal. Chem.* **75,** 627–634.
9. Ni, F. (2004) Recent developments in transferred NOE methods. *Prog. Nucl. Magn. Reson. Spectrosc.* **26,** 517–606.
10. Pervusin, K., Riek, R., Wider, G., and Wuthrich, K. (1997) Attenuated T2 relaxation by mutual cancellation of dipole-dipole coupling and chemical shift anisotropy indicates an avenue to NMR structures of very large biological macromolecules in solution. *Proc. Natl. Acad. Sci. USA* **94,** 12,366–12,371.
11. Fernandez, C. and Wider, G. (2003) TROSY in NMR studies of the structure and function of large biological macromolecules. *Curr. Opin. Struct. Biol.* **13,** 570–580.

12. Pellecchia, M., Meininger, D., Shen, A. L., Jack, R., Kasper, C. B., and Sem, D. S. (2001) SEA-TROSY (solvent exposed amides with TROSY): a method to resolve the problem of spectral overlap in very large proteins. *J. Am. Chem. Soc.* **123,** 4633, 4634.

13. Lin, D., Sze, K. H., Cui, Y., and Zhu, G. (2002) Clean SEA-HSQC: a method to map solvent exposed amides in large non-deuterated proteins with gradient-enhanced HSQC. *J. Biomol. NMR* **23,** 317–322.

14. Kim, S. and Szyperski, T. (2004) GFT NMR experiments for polypeptide backbone and 13Cbeta chemical shift assignment. *J. Biomol. NMR* **28,** 117–130.

15. Frydman, L., Scherf, T., and Lupulescu, A. (2002) The acquisition of multidimensional NMR spectra within a single scan. *Proc. Natl. Acad. Sci. USA* **99,** 15,858–15,862.

16. Weigelt, J., Wikstrom, M., Schultz, J., and van Dongen, M. J. (2002) Site-selective labeling strategies for screening by NMR. *Comb. Chem. High Throughput Screen.* **5,** 623–630.

17. Tolman, J. R., Flanagan, J. M., Kennedy, M. A., and Prestegard, J. H. (1995) Nuclear magnetic dipole interactions in field-oriented proteins: information for structure determination in solution. *Proc. Natl. Acad. Sci. USA* **92,** 9279–9283.

18. Skrynnikov, N. R., Goto, N. K., Yang, D., et al. (2000) Orienting domains in proteins using dipolar couplings measured by liquid-state NMR: differences in solution and crystal forms of maltodextrin binding protein loaded with beta-cyclodextrin. *J. Mol. Biol.* **295,** 1265–1273.

19. Shuker, S. B., Hajduk, P. J., Meadows, R. P., and Fesik, S. W. (1996) Discovering high-affinity ligands for proteins: SAR by NMR. *Science* **274,** 1531–1534.

20. Hajduk, P. J., Sheppard G., Nettesheim, D. G., et al. (1997) Discovery of potent non-peptide inhibitors of stromelysin using SAR by NMR. *J. Am. Chem. Soc.* **119,** 5818–5827.

21. Hajduk, P. J., Olejniczak, E. T., and Fesik, S. W. (1997) One-dimensional relaxation- and diffusion-edited NMR methods for screening compounds that bind to macromolecules. *J. Am. Chem. Soc.* **119,** 12,257–12,261.

22. Lin, M. and Shapiro, M. J. (1996) Mixture analysis in combinatorial chemistry application of diffusion-resolved NMR spectroscopy. *J. Organic Chem.* **61,** 7617–7619.

23. Hajduk, P. J., Dinges, J., Miknis, G. F., et al. (1997) NMR-based discovery of lead inhibitors that block DNA binding of the human papillomavirus E2 protein. *J. Med. Chem.* **40,** 3144–3150.

24. Danielsson, J., Jarvet, J., Damberg, P., and Graslund, A. (2004) Two-site binding of beta-cyclodextrin to the Alzheimer Abeta(1-40) peptide measured with combined PFG-NMR diffusion and induced chemical shifts. *Biochemistry* **43,** 6261–6269.

25. Pelta, M. D., Morris, G. A., Stchedroff, M. J., and Hammond, S. J. (2002) A one-shot sequence for high-resolution diffusion-ordered spectroscopy. *Magn. Reson. Chem.* **40,** S147–S152.

26. Derrick, T. S., McCord, E. F., and Larive, C. K. (2002) Analysis of protein/ligand interactions with NMR diffusion measurements: the importance of eliminating the protein background. *J. Magn. Reson.* **155,** 217–225.

27. Lin, M., Shapiro, M. J., and Wareing, J. R. (1997) Diffusion-edited NMR-affinity NMR for direct observation of molecular interactions. *J. Am. Chem. Soc.* **119,** 5249, 5250.

28. Ponstingl, H. and Otting, G. (1997) NMR assignments, secondary structure and hydration of oxidized Escherichia coli flavodoxin. *Eur. J. Biochem.* **244,** 384–399.

29. Gonnella, N., Lin, M., Shapiro, M. J., Wareing, J. R., and Zhang, X. (1998) Isotope-filtered affinity NMR. *J. Magn. Reson.* **131,** 336–338.

30. Tillett, M. L., Horsfield, M. A., Lian, L. Y., and Norwood, T. J. (1999) Protein-ligand interactions measured by ^{15}N-filtered diffusion experiments. *J. Biomol. NMR* **13,** 223–232.

31. Yuan, P., Marshall, V. P., Petzold, G. L., Poorman, R. A., and Stockman, B. J. (1999) Dynamics of stromelysin/inhibitor interactions studied by 15N NMR relaxation measurements: comparison of ligand binding to the S1-S3 and S'1-S'3 subsites. *J. Biomol. NMR* **15,** 55–64.

32. Clore, G. M. and Gronenborn, A. M. (1982) Theory and applications of the transferred nuclear Overhauser effect to the study of the conformations of small ligands bound to proteins. *J. Magn. Reson.* **48,** 402–417.

33. Campbell, A. P. and Sykes, B. D. (1993) The two-dimensional transferred nuclear Overhauser effect: theory and practice. *Annu. Rev. Biophys. Biomol. Struct.* **22,** 99–122.

34. Meyer, B., Weimar, T., and Peters, T. (1997) Screening mixtures for biological activity by NMR. *Eur. J. Biochem.* **246,** 705–709.

35. Henrichson, D., Ernst, B., Magnani, J. L., Wang, W. T., Meyer, B., and Peters, T. (1999) Bioaffinity NMR spectroscopy: identification of an E-selectin antagonist in a substance mixture by transfer NOE. *Angew. Chem. Intl. Ed.* **38,** 98–102.

36. Herfurth, L., Weimar, T., and Peters, T. (2000) Application of 3D-TOCSY-trNOESY for the assignment of bioactive ligands from mixtures. *Angew. Chem. Int. Ed. Engl.* **39,** 2097–2099.

37. Verdier, L., Gharbi-Benarous, J., Bertho, G., Mauvais, P., and Girault, J. P. (2002) Antibiotic resistance peptides: interaction of peptides conferring macrolide and ketolide resistance with Staphylococcus aureus ribosomes: conformation of bound peptides as determined by transferred NOE experiments. *Biochemistry* **41,** 4218–4229.

38. Adams, E. R., Dratz, E. A., Gizachew, D., et al. (1997) Interaction of human neutrophil flavocytochrome b with cytosolic proteins: transferred-NOESY NMR studies of a gp91phox C-terminal peptide bound to p47phox. *Biochem. J.* **325(Pt. 1),** 249–257.

39. Kleinberg, M. E., Mital, D., Rotrosen, D., and Malech, H. L. (1992) Characterization of a phagocyte cytochrome b558 91-kilodalton subunit functional domain: identification of peptide sequence and amino acids essential for activity. *Biochemistry* **31,** 2686–2690.

40. Kleinjung, J., Petit, M. C., Orlewski, P., et al. (2000) The third-dimensional structure of the complex between an Fv antibody fragment and an analogue of the main immunogenic region of the acetylcholine receptor: a combined two-dimensional NMR, homology, and molecular modeling approach. *Biopolymers* **53,** 113–128.

41. Inooka, H., Ohtaki, T., Kitahara, O., et al. (2001) Conformation of a peptide ligand bound to its G-protein coupled receptor. *Nat. Struct. Biol.* **8,** 161–165.

42. Hynes, R. O. (2002) Integrins: bidirectional, allosteric signaling machines. *Cell* **110,** 673–687.

43. Shimaoka, M. and Springer, T. A. (2003) Therapeutic antagonists and conformational regulation of integrin function. *Nat. Rev. Drug Discov.* **2,** 703–716.

44. Xiong, J. P., Stehle, T., Zhang, R., et al. (2002) Crystal structure of the extracellular segment of integrin alpha Vbeta3 in complex with an Arg-Gly-Asp ligand. *Science* **296,** 151–155.

45. Zwahlen, C., Vincent, S. J. F., Dibari, L., Levitt, M. H., and Bodenhausen, G. (1994) Quenching spin diffusion in selective measurements of transient overhauser effects in nuclear magnetic resonance applications to olignucleotides. *J. Am. Chem. Soc.* **116,** 362–368.

46. Dechantsreiter, M. A., Planker, E., Matha, B., et al. (1999) N-Methylated cyclic RGD peptides as highly active and selective alpha(V)beta(3) integrin antagonists. *Med. Chem.* **42,** 3033–3040.

47. Johnson, M. A., Rotondo, A., and Pinto, B. M. (2002) NMR studies of the antibody-bound conformation of a carbohydrate-mimetic peptide. *Biochemistry* **41,** 2149–2157.

48. Dalvit, C., Fogliatto, G., Stewart, A., Veronesi, M., and Stockman, B. (2001) WaterLOGSY as a method for primary NMR screening: practical aspects and range of applicability. *J. Biomol. NMR* **21,** 349–359.

49. Dalvit, C., Fasolini, M., Flocco, M., Knapp, S., Pevarello, P., and Veronesi, M. (2002) NMR-Based screening with competition water-ligand observed via gradient spectroscopy experiments: detection of high-affinity ligands. *J. Med. Chem.* **45,** 2610–2614.

50. Mayer, M. and Meyer, B. (1999) Characterization of ligand binding by saturation transfer difference NMR spectroscopy. *Angew. Chem. Int. Ed.* **38,** 1784–1788.

51. Klein, J., Meinecke, R., Mayer, M., and Meyer, B. (1999) Detecting binding affinity to immobilized receptor proteins in compound libraries by HR-MAS STD NMR. *J. Am. Chem. Soc.* **121,** 5336, 5337.

52. Tranqui, L., Andrieux, A., Hudry-Clergeon, G., et al. (1989) Differential structural requirements for fibrinogen binding to platelets and to endothelial cells. *J. Cell Biol.* **108,** 2519–2527.

53. Meinecke, R. and Meyer, B. (2001) Determination of the binding specificity of an integral membrane protein by saturation transfer difference NMR: RGD peptide ligands binding to integrin alphaIIbbeta3. *J. Med. Chem.* **44,** 3059–3065.

54. Zhang, L., Mattern, R. H., Malaney, T. I., Pierschbacher, M. D., and Goodman, M. (2002) Receptor-bound conformation of an alpha(5)beta(1) integrin antagonist by (15)N-edited 2D transferred nuclear overhauser effects. *J. Am. Chem. Soc.* **124,** 2862–2863.

55. Fielding, L., Fletcher, D., Rutherford, S., Kaur, J., and Mestres, J. (2003) Exploring the active site of human factor Xa protein by NMR screening of small molecule probes. *Organic Biomol. Chem.* **1,** 4235–4241.

56. Kooistra, O., Herfurth, L., Luneberg, E., Frosch, M., Peters, T., and Zahringer, U. (2002) Epitope mapping of the O-chain polysaccharide of Legionella pneumophila serogroup 1 lipopolysaccharide by saturation-transfer-difference NMR spectroscopy. *Eur. J. Biochem.* **269,** 573–582.

57. Wang, Y. S., Liu, D., and Wyss, D. F. (2004) Competition STD NMR for the detection of high-affinity ligands and NMR-based screening. *Magn. Reson. Chem.* **42,** 485–489.

58. Yan, J., Kline, A. D., Mo, H., Shapiro, M. J., and Zartler, E. R. (2003) The effect of relaxation on the epitope mapping by saturation transfer difference NMR. *J. Magn. Reson.* **163,** 270–276.

59. Jayalakshmi, V. and Krishna, N. R. (2002) Complete relaxation and conformational exchange matrix (CORCEMA) analysis of intermolecular saturation transfer effects in reversibly forming ligand-receptor complexes. *J. Magn. Reson.* **155,** 106–118.

60. Jayalakshmi, V. and Rama, K. N. (2004) CORCEMA refinement of the bound ligand conformation within the protein binding pocket in reversibly forming weak complexes using STD-NMR intensities. *J. Magn. Reson.* **168,** 36–45.

61. Foster, M. P., Wuttke, D. S., Clemens, K. R., et al. (1998) Chemical shift as a probe of molecular interfaces: NMR studies of DNA binding by the three amino-terminal zinc finger domains from transcription factor IIIA. *J. Biomol. NMR* **12,** 51–71.

62. Medek, A., Hajduk, P. J., Mack, J., and Fesik, S. W. (2000) The use of differential chemical shifts for determining the binding site location and orientation of protein-bound ligands. *J. Am. Chem. Soc.* **122,** 1241, 1242.

63. Dornan, J., Taylor, P., and Walkinshaw, M. D. (2003) Structures of immunophilins and their ligand complexes. *Curr. Top. Med. Chem.* **3,** 1392–1409.

64. Hajduk, P. J., Shuker, S. B., Nettesheim, D. G., et al. (2002) NMR-based modification of matrix metalloproteinase inhibitors with improved bioavailability. *J. Med. Chem.* **45,** 5628–5639.

65. Liu, G., Xin, Z., Pei, Z., et al. (2003) Fragment screening and assembly: a highly efficient approach to a selective and cell active protein tyrosine phosphatase 1B inhibitor. *J. Med. Chem.* **46,** 4232–4235.

66. Puius, Y. A., Zhao, Y., Sullivan, M., Lawrence, D. S., Almo, S. C., and Zhang, Z. Y. (1997) Identification of a second aryl phosphate-binding site in protein-tyrosine phosphatase 1B: a paradigm for inhibitor design. *Proc. Natl. Acad. Sci. USA* **94,** 13,420–13,425.

67. Bolon, P. J., Al Hashimi, H. M., and Prestegard, J. H. (1999) Residual dipolar coupling derived orientational constraints on ligand geometry in a 53 kDa protein-ligand complex. *J. Mol. Biol.* **293,** 107–115.

68. Lipsitz, R. S. and Tjandra, N. (2004) Residual dipolar couplings in NMR structure analysis. *Annu. Rev. Biophys. Biomol. Struct.* **33,** 387–413.

69. Giesen, A. W., Homans, S. W., and Brown, J. M. (2003) Determination of protein global folds using backbone residual dipolar coupling and long-range NOE restraints. *J. Biomol. NMR* **25,** 63–71.

70. Wedemeyer, W. J., Rohl, C. A., and Scherag, H. A. (2002) Exact solutions for chemical bond orientations from residual dipolar couplings. *J. Biomol. NMR* **22,** 137–151.

71. Wang, L. and Donald, B. R. (2004) Exact solutions for internuclear vectors and backbone dihedral angles from NH residual dipolar couplings in two media, and their application in a systematic search algorithm for determining protein backbone structure. *J. Biomol. NMR* **29,** 223–242.

72. Huang, X., Moy, F., and Powers, R. (2000) Evaluation of the utility of NMR structures determined from minimal NOE-based restraints for structure-based drug design, using MMP-1 as an example. *Biochemistry* **39,** 13,365, 13,375.

73. Jain, N. U., Noble, S., and Prestegard, J. H. (2003) Structural characterization of a mannose-binding protein-trimannoside complex using residual dipolar couplings. *J. Mol. Biol.* **328,** 451–462.

74. Tian, F., Al Hashimi, H. M., Craighead, J. L., and Prestegard, J. H. (2001) Conformational analysis of a flexible oligosaccharide using residual dipolar couplings. *J. Am. Chem. Soc.* **123,** 485–492.

75. Umemoto, K., Leffler, H., Venot, A., Valafar, H., and Prestegard, J. H. (2003) Conformational differences in liganded and unliganded states of Galectin-3. *Biochemistry* **42,** 3688–3695.

76. Sillerud, L. O. and Larson R. S. (2005) Design and structure of peptide and peptidomimetic antagonists of protein-protein interaction. *Curr. Protein Pept. Sci.* **6,** 151–169.

77. Pellecchia, M., Sebbel, P., Hermanns, U., Wuthrich, K., and Glockshuber, R. (1999) Pilus chaperone FimC-adhesin FimH interactions mapped by TROSY-NMR. *Nat. Struct. Biol.* **6,** 336–339.

78. Sun, W., Yang, J., and Liu, X. Q. (2004) Synthetic two-piece and three-piece split inteins for protein trans-splicing. *J. Biol. Chem.* **279,** 35,281–35,286.

79. David, R., Richter, M. P., and Beck-Sickinger, A. G. (2004) Expressed protein ligation: method and applications. *Eur. J. Biochem.* **271,** 663–677.

80. Fernandez, C., Hilty, C., Bonjour, S., Adeishvili, K., Pervushin, K., and Wuthrich, K. (2001) Solution NMR studies of the integral membrane proteins OmpX and OmpA from Escherichia coli. *FEBS Lett.* **504,** 173–178.

81. Fernandez, C., Adeishvili, K., and Wuthrich, K. (2001) Transverse relaxation-optimized NMR spectroscopy with the outer membrane protein OmpX in dihexanoyl phosphatidylcholine micelles. *Proc. Natl. Acad. Sci. USA* **98,** 2358–2363.

82. McElroy, C., Manfredo, A., Wendt, A., Gollnick, P., and Foster, M. (2002) TROSY-NMR studies of the 91kDa TRAP protein reveal allosteric control of a gene regulatory protein by ligand-altered flexibility. *J. Mol. Biol.* **323,** 463–473.

83. Wienk, H., Maneg, O., Lucke, C., Pristovsek, P., Lohr, F., Ludwig, B., and Ruterjans, H. (2003) Interaction of cytochrome c with cytochrome c oxidase: an NMR study on two soluble fragments derived from Paracoccus denitrificans. *Biochemistry* **42**, 6005–6012.

84. Yuan, C., Li, J., Mahajan, A., Poi, M. J., Byeon, I. J., and Tsai, M. D. (2004) Solution structure of the human oncogenic protein gankyrin containing seven ankyrin repeats and analysis of its structure—function relationship. *Biochemistry* **43**, 12,152–12,161.

85. Leone, M., Zhai, D., Sareth, S., Kitada, S., Reed, J. C., and Pellecchia, M. (2003) Cancer prevention by tea polyphenols is linked to their direct inhibition of antiapoptotic Bcl-2-family proteins. *Cancer Res.* **63**, 8118–8121.

86. Morgan, W. D., Lock, M. J., Frenkiel, T. A., Grainger, M., and Holder, A. A. (2004) Malaria parasite-inhibitory antibody epitopes on Plasmodium falciparum merozoite surface protein-1(19) mapped by TROSY NMR. *Mol. Biochem. Parasitol.* **138**, 29–36.

87. Hajduk, P. J., Meadows, R. P., and Fesik, S. W. (1999) NMR-based screening in drug discovery. *Q. Rev. Biophys.* **32**, 211–240.

88. Hajduk, P. J., Gerfin, T., Boehlen, J. M., Haberli, M., Marek, D., and Fesik, S. W. (1999) High-throughput nuclear magnetic resonance-based screening. *J. Med. Chem.* **42**, 2315–2317.

89. Tugarinov, V., Sprangers, R., and Kay, L. E. (2004) Line narrowing in methyl-TROSY using zero-quantum 1H-13C NMR spectroscopy. *J. Am. Chem. Soc.* **126**, 4921–4925.

90. Bogan, A. A. and Thorn, K. S. (1998) Anatomy of hot spots in protein interfaces. *J. Mol. Biol.* **280**, 1–9.

91. Rodriguez-Mias, R. A. and Pellecchia, M. (2003) Use of selective Trp side chain labeling to characterize protein-protein and protein-ligand interactions by NMR spectroscopy. *J. Am. Chem. Soc.* **125**, 2892, 2893.

92. Dalvit, C., Ardini, E., Flocco, M., Fogliatto, G. P., Mongelli, N., and Veronesi, M. (2003) A general NMR method for rapid, efficient, and reliable biochemical screening. *J. Am. Chem. Soc.* **125**, 14,620, 14,625.

93. Folkers, G. E., van Buuren, B. N., and Kaptein, R. (2004) Expression screening, protein purification and NMR analysis of human protein domains for structural genomics. *J. Struct. Funct. Genomics* **5**, 119–131.

94. Scheich, C., Leitner, D., Sievert, V., et al. (2004) Fast identification of folded human protein domains expressed in E. coli suitable for structural analysis. *BMC. Struct. Biol.* **4**, 4.

95. Kim, S. and Szyperski, T. (2003) GFT NMR, a new approach to rapidly obtain precise high-dimensional NMR spectral information. *J. Am. Chem. Soc.* **125**, 1385–1393.

96. Xia, Y., Zhu, G., Veeraraghavan, S., and Gao, X. (2004) (3,2)D GFT-NMR experiments for fast data collection from proteins. *J. Biomol. NMR* **29**, 467–476.

97. Orekhov, V. Y., Ibraghimov, I., and Billeter, M. (2003) Optimizing resolution in multidimensional NMR by three-way decomposition. *J. Biomol. NMR* **27**, 165–173.

98. Gutmanas, A., Jarvoll, P., Orekhov, V. Y., and Billeter, M. (2002) Three-way decomposition of a complete 3D 15N-NOESY-HSQC. *J. Biomol. NMR* **24**, 191–201.

99. Korzhneva, D. M., Ibraghimov, I. V., Billeter, M., and Orekhov, V. Y. (2001) MUNIN: application of three-way decomposition to the analysis of heteronuclear NMR relaxation data. *J. Biomol. NMR* **21**, 263–268.

100. Orekhov, V. Y., Ibraghimov, I. V., and Billeter, M. (2001) MUNIN: a new approach to multi-dimensional NMR spectra interpretation. *J. Biomol. NMR* **20**, 49–60.

101. Damberg, C. S., Orekhov, V. Y., and Billeter, M. (2002) Automated analysis of large sets of heteronuclear correlation spectra in NMR-based drug discovery. *J. Med. Chem.* **45**, 5649–5654.

102. Deng, Z., Chuaqui, C., and Singh, J. (2004) Structural interaction fingerprint (SIFt): a novel method for analyzing three-dimensional protein-ligand binding interactions. *J. Med. Chem.* **47**, 337–344.
103. Beger, R. D., Buzatu, D. A., Wilkes, J. G., and Lay, J. O. Jr. (2001) (13)C NMR quantitative spectrometric data-activity relationship (QSDAR) models of steroids binding the aromatase enzyme. *J. Chem. Inf. Comput. Sci.* **41**, 1360–1366.
104. Beger, R. D., Freeman, J. P., Lay, J. O. Jr., Wilkes, J. G., and Miller, D. W. (2001) Use of 13C NMR spectrometric data to produce a predictive model of estrogen receptor binding activity. *J. Chem. Inf. Comput. Sci.* **41**, 219–224.
105. Beger, R. D. and Wilkes, J. G. (2001) Developing 13C NMR quantitative spectrometric data-activity relationship (QSDAR) models of steroid binding to the corticosteroid binding globulin. *J. Comput. Aided Mol. Des.* **15**, 659–669.
106. Beger, R. D., Buzatu, D. A., and Wilkes, J. G. (2002) Combining NMR spectral and structural data to form models of polychlorinated dibenzodioxins, dibenzofurans, and biphenyls binding to the AhR. *J. Comput. Aided Mol. Des.* **16**, 727–740.
107. Griffin, J. L. (2004) Metabolic profiles to define the genome: can we hear the phenotypes? *Philos. Trans. R. Soc. Lond. B Biol. Sci.* **359**, 857–871.
108. Homans, S. W. (2004) NMR spectroscopy tools for structure-aided drug design. *Angew. Chem. Int. Ed. Engl.* **43**, 290–300.
109. Pellecchia, M., Sem, D. S., and Wuthrich, K. (2002) NMR in drug discovery. *Nat. Rev. Drug Discov.* **1**, 211–219.
110. Pellecchia, M., Meininger, D., Dong, Q., Chang, E., Jack, R., and Sem, D. S. (2002) NMR-based structural characterization of large protein-ligand interactions. *J. Biomol. NMR* **22**, 165–173.
111. Clore, G. M. and Gronenborn, A. M. (1994) Multidimensional heteronuclear nuclear magnetic resonance of proteins. *Methods Enzymol.* **239**, 349–363.
112. Meadows, R. P., Nettesheim, D. G., Xu, R. X., et al. (1993) Three-dimensional structure of the FK506 binding protein/ascomycin complex in solution by heteronuclear three- and four-dimensional NMR. *Biochemistry* **32**, 754–765.
113. Van Duyne, G. D., Standaert, R. F., Karplus, P. A., Schreiber, S. L., and Clardy, J. (1991) Atomic structure of FKBP-FK506, an immunophilin-immunosuppressant complex. *Science* **252**, 839–842.
114. Van Duyne, G. D., Standaert, R. F., Schreiber, S. L., and Clardy, J. (1991) Atomic structure of the rapamycin human immunophilin FKBP-12 complex. *J. Am. Chem. Soc.* **113**, 7433–7434.

12

Receptor-Binding Sites

Bioinformatic Approaches

Darren R. Flower

Summary

It is increasingly clear that both transient and long-lasting interactions between bio-macromolecules and their molecular partners are the most fundamental of all biological mechanisms and lie at the conceptual heart of protein function. In particular, the protein-binding site is the most fascinating and important mechanistic arbiter of protein function. In this review, I examine the nature of protein-binding sites found in both ligand-binding receptors and substrate-binding enzymes. I highlight two important concepts underlying the identification and analysis of binding sites. The first is based on knowledge: when one knows the location of a binding site in one protein, one can "inherit" the site from one protein to another. The second approach involves the *a priori* prediction of a binding site from a sequence or a structure. The full and complete analysis of binding sites will necessarily involve the full range of informatic techniques ranging from sequence-based bioinformatic analysis through structural bioinformatics to computational chemistry and molecular physics. Integration of both diverse experimental and diverse theoretical approaches is thus a mandatory requirement in the evaluation of binding sites and the binding events that occur within them.

Key Words: Ligand binding; binding site; protein–ligand interaction; computational prediction; drug design; virtual screening; molecular dynamics; ligand docking.

1. Introduction

Whatever may be said of the origins of life, today we live in a protein universe. The diversity of function exhibited by proteins is extraordinary. Enzymes, for example, catalyze most, but not all *(1,2)*, chemical reactions within biological systems. The geometry and structural integrity of cells are maintained by fibrous and globular structural proteins *(3)*. Cell-surface receptors maintain and marshal intercell communication and the interaction between cells and their immediate milieu, effecting signal transduction *(4)*.

From: *Methods in Molecular Biology, vol. 316: Bioinformatics and Drug Discovery*
Edited by: R. S. Larson © Humana Press Inc., Totowa, NJ

As the era of genomics falls before the proteomic and systems biology revolution, it is becoming increasingly clear that both transient and long-lasting interactions between proteins are, seemingly, the most fundamental of all biological mechanisms and that such interactions lie at the conceptual heart of protein function *(5)*. Couple this to the interactions of proteins with small molecules, the province of metabolomics *(6–8)*, and with other biological macromolecules, such as DNA, and it becomes clear that the protein-binding site is the most fascinating and important mechanistic arbiter of protein function *(9,10)*.

It is perhaps easiest to think of the binding site as a very small part of a protein's surface that interacts with an equally small molecule, and, indeed, I focus on this aspect at length herein, but the binding site is also the site of interaction with other proteins or biomacromolecules. In this sense, the size of a binding site is in no way constrained. Equally well, the nature of the molecule being bound, or bound to, will determine the shape and physical properties of a site. This manifests itself in terms of both the amino acids that form a binding site and the overall folding pattern underlying the structure of an individual protein. The particular amino acids lining the binding site give rise to its local, individual shape and, through their chemical interactions, to the site's particular substrate or ligand specificity. The fold, on the other hand, is responsible for the more general shape and size of a binding site. Observed at the level of a genome or a population of genomes, the nature of a protein-binding site is in no way prescribed and, thus, its identification and analysis remain key challenges for both experimental and *in silico* science.

In this review, I examine the nature of binding sites found in both ligand-binding receptors and substrate-binding enzymes. Moreover, I am obliged to focus and do, in the course of my discussion, make reference to the three kinds of binding sites with which I am best acquainted: the G protein-coupled receptor (GPCR), the major histocompatibility complex (MHC), and that of the lipocalins.

The GPCRs form a large and burgeoning set of integral membrane proteins that act as cell-surface receptors responsible for the transduction of a wide array of extracellular signals into some kind of intracellular response *(11)*. GPCRs activate so-called G proteins, a group of ubiquitous guanine nucleotide-binding regulatory proteins. An activated GPCR will associate with the trimeric G protein complex, causing exchange of guanosine 5'-triphosphate for guanosine 5'-diphosphate bound to Gα, followed by dissociation of Gα-guanosine 5'-triphosphate from Gβγ and of both subunits from the receptor. Free Gα then couples to effector enzymes, such as adenylate or guanylate cyclase or phospholipase A2 or C, inhibiting or stimulating production of second messengers, such as cyclic adenosine monophosphate, which, in turn, cause the downstream generation of other messenger molecules, such as arachidonic and phosphatidic acid *(12)*. Moreover, many GPCRs also activate mitogen-activated protein kinases, a process involving GPCR endocytosis and a G protein-mediated pathway involving tyrosine kinase phosphorylation of a large collection of adapter proteins *(13)*. The GPCR is often taken to be the archetypal receptor in drug research and is thus presumed to possess the archetypal binding site as well *(11)*.

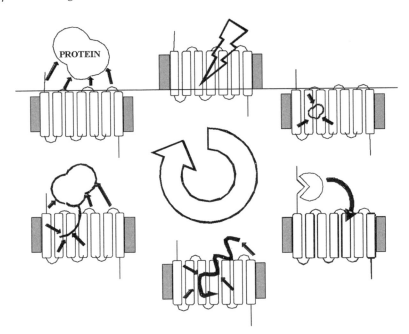

Fig. 1. Diversity in G protein-coupled receptor (GPCR) ligand-binding. Beveled cylinders linked by loops drawn as lines represent transmembrane helices. The membrane is shaded. Solid arrows indicate specific contacts between receptor and ligand. Starting at 12 o'clock and working clockwise, one sees a gradual increase in the size of bound ligands and the complexity of ligand–receptor interactions: first, light interacting with a rhodopsin molecule; second, a small molecule binding to an aminergic GPCR; third, a self-activating GPCR cleaved by a protease; fourth, a peptide binding GPCR; fifth, a small protein, such as a chemokine, binding to a GPCR, exhibiting a mixed binding mode, with interactions from both the transmembrane region and external loops, which is intermediate between that of a peptide and a large protein; sixth, a large protein binding to a GPCR.

GPCRs bind many different types of ligand: large proteins, peptides, and small molecules of as little as a handful of atoms. Certain GPCRs, such as rhodopsin, even interact with light, albeit mediated by a bound retinal molecule. Structurally *(14)*, a GPCR fold comprises seven sequences of 25–35 consecutive residues—typically with a high level of overall hydrophobicity—each representing a transmembrane α-helix, which together span the plasma membrane in an counterclockwise serpentine manner. As shown in **Fig. 1**, within this quasisymmetrical structure—the N-terminus and three loops are extracellular and the C-terminus and three loops are intracellular—evolution has allowed the GPCR to develop a wide variety of binding sites and surfaces.

The products of the MHC play a fundamental part in regulating immune responses. T-cells recognize antigen as peptide fragments complexed with MHC molecules, requiring antigen degradation by proteolytic enzymes prior to complexation *(15)*. The functional role of MHC proteins is thus to bind peptides and "present" these at the cell surface for inspection by T-cell receptors. MHCs are grouped into two classes with related structures *(16,17)*: class I molecules are composed of a heavy chain complexed to β2-microglobulin, and class II molecules consist of two chains (α and β) of similar size. Both classes of MHC molecule have similar three-dimensional (3D) structures: each has two domains, which come together to create a cleft- or groove-shaped peptide-binding site formed from a β-sheet base with sides composed of two α-helices. The principal difference between the two classes is the dimensions of the peptide-binding groove, which, for class I, is constrained to bind 8–10 amino acid peptides but is open at both ends in class II, allowing much larger peptides of varying length to be bound. In most species, but especially clearly in humans, MHC proteins are highly polymorphic, with several hundred genetic variants, or alleles, at each genetic locus, many of which are present at high frequency *(18)*. Different alleles may differ by up to 30 amino acid substitutions. Each class of MHC is represented at several loci: three for class I (in humans, human leukocyte antigen [HLA]-A, B, and -C) and three for class II (in humans, HLA-DR, -DQ, and -DP). The set of linked MHC alleles is called a haplotype. All MHC loci are expressed codominantly: both maternally and paternally inherited sets of alleles are expressed by each cell. In approx 97% of individuals the entire linked MHC complex is inherited without recombination *(19)*. The MHC fold has also been adopted by many other proteins of varying function. Such an example might include CD1, which fulfills a similar role within antigen presentation, but binds lipid, rather than peptide, molecules *(20)*.

Lipocalins *(21–24)* are among the most remarkable of protein families, exhibiting extraordinary diversity at the level of both sequence and function. The family was first defined almost 20 yr ago. Since then, our knowledge of the lipocalins has expanded enormously, with several new family members discovered each year. A typical lipocalin consists of a 160–180 amino acid peptide, folded into eight to nine β-strands, which form a continuously hydrogen-bonded β-barrel with a hydrophobic interior. The family comprises approx 40 distinct small extracellular proteins from a wide variety of tissues with a wide phyletic spread encompassing vertebrate and invertebrate animals, plants, and bacteria. The plasma proteins retinol-binding protein, α-1-acid glycoprotein, and α1-microglobulin; the nasal odorant-binding proteins; the bilin-binding proteins of butterflies; lobster crustacyanin; and temperature-induced lipocalins, which confer a plant its resistance to cold, are all examples of lipocalins. Clinical studies have shown the importance of lipocalins in health and disease; many of them are biomarkers of pregnancy, acute systemic inflammation, renal disorders, nerve growth and regeneration, and proliferation of cancerous cells or allergy. The family is characterized by three molecular recognition properties: binding to cell-surface receptors, the formation of complexes with soluble biomacromolecules, and the binding of small hydrophobic molecules. Lipocalins have historically been regarded as primarily transporters and, from crystallographic results, to possess an archetypal hydrophobic binding site.

From our quick peek at these three types of receptor, one thing is clear. A single binding site can be adapted to fulfill many functional roles, both by adapting its properties and by extending it.

However, the purpose of this work is not to undertake an exhaustive description of binding sites throughout the entire, emerging world of proteins, but to concentrate on their analysis through computational and bioinformatic methods. With a review as wide ranging in scope as this, though, I am obliged to be somewhat restrictive. In particular, I focus on protein-binding sites rather than the catalytic sites of enzyme or abzyme. There are many contemporary reviews on the nature of enzyme-active sites *(25,26)*; these are conflicting, if not totally irreconcilable, views, affording nonetheless a picture of such sites as possessing more similarities than differences. Furthermore, I cannot cite every relevant text, and, to those authors whom I have unwittingly excluded, I apologize.

1.1. On the Nature of Receptor-Binding Sites

Before beginning a more detailed examination of bioinformatic approaches to the analysis of binding sites, let us take the time to step back a little and view the area more generally. What, exactly, is a binding site? As I have already said, there is no obvious or simple definition, but clearly any region of interaction between a protein and some other molecular entity—however small, however large—is a binding site, at least of a sort. This point of interaction may, e.g., be a site of oligomerization, but one is more usually apt to view a binding site as a small, discrete cavity within a much larger protein, which interacts with a small molecule, be it an enzyme substrate or a receptor ligand. The language of chemistry, this is often called host-guest complexation: the protein is the host and the small molecule the guest. The rest of this section concentrates on protein–small molecule interactions, but the points made are easily generalized for other types of interaction.

It is within depressions on the protein surface that the specific binding of small molecules normally occurs; thus, binding sites are often referred to as pockets, cavities, grooves, or clefts. The choice of name is typically dictated by their size: pockets lie at the small end of the spectrum, clefts at the large. What discriminates between a binding site and other regions of a protein surface is a question of important, general interest *(27)*. Purely geometric criteria can be sufficient: enzyme-active sites are, for example, often large, deep clefts *(28,29)*. The size, shape, and burial of a cavity may dictate the type of ligands that can be accommodated. The physicochemical properties of a cavity will also give important insights. Small-molecule binding in surface depressions is ultimately a consequence of the physical principles governing molecular recognition: high affinity can only be gained by adequate steric complementarity and a sufficiently large interaction interface, and specificity is more easily obtained within environments that already impose geometric constraints. Yet, distinguishing a functionally relevant binding site from a cavity without binding properties remains challenging.

A binding site is formed by the 3D arrangement of specific amino acids that confers on a site both its geometrical characteristics—its size and shape—and its characteristic physicochemical properties—how hydrophobic or polar it may be *(30)*. Within such a physicochemical background, a subset of binding site residues will make appropriate amino acid–ligand contacts, whether those interactions are hydrophobic in nature, or mediated by hydrogen bonding, or complementary charge-charge pairing *(31)*. Although these interactions are the property of a particular sequence, the overall geometry—in other words, the size and shape of a binding site—is, generally, a common property of the fold for a given protein, albeit moderated by specific sequence features. The fold, or folding pattern, of a protein is one shared both by close sequence homologs (i.e., proteins that are clearly members of the same protein family) and by other proteins whose sequences are so distant that obvious homology cannot easily be identified between them *(32)*. These so-called structural superfamilies were long ago found to be common, indeed very common. The GPCRs and the lipocalins are, for different reasons, both good examples of this phenomenon. The lipocalins form part of a larger group of proteins called the calycins *(21,23,33,34)*, which also have similar internal ligand-binding sites, but less than obvious sequence similiarity and very different functions, phyletic spread, and cellular localization. Generic, or fold-determined, and specific, or sequence-determined, features of a protein both contribute to the key features of a binding site: on the one hand, its size and shape and, on the other, the nature and geometry of its amino acid side-chain interactions. In this way, one sees that certain folds are adapted to bind specific kinds of ligand; peptide binding by MHCs is a good example of this phenomenon *(17)*. Equally well, however, it is now becoming apparent that as the size of a protein family grows so too does the perceived diversity of chemical structures that it binds, something demonstrated clearly by GPCRs *(35,36)*.

Why are scientists interested in binding sites? Apart from the natural intellectual curiosity so characteristic of scientists, there are also key utilitarian objectives to their study. These are manifest most notably in the discovery of drugs, whether they are therapies to treat human pathologies or those of valued animals, such as farm livestock or companion animals, or antimicrobials whose function is to clear pathogenic organisms without injuring their hosts *(37)*. Drugs are "designed" molecules that bind to proteins, inhibiting or exacerbating their function. I place the word *designed* in quotation marks because many of the most successful, and famous, drugs are natural products: molecules from plant, animal, or microbial sources. By natural products, or secondary metabolites, I really mean compounds that have no explicit role in the internal metabolic economy of the organism that biosynthesized them. There are several competing arguments that offer putative explanations for the existence of such redundant molecules. Arguably, the most appealing of these is evolutionary in nature *(38)*: natural products may confer an augmented opportunity for survival in their producer organisms by binding specifically to macromolecular receptors in other organisms with a resulting physiological action. As a result of this innate capacity for making receptor interactions, as manifest in their overall size and complexity, secondary metabolites will be generally predisposed to make biomacromolecular complexes. One might expect, then, that natural products will perform well in random screening and possess a high probability of high initial activity. Although secondary metabolites can, indeed, be highly potent, their intrinsic complexity makes them synthetically intractable. Natural products will often prove to be either very weak hits, which are seldom attractive for optimization, or very potent and selective compounds that can, with little modification, move straight into clinical trials; cyclosporin *(39)*, FK506 *(40)*, and taxol *(41)* have, for example, all found clinical application.

To understand a ligand-binding site is, in many ways, to understand the ligand. This understanding provides a tool that helps greatly in the elucidation of ligand properties. Although such understanding is no longer the sole pivot on which the success of preclinical drug discovery rests *(42)*, it is only by the proper use of this information that drug design becomes, in any way, systematic and intellectually satisfying, as well as efficient and effective. Of course, the reverse can be equally true: to understand the structures of a set of ligand molecules is to understand, or, at least, to gain insight into the nature of their binding site. This is the basis of pharmacophore mapping *(43)*.

The pharmacophore is an important, unifying concept in drug discovery. It captures the idea that molecules are active at a particular receptor because they possess a set of key functional groups, interacting favorably with this receptor and possessing a geometry complementary to it. A pharmacophore is most usefully defined as an ensemble of interactive functional groups with a defined geometry. A pharmacophore may be derived in several ways: by analogy to a natural substrate or known ligand, by inference from a series of dissimilar biologically active molecules (the so-called active analogue approach), or by direct analysis of the structure of a target protein. Most pharmacophores tend to be fairly simple two-, three-, or four-point (i.e., functional group) pharmacophores, although some incorporate more elaborate features such as best planes and regions of excluded volume. Overspecifying a pharmacophoric pattern through the use of restrictive substructure criteria will limit the overall diversity of identified active molecules. In an ideal pharmacophore, the generality of functional groups does not restrict structural classes while the pharmacophore geometry supplies discriminating power to the search.

Once a pharmacophore model has been derived, there are, in general, two ways to identify molecules that share its features: by *de novo* design, which, at least in an ideal world, generates chemically reasonable, novel hypothetical structures *(44,45)*; and "3D database searching," in which large databases comprising 3D structures are searched for those matching a pharmacophore *(46)*. However, a single pharmacophore is unlikely to recover all active compounds. This is especially true for antagonists and enzyme inhibitors that bind in a number of different ways to block agonist or substrate binding. Each structurally distinct class may make its own individual subset of interactions within the total available within a binding site. Single compounds may also bind to more than one subsite or in several different binding modes. Given the more stringent requirements of receptor activation, agonists may exhibit less diversity in binding *(47)*. Thus, to span the structural diversity and different binding modes exhibited by antagonists and other ligands, many pharmacophores may be required to characterize fully the structural requirements of a given receptor or pharmacological activity. There is always a need, therefore, to test a reasonable number of molecules that fit a pharmacophore model. 3D database searching will ideally identify compounds with properties outside those of the set of molecules used to define the pharmacophore. This allows for the identification of novel chemical structures and molecular features leading to both increased and decreased activity.

Drugs need to balance several competing objectives (*see* **Fig. 2**)—receptor affinity, receptor selectivity, and lack of side effects, which are all mediated by receptors—together

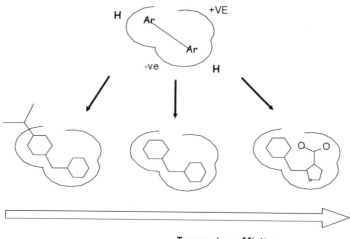

Increasing affinity

Fig. 2. Fitting the pharmacophore. A molecule either will or will not fit a pharmacophore. Although a particular compound may fit the pharmacophore, reflecting receptor complementarity, its activity is not guaranteed. It may possess unfavorable properties, such as extreme lipophilicity. Likewise, it may penetrate excluded volumes or introduce the pairing of like charges. Ranges of activity obtain unexpected enhancements as advantageous additional interactions are made with the receptor. A nominal or toy pharmacophore is shown superposed into an example binding site. Ligands found by the search are of three kinds: (1) molecules that place other groups into excluded volumes and are, as a result, weak or inactive; (2) molecules that fit the minimal requirements of the pharmacophore but introduce no extra interactions; and (3) molecules that fulfill all the pharmacophore's requirements and are complementary to the receptor introducing new groups that make favorable interactions with the binding site.

with other properties, such as lipophilicity and metabolic stability, which are generally not approached from the perspective of a binding site but through physical chemical methods that seek to control global molecular properties, such as lipophilicity *(48)*. However, biology, with which drugs must interact, is largely composed of a collection —albeit a vast collection—of different binding sites. A problem such as plasma protein binding is clearly something that could be addressed by examining drug-to-binding site interaction but is more usually examined in terms of manipulating its global physical properties. Receptor affinity is, however, clearly mediated through a drug's interaction with a binding site; receptor selectivity is mediated by interaction, or lack thereof, with several similar binding sites; and lack of side effects is mediated by binding to both essentially similar, yet functionally distinct, sites and also to dissimilar sites within quite different and unrelated receptors. Of course, binding sites are not restricted to proteins; many drugs bind selectively to other macromolecules, such as the major groove in DNA *(49)*, or, indeed, to supramolecular complexes, such as biological lipid membranes.

Ideas about the structure and physical properties of drug molecules converge in the concept of "drugness" *(50)*. What distinguishes drugs from other molecules, millions of which exist in compound repositories around the world? What determines "drugness"? The set of desirable properties required in a candidate drug? Beyond straightforward physicochemical and, thus, readily evaluated criteria are properties, both structural and physicochemical, that determine a drug's interaction with both the whole organism and the binding site of its biological target *(48)*. Interaction with the whole organism—usually termed DMPK, or ADME/tox, problems—covers a range of biological functions: absorption by the gut, nonspecific drug binding in the blood by human serum albumin or α-1-acid glycoprotein, and the metabolic clearance of compounds. The differing requirements of DMPK and receptor activity often seem in opposition, yet both are required in order to achieve "quality" drugs that are active and can reach an appropriate site of action in a reasonable amount of time and at nontoxic doses. The solution to this dilemma is reaching a balance between potency, mediated through interactions with the binding site, and pharmacokinetic properties. Lipophilicity, for example, is an important physicochemical parameter that, when manipulated properly, can effectively moderate oral absorption, plasma protein binding, and volume of distribution, and strongly influence processes such as pharmacokinetic properties and brain uptake; however, excessive lipophilicity can also increase a compound's vulnerablity to P450 metabolism and clearance *(51)*. One might imagine that binding site-mediated activity is the more difficult problem, but, within pharmaceutical research, one can no longer possibly attack it in isolation.

Increased understanding of the bulk properties of drugs has led to a concomitant increase in the understanding of the types of binding site—so-called beautiful binding sites—most compatible with binding druglike molecules *(52)*. The human genome is composed of both "druggable" receptors—proteins with binding sites that can be bound easily by molecules with the characteristic size, shape, and physicochemical properties consistent with good drugs—and a larger set of receptors that are not "druggable." Thus, one can talk of the "druggable genome" *(53)*, that subset of a genome that is likely to produce ligands with druglike properties. What, then, is a druggable target? The average GPCR, with its small, hydrophobic, internal binding site and important physiological role, is an archetypal druggable receptor *(11)*. Tumor necrosis factor receptor would not be judged such a target, despite its important physiological role, because it contains no easily discernible drug-binding site *(54)*. That is not to say that useful drugs, such as therapeutic antibodies *(55)*, cannot be designed to block its biological activity, yet it remains not obviously druggable. Thus, druggable means proteins exhibiting a hydrophobic binding site of defined proportions, leading to the development of drugs with appropriate properties. As a term, it relates to the structure of the receptor yet also has another component that relates to the provenance of a protein family as a source of successful drug target. Or, put another way, how useful similar or related proteins have been as drug targets. Estimates of the number of druggable receptors vary; whereas current estimates of gene number are converging toward a value in the region of 40,000 *(56)*, the number of "druggable" receptors may be in the region of 2000–4000 *(57)*. About 10% of these have been explored so far, leaving many, many receptors unexamined. Beyond the human genome, other druggable receptors are now being examined. Bacteria, fungi, viruses, and parasites all possess viable targets for drug intervention.

As antibiotic resistance escalates, the search for new antimicrobial compounds, and the number of druggable microbial receptors, will continue to expand.

2. A Primer on the Experimental Characterization of Binding Sites

The previous discussion has highlighted some important concepts that will, it is hoped, illuminate this chapter's discussion of the binding site, but what of binding itself? Let us take a brief, quantitative look at the physical biochemistry of ligand binding to a biomolecular target. Consider a receptor–ligand (RL) complex formed from a receptor (R) binding a ligand (L):

$$R + L \leftrightarrow RL$$

Such interactions frequently obey the law of mass action, which states that the rate of reaction is proportional to the concentration of reactants. The rate of the forward reaction is proportional to $[L][R]$. The rate of the reverse reaction is proportional to $[RL]$ since there is no other species involved in the dissociation. At equilibrium, the rate of the forward reaction is equal to the rate of the reverse reactions, and, hence (using k_1 and k_{-1} as the respective proportionality constants),

$$k_1 [R] [L] = k_{-1} [RL]$$

Rearranging gives the equation:

$$\frac{[R] [L]}{[RL]} = \frac{k_{-1}}{k_1} = K_D = K^{-1}{}_A$$

in which K_A is the equilibrium association constant and K_D is the equilibrium dissociation constant, which also represents the concentration of ligand that occupies 50% of the receptor population at equilibrium. The free energy of binding is related directly to the equilibrium constant

$$\Delta G_{bind} = -RT \ln(K_D)$$

in which ΔG_{bind} is the Gibbs free energy of binding, R is the gas constant, and T is the absolute temperature. The free energy (ΔG) is related to enthalpy (ΔH) and entropy (ΔS) via the well-known Gibbs-Helmhotz equation:

$$\Delta G = \Delta H - T\Delta S$$

Assuming linearity, the enthalpy and entropy term can be obtained using the van't Hoff relation:

$$\ln K_D = \frac{\Delta H}{RT} - \frac{\Delta S}{R}, \quad \frac{d(\ln K_D)}{dT} = \frac{\Delta H}{RT^2}$$

The potential usefulness of this is obvious: plotting $\ln(K_D)$ vs $1/T$ should describe a straight line with slope equal to ($\Delta H/R$) and y intercept of ($\Delta S/R$). van't Hoff plots only identify part of the binding enthalpy: that part directly related to the observed measurement signal. This means that only for a direct transformation from a defined initial state to a final state is the extracted enthalpy equivalent to ΔH_{bind}, as obtained by other methods, such as isothermal titration calorimetry (ITC). No intermediate states are allowed nor should other steps be involved. ΔG typically has only moderate temperature dependence within biological systems; thus, a truly accurate and reliable estimate of enthalpy and entropy is seldom possible using van't Hoff plots.

Energy is that property of a system that invests it with the ability to do work or produce heat. Formally, enthalpy is defined by

$$H = U + PV$$

in which U is the total internal energy of a system, P is the pressure, and V is the volume. Under conditions of constant pressure, ΔH is the heat absorbed by a system from its surroundings, and, for a molecular system, it is a function of both its kinetic and potential energies. Entropy is often described as a measure of *disorder* within a molecular system. Increasing entropy is better described as the partitioning of the energy of a system into an increasing number of explicit microstates, which are themselves a function of the position and momentum of each constituent atom *(58)*. It is often difficult to decompose fully enthalpies and entropies into readily identifiable separate molecular contributions. Favorable enthalpic contributions to the free energy can include complementary electrostatic contributions, such as salt bridges, hydrogen bonds, dipole–dipole interactions, and interactions with metal ions; and van der Waals interactions between ligand and receptor atoms. Entropic contributions can include global properties of the system, such as the loss of three rotational and three vibrational degress of freedom on binding, and local properties, such as conformational effects, including the loss of internal flexibility in both protein and ligand. Unfavorable entropic contributions from the increased rigidity of backbone and side-chain residues on ligand binding within the binding pocket are, in part, offset by favorable increases in conformational freedom at nearby residues *(59)*. Strictly, all protein–ligand binding also involves multiple interactions with the solvent, typically a weakly ionic aqueous solution, and is a multicomponent process, rather than a binary one such as dimerization. These solvent interactions lead to solvation, desolvation, and hydrophobic effects, each with both an enthalpic and an entropic component.

As affinity rises, the phenomenon of enthalpic cooperativity, or so-called enthalpy–entropy compensation *(60)*, becomes more important. Where multiple, weak noncovalent interactions hold a molecular complex together, the enthalpy of all of the individual intermolecular bonding interactions is reduced by extensive intermolecular motion. As additional interaction sites generate a complex that is more strongly bound, intermolecular motion is dampened, with all individual interactions becoming more favorable. The trade-off between intermolecular motion and enthalpic interactions accounts for the way in which entropy and enthalpy compensate for each other.

2.1. Spectroscopic and Calorimetric Methods of Binding Analysis

Experimentally, the measurement of equilibrium dissociation constants has most often been addressed using radioligand binding assays, although they are, in their turn, beginning to give way to more sophisticated and convenient instrumental technology, principally surface plasmon resonance (SPR) *(61)*, but also a variety of other methods, such as ITC *(62)*. Saturation analysis measures equilibrium binding at various radio-ligand concentrations to determine receptor number (usually denoted B_{max}) and affinity (K_D). Competitive binding experiments measure receptor-ligand binding at a single concentration of labeled ligand in the presence of various concentrations of unlabeled ligand. Competition experiments can be either homologous (in which the labeled and unlabeled ligands are the same) or, more commonly, heterologous (in which labeled and unlabeled ligands are different) inhibition assays.

IC$_{50}$ values, as obtained from a competitive radioligand assay *(63)*, are among the most frequently reported affinity measures. The value given is the concentration required for 50% inhibition of a labeled standard by the test ligand. Therefore, nominal binding affinity is inversely proportional to the IC$_{50}$ value. IC$_{50}$ values may vary among experiments, depending on the intrinsic affinity and concentration of the standard radiolabeled reference compound, as well as the intrinsic affinity of the test molecule. The K_D of the test peptide can be obtained from the IC$_{50}$ value using the relationship derived by Cheng and Prusoff *(64)*:

$$K^i_D = \frac{IC_{50}}{\left(1 + \frac{[L^S_{tot}]}{K^S_D}\right)}$$

in which K^i_D is the dissociation constant for the inhibitor or test ligand, K^S_D is the dissociation constant for the radiolabeled standard, and $[L^S_{tot}]$ is the total concentration of the radiolabel. This relation holds at the midpoint of the inhibition curve under two principal constraints: the total amount of radiolabel is much greater than the concentration of bound radiolabel, and the concentration of bound test compound is much less than the IC$_{50}$. This relation, although an approximation, holds well under many assay conditions.

Although radioligand assays are well known, there are innumerable alternative methodologies, able to offer both increased operator convenience and experimental tractability. In the case of enzyme reactions, the influence on enzyme kinetics is followed by means of a readily detectable physical property (e.g., absorption, fluorescence, or fluorescence polarization of one of the reaction partners). There are, however, also methods that can deliver fuller insights into the underlying thermodynamics, kinetics, and contributions made by different molecular components. The two key players here are SPR *(61)* and ITC *(62)*.

SPR is an important and increasingly widely used technique *(65)*. It is able to measure biomolecular interactions in real time in a label-free environment *(66)*. An interactant is immobilized to the sensor surface while the other interactant is free in solution and passed over the surface, allowing SPR to detect the binding of a ligand to a protein, which is anchored to a solid support, or of a protein to a ligand, which is attached to the support by a linker group. The technique allows all types of molecular interaction to be measured, including protein–protein, DNA–protein, and lipid–protein. Moreover, "on" and "off" rates can be accessed using this method. Other methods, such as densimetric and ultrasonic velocimetric titration measurements *(67)*, are also important, giving insights into specific molecular events, such as hydration changes.

Steady-state fluorescence spectroscopy *(68)* is also widely used in the study of biomolecular interactions and kinetics and relies on measuring fluorescence change at a given wavelength. Time-resolved fluorescence spectroscopy measures the time dependence of fluorescence intensity after excitation and is far more sensitive to alterations in conformational changes or interactions made by fluorescent residues—tryptophan, tyrosine, and phenylalanine—than steady-state intensity measurements. Using polarized light allows time-resolved fluorescence anisotropy measurements, which can provide useful information about local residue freedom as well as global protein motion. Mass spectrometry also offers some interesting insights into the nature of binding affinity by investigating the dissociation of a protein–ligand complex as a function of, say, acceleration voltage *(69)*. Atomic force microscopy can determine the strength of intermolecular interactions by a controlled mechanical rupture of a particular protein–ligand complex *(70)*. Every relevant spectroscopic technique provides, to a greater or lesser degree, valuable information complementary to that of other methods. It is only through a full and complete combination of several such techniques that the intricate puzzle of protein–ligand interaction can be carefully reconstructed.

However, if one seeks a single methodology for obtaining relevant thermodynamic properties of binding reactions, the current leader is undoubtedly ITC, which is rapidly becoming the method of choice for such studies *(62,71–73)*. The main reason for this is that ITC simultaneously generates global values for two parameters: the equilibrium constant and, thus, the free energy of binding (ΔG), which it computes from the shape of the titration curve. However, ITC also measures enthalpy (ΔH), which it derives from the integrated heat of reaction; entropy (ΔS), which is related to the difference in ΔG and ΔH; and also the heat capacity (ΔCp) of the system. In ITC, a ligand is added stepwise at constant temperature to a solution of receptor and the overall heat of the reaction is recorded. ITC is an example of a variety of microcalorimetry methods, of which differential scanning calorimetry (DSC) is another well-known example. What sets ITC apart is its ability to measure both affinity and its thermodynamic contributions directly from heat changes during the binding process. Because such changes are observed during most binding reactions, ITC is broadly applicable, with applications ranging from chemical and biochemical binding to enzyme kinetics. ITC is both rapid and sensitive, but above all it is a direct method without the need for chemical modification or immobilization. It is the only technique that measures enthalpy directly, eliminating the requirement for van't Hoff analysis, which is often time-consuming and prone to error. However, interpretation of derived parameters remains a pivotal challenge. Moreover, reliable analysis of the titration curve requires dissociation constants more than $10^{-9} M$. To measure more affine compounds, the detection range must be extended by displacing lower-affinity ligands.

For most biological systems, multiple ITC measurements conducted over a range of temperatures exhibit a pronounced temperature dependence for both ΔH and $T\Delta S$. However, ΔCp is essentially temperature independent in the range associated with biological reactions and is generally negative for protein–ligand complexes. Thus, the complex has a lower heat capacity than the sum of free ligand and protein. As temperature increases, ligand binding becomes both more exothermic and less entropically favorable.

As already stated, ITC is well suited to the analysis of association between biomolecules, but it is complemented by DSC *(74)*, which can provide a more comprehensive description of the associated thermodynamics, enabling a better decomposition of different components of the enthalpy and entropy, such as those composed of contributions from the binding reaction proper, from conformational changes of the component molecules during association, from changes in molecule/solvent interactions, and also in the state of protonation. DSC also provides more information on heat capacity changes and can give important insights into the conformational changes seen in biological systems. In DSC, the system is heated at a uniform rate under nearly adiabatic conditions and the resulting temperature change is recorded. Any deviation from constant heat absorption usually demonstrates that intramolecular packing has altered or indicates conformational rearrangements or structural fluctuations.

3. Sequence-Based Approaches to Prediction of Binding Sites

Evolution underlies modern-day biology in much the same way that God underpinned medieval theology: it is now a concept that is accepted so universally that its veracity is seldom, if ever, questioned, and what is true of biology is equally true of bioinformatics. Evolution is fundamental to conceptual interpretations of macromolecular sequence data and their place within the hierarchy of biological explanation. Increasingly, however, methods that are at least nominally based on evolutionary arguments are also proving to be useful practically, rather than simply providing intellectually satisfying retrodictive rationales. Thus, much of bioinformatics reduces to questions of detecting the evolutionary conservation of functionally important sequence patterns: patterns that determine and maintain the stability of a protein's tertiary structure, patterns of interacting residues that determine and constrain protein folding, or the identification of important residues in a binding site.

Geometrical constraints or constraints imposed by fundamental limitations of chemical reactivity may greatly restrict the way in which enzymes are able to undertake the elementary steps of a particular reaction, requiring a strictly defined spatial arrangement of the chemically unique reaction partners. This means that determinants of molecular recognition must be highly conserved in their relative orientation. This can occur through either convergent or divergent evolutionary processes *(75)*. In divergent evolution, an ancestral binding or catalytic site remains broadly fixed, while in the population of descendent sequence, surrounding regions experience sequence drift or functional specialization, which may or may not affect specificity. In convergent evolution, originally distinct sequences, without readily discernible homology, alter in time, ultimately attaining a similar structure but via alternative routes and against an otherwise unrelated sequence backdrop (*see* **Fig. 3**).

When patterns responsible for molecular recognition are conserved between the binding sites of proteins that are related in some way to each other, it is often possible to localize binding sites by searching for similarities either in the primary sequence or in their tertiary structure. This, of course, presupposes that one has knowledge of binding site localization. This may be obtained from analysis of mutants, either derived intentionally by mutagenesis experiments or from natural mutants or sequence variants

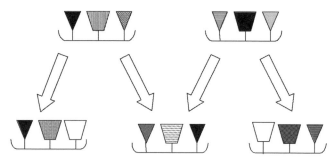

Fig. 3. Convergent vs divergent evolution. Two binding sites undergo gene duplication and then subsequent divergent evolution. Under different evolutionary pressures, two protein offspring converge on a common structure, while other duplicants face substantially different pressures and arrive at distinctly different structures. Of course, such a simplified view of evolution, although usefully illustrative, is highly simplistic. Evolutionary pressures are felt by the whole organism, not by individual proteins. Moreover, proteins must balance functional constraints, driving evolutionary change, with issues of stability, genetic drift, and the metabolic constraints imposed by the organism in synthesizing them. Many of these conflicting constraints are resolved by the innate functional degeneracy, at the level of metabolism, signaling, and so on, of the complex organism.

or from chemical labeling or some related experimental technique. In this way, it may be possible to "inherit" a binding site from one sequence to another or from one structure to another. This is by far the most popular approach to binding site prediction. This process is performed either at the level of sequence homology or by establishing structural similarities, such as searching for geometrically constrained constellations of catalytic residues, requiring a sequence and/or a structural search to be preformed. Such searches are often implicit in sequence searches or the formation of multiple sequence alignments (MSAs), assuming, of course, that equivalent, or at least similar, residues can be found at the correct alignment positions. However, more explicit methods are beginning to emerge *(76,77)*.

Traditionally, bioinformatics assigns functional data by searching for relatives in sequence databases *(78)*. Analysis, in any depth, of sequence searching is clearly well beyond the scope of the current work. Nonetheless, operationally speaking at least, it is fair to say that the MSA, the ultimate product of sequence searching, lies at the heart of bioinformatics. The MSA is something that is at once practically useful and intellectually powerful; it is conceptually unifying, and with it, one can achieve so much (*see* **Fig. 4**).

When attempts are made to identify binding sites, one may search for either clearly conserved individual sequence motifs, such as the sequence motifs that characterize dehydrogenase sites *(79)*, or sets of essentially isolated residues, such as the HIS-ASP-SER catalytic triad of protease and so on *(80)*. The first type of motif can be searched for directly, whereas the second type of motif requires subsidiary data in order to identify them properly. Proteins of related function often share a comparable binding site, and, thus, the binding site of a new sequence or structure may be detected by comparison

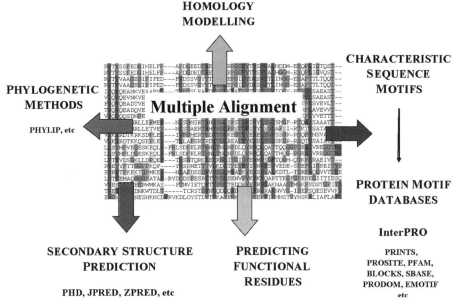

Fig. 4. Multiple Sequence Alignments allow one to predict 3D structure, either through homology modeling or via *de novo* prediction of secondary structure; to undertake phylogenetic analysis; to identify functionally important residues; and to identify important motifs and, thus, develop discriminators for the membership of protein families.

with other proteins of the same function. The first step in identifying a binding site by homology is to identify the protein family to which a sequence belongs. The definition of a protein family, the principal step in the annotation of macromolecular sequence data, proceeds via an iterative process of similarity searching in sequence, structure, and motif databases to generate a sequence corpus, which represents the whole sequence set comprising the family *(48)*. Motif databases, of which there are many, contain distilled descriptions of protein families that can be used to classify other sequences in an automated fashion. There are several ways to characterize motifs: through human inspection of sequence patterns, by using software to extract motifs from a multiple alignment, or by using a program such as MEME to generate motifs directly from a set of unaligned sequences *(81)*. A motif or, more likely, a set of motifs defining the family can then be deposited in one of the many motif databases, such as PRINTS *(82)*, or secondary, or derived, motif databases, such as INTERPRO *(83)*.

With either convergent or highly divergent evolution, important structural and functional relationships are only detectable from 3D structure, which is typically more conserved than sequence similarity *(84)*. Because function and binding typically exhibit an intimate linkage, elucidating functionality and the identification of binding pockets are often highly interrelated tasks. Various algorithms are available for comparing protein structures in 3D to recognize structurally related proteins *(32)*. Such programs are efficient enough to perform rapid searches of entire structural databases such as the

Protein Data Bank (PDB). The results of mutual comparisons for all known protein structures are themselves stored in databases that provide classifications of protein structures, in part with functional annotations. Likewise, a comparison of pockets on the surface of different proteins may allow one to detect functional relationships. Accordingly, comparisons based on similarity with well-characterized proteins of known structure and function can provide an additional route to the identification of binding sites. It is, therefore, often advisable to go beyond the comparison of protein folds or global structural motifs in order to look at local structural motifs, such as catalytic triads, which are able to capture the essence of the biochemical function *(85–87)*.

Thus, there are three main ways in which to obtain information about a binding site when confronted by a newly determined sequence or structure. First, as already described, the principal method of identifying the location of a binding site is by "inheriting" its experimentally defined location in one structure or sequence to another structure of sequence, modifying it as necessary. Secondly, one can use an artificial intelligence technique to "predict" the location of a binding site *(88)*. Third, one can use phylogenetic techniques to "infer" the location of function-critical residues *(89)*.

Recently, there has been a move to adapt artificial intelligence techniques, such as artificial neural networks (ANNs) or hidden Markov models, each a mainstay of bioinformatic prediction methodology in other disciplines, to the search for binding sites. The potential usefulness of this is becoming particularly important as genomics efforts, both sequence and structural, begin to generate large numbers of unannotated protein sequences and X-ray structures. Gutteridge et al. *(88)* trained an ANN to use both sequence and structural data to identify catalytic residues in enzymes. The ANN output and spatial clustering of highly scored residues then predicts the binding site location. In a test set, more than 69% of sites were predicted accurately, and another 25% were partially correct, with failures mainly owing to poor automatic sequence alignments. Gadiraju et al. *(90)* developed software that searches genomic sequences with information theory-based weight matrices in order to identify binding sites. Scans of human genome assemblies required 4–6 h for transcription factor-binding sites and 10–19 h for splice sites. Some of the sites identified were transcription factor-binding sites, including PXR/RXRα, AHR, and nuclear factor-κB p50/p65, and RNA-binding sites, including splice donor, acceptor, and SC35 recognition sites. Chou and Cai *(91)* made use of a covariant discriminant algorithm to identify enzyme-active sites, using the serine hydrolase family as an example. They report cross-validated accuracies of 99% for 88 enzymes and likewise for an independent test set of 50. Keil et al. *(92)* used an ANN to predict binding site locations based on the physical and chemical properties of overlapping molecular surface patches. Their ANN was able to categorize patches as nonbinding, protein–ligand, protein–protein, or protein–DNA.

In the absence of experimental evidence for the location of a binding site, an approach alternative to either a search-based inheritance of binding site locations or an artificial intelligence prediction is the use of evolutionary or phylogenetic methods to identify function-critical residues. In this way, a set of residues is predicted to be key to the correct function of the protein, presumably by participating in protein–ligand interactions within the binding site. A multiple alignment is required, within which strictly conserved residues can be regarded as functional; however, conservation patterns are often more complicated, necessitating the development of a tranche of sophisticated techniques. The first such algorithm was developed by Casari et al. *(89)*, who used a simple yet powerful representation of both whole sequences and individual residues as vectors in a general sequence space. Projections into a lower-dimensional space revealed residue groups specific for individual subfamilies that were likely to be involved directly in function. Lichtarge et al. *(93)* developed an evolutionary trace methodology and applied it to Src homology (SH) 2 and SH3 domains, for which many relatively short sequences are available. The method extracts functionally important residues from sequence conservation patterns in homologous proteins and maps them onto a protein surface to identify functional interfaces. Crowder et al. *(94)* subjected 330 aligned sequences of RNA-binding domains to covariance analysis, which revealed a single network of covariant amino acid pairs comprising the buried core of the protein and an important surface patch. Mirny and Gelfand *(95)* used the concept of orthologs and paralogs to identify residues determining specificity for protein–DNA and protein–ligand recognition. Li et al. *(96)* extended this approach and used it to predict the specificity-determining residues that enable different protein kinases to recognize their substrates. Finally, Bradford and Westhead *(97)* analyzed how conservation patterns at an interface differ from the noninterface surface in seven pairs of proteases and inhibitors. For the proteases, an interface could be distinguished from the noninterface region by its degree of conservation. However, the distinction between the interface and noninterface was not clear for the inhibitors. Indeed, in five cases, the interface was more variable than the rest of the molecule. This may cause problems for binding site prediction, which assumes that the biggest cluster of conserved surface residues corresponds to an interface.

4. Structural Approaches

Protein function is often synonymous with processes of ligand recognition, which usually occur in defined binding sites on the protein surface. Analysis of binding sites in structural terms seeks to identify similarity of function that is broadly independent of any homology apparent at the levels of sequence and fold and extends beyond the search for conserved structural and/or sequence motifs. Although a full examination of the many and varied approaches to either the experimental or theoretical determination of binding sites is beyond the scope of this chapter, it is both informative and useful to adumbrate certain salient points in this regard. Let us briefly examine three principal approaches: experimental methods, focusing on X-ray crystallography; so-called homology, or knowledge-based, modeling; and constraint-based *de novo* modeling.

X-ray crystallography has been around for a long time now. Although technical innovations are constantly accelerating the process of producing fully refined crystal structures, crystallography has had a reputation for being inherently slow. This has discouraged many from using this technology. However, in a decade or two I am confident that this situation will have changed out of all recognition with time, money, and talent pouring into the newly emergent discipline of structural genomics. This clearly reflects the general recognition of how important protein structures are within biomedical research

(98). The genome sequences from a tranche of prokaryotic and eukaryotic organisms are now available, including, most excitingly, the human genome. There are well in excess of 150 completed genome sequences, with more appearing with frightening regularity *(99)*. This is clearly a huge quantity of information—a mountain, indeed a veritable Everest, to dwarf the informational molehills of preceding decades. With access to the sequences of hundreds of complete genomes, the principal objective of structural genomics is to generate a comprehensive overview of the universe of protein folds. Currently, more than 3000 distinct, solved protein structures are available in the public domain *(100)*. Within the next 5–10 yr, structural genomics, in the guise of high-throughput multidimensional nuclear magnetic resonance (NMR) spectroscopy and X-ray crystallography, is expected to produce something on the order of 10^4 experimentally determined protein structures, so one or more example experimental structures will be available for every protein sequence family. Protein homology modeling could then produce structural models for almost all proteins observed in nature. Whatever the real success of such endeavors proves to be, they will greatly increase the total amount of protein structural information available *(101)*.

Any reasonable division of a genome into structurally distinct protein families will necessitate many hundred protein structure determinations. Structural genomics will require new ways to automate experimental structure determination. X-ray crystallography has traditionally progressed through several stages, from the very biochemical to the abstractly mathematical *(102)*. Having identified a protein of interest, one needs to produce sufficient pure protein to perform the search for appropriate crystallization conditions. Once one has crystals of the protein, one needs to collect X-ray diffraction data from these crystals and the "solve" structure. This involves solving the phase problem: recovering the electron density within the unique part of the lattice by combining the intensities of diffracted X-rays with the phase, the other component of the Fourier transform that links real molecular electron density and the experimentally determined diffraction pattern. The final stage requires building and refining a protein model within the electron density and ultimately refining this crude model to optimize its ability to re-create the diffraction pattern. The production of protein is probably the most generic aspect of structural genomics, although few people want quite such pure protein in such large amounts. The development of many different high-throughput protein production systems is currently under way in both academic and commercial organizations. These include in vitro, or cell-free, systems as well as examples based on well-understood microbial systems, such as *Escherichia coli* *(103)*. Selenium incorporation allows the phasing of the protein diffraction pattern using multiwavelength anomalous diffraction, the so-called MAD technique, which offers a general approach for the elucidation of atomic structures *(104)*.

Once one has sufficient protein, the next stage in crystallography is obtaining crystals. This is one of the two main problems remaining in X-ray crystallography. Although the phase problem is slowly yielding to various different forms of attack, crystallization remains very much a black art. The process of growing protein crystals is still poorly understood and still requires a trial-and-error process to determine the relatively few idiosyncratic conditions of pH, ionic strength, and precipitant and buffer concentrations necessary for the growth of diffraction-quality crystals. However, even this recalcitrant discipline is yielding to the power of robotics and informatics *(105)*. Robust multivariate statistics have been used to relate variations in experimental conditions, within experimentally designed crystallization trials, to their results *(106)*. Although these mathematical models cannot explain crystallization mechanisms, they do provide a powerful pragmatic tool allowing the setting up of crystallization trials in a more rational and more confident manner.

Until recently, crystal mounting has seemed to be the aspect of crystallography least suitable for automation. The process of mounting a protein crystal such that it can sit comfortably in an X-ray beam is a highly interactive process requiring a prodigious feat of manual manipulation, personal dexterity, and physical adroitness. Although one may learn the techniques involved, it is by no means easy. However, the system developed by Muchmore et al. *(107)* addresses most of these issues through a combination of cryogenic temperatures, intelligent software, and a high degree of robotic control. Although the systems that they describe have a rather Heath Robinson appearance, they are no worse than the setups used in other high-throughput regimes within the drug industry.

The diffraction pattern is obtained by allowing a focused beam of X-rays to pass through a crystal. Each spot on the diffraction pattern represents an intensity and has associated with it another quantity, the phase, that when combined with it through a Fourier transform yields an electron density map. Unlike small-molecule crystals, in which phases can be determined directly from relationships between intensities, proteins require more approximate solutions. However, in the context of structural genomics, most are undesirable. Molecular replacement requires an existing 3D model of a homologous protein, whereas multiple isomorphous replacement requires a trial-and-error search for heavy atom derivatives. MAD phasing, as mentioned, is a much better alternative. Another approach is the development of so-called direct methods. Miao et al. *(108)* developed an interesting approach. They propose the use of ultrashort, intense X-ray pulses to record diffraction data in combination with direct phase retrieval. Their approach relies on the production of femtosecond X-ray pulses generated by free electron X-ray lasers with a brilliance 10^8 times that of current synchrotons. They combine these with clever manipulation of the diffraction data for single specimens to produce an accurate, phased, and interpretable electron density map. As we have seen, many of the advances in the biochemical and biophysical stages of the crystallographic process —protein production and crystallization—will be greatly enhanced by automation. Other technical advances will solve or side step many of the inherently intractable problems of crystallography, such as the phase problem.

Thus far, I have discussed soluble, globular proteins, but what of membrane proteins? Because they exist within a complex environment containing both a lipid and an aqueous phase, such proteins present distinctly different problems for automation and high-throughput crystallography. Integral membrane proteins are generally large and often form multimeric complexes. Together with the practical problems associated with preparing samples containing biological membranes, it has not proved possible to study them successfully using multidimensional NMR. Consequently, most structural information has come from crystallographic techniques: X-ray crystallography for those cases in which it has proved possible to produce true 3D crystals—for example, the photosynthetic reaction center *(109)* or porin *(110)*—and electron crystallography, which combines image analysis from electron microscopy with electron diffraction data to study two-dimensional (2D) crystalline arrays. This technique was used to solve the structure of bacteriorhodopsin at 3.5 Å *(111)*.

The greatest obstacles to the successful determination of membrane protein structures remain technical: problems with the overexpression, purification, and concentration of membrane proteins *(112)* and with the preparation of 3D crystals for X-ray studies or 2D electron crystallography *(113)*. For the time being, both remain daunting challenges, although continuing innovation *(114,115)* does offer hope for the future. Much work still needs to be done to overcome the immense technical difficulties inherent in the crystallographic study of membrane protein, but work is beginning.

For example, the semiacademic MePNeT initiative (www.mepnet.org/), which is supported commercially by more than 30 pharmaceutical, biotech, and startup companies (including AstraZeneca, Boehringer Ingelheim, Glaxosmithkline, and Novo Nordisk), has selected the best validated and most advanced methods to express 100 GPCRs in three systems: *E. coli, Pichia pastoris*, and Semliki Forest Virus-infected cells. It is perhaps worth drawing a parallel with X-ray crystallography: 20 yr ago solving the structure of a soluble protein was a rare and major event, the number of skilled macromolecular crystallographers was limited, and the number of properly equipped laboratories was small. Today, several X-ray crystal structures are solved every day in one of hundreds of laboratories around the world staffed by a large community of trained crystallographers. Notwithstanding the capricious nature of protein crystallization, structure solution has become almost commonplace. As technical problems are solved and the necessary skills become more widespread, the crystallographic study of membrane proteins will become similarly routine.

The main alternative method to the experimental structural approaches of X-ray crystallography and multidimensional NMR is protein homology modeling. It is now more than 35 yr since the first published example of this much misunderstood discipline: the modeling of the unknown structure of one protein based on the known structure of another protein with a closely related sequence. Browne et al. *(116)* modeled the structure of lactalbumin on the known structure of lysozyme. In the intervening years, as the number of known sequences and structures has increased exponentially, albeit at different rates, homology modeling has increased dramatically in popularity.

Methods such as COMPOSER *(117)*, and especially MODELER *(118)*, have largely automated the more routine aspects of homology modeling, freeing the seasoned practitioner to concentrate on the science involved and not waste his or her time on tedious and frustrating technicalities. However, other attempts at automation, particularly Web servers, such as SWISS-MODEL *(119)*, have created the impression that the whole process can be completely automated without the need for human intellectual input of any kind. Unfortunately, this is regrettably utterly untrue. Despite the belief that it is otherwise, homology modeling, at least when undertaken by experts, is as rigorous and difficult an undertaking as any other aspect of science. Yet, like so many computational methods, it is easy for the naïve user to generate models of pleasing veris-imilitude but little rigorous value. Although it may sometimes still be useful to generate such models, and it is always the case that a model need only answer the question that is asked, even an approximate model generated for the purpose of visualization and illustration should really be generated properly using robust methodology.

Complementary to the discipline of homology modeling, is the area of *de novo* modeling, perhaps best typified by the modeling of GPCRs. Rather than base a model on a known structure or structures, such methods use fundamental structural princi-ples, such as the conformation of secondary structure elements *(120,121)*, together with a variety of physical, chemical, and biological data, such as chemical labeling and infor-mation from mutagenesis experiments, to build a structural model constrained by these data. Models of GPCRs have, for example, been constructed by taking the sequences of the seven most hydrophobic sections of their sequences, which correspond to the transmembrane regions of the receptor, and building them as ideal α-helices. This set of amphipathic helices is then docked together, using the structure of bacteriorhodop-sin as a scaffold, so that their hydrophobic faces are orientated into the membrane phase and their hydrophilic faces—and functionally important residues—point into the lumen of the protein. Bundle *(122)* and Panda *(123)* are programs devised to facilitate the auto-mated or unsupervised construction of 3D models based on different kinds of experi-mental constraints.

As the volume of available information about GPCRs, deriving from innumerable experimental structure-function studies, has grown to include site-directed mutagene-sis, chemical labeling, crosslinking studies, fluorescence quenching, and a wealth of structure-activity data on congeneric series of ligands, to name but a few, there has been a shift in emphasis away from the ad hoc modeling of early days to more rigorous approaches based on the integration of many data sources and the satisfaction of con-straints, used singly or in clever combinations, imposed directly and indirectly by the data. The most widely used data come from site-directed mutagenesis of individual receptors. Such information can be used, on the one hand, to validate a receptor model and, on the other, to refine and improve it.

4.1. Binding Sites: Experimental and Theoretical Determination

As discussed, there are several approaches to identifying or predicting the location of a binding site. One can search sequences for motifs or search structures for geometrically defined patterns of residue, or one can use artificial intelligence techniques to predict *de novo* putative active sites, or use evolutionary and related techniques to locate residues critical to function. In this way, one can inherit or infer the position of a binding site. The certainty, or rather lack of certainty, with which one can copy sites from one molecule to another is currently a limiting factor in the large-scale use of structural genomics, and the techniques of homology modeling implicit within it, in the identification of key biologi-cal targets.

Having thus determined a binding site, confidently or not, one can then ask several pertinent questions: How does one go on to characterize a binding site? Does the cur-rent model represent the optimum structure? If not, how can it be optimized? Should

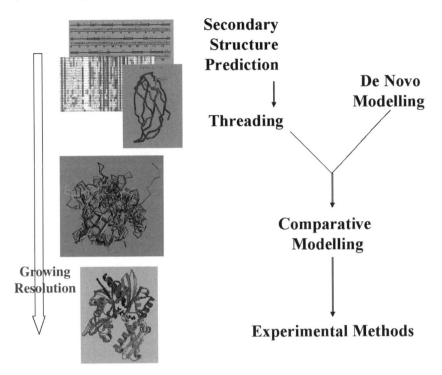

Secondary Structure Prediction

De Novo Modelling

Threading

Comparative Modelling

Growing Resolution

Experimental Methods

Fig. 5. Nominal resolution of protein models. Low-resolution models are inherently fuzzy and imprecise. As one gains more and more relevant information, the model becomes more accurate and its resolution improves. Very low-resolution models correspond to predictions of a protein's secondary structure. Models produced by threading, although possessing a greater degree of tertiary verisimilitude, can be little better. Likewise, the *de novo* modeling of membrane proteins, based, in the main, on topological constraints imposed by the two-dimensional geometry of the membrane phase and some understanding of interacting residues, can be equally imprecise. The highest resolution comes from models derived by X-ray. However, the prevalent view assumes that experimental structures are not models but reality. Both X-ray and nuclear magnetic resonance attempt to model sets of constraints, such as the difference between observed and calculated structure factors, and are prone to all manner of random and systematic errors. Intermediate between these extremes is the area of comparative protein modeling. This improvement in model quality gives rise to a corresponding improvement in its predictivity. The level of detail one draws from one's analysis should match the level of detail, the resolution, or the fuzziness of the model—general and qualitative at early stages, highly specific and quantitative later on. Using appropriate information in the appropriate way and at the appropriate time allows one to get the most from one's model. Overinterpretation at an early stage can be misleading; at every stage, it is experimental validation that drives the process of model refinement.

one look at a static representation of the site or should one look at a dynamic representation? Certain of these aspects are discussed in much greater detail subsequently, but first a brief diversion is necessary. This diversion is not a detour; however, it tracks through a variety of important issues. Some of these other issues are perhaps more fundamental than others, at least in the sense that they are limiting; if they are not addressed properly, then it is unlikely that other analytical or simulation methods will be able to compensate effectively for their deficiencies.

An homology model typically represents one of a number—and this may be potentially a large number—of alternative structures. The process of building a homology model, irrespective of the precise technique employed, involves the identification of one, and usually many more than one, related structures, which are then superposed in three dimensions *(124)*, so that as many as possible of the structures are aligned *(125)*. This effectively partitions the structural alignment into structurally conserved regions with a low root-mean-squared deviation (RMSD) and variable regions—typically, but not exclusively, loop regions outside elements of secondary structure—of different length and conformation that cannot be appropriately superimposed. Structurally conserved regions usually correspond to conserved sequence patterns or motifs, and variable regions to those parts of the sequence that show the greatest dissimilarity within an MSA. An homology model will, more or less exclusively, share a common fold with a conserved common core of secondary structure elements but otherwise may have radically different loop conformations and loop sizes. A model may show only a small number of conserved residues, which will often be fixed in their conformation. The rest of the model may contain a large set of residues for which a defined rotameric state cannot be inherited from an existing structure or structures. It has long been known that the positions of the set of Cα carbons, which is often referred to as the Cα trace, is sufficient to define the position of the whole protein backbone and Cβ carbons *(126–139)*. However, the difficulty inherent in correctly positioning the rotamers of each amino acid side chain is of a wholly different order, leading to the development of a large number of different methods that address this issue *(140–169)*.

The veracity of such prediction methods is usually benchmarked against crystal structure data. However, as any thinking crystallographer will tell you, X-ray crystallography produces structures that, despite a feeling of overwhelming verisimilitude, are still only models. Although it is common for what Professor Sir Tom Blundell is wont to call "lookers" (theoretical analysts of crystal structures) to assume, subconsciously if not consciously, that a crystal structure lodged in the PDB is a fixed and immutable thing possessed of transcendent inerrancy, this is unfortunately far from the truth. DePristo, one of crystallography's young turks, incidentally working as an acolyte within Blundell's group, has shown—conclusively in my view—that even high-resolution crystal structures can be modeled to equal accuracy by an ensemble of similar but distinct structural models, exhibiting a spectrum of different side-chain conformations and a set of distinct backbone conformations *(170–173)*.

Clearly, the need to identify the correct rotameric state is crucial to the accurate description of a binding site and its potential interaction with a ligand, be that a small molecule or a large protein. The exact geometry of side-chain interaction may be crucial to ligand binding or to the stereospecificity of a reaction. Getting this step wrong may lead one to identify the wrong ligand in a virtual screening experiment or to produce incorrect and inaccurate simulations using molecular dynamics (MD). Highly accessible residues are likely to suffer little constraint and are equally likely to be flexible, perhaps adopting a range of conformations. Many prediction methods will return a ranked list of side-chain conformations and/or alternative sets of residues that represent different solutions to the combinatorial problem of side-chain placement. Because the number of solutions that possess equal or nearly equal likelihood is often large, it is often necessary to cluster these solutions and, thus, select exemplar conformations. Although it may be possible to reduce the total number of alternatives to such representative ensembles *(174–179)* and, thus, allow the task of using such data to become tractable, no current method is able to perform this identification with satisfactory accuracy. As described subsequently, this problem is compounded by the fact that the conformation of the binding site, including, but not limited to, the rotameric state adopted by its side chains, may be significantly affected, and in an unpredictable manner, by the presence of a ligand.

Assuming, for the moment at least, that it has proved possible both to recognize the location or a binding site, in terms of its constituent amino acids, and to identify one or a few rotameric states for each side chain within the binding site—equating to a limited ensemble of receptor models—then it should also now become possible to examine, and further optimize, the structure of the binding site in terms of its underlying physical and, thus, biological properties, such as hydrogen bonding and ionization state.

Except at very high resolution, protein crystallography does not routinely produce electron density maps of sufficient quality to position accurately hydrogen atoms. Moreover, the scattering of X-rays by carbon, oxygen, and nitrogen atoms is essentially the same at the resolutions and data quality typical of modern macromolecular crystallography and, therefore, it is difficult to distinguish correctly among such atoms. This means that it is difficult to orientate the side chains of Asn, Gln, and His properly. Indeed, they appear symmetrical in the electron density and their rotameric state is often judged solely on the basis of hydrogen-bonding patterns. In very well-resolved protein structures and those structures for which neutron diffraction data are available, it has been observed that almost all buried hydrogen bond donors and acceptors are satisfied. On this basis, several researchers, seeking to identify the most favorable set of residue conformations in terms of the fulfillment of potential hydrogen bonding, have tried to develop automated methods able to compare symmetry-related alternate rotameric states within the binding site and place polar hydrogens optimally. This is particularly important for any subsequent analysis of ligand–protein interaction.

The assignment of hydrogen bonds to a particular residue is most secure when surrounding groups include either obligate hydrogen-bond donors (such as a peptide NH group) or obligate acceptors (such as a carboxyl group). In most cases, however, the local environment contains only ambiguous donors or acceptors, such as hydroxyl, histidine, and nonpeptide amide groups, or water molecules. Histidine residues have a particular assignment problem: a flip of the side-chain ring exchanges carbon and nitrogen at the ortho- and metapositions, leading to a choice between a polar or charged NH and a carbon that does form a hydrogen bond. Nonetheless, the orientation of the ring can also be ambiguous. This requires an analysis of the whole local network of hydrogen bonds. Moreover, there may be several equally favorable solutions to the hydrogen placement process, requiring extra ad hoc requirements, such as hydrogen bond energies, to distinguish them.

A number of automated algorithms have been devised to address the issue of hydrogen placement and ring flips. For example, Network *(180)* analyzes protein hydrogen-bond networks, dividing potential interacting donors and acceptors pairs into groups, but does not allow for amide or histidine flips. A search is performed on each such group to find the arrangement with the greatest number of hydrogen bonds. The polar hydrogens of histidine are treated specifically, and the polar hydrogens of serine, threonine, tyrosine, and lysine, and the amino terminus are also considered. Protonation states are also allowed to change if this results in the fulfillment of additional hydrogen bonds. HBPLUS *(181)* swaps the symmetry-related states of histidine, glutamine, and asparagine residues, so that the number of unsatisfied buried H-bonding groups is minimized. Although the program fails to account for pairs or larger interacting groups, it classifies all alternative orientations into a small set of categories ranging from highly favored to highly suspect.

A hydrogen placement procedure, which acts by optimizing the total hydrogen bond energy of the network and deals with ring flips; hydrogen addition; and the prediction of the ionization states of His, Asp, and Glu residues, has been implemented in the multifunctional graphics and modeling system WhatIf *(182)*. Where appropriate, the method also accounts for crystal symmetry. WhatIf also assigns hydrogen positions for all high-occupancy water molecules, takes account of hydrogen bonds between subunits related by crystal symmetry, and is biased against flips in marginal cases. Although the program performs a thorough analysis of hydrogen-bond networks, reaching a decision for every ambiguous polar group, its results are not easily evaluated because no estimates of confidence are given. Moreover, the inclusion of hydrogens on water molecules, which is required for accurate amide assignment, makes the problem explode combinatorially, requiring an approximate solution using simulated annealing rather than a closed form solution or one obtained by an exhaustive search of all possibilities.

The confident placement of water molecules is seldom a reliable feature of crystal structures. *Structural* or *bound* waters are those solvent molecules that are resolved by crystallography, are not readily exchanged with waters from the bulk solvent phase, have a long measurable lifetime, and are typically conserved between similar structures. They can be distinguished from displaceable water molecules, which are often artifacts of the crystallography model building; the R-factor, the fit between calculated and observed X-ray intensities, can usually be improved by the liberal addition of water molecules. Structural waters are also an important part of a binding site and can participate in optimizable hydrogen-bonded networks. WaterScore is a recent program developed to identify such waters from the comparison of protein structures *(183)*, but there are many others *(184–188)*. Various assumptions can be used to identify structural waters, such as their conservation between different structures and the observation that they are not easily displaced during MD simulations. The confident identification of *bound* water molecules has led to the development of programs *(189–195)* that seek to solvate protein surfaces, including binding sites, using a knowledge-based approach. Such informed solvation can be useful in attempts to accelerate solvent equilibration in MD simulations.

Most recently, Word et al. *(196)* have investigated this issue using contact dot methodology *(197)* and produced the program *reduce*. The method is able to optimize the hydrogen-bonding networks and assign glutamine, asparagine, and histidine flips. The use of programs such as *reduce* or WhatIf, would, in principal, improve assignments for the majority of structures. Indeed, when treated in this way, the quality of the vast majority of tested protein structures can be improved, and the degree of improvement is inversely proportional to resolution. Together with the results of DePristo and colleagues, this suggests that the systematic, and perhaps automatic, reevaluation of most protein structures within the PDB is an achievable objective, something that might yet rank alongside the development of automated structure verification software *(198–200)* as a positive and synergistic benefit of structural bioinformatics' interaction with X-ray crystallography.

Several researchers have addressed explicitly the improvements in pK_a calculations that an optimized hydrogen bond network can offer. For example, Nielsen et al. *(201)* have sought to use optimized hydrogen bond networks, including asparagine, glutamine, and histidine flips, to improve the quality of pK_a calculations performed by programs such as DelPhi and applied their method to certain well-characterized proteins, such as superoxide dismutase, lysozyme, and bovine pancreatic trypsin inhibitor. They found that optimized networks improved electrostatic calculations in or near enzyme-active sites for about one-fourth of all enzymes in the PDB. This compares with WhatIf, which found that about 85% of structures examined were improved by their calculations. More recently, Nielsen and Vriend *(202)* have performed pK_a calculations using finite difference solutions to the Poisson-Boltzmann (PB) equation, which require energy calculations performed for many different protein protonation states. These are usually modeled by altering the charges on certain atoms, or by adding or removing hydrogens, and occasionally by optimizing the local positions of protons. Nielsen and Vriend *(202)* globally optimize the hydrogen-bond network for each protonation state used, giving significant improvements in accuracy for calculated pK_a values.

The ionization constant, K_a, is a measure of the acidity of a compound, i.e., its ability to donate a proton. A more convenient way of expressing such a scale is to use pK_a, which equals $-\log_{10}(K_a)$. For weak acids and bases, such as the 20 natural amino acids, pK_a values range from 4.5 for the side-chain carboxyl of aspartate to 12.0 for side-chain guanidinium group of arginine. Side-chain residues within proteins have pK_a values that are moderated by their microenvironments, the nature of their near neighbors, the extent of hydrogen bonding, and so forth and can take on a range of values quite different from those quoted in undergraduate textbooks. These values can be measured experimentally using a variety of methods, such as NMR, or calculated from the 3D structure of a protein using a variety of methods, such as the linearized PB equation.

Recently, Forsyth et al. *(203)* reviewed 212 experimental carboxyl pK_a values (97 glutamate and 115 aspartate) from 24 structurally characterized proteins. Overall average pK_a values for active-site point (ASP) were 3.4 ± 1.0; for basic ($pI > 8$) proteins, the average pK_a value was 3.9 ± 1.0; and for acidic ($pI < 5$) proteins, the average pK_a was 3.1 ± 0.9. Overall average pK_a values for GLU were 4.1 ± 0.8, and average pK_a values for glutamates are approx 4.2 in both acidic and basic proteins. Likewise, Edgcomb and Murphy *(204)* recently reviewed the literature values of pK_as for titratable histidines; average pK_a values for titratable HIS were 6.6 ± 0.9. There is no similar, systematic survey for the basic amino acids, lysine and arginine, although Harris and Turner *(205)* have recently reviewed perturbed pK_a values for all amino acids in enzyme-active sites. However, there is anecdotal evidence, and a brief review of the literature would suggest that lysine and arginine display a similar range and diversity of pK_a values.

Solvent accessibility has long been thought to exert a profound influence on pK_a values. Exposed carboxyl group pK_a values exhibit narrow distributions compared to buried acidic residues, which range by up to 5 pH units. Likewise, the variability in histidine pK_a values also increases when the majority of its side chain is buried. Hydrogen bonding is also considered a key factor. Whereas pK_a values for glutamates show no real correlation with the degree of hydrogen bonding, mean pK_a values for aspartates are inversely proportional to the number of H-bonds. Interestingly, values for binding site glutamates and aspartates are often well outside normal ranges; in a study by Forsyth et al. *(203)*, 10 pK_a values greater than 5.5 were found, most involved in binding, and these groups were buried and accepted, at most, one H-bond.

There is clearly no simple, ready explanation for the pK_a values taken by ionizable groups within proteins; it is presumably a subtle environmental effect, but no quantitative relationships among the heterogeneous polar, apolar, and mixed environments experienced by different ionizable groups and their pK_a values is apparent from available data. However, the ionization or protonation of amino acid residues buried within proteins is often rationalized on the contradictory basis of either a hydrophobic environment, which raise the ionization constant of both acidic and basic residues, or charge-charge interactions, which raises the ionization constant for the pairing of like charges but decrease it on the formation of intermolecular salt bridges. Salt bridges in proteins occur when differently charged residues are close enough to experience strong electrostatic attraction. Their net electrostatic free energy is divided among three components: coulombic charge-charge interactions, charge–dipole interactions, and charge desolvation. Favorable charge-charge interaction is often opposed by unfavorable charge desolvation.

In the case of carboxyls, calculated electrostatic potentials show only very modest correlations with experimentally derived pK_a values. Moreover, these correlations are not improved by accounting for desolvation effects, such as terms accounting for accessible surface areas. This has led to the deployment of much more sophisticated calculational strategies. During the past 25 yr, protein pK_a calculations have generated much interest and have improved in accuracy *(202,206–210)*. Current pK_a calculation packages usually calculate electrostatic energies using the PB equation, although different approaches have been proposed *(211,212)*. Implementations of various PB equation solvers are available, including DelPhi II *(213)*, UHBD *(214)*, and APBS *(215)*.

In pK_a calculations, three kinds of energies are needed: background interaction energies, energies of desolvation, and site-to-site electrostatic interaction energies between pairs of titratable groups. The first two terms, desolvation energies and background interaction energies, allow calculation of how the protein environment affects the "intrinsic pK_a": the pK_a value of a titratable group when all the other titratable groups are fixed in their neutral state. Combining knowledge of intrinsic pK_a values for each titratable residue with site-to-site interaction energies allows calculation of the energy of every protein protonation state at a particular pH. For proteins with greater than 35 titratable groups, such calculations become intractable when using the Boltzmann formalism.

Generally speaking, current computational methods are usually prone to significant uncertainties resulting from both insufficiently accurate structural information and the unwarranted use of various simplifying assumptions. With only a few exceptions, the majority of articles report studies that look at one or a few proteins. They generally report satisfactory results but use a heterogeneous population of parameter values and assumptions. This makes a proper evaluation of their success very difficult. Larger-scale, comparative analysis for many proteins has seldom, if ever, been attempted.

I have already had cause to mention the flexibility of binding sites as a limiting factor in determining the constellation of residue conformations and rotameric states produced by experimental or model building exercises. The mutual dependence of ligand and protein conformation is an important example of this. The structure of a ligand–receptor complex is not the consequence of an inflexible docking of one rigid molecule with another rigid molecule. Rather, both are flexible: the small molecule or peptide bound by the protein does not necessarily bind in its minimum conformation as might be determined in solution. Neither is the conformation adopted by the bound ligand necessarily that which might be seen in high-resolution small-molecule crystal structures. Likewise, the protein does not necessarily retain the same side-chain rotamers as in its apo form, nor are these rotamers necessarily those of its lowest energy conformation. Rather, the structure of the complex is close to the minimum energy conformation of the system composed of the combined molecules. The small-molecule guest adapts to the constraints imposed by its macromolecular host, and, to some degree at least, vice versa.

A number of investigators have described this phenomenon. For example, Nicklaus et al. (*216*) compared computationally generated small-molecule structures with their conformations derived by crystallography and for the best performing structure generation method, which generated multiple conformers per molecule, identified only a 60% agreement. For single conformer generation, this value fell to 38%. In a later study, Nicklaus et al. (*217*) compared the experimental conformation of 33 compounds present in both the PDB and Cambridge Structural Database of small-molecule X-ray structures with the global energy minimum conformation generated by the molecular mechanics program CHARMm. The protein-bound conformation differed from the small-molecule crystal structure and from the global energy minimum, with the amount of difference roughly proportional to the number of freely rotatable bonds within the molecule. For most compounds, the global minimum conformational energy is well below that for both protein-bound and small-molecule crystal conformations. In an updated and extended study, Bostrom et al. (*218*) examined the conformational energies needed by ligands in 33 ligand–protein complexes to adopt their bioactive conformations. For about 70% of the complexes, differences in calculated energies were ≤3 kcal/mol.

In a more specific study, Moodie and Thornton (*219*) examined the effect on nucleotide conformation of binding to protein, by comparing the X-ray crystal structures of free and protein-bound nucleotides. Nucleotides were found to bind in low-energy conformations, not significantly different from their "free" conformations except that they adopted an extended conformation in preference to the "closed" structure predominantly observed by free nucleotide. Most recently, Fradera et al. (*220*) analyzed how the conformation of representative protein-binding sites is dependent on the bound ligand and found that the ligand induces small, but significant, structural alterations in the site that can, in turn, lead to important changes in the molecular recognition properties of the protein.

4.2. Analyzing and Visualizing a Binding Site

How does one analyze and characterize the structure of a binding site, once a protein's tertiary structure has been derived? We have already seen how such a question might be approached when only sequence data are available to us. When 3D structural information is available, however, there are two main alternatives: the location of the binding site can be either known or unknown. When a site is known, one's depth of knowledge can still be very variable. One may only have some slight indication, perhaps from other experimental evidence, such as mutagenesis, where the site is located, or one may have a fully defined binding site with a set of cocrystal structures illuminating the nature of ligand binding. At one extreme, where one has a situation characterized by a paucity of information, one requires an analysis similar to that described in the *structural* sequence-only case. Historically, the function of the target is likely to be known, but, as noted, increasingly it can be seen that structural genomics generates protein structures whose function remains unknown *(221)*. Even for proteins that have been well characterized biochemically, their function may not be understood in terms of structure *(222)*. At the other extreme, where binding is very well characterized, techniques of virtual screening and/or MD, as discussed in subsequent sections, will be of the greatest use. The most commonly encountered situation is an intermediate one: enough is known to make analysis tractable and rewarding, but the system is not so fully explored as to be characterized to death, though these older, rarer systems are nonetheless useful for the development and validation of new methodologies.

Such an intermediate situation requires a careful analysis of the protein structure, because the principle prerequisite for tight binding between ligand and receptor is specific interactions formed between protein and ligand atoms in the binding site. These contacts, as such interactions are often known, are typically noncovalent in nature and are mediated by ionic interactions, hydrogen bonds, and van der Waals forces. Their sum should exceed unfavorable contributions such as desolvation or the freezing out of translational and rotational degrees of freedom. There is now a plethora of sophisticated computational techniques that have been developed to address the issue of identifying areas able to make favorable interactions with potential ligands. These form a spectrum that extends from the purely geometric, through the mapping of physical problems, such as electrostatic or hydrophobic potentials; simple interaction potential mappings with atoms or pseudoatoms, such as CoMFA *(223)*; functional group mapping, as evidenced by GRID *(224)*, to multicopy minimization of functional groups *(225)*, and, ultimately, to sophisticated docking algorithms *(226,227)*.

Visualization of the surface of a protein molecule is one of the most basic and yet also one of the most luculent approaches to binding site analysis: just as there are many ways to calculate the quantitative solvent accessibility of a molecular surface *(228)*, there are many ways to generate and visualize alternative molecular representations. The simplest is to place spheres of appropriate van der Waals radii centered on each atom. This can then be expanded by the radius of a solvent sphere to form the accessible surface. More complex surfaces such as a Connolly surface, obtained by rolling a sphere over the surface, are formed of both convex accessible patches and concave reentrant regions (*229*). Various other methods have been devised to allow subtle variations of these types of surface to be generated and triangulated (*230,231*).

Once a structural representation of an accessible or a Connolly surface has been defined, texture mapping can be used to simultaneously reduce geometric complexity; enhance realism, and allow significant quantities of molecular data to be visualized, inspected, and interpreted. Texture mapping can produce highly accurate renderings of complex isodensity contours and facilitate volume rendering of large, 3D density distributions. A useful approach for visual analysis of a binding site is to map underlying physical properties onto a protein molecular surface representation (*232*). Popular properties for display would include hydrophobicity and electrostatic potentials. An interesting alternative, available when one has access to multiple alignments linked to a representative protein structure, is the projection of sequence variability on the surface. Such visualization tools can allow one to identify a binding site from an unusual concentration of extreme properties—whether they are hydrophobicity or hydrophilicity, positive or negative electrostatic potential, or high sequence variability—within the average background surface distribution.

Electrostatic potential is a common display property often obtained by solving the PB equation (*233*), for which, as I have said, many programs are now available (e.g., UHBD (*214*), DELPHI (*215*)). Several molecular graphics programs can then color code appropriate protein surface representations. One of the most popular is GRASP (*234*), which also contains a robust PB solver and can thus be used for electrostatic-potential surface mapping. The online service GRASS preserves parts of its functionality enabling users to display electrostatic properties and hydrophobicity measures projected onto surface representations. Other methods for generating hydrophobicity maps have also been developed (*235*), in which the binding energy of a nonpolar probe sphere is calculated using a combination of a Lennard-Jones potential and the electrostatic desolvation energy. A comparison using 10 diverse protein–ligand complexes revealed a high predictive power with respect to nonpolar binding. Another well-used method for evaluating hydrophobic potential is the HINT methodology (*236*).

During potential mapping, a surface would, typically, be scanned for regions that make significant interactions with a particular probe or set of probes, whether they are simple atoms or pseudoatoms, larger fragments, functional groups, or even whole ligand molecules. This will allow regions whose interaction with functional groups is energetically favored to be identified. This will, in turn, allow a functional map characterizing the binding site to be generated, which may also be able to guide the positioning of potential ligands.

However, because binding sites are often located within surface depressions, many computational strategies or algorithms have been developed that are able to detect geometrical indentations, such as pockets, pits, or cavities, on the surface of proteins, as an aid to the identification of putative binding sites. Many such programs have been developed. LIGSITE *(237)* evolved from the earlier program POCKET *(238)*. By placing a protein into a grid, it evaluates the extent of burial for all lattice points outside the protein. Burial at a given point is found by scanning all adjacent grid points for enclosure by protein atoms, with highly buried lattice points clustered to identify cavities. LIGSITE was tested with 10 complexes and in each case correctly identified the location of the binding site *(237)*.

The PROtein POcket Search, or APROPOS, method identifies pockets by comparing surfaces generated at different levels of resolution, i.e., an envelope surface describing the global shape of the protein and a suitably detailed surface reflecting the local structure. Based on tests with more than 300 proteins, the method was reported to locate binding sites with high reliability *(239)*. The program CAST is a further, more recent example of a method that implements an α-shape description of a protein surface *(240)*.

In the Putative Active Site with Spheres (PASS) algorithm, a protein is first coated with a layer of spherical probes. After filtering probes to eliminate those that clash with the protein, those not sufficiently buried, or those located too close to a more buried probe, a new layer of probes is grown onto the scaffold of previous probes and filtered again *(241)*. Growing and filtering are repeated until no new probes survive the filters. For all surviving spheres, probe weights are computed. These are proportional to the number of local probe spheres and their extent of burial. Probes with high weights are then clustered, identifying ASPs, which should represent the centers of potential binding sites. For 20 structures, PASS could identify binding sites in 12 cases as top-ranked ASPs and in 16 cases as one of the top three *(241)*.

Tools relying solely on geometrical criteria to locate binding sites are able to find all significant surface depressions but cannot easily discriminate sites of functional significance from other cavities. To do so, one is obliged to "score" the various pockets and depressions using some kind of interaction energy function. Various methods are available for this function. One of the simplest approaches uses an energy function to identify regions favorable for interaction with particular ligand functional groups. Frequently, methods of this kind use a discrete 3D lattice to position probe atoms or groups within the binding site. The archetypal program of this class is GRID *(224)*. It places probes such as methyl, hydroxyl, ammonium, or carbonyl at regularly spaced grid points within the active site. An energy function is used, at each grid point, to calculate the interaction energy between the probe and the protein and from this a functional map of the binding site is constructed. This indicates the most favorable regions for placing ligand groups with similar properties to the probes. Visualization of the maps by contouring at appropriate energy levels can identify hot spots. Since the first introduction of GRID, new types of probes and energy functions have been developed to enhance further the reliability of the method *(242–244)*. Similar methodology, such as CoMFA *(223)*, CoMSIA *(245)*, or PIPSA *(246)*, can be used to analyze binding sites. It is worth noting, though, that in principle any scoring function could be applied to perform hotspot analysis.

An obvious extension of this methodology allows one to analyze and classify sets of related molecules, including large protein families or proteins that exhibit significant polymorphism. Molecular interaction fields, such as those generated by GRID, can be computed for each model and then analyzed using a chemometrical method, such as principal component analysis and consensus principal component analysis (CPCA). This classification does not rely on protein sequence similarities, because descriptors are derived from 3D binding site information computed using molecular interaction fields. In an initial study *(247)*, the method was applied to nine structures of three homologous serine proteases: thrombin, trypsin, and factor Xa. The regions identified as being important for selectivity were in excellent agreement with available experimental data and inhibitor structure–activity relationships. Subsequently, this method has been refined and applied to a variety of protein groups. Ridderstrom et al. *(248)* undertook a selectivity analysis using the GRID/CPCA strategy on four human cytochrome P450 2C homology models: CYP2C8, 2C9, 2C18, and 2C19. Their analysis identified CYP2C8 as the most distinct structure with function determining amino acids at positions 114, 205, and 476. Terp et al. *(249)* used the method to investigate regions of selectivity in matrix metalloproteinases. Ji et al. *(250)* used molecular interaction fields to analyze selectivity differences between isoforms of nitric oxide synthase. Naumann and Matter *(251)* clustered 26 X-ray structures of eukaryotic protein kinases into subfamilies with similar protein-ligand interactions in the adenosine triphosphate-binding site. Their classification, which they called a "target family landscape," identified a common binding pattern and specific interaction sites for particular kinase subfamilies. Myshkin and Wang *(252)* used the GRID/CPCA methodology to explore selectivity issues in Eph receptor tyrosine kinases. Kurz et al. *(253)* used this approach to explore specificity of interaction in fatty acid-binding proteins, a member of the calycin superfamily, which also contains the lipocalins. Doytchinova et al. *(254)* extended the technique combining GRID with CoMSIA and CPCA with hierarchical clustering to generate a robust, consensus clustering of more than 1500 human class I MHC alleles.

One of the most interesting methodologies to emerge recently is the multicopy simultaneous search (MCSS) approach *(255)*, originally developed by Miranker *(256)*. MCSS uses a molecular mechanics formalism to place large numbers of small functional groups —simple ketones or hydroxyls—at favorable positions within a protein's active site. Instead of using probe atoms on a regular grid, several thousand probe groups are randomly distributed over the binding site and then energy minimized. During these calculations, the protein interacts with the whole swarm of ligands while each of the functional groups only sees the protein and not each other. The probes can thus cluster in local minima, allowing identification of the most favorable interaction sites.

Dynamic Ligand Design is a truly elegant extension of this approach with powerful conceptual appeal *(257)*. The results of the MCSS are turned into molecules under the influence of a pseudopotential function that joins atoms correctly accounting for stereochemistry. Their potential energy function allows atoms to sample a parameter space that includes both the Cartesian coordinates and atom type. Thus, atoms can mutate into different element types and hybridizations. Subsequently, a modified version of the method was developed that used a new potential energy function, optimization by simulated annealing, and evaluation using a thermodynamic cycle *(258)*. Other extensions to the methodology include flexibility of the protein target, which contrasts with standard MCSS, which has the protein kept rigid *(259)*.

DrugScore potentials can also be used in this way *(260)*. Its ability to predict hot spots was determined for 158 protein–ligand complexes. Depending on the atom-type classification, overall prediction rates of 74 and 85% were obtained. However, a note of warning for computational functional group mapping techniques comes from work undertaken by crystallographers that addresses experimental solvent-like functional group interaction with proteins. In one sense, this can be seen as an attempt to use an experiment to benchmark computation, although from a teleonomic perspective, techniques such as GRID are not intended to reproduce this kind of system but, rather, to indicate likely points of favorable interaction within designed ligands.

Ringe and Mattos *(261)* represented different functional groups by different solvents —benzene for aromatic groups, dimethyl formamide for peptides, and so on—with about six probes locating most major binding regions on the protein surface. They analyzed the surface of the enzyme elastase, finding three hot spots, including the active site. English et al. *(262,263)* used X-ray crystallography to determine the high-resolution crystal structures of thermolysin soaked in high concentrations of the cosolvents acetone, acetonitrile, phenol, and isopropanol. Analysis of the solvent positions showed little correlation with interaction energies computed using a molecular mechanics force field or with favorable positions defined using GRID. However, the experimentally determined solvent positions were consistent with the structures of known protein-ligand complexes of thermolysin. Indeed, the structure of the protein complex was essentially the same as the native enzyme. Byerly et al. *(264)* used NMR to analyze the *E. coli* peptide deformylase, identifying points of interaction with several simple organic solvents (acetone, dimethyl sulfoxide, ethanol, isopropanol) from local perturbation of amide chemical shifts. These groups map to the active site and an additional surface pocket. Joseph-McCarthy et al. *(265)* used the structure of RNase A with two bound formates (carboxyl mimics) to benchmark MCSS in terms of experimentally determined formate and water positions. Together, these results suggest that existing potential energy functions are not accurate enough to model correctly protein-ligand interactions even for the simplest ligands. Yet this approach is, as we have seen, still widely used.

Rule- or knowledge-based approaches are a different class of methods that make use of the directional information stored in accumulated crystallographic data through the derivation of rules for preferred ligand–protein patterns of interaction. An example is the so-called composite crystal-field approach *(266)*. Here, small-molecule crystal data, as exemplified by the Cambridge Structural Database, were analyzed statistically for intermolecular contact geometries of various functional groups, producing scatter plots of the experimental distributions. These plots can, in turn, be used to guide the placement of functional groups within a binding site. LUDI, a program for *de novo* design, has translated a statistical analysis of nonbonded interactions into rules for the calculation of "interaction sites" *(267,268)*, which are discrete positions and vectors in space suitable for forming hydrogen bonds or filling hydrophobic pockets.

SUPERSTAR has been developed to identify interaction sites in proteins using information from the database ISOSTAR *(269,270)*. A binding site is first decomposed into structural fragments, and then the distribution of selected probes is superimposed around these fragments. A 3D map then indicates the probability of probe placement at different positions. For a test set of 122 protein-ligand complexes, SUPERSTAR detects the correct atom type for solvent-inaccessible ligand atoms in 82–90% of cases. Similar concepts, although based on data from 83 high-resolution protein structures from the PDB, are used by X-SITE *(271)*. Spatial contact distributions were derived from 163 triatomic fragments to highlight favorable binding site interactions.

Several approaches have used docking to help identify potential binding sites. Bliznyuk and Gready *(272,273)* performed a grid search of van der Waals energy surrounding a protein and subsequently used Fast Fourier Transform techniques to scan the surface for possible ligand orientations, which were then energy minimized. Top-ranked orientations were evaluated using PB calculations. Ruppert et al. *(274)* used a function parameterized on experimental ligand-binding energies to score probes coating their protein for affinity at each position. The binding site was then detected by clustering high-binding probes. The PROFEC (Pictorial Representation of Free-Energy Changes) approach of Radmer and Kollman *(275)* or variants generated by Pearlman and Charifson *(276)* (One-Window Free-Energy Grid [OWFEG]) are based on free-energy-perturbation (FEP) calculations. Two molecular dynamic trajectories are used to determine free-enthalpy changes resulting from the placement of an atom or group at different locations around an inhibitor, both in solution and at the protein-binding site.

4.3. Virtual Screening Approaches to Receptor–Ligand Interaction

Virtual screening is now becoming a technique of central importance within preclinical drug discovery. Virtual screening, as the term is most often used and understood, involves using a model of a protein-binding site to predict, quantitatively or qualitatively, some appropriate measure of receptor binding—in other words, to discriminate between a small set of ligands with appreciable affinity for that binding site and the bulk of organic molecules lacking affinity.

Two types of virtual screening are available. One derives directly from cheminformatics applications within drug discovery and is based on empirical molecular mechanics energies to score host-guest complexes. The other type originates from structural bioinformatics. It uses a threading approach to estimate binding using an atomic pair potential to score the complementarity of ligand–receptor interactions.

There are two linked and unsolved problems frustrating attempts to develop virtual screening methodologies: the accurate automatic docking of ligands and the accurate quantitative prediction of ligand affinity. Although many methods for automated ligand docking have been suggested *(277–279)*, and there have been some successful applications *(280,281)*, their overall performance, although improving, remains capricious and comparatively poor. Likewise, it remains difficult to predict binding affinities reliably using protein–ligand complexes, even where experimental structures are available *(282–284)*. Solving problems such as these remains a significant future challenge for bioinformatics.

As a process, virtual screening can be divided into four stages (*see* **Fig. 6**). The first stage is composed of two independent parts, which may be undertaken contemporaneously or sequentially. One of these parts concerns the preselection of potential ligand molecules. Such molecules can be selected either by applying rigorous criteria to exist-

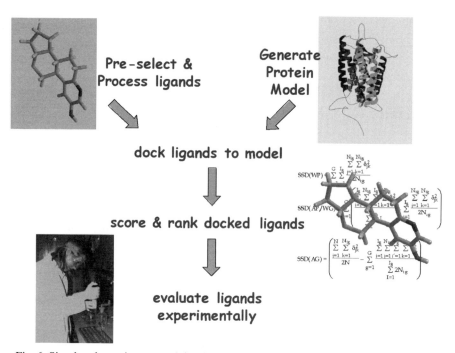

Pre-select &
Process ligands

Generate
Protein
Model

dock ligands to model

score & rank docked ligands

evaluate ligands
experimentally

Fig. 6. Simple schematic summarizing key subprocess in virtual screening. Small molecules are screened and the best selected. At the same time, a binding site model is constructed. The screened set of small molecules is docked to the target binding site. These are then scored and ranked, and the top hits, or representatives thereof, are screened for activity.

ing compound collections or by applying complex and subtle rules in the design of new combinatorial libaries. Such rules or selection criteria come in many guises. They may reflect the properties of successful, marketed drugs or the known structural preferences exhibited by the ligands of related receptors. A thorough discussion of such approaches is beyond both the scope and purpose of the current work, but a brief adumbration seems appropriate.

Selection criteria are often called Lipinski analysis *(285)*: the use of upper and/or lower bounds on quantities such as molecular weight (MW) or Log P to help tailor the putative in vivo properties of drugs. Lipinski's rule of 5 predicts that effective intestinal absorption is more probable when there are fewer than five H-bond donors, less than 10 H-bond acceptors, MW is less than 500, and the calculated Log P is lower than 5. A more careful experimental analysis of orally available marketed drugs indicates slight differences to the Lipinski criteria, albeit for a set of small, relatively old drugs, but this analysis certainly confirms similar overall property patterns *(286)*. However, these criteria are very focused on oral human drugs: the current "holy grail" of most preclinical drug discovery. However, the properties of molecules can be very different. For agrochemicals—pesticides and herbicides—plant bioavailability arises through potency, stability, and passive transport. To achieve this for small-molecule agrochemicals,

MW should be between 200 and 500, clog P should be less than 4, and the number of H-bonding groups should be less than 3. Although these criteria do not differ greatly from the rule of 5, the requirement for an acidic pK_a is a significant difference. Orally bioavailable human drugs are biased toward lipophilic basic amines, which as acidic compounds, with their increased nonspecific binding by human serum albumin and other plasma proteins, are significantly underrepresented. The desire to progress beyond these relatively simple and eminently explicable selection thresholds has led many to search for leadlikeness criteria. Leads must meet variable, project-dependent selection criteria, which include validated biological activity in primary and secondary screens, normally against known targets, for a series of related compounds; patentability; and a promising initial DMPK profile. Historical analysis of leads is difficult, complicated by the clear biases in the extant literature, and by the intrinsic complexity of the optimization process itself. Although the two chemical spaces overlap, there seems to be a real difference between lead and drug. Leadlike compounds typically have 1–5 rings, 2–15 rotatable bonds, MW less than 400, less than 9 acceptors, less than 3 donors, and a log P range of 0.0–3.0. On average, drugs have 2 less rotatable bonds, MW 100 lower, and a reduction in log P of 0.5–1.0 log units compared to leads. High-throughput screening identifies lead compounds with higher MW, higher lipophilicity, and lowered solubility. Driven to enhance receptor affinity, medicinal chemistry optimization tends to exacerbate all of these trends, as leads progress inexorably toward clinical candidates. Thus, one of the main objectives in the identification of leadlike compounds for screening is the need for smaller, less lipophilic compounds that, on optimization, will produce compounds that retain druglike properties.

The other part of this initial stage is the creation of a binding site model. Most virtual screening efforts tend to focus on experimentally derived binding site models, but many biologically important receptor targets do not yet have structures derived by X-ray crystallography and multidimensional NMR. In particular, these include many membrane proteins, such as GPCRs and ion channels. Overcoming the intrinsic problems of modeling GPCRs, or other membrane proteins, will not be straightforward. As we have seen, there are attempts to address this through membrane protein structural genomics. Another promising route is the development of methods for large-scale comparative modeling. Several problems need to be solved:

1. The development of sensitive α-helical amino acid pair-potential functions that will enhance the performance of structure–sequence matching when sequence-sequence matches is not strong enough to guide homology modeling adequately.
2. The correlation of the size and shape of bound ligands with sequence variation within a family, to predict more accurately the size and shape of particular GPCRs.
3. The obtainment of accurate predictions of nonmembrane-embedded structures, such as interconnecting loops that link transmembrane helices.

Although the structure of rhodopsin, the only experimental GPCR structure, provides a useful template for the small-molecule binding sites of a subset of GPCRs, it is a poor model for the loops. Loop conformations vary greatly within and between GPCR families, yet fulfill vital roles in the binding of large and medium ligands such as proteins and peptides.

Moreover, there is a general issue in modeling membrane receptors of which the GPCR-binding site is the key exemplar. Generally, initial model generation for virtual screening will need to identify both agonist-bound and antagonist-bound conformations against which to dock candidate ligands. Experience from pharmaceutical drug discovery shows that it is easier to find antagonists, which block binding, than it is to find agonists, which need to mimic precisely the requirements of endogenous ligand binding. Even an inaccurate model will prove capable of identifying antagonists, but an extremely more accurate model is required for an agonist-binding site. Recent work has allowed a conserved helix bundle assembly to be identified for most GPCRs in their antagonist-bound state *(287,288)*.

The second stage of the conceptual virtual screening protocol involves docking a limited number of "most different" conformations of each small molecule to an ensemble of macromolecular models. The initial screening or design will have generated a restricted list of more drug- or leadlike molecules. By using data on ligands from homologous receptors, this list may also be tailored to be ligand-like. Solutions to the docking problem must take into account the flexibility of both ligand and protein, and if one is docking against either a homology or an experimental model, then one must also take into account errors and uncertainties in the binding site structure. For each of the candidate molecules selected for docking, several ligand conformations will usually be searched against a limited number of receptor conformations. This leads to a combinatorial explosion in the number of possible ways of docking an individual molecule, each of which must be evaluated. Many sophisticated methods for conformational searching are known, and many are implemented in most major proprietary molecular modeling software. The goal here is to address the issue of "most different" conformations. Using ligands from 32 complex structures, Bostrom *(289)* assessed several programs (Catalyst, Confort, OMEGA, Flo99, and MacroModel) for their ability to find bioactive conformations during the generation of conformational ensembles. MacroModel outperformed the other methods, whereas Catalyst and Confort performed least well. Omega, a new rule-based method, was orders of magnitude faster than the other methods, yet gave reasonable results. Very flexible ligands with 8+ rotatable bonds never returned correct bioactive conformations. More recently, robust multivariate statistics, in the form of D-optimal design, were used to evaluate OMEGA's ability to generate bioactive conformations *(290)*. A data set of 36 high-resolution complexes was analyzed. Twenty-eight bioactive conformations were retrieved when using a low-energy cutoff (5 kcal/mol), a low RMSD value (0.6 A) for duplicate removal, and a maximum of 1000 output conformations. Again, bioactive conformers of highly flexible ligands were not identified.

As a process, docking is a sampling exercise, and as such, it is necessary to cover as much of the sample space as possible in as efficient a manner as one can achieve. It is seldom possible to attack this problem in a satisfactory manner, leading to a trade-off between time and combinations of conformation and orientation searched. To deal with this, powerful computational optimization algorithms, such as Monte Carlo or genetic algorithms, are now often employed. The work of Anderson et al. *(291)* is a recently reported attempt to bypass some of these problems. They defined a minimum set of flexible residues within the active site, thus effectively increasing the docking site from a single conformation to an ensemble with a concomitant decrease in the bias that is inherent in the use of a single, rigid protein conformation. It is not the first, nor likely to be the last, attempt to do something of this sort *(174,175,292)*.

Likewise, probing of the active site can have a major impact on the quality of dockings. There are two main approaches to this problem. One uses some type of pregenerated set of favorable interaction points within the binding site and tries to fit molecules to this, in a way analogous to the fitting of molecules into an initial electron density map in X-ray crystallography *(293)*. As we have seen, there are many ways to identify these points of interaction, such as GRID *(224)* or MCSS *(225)*.

The alternative strategy is to evaluate a potential docking using some form of molecular mechanics energy evaluated between docked ligand and receptor. In either case, one would attempt to evaluate and score, for each molecule, several different docking conformations and orientations. The potential energy function used to evaluate docking within a particular docking run need not be the same as that used to score different dockings.

Each conformation of each candidate ligand can be docked against one or more protein models. The docking itself involves orientating, i.e., rotating and translating, the small molecule relative to the larger molecule. Each orientation is sometimes referred to as a pose. Were one to attempt a brute force solution to this problem, then one would perform a grid search over the whole molecule or just a binding site if it has been defined. At each grid point one would need to generate a large number of rotations of the molecule, evaluating each one. A recent method developed in Graham Richards laboratory's *(294,295)* addresses this kind of brute force solution directly but makes use of an elegant trick, so obvious yet so clever, to make it tractable. Using k-means clustering, small-molecule structures are approximated by an ascending hierarchy of points, starting with one point and progressing to the number of atoms in the molecule. At each clustering level, this point set is translated and rotated at each grid point within the lattice within which the protein is embedded. However, for each cycle only grid points at which a negative energy was found in the previous cycle are analyzed. In this way, the number of points diminishes in an exponential fashion, reducing the total number of computations to a tiny fraction of those required by a naïve grid search. A later variant of the method looked at searching for different conformations of the ligand, again making use of a reduced representation: for low numbers of points, many different conformations are represented by the same point set and, hence, the number of calculations is reduced; it is only when the number of points approaches the number of atoms in the molecule that the number of conformers becomes an issue. The approach is replete with promise but clearly requires much more work before that promise is realized.

The third stage of virtual screening involves scoring and, thus, ranking the final docked orientations of candidate molecules. There are several key advantages to virtual screening vs high-throughput screening: apart from the pecuniary advantage of computer screening vs multi-million-dollar robotic assays, the relative celerity of the process tends to drive its use. To that end, and in order to evaluate effectively thousands upon thousand of compounds, screening methods tend to be fast and empirically based, rather than more time-consuming methods, such as MDD. Scoring functions are normally used in the context of docking to estimate binding affinities (for a brief review of currently used scoring functions, *see* **ref. 296**). Many docking methods, such as AutoDock *(297,298)*, ICM *(299)*, DOCK *(300,301)*, or ProDock *(302)*, make use of grid representations to speed up the energy evaluation during the docking process.

Developed by Bohm *(303)*, the archetypal empirical scoring function (SCORE1), which accounted for hydrogen bonds, ionic interactions, buried nonpolar surface regions, and the loss of molecular mobility, produced a cross-validated standard deviation of 9.3 kJ/mol for an initial training set of 45 receptor–ligand complexes. A second scoring function (SCORE2) *(304)*, which added contributions from the burial of hydrogen bonds and additional terms for aromatic and unfavorable electrostatic interactions, reduced the standard deviation to 8.8 kJ/mol for a training set of 82 receptor–ligand complexes. Eldridge et al. *(305)* described a similar approach that uses 82 complexes and a different description of intramolecular flexibility.

Many virtual screening methodologies are currently in use, all with their own advantages and disadvantages. Most attempt to overcome the limitations of computer time by using very simple methodologies that allow each virtual small-molecule structure to be docked and scored very quickly. Examples of these include GOLD *(306)* and DOCK *(301)*. Of course, virtual screening methods exhibit a wide range of alternative methodologies of increasing complexity, from simple rule-based scoring to what are essentially forms of relatively time-consuming atomistic MD simulations such as Linear Interaction Energies (LIE) *(307)*.

The relative success of FRESNO *(308,309)* in the prediction of binding affinities for MHC-peptide interactions suggests that optimization of the screening function, within a chemical area or protein family, rather than the use of totally generic screening functions, may be a better route to success. The authors of FRESNO used a training set comprising five experimentally determined HLA-A*0201 peptide complexes and 37 modeled H-2Kk complexes to reparameterize Eldridge et al.'s *(305)* scoring function. McMartin and Bohacek *(310)* used nine thermolysin-inhibitor complexes to parameterize a simple scoring function composed of hydrogen bond number and hydrophobic contacts. Kasper et al. *(311)* used a training set of 11 peptide–chaperone DnaK complexes to parameterize their scoring function.

The inability to predict quantitative binding constants using simulation approaches has led many to combine calculations with some type of statistics in order to leverage model predictivity. Regression-based empirical scoring functions assume that the total ΔG can be approximated by a summation of individual contributions, with the weights or coefficients in the regression equation being determined by multiple linear regression, partial least squares regression, or an artificial intelligence approach, such as an ANN, using an initial training set of receptor–ligand crystal complexes and corresponding experimental binding affinities. All regression-based methods, their transferability to new congeneric series, and the accuracy of any results obtained are thus highly contingent on the initial choice of training set. Because of their derivation, regression-based methods favor particular types of interaction, typically the most frequently observed in crystal structures.

The VALIDATE methodology of Head et al. *(312)* uses terms accounting for steric and electrostatic energies from AMBER, a calculated Log P term, polar and nonpolar surface surfaces, and an intramolecular flexibility term, with weights obtained using a training set of 55 receptor-ligand complexes. One of the most interesting of these approaches is PrGen *(313,314)*. This approach uses correlation-coupled minimization to optimize the receptor–ligand interactions for a series of ligands of known affinity so that the model becomes predictive both within and, it is hoped, beyond the training set.

The development of atomic-level knowledge-based scoring functions is based on observed frequency distributions of typical interactions: in any system, only those interactions close to the frequency maxima in the data set will be considered favorable. This approach is well known in the field of protein-fold prediction. Using the "inverse Boltzmann law," frequency distributions of interatomic interactions are converted into "knowledge-based potentials" or "potentials of mean force." An example of this approach is the BLEEP scoring function *(315)*, derived from 820 receptor–ligand atompair distributions. For 90 complexes a correlation coefficient of 0.74 was achieved for experimental binding affinities.

Finally, the fourth stage of virtual screening is to analyze and postprocess the results of the scored and ranked docked candidate molecules. In an ideal world, a virtual screening effort would produce a tiny handful of extravagantly active molecules that can be rapidly optimized for selectivity and bioavailability and other DMPK properties. Desirable as this situation may be, it is just as unlikely. More often, one has an array of weakly active, yet equipotent, molecules. What can be done with these? If they are small enough in number, or one's screens have the necessary capacity, they can all be screened. Alternatively, one can cluster them into chemically similar groups and evaluate a sparse sampling of molecules, and, for active compounds, retesting any structural relatives. One can rank them in different ways using a wider range of criteria, selecting the best hits.

Clearly the more resources, in terms of both human and computer time, one is prepared to employ in generating and evaluating possible dockings, the more likely a good solution will be obtained. Likewise, the more sophisticated and, thus, generally, time-consuming one's methods are for evaluating the scoring phase of the virtual screening process, the more likely screening will be accurate. If one wishes to dock a few dozen small-molecule structures, then one can afford to expend a great deal of time on this process, but if the goal is to dock a large virtual library, then the practical limitations of computer time will reduce this to a minimum. Recently, Richards and colleagues *(316,317)* have made use of Internet-based, peer-to-peer distributed computing technology or screensaver technology, of the type made famous by seti@home, to prosecute virtual screening of a number of cancer targets and anthrax virulence factors. This is, essentially, a PC compute farm, but on a truly massive scale. However, access to this technology is unlikely to become widely available.

Consideration of several scoring functions simultaneously, consensus screening, is a practical strategy for improving the quality of the discrimination between ligands and nonligands. There have been some attempts recently to combine the results of these different approaches, of which CScore, distributed by Tripos, is perhaps the best known. My own experience with such software suggests that any improvement that might come from using data fusion methodologies such as this are strongly tempered by the nature of the problem one is trying to solve. It may increase the gain of true positives in a particular screening experiment, but it has much less success in producing an improved quantitative correlation with experimental data. So and Karplus *(318)* have described a somewhat similar approach, that is specifically designed to produce more accurate quantitative data. They evaluated a variety of different methods using 30 glycogen phosphorylase inhibitors as their test set. The methods that they employed covered a variety of 2D and 3D quantitative structure activity relationship methodologies, as well as structure-based design tools such as LUDI. A jury method used to combine the different independent predictions led to a significant increase in predictivity. Their averaged predictions indicated that combining different methods was superior to individual results.

Charifson et al. *(319)* used a logical AND to combine scores from ChemScore *(305)*, DOCK *(301)*, and the "piecewise linear potential" function *(320)*. In a test using three target enzymes, their consensus scoring allowed recovery of known inhibitors with improved accuracy. Using seven different target proteins for virtual screening, Stahl and Rarey *(321)* combined terms from PLP score *(319)* and SCORE1 *(303)*, implementing this within FlexX to achieve robust enrichment. Terp et al. *(322)* correlated eight scoring functions with experimental binding affinities for 120 protein–ligand complexes using partial least squares, yielding quantitative affinity predictions.

4.4. MD Approaches to Receptor–Ligand Docking

One can use a quite different approach to predict ligand–receptor binding through the use of atomistic MD simulations, which can calculate the ΔG_{bind} for a given molecular system. It has the advantage that, in principal, there is no reliance on known binding data, because it attempts the *de novo* prediction of all relevant parameters given knowledge of the system's starting structure, be that an experimental structure or a convincing homology model of ligand–receptor complex. Unlike other methods, such as virtual screening, MD can, in principal at least, account for both explicit solvation and the intrinsic flexibility of both receptor and ligand. Thus, and in contrast to virtual screening, molecular dynamics addresses a dynamic, rather than static, picture of biomolecular systems.

The underlying physics, or physical chemistry, of molecular interactions is, of course, a vast, and somewhat impenetrable, subject, at least for the uninitiated. In statistical mechanics terms, free energy (ΔG) is defined in terms of the partition function. However, for most types of calculation such a "theoretical" definition has limited utility in a practical sense. What is more easily calculated, however, is the free energy difference between two states. Several simulation methods exist that can evaluate free energies. Each method is based on different assumptions and offers differing levels of approximation.

Viewed from the standpoint of thermodynamics, the effective prediction of ΔG_{bind} for receptor–ligand complexation is best obtained from either thermodynamic integration or FEP calculations. These approaches use the relationship between the free energy of the system under consideration and the ensemble average of an energy function describing that system. The energy of the system is described as a function of the coordinates of the particles in configuration space.

In an isobaric and isothermal reaction, the difference between enthalpy (ΔH) and free energy (ΔG) is related to the product of changes in pressure (ΔP) and volume (ΔV), which is negligible for processes in solution, so free enthalpies can also be obtained. In FEP methodology, for example, the free energy is calculated at discrete intervals j using the expressions

$$G_{\lambda(j+1)} - G_{\lambda(j)} = -RT \ln < e^{V_{\lambda(j+1)}} - V_{\lambda(j)} > \lambda(j+1)$$

$$\Delta G = G_1 - G_0 = \sum_j G_{\lambda(j+1)} - G_{\lambda(j)}$$

in which G_1 and G_0 are the free energies of the two states and V is the potential energy of the system. In thermodynamic integration, the free energy of the system is calculated by

$$\Delta G = G_1 - G_0 = \int_0^1 d\lambda \, \langle dV/d\lambda \rangle$$

To solve this equation numerically, one must transform it, from a continuous integration over a

$$\frac{\delta H}{\delta \lambda} \sim \frac{\delta H}{\Delta \lambda}$$

continuum of indivisible steps, to a discrete integration over a set of individual steps. In slow growth methods, one assumes that steps are very close and one can approximate

$$\Delta G = H_{\lambda = 0} - H_{\lambda = 1}$$

MD simulation is, itself, a technique to compute the equilibrium position of a classic multiple-body system. It is assumed that the atoms of the system are constrained by an interatomic potential energy force field. Each of the N atoms in the simulation is treated as a point mass and Newton's equations are integrated to compute their motion. This can be written in the formalism of Hamiltonian mechanics as

$$x = JdH(x)$$

in which J is the identity matrix of rank 2; and $H = T + U$, in which T is the kinetic energy and U is the potential energy. One needs to provide the initial configuration of the system at $t = 0$, i.e., the coordinates of all atoms in a six-dimensional hyperspace. Thus, at regular time intervals, one resolves the classic equation of motion represented by the N equations implicit here. The gradient of the potential energy function is used to calculate the forces on the atoms while the initial velocities on the atoms are generated randomly. At this point new positions and velocities are computed and the atoms moved to these new positions. To measure an observable quantity, one must be able to express this as the position in a phase space of dimension $6 \times N$. The information within the system is largely contained within the potential energy function, which takes the form of a simple penalty function for most simulations of biomolecules.

For large molecular systems comprising thousands of atoms, many of the more sophisticated modeling techniques, which often describe the potential energy surface in terms of quantum mechanics, are too demanding of computer resources to be useful. The Born-Oppenheimer approximation states that the Schrodinger Equation for a molecule can be separated into a part describing the motions of the electrons and a part describing the motions of the nuclei and that these two motions can be studied independently. One can then think of molecules as mechanical assemblies made up of simple elements such as balls (atoms), rods or sticks (bonds), and flexible joints (bond angles and torsion angles). Terms that describe the van der Waals, electrostatic, and possibly hydrogen-bonding interactions between atoms supplement molecular mechanics force fields.

Questions remain, however, regarding the general applicability of molecular dynamic simulation techniques for studying the dizzying complexity of macromolecular systems of any size or biological interest. Obvious limitations are manifold: restricted sampling of configuration space or the accuracy of current force fields or MD's dependence on particular simulation protocols, to name but a few. Long simulation runs are needed and current techniques allow only small differences in structure of the ligands if reliable predictions of ΔG are to be made. Broadly speaking, there are two main routes to addressing the formidable problems associated with MD techniques. One is the use of tightly coupled supercomputing to increase massively the computing resources available. This is required because distributed computing of the screen-saver type is not applicable to this problem; distributed computing is discussed in more detail subsequently. The other approach is to introduce approximations. Approximations are of two kinds: simplifying constraints within simulations themselves and more fundamental approximations in the underlying simulation methodology. Constrained simulations take many forms but typically use constraints and/or restraints to reduce the effective degrees of freedom within a system. This usually takes the form of "freezing" atoms, either by dampening their movements or by making them immobile. Sometimes these constraints and restraints are combined by creating concentric spheres centered on the binding site, which is allowed to move freely, outside of which there is a zone where atom movements are restrained, and outside of this is a properly frozen zone where atom positions are fixed. The problem with such strategies is obvious: how does one constrain a system appropriately? If one knows the answer in advance, then one may choose, perhaps by a process of trial and error, suitable constraints and restraints to obtain that answer. Developing a truly predictive system using ad hoc constraints is much more difficult.

In terms of simulation methodology, many techniques that use approximations exist. A notable example was introduced by Aqvist and co-workers *(303)*. To circumvent the inherent computing resource problems endured by thermodynamic integration or FEP, Aqvist used large, diverse sets of ligand-receptor complexes to develop and refine a semiempirical method, which is usually referred to as the LIE approach. Absolute ΔG_{bind} values were calculated for two states: ligand and protein-ligand complex, both simulated in water. Mean values for the electrostatic and van der Waals components of ΔG_{bind} were then obtained from these simulations, and weighting parameters for these two contributions were obtained by regression against known binding affinities. However, the required scaling of the individual weights is contingent on the conditions used in the simulation, which would seem to limit the universality of the method. Nonetheless, and on a pragmatic level, the ability to train this method makes it appropriate to investigate binding to a particular receptor. Liaison, a program distributed by Schrodinger, combines molecular mechanics LIE methodology with a statistical model-building capacity to generate models of ligand affinity within defined ligand receptor series.

Another set of approaches assumes that ΔG_{bind} can be decomposed into a simple sum of contributions, a so-called master equation, that can be defined physicochemically so as to avoid cross terms. All contributions to ΔG_{bind} are derived from one or a few generic structures rather than average values from an ensemble. Electrostatic contributions in the presence of water can be determined from a continuum solvent model through a numerical solution of a linear PB equation. By considering a simple model, including discrete atomic point charges, of the ligand, receptor, and receptor–ligand complex as regions with a low dielectric constant embedded in a higher dielectric medium, polar interaction energies can be calculated with respect to the solvent. A nonpolar contribution to the desolvation energy is assumed to be proportional to the accessible surface area lost from both molecules on complexation. Entropic contributions are factored as the loss of overall molecular motion as well as intramolecular flexibility. Many methods have used this approach to predict ΔH_{bind} *(323–325)*. Similarly, Zou et al. *(326)* used the "generalized Born Model" (GB) of Still et al. *(327)* for the calculation of polar interaction energies.

Molecular mechanics/GBSA (generalized Born surface area) is a widely used strategy of this type for calculating the binding free energy *(328,329)*. It combines molecular mechanical interaction energies with solvation terms based on implicit solvation models, which can be obtained from the GB approach and a surface-dependent term or using the PB equation. Both contributions are average values taken from a sampled MD trajectory with explicit consideration of waters and counterions. Entropic contributions are obtained from a normal mode or quasi-harmonic analysis of the trajectory. Receptor–ligand complexes with significant structural differences may be studied effectively using this technique. The free energies for the complex, isolated ligand, and isolated receptor, are calculated for snapshot structures taken from the molecular dynamic trajectory. The binding free energy is calculated as follows:

$$\Delta G_b = G(\text{complex}) - G(\text{free receptor}) - G(\text{free ligand})$$

$$G(\text{molecule}) = \langle E_{MM} \rangle + \langle G_{sol} \rangle - TS$$

in which ΔG_b is the binding free energy in water, E_{MM} is the molecular mechanical energy, G_{sol} is the solvation energy, and $-TS$ is the entropy contribution to the solvation. Angle brackets denote the average for a set of structures along a molecular dynamic trajectory. The molecular mechanics energy, E_{MM}, represents the internal bonded energy (E^{bonded}), electrostatic (E_{int}^{ele}), and van der Waals (E_{int}^{vdW}) interactions; and the solvation energy, G_{sol}, is divided into two parts, the electrostatic (G_{sol}^{ele}) and the hydrophobic (G_{sol}^{np}) contributions:

$$E_{MM} = E^{\text{bonded}} + E_{int}^{ele} + E_{int}^{vdW}$$

$$G_{sol} = G_{sol}^{ele} + G_{sol}^{np}$$

The molecular mechanics energy, E_{MM}, is calculated using an empirical force field. The electrostatic contribution to the solvation free energy, G_{sol}^{ele}, is calculated by the GB method *(327)*. Studies have shown that there is a good correspondence between GB and finite-difference PB calculations *(330,331)*, although the latter has been used more frequently to calculate the electrostatic solvation free energy. The hydrophobic contribution, G_{isol}^{np}, is estimated empirically based on solvent-accessible surface area. When calculating the binding free energy difference, it may be assumed that the standard entropy change is similar for both models and can therefore be assumed to cancel.

The growth of computer power during the last two decades has allowed the study of biologically interesting systems including small and medium proteins using atomistic MD methodology. However, researchers are still faced with problems concerning the validity of their models and the relatively short time scales that can be reached on current serial machines. Many approaches have been tried to circumvent these problems, but only with limited success, because almost any attempt to reach longer time scales will result in more approximations in the model. Previous attempts to utilize MD and other atomistic simulation methods to investigate receptor–ligand interactions have foundered on technical limitations within present computing methods. Although many methods link thermodynamic properties to simulations, they take an unrealistically long time. A basic simulation yielding a free energy of binding requires something like 10 ns of simulation. On the average desktop serial workstation, this requires a compute time on the order of 300 h/ns. To simulate as few as a dozen flexible molecules might entirely occupy a machine for several years. To circumvent these technical limitations, one recourse might be to take advantage of high-performance, massively parallel implementations of MD codes running on large supercomputers with 128, 256, or 512 nodes. Another, complementary way to circumvent this problem is to make use of "grid computing." This refers to an ambitious and exciting global effort to develop an environment in which individual users can access computers, databases, and experimental facilities simply and transparently, without having to consider where those facilities are located.

Difficulties inherent in analyses of protein–ligand complex using simulation are demonstrated well by the application of MD approaches to the MHC–peptide system. Small in biomolecular terms, it is nonetheless prohibitively problematic in terms of computing methodology. Delisi and colleagues were among the first to apply molecular dynamics to peptide–MHC binding, and have subsequently developed a series of different methods *(332–336)*. Part of this work has concentrated on accurate docking using molecular dynamics and part on determining free energies from peptide–MHC complexes. Rognan and colleagues have, over a long period, also made important contributions to this area *(337–342)*. In their work, dynamic properties of the solvated protein–peptide complexes, such as atomic fluctuations, solvent-accessible surface areas, and hydrogen-bonding patterns, correlated well with available binding data. They have been able to discriminate between binders that remain tightly anchored to the MHC molecule from nonbinders that are significantly weaker. Other work by this group *(343–345)* has concentrated on the design of nonnatural ligands for MHC molecules, demonstrating the generality of molecular dynamic approaches to problems of MHC binding. Other work in the area has come from those interested in using the methodology to analyze and predict features of peptide–MHC complexes. These methods have examined class I *(346,347)* and class II *(348)*, as well as investigated the effect of peptide identity on the dynamics of T-cell interaction *(349)*. Recently, Wan et al. *(350)* have applied massively parallel supercomputing technology to the simulation of the peptide–MHC complex using an implementation of the AMBER force field within the LAMMPS program, which was developed to scale well on multiprocessor machines. Unlike other attempts to simulate MHCs, these investigators have performed long-duration unconstrained simulations, in short turnaround times, demonstrating, beyond reasonable doubt, that only full, rather than truncated, models can return accurate dynamic and time-averaged properties.

5. Discussion

Generally speaking, currently available methods for the identification and analysis of binding sites are useful computational tools able to exploit protein structural data in order to facilitate the design of molecules. Whichever particular method is selected for binding site analysis, the results typically support interactive design work and provide suggestions for the modulation of ligand properties. The process—structure-based drug design—seeks to identify or construct ligands that can bind with high affinity to a structurally defined binding site of a target protein. It is thus important to analyze properly a binding site by mapping those characteristics that are essential for molecular recognition. Successful examples of structure-based design include ligands for carbonic anhydrase *(351)* and DNA-gyrase *(352)*. These and other examples provide compelling evidence for the hierarchical, stepwise application of such techniques to be regarded as a strategy of proven worth. Nevertheless, a considerable set of limiting factors still precludes the development of a reliable, fully automated approach leading from a target structure all the way to a drug. Careful use of the methods and an equally careful interpretation of the results are still required. Success is also still dependent on the nature and quality of experimental data, whether structural or functional.

Many current limitations result from simplifications made to keep algorithms tractable given present-day computing resources, while others clearly reflect persisting problems in understanding and modeling fundamental processes of biomolecular recognition. Problems of protein flexibility, solvent interactions, the dynamic synergism between ligand and receptor, or the proper consideration of the cellular environment all remain important stumbling blocks. Researchers are presently unable to quantify binding accurately using theory alone. For this reason, knowledge-based methods may represent the best approach for the foreseeable future, taking advantage, as they do, of the growing volume of experimental data and account, implicitly at least, for many effects that are not yet properly understood. Yet different methods have different strengths and weaknesses, and it is often advisable to combine several methods when tackling a particular system.

A combination of approaches, including both inheritance of locations and *de novo* prediction, has allowed and fomented the development of databases that archive information about binding sites. The first and arguably most important database of protein ligand receptor complexes is the PDB *(353,354)*, now run by the Research Collaborative for Structural Biology. This stores the raw coordinates of almost all published protein structures. Other databases have taken the contents of the PDB and imposed manually or automatically derived structural hierarchies aimed at simplifying and systematizing the ever-expanding structural universe of proteins. The two most important examples of such databases are CATH *(355,356)* and SCOP *(357)*. ISOSTAR *(358)* is a database of nonbonded interaction geometries that contains approx 10,000 distributions of about 40 different types of contact groups (such as ammonium nitrogen atoms, carbonyl oxygen atoms, and methyl carbon atoms) around about 300 central groups. Data mining for protein-ligand complexes can be undertaken using RELIBASE (receptor–ligand database) *(359,360)*. It contains all structures in the PDB as well as additional data including ligand atom and bond types, substructures, and crystal packing. CAVBASE *(361)* is a recently developed database system focusing on the automated detection of similar binding site structure. It uses the LIGSITE methodology *(237)* to identify, excise, and store protein surface cavities. For two example proteins, chorismate mutases and serine proteases, CAVBASE returned proteins of similar function as the best ranked hits even when they showed no significant sequence similarity *(362)*. The eF-site (electrostatic surface of functional site) is another molecular surface database *(363)*, which is composed of four subdatabases: eF-site/antibody (corresponding to the antigen-binding sites of antibodies with the same orientations), eF-site/prosite (corresponding to the molecular surfaces for the individual motifs in the PROSITE database), eF-site/P-site (corresponding to phosphate-binding sites), and eF-site/ActiveSite (corresponding to active-site surfaces for the representatives of the individual protein family). Many other databases, relevant in theme to the present discussion, are also available: other structural databases *(364–367)*, databases storing quantitative measures of receptor ligand affinity *(368–371)*, and also more qualitative databases containing data on protein-protein interactions *(372,373)*.

Although such databases may provide initial hints about function and binding site location, the relationship between structure and function is by no means simple and straightforward. A similar fold does not necessarily imply a similar biochemical function, and proteins with different folds can also show the same function and catalytic mechanism; the lipocalins are an interesting example of a low-homology protein family, notorious for the difficulty in assigning family membership, embedded in a larger structural superfamily, the calycins, which seems even more tenuous at the sequence level. As a starting point for the analysis of binding sites, it is often necessary to retrieve all structural information that is available concerning the system of interest, requiring databases supporting fast, flexible, and efficient user interfaces and tools for the retrieval, visualization, and analysis of data concerning protein–ligand complexes.

To understand the binding site is to understand binding, and to understand binding is to understand the binding site. It is the binding site, after all, that specifies the structural and physicochemical constraints that must be met by any putative ligand *(374)*, yet within an evolutionary, teleonomic context, it is also the properties of the ligand that determine the nature of the binding site. The purpose of this chapter has been to examine the different methodologies that have been used to analyze, visualize, and predict binding sites, rather than to discuss in detail the nature of such analyses. However, some things are clear. Ligand-binding sites are generally hydrophobic depressions, ranging in size and concavity, depending on the nature of the molecule bound. Moreover, typically, yet not without exception, interfaces between subunits show distinct differences in their geometrical properties compared to ligand-binding sites. For example, protein-protein interactions occur between flat areas of protein surface, whereas specific interactions of smaller ligands take place in pockets in the surface.

6. Conclusion

There are two concepts that underlie our faltering steps to identify and analyze binding sites. The first is based on knowledge: when we know the location of a binding site in one protein, then identifying that either the sequence or structure of another protein is similar to it allows us to "inherit" the site from the first protein to the second. This may involve a direct search for a clearly related sequence or structure, or a search for more abstract motifs or geometric pattern of residues interacting in 3D. The second approach involves the *a priori* prediction of a binding site from a sequence or a structure. This may involve an artificial intelligence or phylogenetic method operating on a sequence or a structural analysis operating at the level of the physicochemical properties of the site and of potential interactions with ligands in 3D. Inherent uncertainty, such as the dependence of binding site conformation on the presence of a ligand, can be addressed either by dynamic methods able to predict these changes, such as high-performance MD, or by trying to build this uncertainty into search models, so that ligands are detected even when the binding site is represented by a suboptimal model. Thus, the full and complete analysis of binding sites will necessarily involve the full range of informatic techniques ranging from sequence-based bioinformatic analysis through structural bioinformatics to computational chemistry and molecular physics. Integration of both diverse experimental and diverse theoretical approaches is thus a mandatory requirement in the evaluation of binding sites and the binding events that occur within them.

References

1. Lilley, D. M. (2003) The origins of RNA catalysis in ribozymes. *Trends Biochem. Sci.* **28,** 495–501.
2. Nicolaou, K. C., Zipkin, R. E., and Petasis, N. A. (1982) The endiandric acid cascade—electrocyclizations in organic-synthesis 3. Biomimetic approach to endiandric acids-A-acid-G—synthesis of precursors. *J. Am. Chem. Soc.* **104,** 5558–5560.
3. Ingber, D. E. (2003) Tensegrity I. Cell structure and hierarchical systems biology. *J. Cell Sci.* **116,** 1157–1173.
4. Ingber, D. E. (2003) Tensegrity II. How structural networks influence cellular information processing networks. *J. Cell Sci.* **116,** 1397–1408.
5. Nooren, I. M. and Thornton, J. M. (2003) Diversity of protein-protein interactions. *EMBO J.* **22,** 3486–3492.
6. Weckwerth, W. (2003) Metabolomics in systems biology. *Annu. Rev. Plant Biol.* **54,** 669–689.
7. Watkins, S. M. and German, J. B. (2002) Metabolomics and biochemical profiling in drug discovery and development. *Curr. Opin. Mol. Ther.* **4,** 224–228.
8. Fiehn, O. (2002) Metabolomics: the link between genotypes and phenotypes. *Plant Mol. Biol.* **8,** 155–171.
9. Van Regenmortel, M. H. (2002) A paradigm shift is needed in proteomics: 'structure determines function' should be replaced by 'binding determines function.' *J. Mol. Recognit.* **15,** 349–351.

10. Van Regenmortel, M. H. (2002) Reductionism and the search for structure-function relationships in antibody molecules. *J. Mol. Recognit.* **15,** 240–247.
11. Flower, D. R. (1999) Modelling G-protein-coupled receptors for drug design. *Biochim. Biophys. Acta* **1422,** 207–234.
12. Watson, S. and Arkinstall, S. (1994) *The G Protein Linked Receptors Facts Book.* Academic, New York.
13. Lefkowitz, R. J. (1998) G protein–coupled receptors III: new roles for receptor kinases and arrestins in receptor signalling and desensitization. *J. Biol. Chem.* **273,** 18,677–18,680.
14. Palczewski, K., Kumasaka, T., Hori, T., et al. (2000) Crystal structure of rhodopsin: a G protein-coupled receptor. *Science* **289,** 739–745.
15. Flower, D. R. (2003) Towards in silico prediction of immunogenic epitopes. *Trends Immunol.* **24,** 667–674.
16. Flower, D. R., McSparron, H., Blythe, M. J., et al. (2003) Computational vaccinology: quantitative approaches. *Novartis Found. Symp.* **254,** 102–120.
17. Doytchinova, I. A. and Flower, D. R. (2002) Quantitative approaches to computational vaccinology. *Immunol. Cell. Biol.* **80,** 270–279.
18. Garrigan, D. and Hedrick, P. W. (2003) Perspective: detecting adaptive molecular polymorphism: lessons from the MHC. *Evol. Int. J. Organic Evol.* **57,** 1707–1722.
19. Doytchinova, I. A., Taylor, P., and Flower, D. R. (2003) Proteomics in vaccinology and immunobiology: an informatics perspective of the immunone. *J. Biomed. Biotechnol.* **2003,** 267–290.
20. Roura-Mir, C. and Moody, D. B. (2003) Sorting out self and microbial lipid antigens for CD1. *Microbes Infect.* **5,** 1137–1148.
21. Flower, D. R., North, A. C., and Sansom, C. E. (2000) The lipocalin protein family: structural and sequence overview. *Biochim. Biophys. Acta* **1482,** 9–24.
22. Akerstrom, B., Flower, D. R., and Salier, J. P. (2000) Lipocalins: unity in diversity. *Biochim. Biophys. Acta* **1482,** 1–8.
23. Flower, D. R. (1996) The lipocalin protein family: structure and function. *Biochem. J.* **318,** 1–14.
24. Flower, D. R., North, A. C., and Attwood, T. K. (1993) Structure and sequence relationships in the lipocalins and related proteins. *Protein Sci.* **2,** 753–761.
25. Benkovic, S. J. and Hammes-Schiffer, S. (2003) A perspective on enzyme catalysis. *Science* **301,** 1196–1202.
26. Garcia-Viloca, M., Gao, J., Karplus, M., and Truhlar, D. G. (2004) How enzymes work: analysis by modern rate theory and computer simulations. *Science* **303,** 186–195.
27. Ringe, D. (1995) What makes a binding site a binding site. *Curr. Opin. Struct. Biol.* **5,** 825–829.
28. Liang, H., Edelsbrunner, C., and Woodward, G. (1998) Anatomy of protein pockets and cavities: measurement of binding site geometry and implications for ligand design. *Protein Sci.* **7,** 1884–1897.
29. Laskowski, R. A., Luscombe, N. M., Swindells, M. B., and Thornton, J. M. (1996) Protein clefts in molecular recognition and function. *Protein Sci.* **5,** 2438–2452.
30. Sine, S. M. (2002) The nicotinic receptor ligand binding domain. *J. Neurobiol.* **53,** 431–446.
31. Marti, D. N. and Bosshard, H. R. (2003) Electrostatic interactions in leucine zippers: thermodynamic analysis of the contributions of Glu and His residues and the effect of mutating salt bridges. *J. Mol. Biol.* **330,** 621–637.
32. Holm, L. and Sander, C. (1994) Searching protein structure databases has come of age. *Proteins* **19,** 165–173.

33. Flower, D. R., North, A. C., and Attwood, T. K. (1991) Mouse oncogene protein 24p3 is a member of the lipocalin protein family. *Biochem. Biophys. Res. Commun.* **180,** 69–74.

34. Flower, D. R. (1993) Structural relationship of streptavidin to the calycin protein superfamily. *FEBS Lett.* **333,** 99–102.

35. Fredriksson, R., Lagerstrom, M. C., Lundin, L. G., and Schioth, H. B. (2003) The G-protein-coupled receptors in the human genome form five main families: phylogenetic analysis, paralogon groups, and fingerprints. *Mol. Pharmacol.* **63,** 1256–1272.

36. Fredriksson, R., Hoglund, P. J., Gloriam, D. E., Lagerstrom, M. C., and Schioth, H. B. (2003) Seven evolutionarily conserved human rhodopsin G protein-coupled receptors lacking close relatives. *FEBS Lett.* **554,** 381–388.

37. Flower, D. R. (ed.). (2002) *Drug Design: Cutting Edge Approaches*, Royal Society of Chemistry, Cambridge, UK.

38. Stone, M. J. and Williams, D. H. (1992) On the evolution of functional secondary metabolites (natural products). *Mol. Microbiol.* **6,** 29–34.

39. Hamawy, M. M. (2003) Molecular actions of calcineurin inhibitors. *Drug News Perspect.* **16,** 277–282.

40. Plosker, G. L. and Foster, R. H. (2000) Tacrolimus: a further update of its pharmacology and therapeutic use in the management of organ transplantation. *Drugs* **59,** 323–389.

41. Oberlies, N. H. and Kroll, D. J. (2004) Camptothecin and taxol: historic achievements in natural products research. *J. Nat. Prod.* **67,** 129–135.

42. Service, R. F. (2004) Surviving the blockbuster syndrome. *Science* **303,** 1796–1799.

43. Marriott, D. P., Dougall, I. G., Meghani, P., Liu, Y. J., and Flower, D. R. (1999) Lead generation using phamacophore mapping and three dimensional database searching: application to muscarinic M(3) receptor antagonists. *J. Med. Chem.* **42,** 3210–3216.

44. Honma, T. (2003) Recent advances in de novo design strategy for practical lead identification. *Med. Res. Rev.* **23,** 606–632.

45. Klebe, G. (2000) Recent developments in structure-based drug design. *J. Mol. Med.* **78,** 269–281.

46. Martin, Y. C. (1992) 3D database searching in drug design. *J. Med. Chem.* **35,** 2145–2154.

47. Green, D. V. (2003) Virtual screening of virtual libraries. *Prog. Med. Chem.* **41,** 61–97.

48. Flower, D. R. (2002) Molecular informatics: sharpening drug design's cutting edge, *in Drug Design: Cutting Edge Approaches* (Flower, D. R., ed.), Royal Society of Chemistry, Cambridge, UK, pp. 1–52.

49. Chaires, J. B. (1998) Drug–DNA interactions. *Curr. Opin. Struct. Biol.* **8,** 314–320.

50. Lipinski, C. A. (2000) Drug-like properties and the causes of poor solubility and poor permeability. *J. Pharmacol. Toxicol. Methods* **44,** 235–249.

51. van de Waterbeemd, H., Smith, D. A., and Jones, B. C. (2001) Lipophilicity in PK design: methyl, ethyl, futile. *J. Comput. Aided Mol. Des.* **15,** 273–286.

52. Teague, S. J., Davis, A. M., Leeson, P. D., and Oprea, T. (1999) The design of leadlike combinatorial libraries. *Angew Chem. Int. Ed. Engl.* **38,** 3743–3748.

53. Hopkins, A. L. and Groom, C. R. (2002) The druggable genome. *Nat. Rev. Drug Discov.* **1,** 727–730.

54. Idriss, H. T. and Naismith, J. H. (2000) TNF alpha and the TNF receptor superfamily: structure-function relationship(s). *Microsc. Res. Tech.* **50,** 184–195.

55. Hudson, P. J. and Souriau, C. (2001) Recombinant antibodies for cancer diagnosis and therapy. *Expert Opin. Biol. Ther.* **1,** 845–655.

56. Harrison, P. M., Kumar, A., Lang, N., Snyder, M., and Gerstein, M. (2002) A question of size: the eukaryotic proteome and the problems in defining it. *Nucleic Acids Res.* **30,** 1083–1090.

57. Swindells, M. B. and Overington, J. P. (2002) Prioritizing the proteome: identifying pharmaceutically relevant targets. *Drug Discov. Today* **7**, 516–521.
58. Lambert, F. L. (2002) "Entropy Is Simple, Qualitatively." *J. Chem. Educ.* **79**, 1241–1246.
59. Bingham, R. J., Findlay, J. B., Hsieh, S. Y., et al. (2004) Thermodynamics of binding of 2-methoxy-3-isopropylpyrazine and 2-methoxy-3-isobutylpyrazine to the major urinary protein. *J. Am. Chem. Soc.* **126**, 1675–1681.
60. Calderone, C. T. and Williams, D. H. (2001) An enthalpic component in cooperativity: the relationship between enthalpy, entropy, and noncovalent structure in weak associations. *J. Am. Chem. Soc.* **123**, 6262–6267.
61. Roos, H., Karlsson, R., Nilshans, H., and Persson, A. (1998) Thermodynamic analysis of protein interactions with biosensor technology. *J. Mol. Recognit.* **11**, 204–210.
62. Pierce, M. M., Raman, C. S., and Nall, B. T. (1999) Isothermal titration calorimetry of protein-protein interactions. *Methods* **19**, 213–221.
63. Marshall, K. W., Liu, A. F., Canales, J., et al. (1994) Role of the polymorphic residues in HLA-DR molecules in allele-specific binding of peptide ligands. *J. Immunol.* **152**, 4946–4953.
64. Cheng, Y. and Prusoff, W. H. (1973) Relationship between the inhibition constant (K1) and the concentration of inhibitor which causes 50 per cent inhibition (I50) of an enzymatic reaction. *Biochem. Pharmacol.* **22**, 3099–3108.
65. Van Regenmortel, M. H. (2003) Improving the quality of BIACORE-based affinity measurements. *Dev. Biol. (Basel)* **112**, 141–151.
66. Cooper, M. A. (2003) Label-free screening of bio-molecular interactions. *Anal. Bioanal. Chem.* **377**, 834–842.
67. Chalikian, T. V. and Filfil, R. (2003) How large are the volume changes accompanying protein transitions and binding? *Biophys. Chem.* **104**, 489–499.
68. Tetin, S. Y. and Hazlett, T. L. (2000) Optical spectroscopy in studies of antibody-hapten interactions. *Methods* **20**, 341–361.
69. Aebersold, R. and Mann, M. (2003) Mass spectrometry-based proteomics. *Nature* **422**, 198–207.
70. Alonso, J. L. and Goldmann, W. H. (2003) Feeling the forces: atomic force microscopy in cell biology. *Life Sci.* **72**, 2553–2560.
71. Jelesarov, I. and Bosshard, H. R. (1999) Isothermal titration calorimetry and differential scanning calorimetry as complementary tools to investigate the energetics of biomolecular recognition. *J. Mol. Recognit.* **12**, 3–18.
72. Holdgate, G. A. (2001) Making cool drugs hot: isothermal titration calorimetry as a tool to study binding energetics. *Biotechniques* **31**, 164–166.
73. Cliff, M. J. and Ladbury, J. E. (2003) A survey of the year 2002 literature on applications of isothermal titration calorimetry. *J. Mol. Recognit.* **16**, 383–391.
74. Weber, P. C. and Salemme, F. R. (2003) Applications of calorimetric methods to drug discovery and the study of protein interactions. *Curr. Opin. Struct. Biol.* **13**, 115–121.
75. Rost, B. (1997) Protein structures sustain evolutionary drift. *Struct. Fold Des.* **2**, S19–S24.
76. Aloy, P., Querol, E., Aviles, F. X., and Sternberg, M. J. (2001) Automated structure-based prediction of functional sites in proteins: applications to assessing the validity of inheriting protein function from homology in genome annotation and to protein docking. *J. Mol. Biol.* **311**, 395–408.
77. Cammer, S. A., Hoffman, B. T., Speir, J. A., et al. (2003) Structure-based active site profiles for genome analysis and functional family subclassification. *J. Mol. Biol.* **334**, 387–401.

78. Andrade, M. A. and Sander, C. (1997) Bioinformatics: from genome data to biological knowledge. *Curr. Opin. Biotechnol.* **8,** 675–683.
79. Kleiger, G. and Eisenberg, D. (2002) GXXXG and GXXXA motifs stabilize FAD and NAD(P)-binding Rossmann folds through C(alpha)-H. . . O hydrogen bonds and van der waals interactions. *J. Mol. Biol.* **323,** 69–76.
80. Artymiuk, P. J., Poirrette, A. R., Grindley, H. M., Rice, D. W., and Willett, P. (1994) A graph-theoretic approach to the identification of three-dimensional patterns of amino acid side-chains in protein structures. *J. Mol. Biol.* **243,** 327–344.
81. Bailey, T. L. and Elkan, C. (1995) The value of prior knowledge in discovering motifs with MEME. *Proc. Int. Conf. Intell. Syst. Mol. Biol.* **3,** 21–29.
82. Attwood, T. K., Bradley, P., Flower, D. R., et al. (2003) PRINTS and its automatic supplement, prePRINTS. *Nucleic Acids Res.* **31,** 400–402.
83. Mulder, N. J., Apweiler, R., Attwood, T. K., et al. (2003) The InterPro Database, 2003 brings increased coverage and new features. *Nucleic Acids Res.* **31,** 315–318.
84. Orengo, C. A., Todd, A. E., and Thornton, J. M. (1999) From protein structure to function. *Curr. Opin. Struct. Biol.* **9,** 374–382.
85. Thornton, J. M., Todd, A. E., Milburn, D., Borkakoti, N., and Orengo, C. A. (2000) From structure to function: approaches and limitations. *Nat. Struct. Biol.* **7,** 991–994.
86. Wallace, A. C., Borkakoti, N., and Thornton, J. M. (1997) TESS: a geometric hashing algorithm for deriving 3D coordinate templates for searching structural databases: application to enzyme active sites. *Protein Sci.* **6,** 2308–2323.
87. Russell, R. B. (1998) Detection of protein three-dimensional side-chain patterns: new examples of convergent evolution. *J. Mol. Biol.* **279,** 1211–1227.
88. Gutteridge, A., Bartlett, G. J., and Thornton, J. M. (2003) Using a neural network and spatial clustering to predict the location of active sites in enzymes. *J. Mol. Biol.* **330,** 719–734.
89. Casari, G., Sander, C., and Valencia, A. (1995) A method to predict functional residues in proteins. *Nat. Struct. Biol.* **2,** 171–178.
90. Gadiraju, S., Vyhlidal, C. A., Leeder, J. S., and Rogan, P. K. (2003) Genome-wide prediction, display and refinement of binding sites with information theory–based models. *BMC Bioinf.* **4,** 38–45.
91. Chou, K. C. and Cai, Y. D. (2004) A novel approach to predict active sites of enzyme molecules. *Proteins* **55,** 77–82.
92. Keil, M., Exner, T. E., and Brickmann, J. (2004) Pattern recognition strategies for molecular surfaces: III. Binding site prediction with a neural network. *J. Comput. Chem.* **25,** 779–789.
93. Lichtarge, O., Bourne, H. R., and Cohen, F. E. (1996) An evolutionary trace method defines binding surfaces common to protein families. *J. Mol. Biol.* **257,** 342–358.
94. Crowder, S., Holton, J., and Alber, T. (2001) Covariance analysis of RNA recognition motifs identifies functionally linked amino acids. *J. Mol. Biol.* **310,** 793–800.
95. Mirny, L. A. and Gelfand, M. S. (2002) Using orthologous and paralogous proteins to identify specificity-determining residues in bacterial transcription factors. *J. Mol. Biol.* **321,** 7–20.
96. Li, L., Shakhnovich, E. I., and Mirny, L. A. (2003) Amino acids determining enzyme-substrate specificity in prokaryotic and eukaryotic protein kinases. *Proc. Natl. Acad. Sci. USA* **100,** 4463–4468.
97. Bradford, J. R. and Westhead, D. R. (2003) Asymmetric mutation rates at enzyme-inhibitor interfaces: implications for the protein-protein docking problem. *Protein Sci.* **12,** 2099–2103.
98. Burley, S. K. (2000) An overview of structural genomics. *Nat. Struct. Biol.* **7,** 932–934.

99. Paine, K. and Flower, D. R. (2002) Bacterial bioinformatics: pathogenesis and the genome. *J. Mol. Microbiol. Biotechnol.* **4,** 357–365.

100. Berman, H. M., Westbrook, J., Feng, Z., et al. (2000) The protein data bank. *Nucleic Acids Res.* **28,** 235–242.

101. Berman, H. M., Bhat, T. N., Bourne, P. E., et al. (2000) The protein data bank and the challenge of structural genomics. *Nat. Struct. Biol.* **7,** 957–959.

102. McReee, D. (1999) *Practical Protein Crystallography,* 2nd ed., Academic, New York.

103. Betton, J. M. (2003) Rapid translation system (RTS): a promising alternative for recombinant protein production. *Curr. Protein Pept. Sci.* **4,** 73–80.

104. Bae, J. H., Alefelder, S., Kaiser, J. T., et al. (2001) Incorporation of beta-selenolo[3,2-b] pyrrolyl-alanine into proteins for phase determination in protein X-ray crystallography. *J. Mol. Biol.* **309,** 925–936.

105. Chayen, N. E., Boggon, T. J., Cassetta, A., et al. (1996) Trends and challenges in experimental macromolecular crystallography. *Q Rev. Biophys.* **29,** 227–278.

106. Sedzik, J. and Norinder, U. (1997) Statistical analysis and modelling of crystallization outcomes. *J. Appl. Crystallogr.* **30,** 502–506.

107. Muchmore, S. W., Olson, J., Jones, R., et al. (2000) Automated crystal mounting and data collection for protein crystallography. *Struct. Fold. Des.* **8,** R243–R246.

108. Miao, J., Hodgson, K. O., and Sayre, D. (2001) An approach to three-dimensional structures of biomolecules by using single-molecule diffraction images. *Proc. Natl. Acad. Sci. USA* **98,** 6641–6645.

109. Deisenhofer, J., Epp, O., Miki, K., Huber, R., and Michel, H. (1985) Structure of the protein subunits in the photosynthetic reaction centre of rhodopseudomonas viridis at 3 angstroms resolution. *Nature* **318,** 618–620.

110. Weiss, M. S. and Schulz, G. E. (1992) Structure of porin refined at 1.8 angstroms resolution. *J. Mol. Biol.* **227,** 493–502.

111. Henderson, R., Baldwin, J. M., Ceska, T. A., Zemlin, F., Beckmann, E., and Downing, K. H. (1990) Model for the structure of bacteriorhodopsin based on high-resolution electron cryo-microscopy. *J. Mol. Biol.* **213,** 899–921.

112. Grisshammer, R. and Tate, C. G. (1995) Overexpression of integral membrane proteins for structural studies. *Q. Rev. Biophys.* **28,** 315–422.

113. Kuhlbrandt, W. (1992) Two-dimensional crystallization of membrane proteins. *Q. Rev. Biophys.* **25,** 1–49.

114. Grisshammer, R. and Tucker, J. (1997) Quantitative evaluation of neurotensin receptor purification by immobilized metal affinity chromatography. *Protein Express. Purif.* **11,** 53–60.

115. Wilson-Kubalek, E. M., Brown, R. E., Celia, H., and Milligan, R. A. (1998) Lipid nanotubes as substrates for helical crystallization of macromolecules. *Proc. Natl. Acad. Sci. USA* **95,** 8040–8045.

116. Browne, W. J., North, A. C., Phillips, D. C., Brew, K., Vanaman, T. C., and Hill, R. L. (1969) A possible three-dimensional structure of bovine alpha-lactalbumin based on that of hen's egg-white lysozyme. *J. Mol. Biol.* **42,** 65–86.

117. Topham, C. M., Thomas, P., Overington, J. P., Johnson, M. S., Eisenmenger, F., and Blundell, T. L. (1990) An assessment of COMPOSER: a rule-based approach to modelling protein structure. *Biochem. Soc. Symp.* **57,** 1–9.

118. Sali, A. and Blundell, T. L. (1993) Comparative protein modelling by satisfaction of spatial restraints. *J. Mol. Biol.* **234,** 779–815.

119. Schwede, T., Kopp, J., Guex, N., and Peitsch, M. C. (2003) SWISS-MODEL: an automated protein homology-modeling server. *Nucleic Acids Res.* **31,** 3381–3385.

120. Pauling, L., Corey, R. B., and Branson, H. R. (1951) The structure of proteins: two hydrogen-bonded helical configurations of the polypeptide chain. *Proc. Natl. Acad. Sci. USA* **37,** 205–211.
121. Pauling, L. and Corey, R. B. (1951) The structure of hair, muscle, and related proteins. *Proc. Natl. Acad. Sci. USA* **37,** 251–256.
122. Filizola, M., Perez, J. J., and Cartenifarina, M. (1998) Bundle—a program for building the transmembrane domains of G-protein-coupled receptors. *J. Comput. Aided Mol. Des.* **12,** 111–118.
123. Herzyk, P. and Hubbard, R. E. (1995) Automated method for modelling seven-helix transmembrane receptors from experimental data. *Biophys. J.* **69,** 2419–2442.
124. Flower, D. R. (1999) Rotational superposition: a review of methods. *J. Mol. Graph Model.* **17,** 238–244.
125. Subbarao, N. and Haneef, I. (1991) Defining topological equivalences in macromolecules. *Protein Eng.* **4,** 877–884.
126. Claessens, M., Van Cutsem, E., Lasters, I., and Wodak, S. (1989) Modelling the polypeptide backbone with 'spare parts' from known protein structures. *Protein Eng.* **2,** 335–345.
127. Reid, L. S. and Thornton, J. M. (1989) Rebuilding flavodoxin from C alpha coordinates: a test study. *Proteins* **5,** 170–182.
128. Correa, P. E. (1990) The building of protein structures from alpha-carbon coordinates. *Proteins* **7,** 366–377.
129. Holm, L. and Sander, C. (1991) Database algorithm for generating protein backbone and side-chain co-ordinates from a C alpha trace application to model building and detection of co-ordinate errors. *J. Mol. Biol.* **218,** 183–194.
130. Levitt, M. (1992) Accurate modeling of protein conformation by automatic segment matching. *J. Mol. Biol.* **226,** 507–533.
131. Luo, Y., Jiang, X., Lai, L., Qu, C., Xu, X., and Tang, Y. (1992) Building protein backbones from C alpha coordinates. *Protein Eng.* **5,** 147–150.
132. Bassolino-Klimas, D. and Bruccoleri, R. E. (1992) Application of a directed conformational search for generating 3-D coordinates for protein structures from alpha-carbon coordinates. *Proteins* **14,** 465–474.
133. Payne, P. W. (1993) Reconstruction of protein conformations from estimated positions of the C alpha coordinates. *Protein Sci.* **2,** 315–324.
134. Mandal, C. and Linthicum, D. S. (1993) PROGEN: an automated modelling algorithm for the generation of complete protein structures from the alpha-carbon atomic coordinates. *J. Comput. Aided Mol. Des.* **7,** 199–224.
135. Mathiowetz, A. M. and Goddard, W. A. 3rd. (1995) Building proteins from C alpha coordinates using the dihedral probability grid Monte Carlo method. *Protein Sci.* **4,** 1217–1232.
136. Mendes, J., Nagarajaram, H. A., Soares, C. M., Blundell, T. L., and Carrondo, M. A. (2001) Incorporating knowledge-based biases into an energy-based side-chain modeling method: application to comparative modeling of protein structure. *Biopolymers* **59,** 72–86.
137. Kazmierkiewicz, R., Liwo, A., and Scheraga, H. A. (2003) Addition of side chains to a known backbone with defined side-chain centroids. *Biophys. Chem.* **100,** 261–180.
138. Iwata, Y., Kasuya, A., and Miyamoto, S. (2002) An efficient method for reconstructing protein backbones from alpha-carbon coordinates. *J. Mol. Graph Model.* **21,** 119–128.
139. Adcock, S. A. (2004) Peptide backbone reconstruction using dead-end elimination and a knowledge-based forcefield. *J. Comput. Chem.* **25,** 16–27.
140. Lee, C. and Subbiah, S. (1991) Prediction of protein side-chain conformation by packing optimization. *J. Mol. Biol.* **217,** 373–388.

141. Lasters, I. and Desmet, J. (1993) The fuzzy-end elimination theorem: correctly implementing the side chain placement algorithm based on the dead-end elimination theorem. *Protein Eng.* **6,** 717–22.

142. Wilson, C., Gregoret, L. M., and Agard, D. A. (1993) Modeling side-chain conformation for homologous proteins using an energy-based rotamer search. *J. Mol. Biol.* **229,** 996–1006.

143. Dunbrack, R. L. Jr. and Karplus, M. (1993) Backbone-dependent rotamer library for proteins: application to side-chain prediction. *J. Mol. Biol.* **230,** 543–574.

144. Tanimura, R., Kidera, A., and Nakamura, H. (1994) Determinants of protein side-chain packing. *Protein Sci.* **3,** 2358–2365.

145. Dunbrack, R. L. Jr. and Karplus, M. (1994) Conformational analysis of the backbone-dependent rotamer preferences of protein sidechains. *Nat. Struct. Biol.* **1,** 334–340.

146. Goldstein, R. F. (1994) Efficient rotamer elimination applied to protein side-chains and related spin glasses. *Biophys. J.* **66,** 1335–1340.

147. Keller, D. A., Shibata, M., Marcus, E., Ornstein, R. L., and Rein, R. (1995) Finding the global minimum: a fuzzy end elimination implementation. *Protein Eng.* **8,** 893–904.

148. Lasters, I., De Maeyer, M., and Desmet, J. (1995) Enhanced dead-end elimination in the search for the global minimum energy conformation of a collection of protein side chains. *Protein Eng.* **8,** 815–822.

149. Ogata, K. and Umeyama, H. (1997) Prediction of protein side-chain conformations by principal component analysis for fixed main-chain atoms. *Protein Eng.* **10,** 353–359.

150. Dunbrack, R. L. Jr. and Cohen, F. E. (1997) Bayesian statistical analysis of protein side-chain rotamer preferences. *Protein Sci.* **6,** 1661–1681.

151. Bower, M. J., Cohen, F. E., and Dunbrack, R. L. Jr. (1997) Prediction of protein side-chain rotamers from a backbone-dependent rotamer library: a new homology modeling tool. *J. Mol. Biol.* **267,** 1268–1282.

152. Ogata, K. and Umeyama, H. (1997) Prediction of protein side-chain conformations by principal component analysis for fixed main-chain atoms. *Protein Eng.* **10,** 353–359.

153. De Maeyer, M., Desmet, J., and Lasters, I. (1997) All in one: a highly detailed rotamer library improves both accuracy and speed in the modelling of sidechains by dead-end elimination. *Fold Des.* **2,** 53–66.

154. Tuffery, P., Etchebest, C., and Hazout, S. (1997) Prediction of protein side chain conformations: a study on the influence of backbone accuracy on conformation stability in the rotamer space. *Protein Eng.* **10,** 361–372.

155. Huang, E. S., Koehl, P., Levitt, M., Pappu, R. V., and Ponder, J. W. (1998) Accuracy of side-chain prediction upon near-native protein backbones generated by Ab initio folding methods. *Proteins* **33,** 204–217.

156. Leach, A. R. and Lemon, A. P. (1998) Exploring the conformational space of protein side chains using dead-end elimination and the A* algorithm. *Proteins* **33,** 227–239.

157. Mendes, J., Soares, C. M., and Carrondo, M. A. (1999) Improvement of side-chain modeling in proteins with the self-consistent mean field theory method based on an analysis of the factors influencing prediction. *Biopolymers* **50,** 111–131.

158. Mendes, J., Baptista, A. M., Carrondo, M. A., and Soares, C. M. (1999) Improved modeling of side-chains in proteins with rotamer-based methods: a flexible rotamer model. *Proteins* **37,** 530–543.

159. Samudrala, R., Huang, E. S., Koehl, P., and Levitt, M. (2000) Constructing side chains on near-native main chains for ab initio protein structure prediction. *Protein Eng.* **13,** 453–457.

160. Xiang, Z. and Honig, B. (2001) Extending the accuracy limits of prediction for side-chain conformations. *J. Mol. Biol.* **311,** 421–430.

161. Mendes, J., Nagarajaram, H. A., Soares, C. M., Blundell, T. L., and Carrondo, M. A. (2001) Incorporating knowledge-based biases into an energy-based side-chain modeling method: application to comparative modeling of protein structure. *Biopolymers* **59**, 72–86.

162. Looger, L. L. and Hellinga, H. W. (2001) Generalized dead-end elimination algorithms make large-scale protein side-chain structure prediction tractable: implications for protein design and structural genomics. *J. Mol. Biol.* **307**, 429–445.

163. Liang, S. and Grishin, N. V. (2002) Side-chain modeling with an optimized scoring function. *Protein Sci.* **11**, 322–331.

164. Liu, Z., Jiang, L., Gao, Y., Liang, S., Chen, H., Han, Y., and Lai, L. (2003) Beyond the rotamer library: genetic algorithm combined with the disturbing mutation process for up-building protein side-chains. *Proteins* **50**, 49–62.

165. Gordon, D. B., Hom, G. K., Mayo, S. L., and Pierce, N. A. (2003) Exact rotamer optimization for protein design. *J. Comput. Chem.* **24**, 232–243.

166. Desmet, J., Spriet, J., and Lasters, I. (2002) Fast and accurate side-chain topology and energy refinement (FASTER) as a new method for protein structure optimization. *Proteins* **48**, 31–43.

167. Bolon, D. N., Marcus, J. S., Ross, S. A., and Mayo, S. L. (2003) Prudent modeling of core polar residues in computational protein design. *J. Mol. Biol.* **329**, 611–622.

168. Canutescu, A. A., Shelenkov, A. A., and Dunbrack, R. L. Jr. (2003) A graph-theory algorithm for rapid protein side-chain prediction. *Protein Sci.* **12**, 2001–2014.

169. Peterson, R. W., Dutton, P. L., and Wand, A. J. (2004) Improved side-chain prediction accuracy using an ab initio potential energy function and a very large rotamer library. *Protein Sci.* **13**, 735–751.

170. Shetty, R. P., De Bakker, P. I., DePristo, M. A., and Blundell, T. L. (2003) Advantages of fine-grained side chain conformer libraries. *Protein Eng.* **16**, 963–969.

171. DePristo, M. A., De Bakker, P. I., Shetty, R. P., and Blundell, T. L. (2003) Discrete restraint-based protein modeling and the Calpha-trace problem. *Protein Sci.* **12**, 2032–2046.

172. DePristo, M. A., de Bakker, P. I., Lovell, S. C., and Blundell, T. L. (2003) Ab initio construction of polypeptide fragments: efficient generation of accurate, representative ensembles. *Proteins* **51**, 41–55.

173. de Bakker, P. I., DePristo, M. A., Burke, D. F., and Blundell, T. L. (2003) Ab initio construction of polypeptide fragments: accuracy of loop decoy discrimination by an all-atom statistical potential and the AMBER force field with the Generalized Born solvation model. *Proteins* **51**, 21–40.

174. Lorber, D. M. and Shoichet, B. K. (1998) Flexible ligand docking using conformational ensembles. *Protein Sci.* **7**, 938–950.

175. Claussen, H., Buning, C., Rarey, M., and Lengauer, T. (2001) FlexE: efficient molecular docking considering protein structure variations. *J. Mol. Biol.* **308**, 377–395.

176. Kumar, S. and Nussinov, R. (2002) Relationship between ion pair geometries and electrostatic strengths in proteins. *Biophys. J.* **83**, 1595–1612.

177. Lorber, D. M., Udo, M. K., and Shoichet, B. K. (2002) Protein-protein docking with multiple residue conformations and residue substitutions. *Protein Sci.* **11**, 1393–1408.

178. Evers, A., Gohlke, H., and Klebe, G. (2003) Ligand-supported homology modelling of protein binding-sites using knowledge-based potentials. *J. Mol. Biol.* **334**, 327–345.

179. Kallblad, P. and Dean, P. M. (2003) Efficient conformational sampling of local side-chain flexibility. *J. Mol. Biol.* **326**, 1651–1665.

180. Bass, M. B., Hopkins, D. F., Jaquysh, W. A., and Ornstein, R. L. (1992) A method for determining the positions of polar hydrogens added to a protein structure that maximizes protein hydrogen bonding. *Proteins* **12,** 266–277.
181. McDonald, I. K. and Thornton, J. M. (1995) The application of hydrogen bonding analysis in X-ray crystallography to help orientate asparagine, glutamine and histidine side chains. *Protein Eng.* **8,** 217–224.
182. Hooft, R. W., Sander, C., and Vriend, G. (1996) Positioning hydrogen atoms by optimizing hydrogen-bond networks in protein structures. *Proteins* **26,** 363–376.
183. Garcia-Sosa, A. T., Mancera, R. L., and Dean, P. M. (2003) WaterScore: a novel method for distinguishing between bound and displaceable water molecules in the crystal structure of the binding site of protein-ligand complexes. *J. Mol. Model* **9,** 172–182.
184. Poornima, C. S. and Dean, P. M. (1995) Hydration in drug design. 2. Influence of local site surface shape on water binding. *J. Comput. Aided Mol. Des.* **9,** 513–520.
185. Poornima, C. S. and Dean, P. M. (1995) Hydration in drug design. 3. Conserved water molecules at the ligand-binding sites of homologous proteins. *J. Comput. Aided Mol. Des.* **9,** 521–531.
186. Raymer, M. L., Sanschagrin, P. C., Punch, W. F., Venkataraman, S., Goodman, E. D., and Kuhn, L. A. (1997) Predicting conserved water-mediated and polar ligand interactions in proteins using a K-nearest-neighbors genetic algorithm. *J. Mol. Biol.* **265,** 445–464.
187. Rarey, M., Kramer, B., and Lengauer, T. (1999) The particle concept: placing discrete water molecules during protein-ligand docking predictions. *Proteins* **34,** 17–28.
188. Meiering, E. M. and Wagner, G. (1995) Detection of long-lived bound water molecules in complexes of human dihydrofolate reductase with methotrexate and NADPH. *J. Mol. Biol.* **247,** 294–308.
189. Pitt, W. R. and Goodfellow, J. M. (1991) Modelling of solvent positions around polar groups in proteins. *Protein Eng.* **4,** 531–537.
190. Wade, R. C., Bohr, H., and Wolynes, P. G. (1992) Prediction of water binding-sites on proteins by neural networks. *J. Am. Chem. Soc.* **114,** 8284–8285.
191. Pitt, W. R., Murrayrust, J., and Goodfellow, J. M. (1993) Aquarius2—knowledge-based modeling of solvent sites around proteins. *J. Comp. Chem.* **14,** 1007–1018.
192. Roe, S. M. and Teeter, M. M. (1993) Patterns for prediction of hydration around polar residues in proteins. *J. Mol. Biol.* **229,** 419–427.
193. Goodfellow, J. M., Pitt, W. R., Smart, O. S., and Williams, M. A. (1995) New methods for the analysis of the protein solvent interface. *Comp. Phys. Commun.* **91,** 321–329.
194. Ehrlich, L., Reczko, M., Bohr, H., and Wade, R. C. (1998) Prediction of protein hydration sites from sequence by modular neural networks. *Protein Eng.* **11,** 11–19.
195. Raymer, M. L., Sanschagrin, P. C., Punch, W. F., Venkataraman, S., Goodman, E. D., and Kuhn, L. A. (1997) Predicting conserved water-mediated and polar ligand interactions in proteins using a K-nearest-neighbors genetic algorithm. *J. Mol. Biol.* **265,** 445–464.
196. Word, J. M., Lovell, S. C., Richardson, J. S., and Richardson, D. C. (1999) Asparagine and glutamine: using hydrogen atom contacts in the choice of side-chain amide orientation. *J. Mol. Biol.* **285,** 1735–1747.
197. Word, J. M., Lovell, S. C., LaBean, et al. (1999) Visualizing and quantifying molecular goodness-of-fit: small-probe contact dots with explicit hydrogen atoms. *J. Mol. Biol.* **285,** 1711–1733.
198. Laskowski, R. A., MacArthur, M. W., Moss, D. S., and Thornton, J. M. (1993) PROCHECK: a program to check the stereochemical quality of protein structures. *J. Appl. Crystallogr.* **26,** 283–291.

199. Pontius, J., Richelle, J., and Wodak, S. (1996) Deviations from standard atomic volumes as a quality measure for protein crystal structures. *J. Mol. Biol.* **264,** 121–136.

200. Hooft, R. W. W., Sander, C., and Vriend, G. (1997) Objectively judging the quality of a protein structure from a Ramachandran plot. *CABIOS* **13,** 425–430.

201. Nielsen, J. E., Andersen, K. V., Honig, B., et al. (1999) Improving macromolecular electrostatics calculations. *Protein Eng.* **12,** 657–662.

202. Nielsen, J. E. and Vriend, G. (2001) Optimizing the hydrogen-bond network in Poisson-Boltzmann equation-based pK(a) calculations. *Proteins* **43,** 403–412.

203. Forsyth, W. R., Antosiewicz, J. M., and Robertson, A. D. (2002) Empirical relationships between protein structure and carboxyl pKa values in proteins. *Proteins* **48,** 388–403.

204. Edgcomb, S. P. and Murphy, K. P. (2002) Variability in the pKa of histidine side-chains correlates with burial within proteins. *Proteins* **49,** 1–6.

205. Harris, T. K. and Turner, G. J. (2002) Structural basis of perturbed pKa values of catalytic groups in enzyme active sites. *IUBMB Life* **53,** 85–98.

206. Warshel, A. (1981) Calculations of enzymatic reactions: calculations of pKa, proton transfer reactions, and general acid catalysis reactions in enzymes. *Biochemistry* **20,** 3167–3177.

207. Bashford, D. and Karplus, M. (1990) pKa's of ionizable groups in proteins: atomic detail from a continuum electrostatic model. *Biochemistry* **29,** 10,219–10,225.

208. Gilson, M. K. (1993) Multiple-site titration and molecular modeling: two rapid methods for computing energies and forces for ionizable groups in proteins. *Proteins* **15,** 266–282.

209. Demchuk, E., Mueller, T., Oschkinat, H., Sebald, W., and Wade, R. C. (1994) Receptor binding properties of four-helix-bundle growth factors deduced from electrostatic analysis. *Protein Sci.* **3,** 920–935.

210. Nielsen, J. E., Borchert, T. V., and Vriend, G. (2001) The determinants of alpha-amylase pH-activity profiles. *Protein Eng.* **14,** 505–512.

211. Mehler, E. L. and Guarnieri, F. (1999) A self-consistent, microenvironment modulated screened coulomb potential approximation to calculate pH-dependent electrostatic effects in proteins. *Biophys. J.* **77,** 3–22.

212. Sandberg, L. and Edholm, O. (1999) A fast and simple method to calculate protonation states in proteins. *Proteins* **36,** 474–483.

213. Nicholls, A. and Honig, B. (1991) A rapid finite difference algorithm, utilizing successive over-relaxation to solve the Poisson-Boltzmann equation. *J. Comput. Chem.* **12,** 435–445.

214. Madura, J. D., Briggs, J. M., Wade, R. C., et al. (1995) Electrostatics and diffusion of molecules in solution: simulations with the University of Houston Brownian Dynamics program. *Comput. Phys. Commun.* **81,** 57–95.

215. Baker, N. A., Sept, D., Joseph, S., Holst, M. J., and McCammon, J. A. (2001) Electrostatics of nanosystems: application to microtubules and the ribosome. *Proc. Natl. Acad. Sci. USA* **98,** 10,037–10,041.

216. Nicklaus, M. C., Milne, G. W., and Zaharevitz, D. (1993) Chem-X and CAMBRIDGE: comparison of computer generated chemical structures with X-ray crystallographic data. *J. Chem. Inf. Comput. Sci.* **33,** 639–646.

217. Nicklaus, M. C., Wang, S., Driscoll, J. S., and Milne, G. W. (1995) Conformational changes of small molecules binding to proteins. *Bioorg. Med. Chem.* **3,** 411–428.

218. Bostrom, J., Norrby, P. O., and Liljefors, T. (1998) Conformational energy penalties of protein-bound ligands. *J. Comput.-Aided Mol. Des.* **12,** 383–936.

219. Moodie, S. L. and Thornton, J. M. (1993) A study into the effects of protein binding on nucleotide conformation. *Nucleic Acids Res.* **21,** 1369–1380.

220. Fradera, X., De La Cruz, X., Silva, C. H., Gelpi, J. L., Luque, F. J., and Orozco, M. (2002) Ligand-induced changes in the binding sites of proteins. *Bioinformatics* **18**, 939–948.

221. Terwilliger, T. C., Park, M. S., Waldo, G. S., et al. (2003) The TB structural genomics consortium: a resource for Mycobacterium tuberculosis biology. *Tuberculosis* **83**, 223–249.

222. Whisstock, J. C. and Lesk, A. M. (2003) Prediction of protein function from protein sequence and structure. *Q. Rev. Biophys.* **36**, 307–340.

223. Cramer, R. D. 3rd, Patterson, D. E., and Bunce, J. D. (1989) Recent advances in comparative molecular field analysis (CoMFA). *Prog. Clin. Biol. Res.* **291**, 161–165.

224. Goodford, P. J. (1985) A computational procedure for determining energetically favorable binding sites on biologically important macromolecules. *J. Med. Chem.* **28**, 849–857.

225. Takano, Y., Koizumi, M., Takarada, R., Kamimura, M. T., Czerminski, R., and Koike, T. (2003) Computer-aided design of a factor Xa inhibitor by using MCSS functionality maps and a CAVEAT linker search *J. Mol. Graph. Model.* **22**, 105–114.

226. Bliznyuk, A. A. and Gready, J. E. (1998) Identification and energetic ranking of possible docking sites for pterin on dihydrofolate reductase. *J. Comput. Aided Mol. Des.* **12**, 325–333.

227. Bliznyuk, A. A. and Gready, J. E. (1999) Simple method for locating possible ligand binding sites on protein surfaces. *J. Comput. Chem.* **20**, 983–988.

228. Flower, D. R. (1997) SERF: a program for accessible surface area calculations. *J. Mol. Graph. Model.* **15**, 238–244.

229. Connolly, M. L. (1983) Solvent-accessible surfaces of proteins and nucleic acids. *Science* **221**, 709–713.

230. Silla, E., Villar, F., Nilsson, O., Pascual-Ahuir, J. L., and Tapia, O. (1990) Molecular volumes and surfaces of biomacromolecules via GEPOL: a fast and efficient algorithm. *J. Mol. Graph.* **8**, 168–172.

231. Connolly, M. L. (1985) Molecular-surface triangulation. *J. Appl. Crystallogr.* **18**, 499–505.

232. Heiden, W., Moeckel, G., and Brickmann, J. (1993) A new approach to analysis and display of local lipophilicity/hydrophilicity mapped on molecular surfaces. *J. Comput. Aided Mol. Des.* **7**, 503–514.

233. Honig, B. and Nicholls, A. (1995) Classical electrostatics in biology and chemistry. *Science* **268**, 1144–1149.

234. Nicholls, A., Sharp, K. A., and Honig, B. (1991) Protein folding and association: insights from the interfacial and thermodynamic properties of hydrocarbons. *Proteins* **11**, 281–296.

235. Scarsi, M., Majeux, N., and Caflisch, A. (1999) Hydrophobicity at the surface of proteins. *Proteins* **37**, 565–575.

236. Kellogg, G. E., Semus, S. F., and Abraham, D. J. (1991) HINT: a new method of empirical hydrophobic field calculation for CoMFA. *J. Comput. Aided Mol. Des.* **5**, 545–552.

237. Hendlich, M., Rippmann, F., and Barnickel, G. (1997) LIGSITE: automatic and efficient detection of potential small-molecule binding sites in proteins. *J. Mol. Graph. Model.* **15**, 359–363.

238. Levitt, D. G. and Banaszak, L. J. (1992) POCKET: a computer graphics method for identifying and displaying protein cavities and their surrounding amino acids. *J. Mol. Graph.* **10**, 229–234.

239. Peters, K. P., Fauck, J., and Frommel, C. (1996) The automatic search for ligand binding sites in proteins of known three-dimensional structure using only geometric criteria. *J. Mol. Biol.* **256**, 201–213.

240. Liang, J., Edelsbrunner, H., and Woodward, C. (1998) Anatomy of protein pockets and cavities: measurement of binding site geometry and implications for ligand design. *Protein Sci.* **7**, 1884–1897.

241. Brady, G. P. Jr. and Stouten, P. F. (2000) Fast prediction and visualization of protein binding pockets with PASS. *J. Comput. Aided Mol. Des.* **14**, 383–401.
242. Boobbyer, D. N., Goodford, P. J., McWhinnie, P. M., and Wade, R. C. (1989) New hydrogen-bond potentials for use in determining energetically favorable binding sites on molecules of known structure. *J. Med. Chem.* **32**, 1083–1094.
243. Wade, R. C. and Goodford, P. J. (1993) Further development of hydrogen bond functions for use in determining energetically favorable binding sites on molecules of known structure. 2. Ligand probe groups with the ability to form more than two hydrogen bonds. *J. Med. Chem.* **36**, 148–156.
244. Wade, R. C., Clark, K. J., and Goodford, P. J. (1993) Further development of hydrogen bond functions for use in determining energetically favorable binding sites on molecules of known structure. 1. Ligand probe groups with the ability to form two hydrogen bonds. *J. Med. Chem.* **36**, 140–147.
245. Klebe, G., Abraham, U., and Mietzner, T. (1994) Molecular similarity indices in a comparative analysis (CoMSIA) of drug molecules to correlate and predict their biological activity. *J. Med. Chem.* **37**, 4130–4146.
246. Blomberg, N., Gabdoulline, R. R., Nilges, M., and Wade, R. C. (1999) Classification of protein sequences by homology modeling and quantitative analysis of electrostatic similarity. *Proteins* **37**, 379–387.
247. Kastenholz, M. A., Pastor, M., Cruciani, G., Haaksma, E. E., and Fox, T. (2000) GRID/CPCA: a new computational tool to design selective ligands. *J. Med. Chem.* **43**, 3033–3044.
248. Ridderstrom, M., Zamora, I., Fjellstrom, O., and Andersson, T. B. (2001) Analysis of selective regions in the active sites of human cytochromes P450, 2C8, 2C9, 2C18, and 2C19 homology models using GRID/CPCA. *J. Med. Chem.* **44**, 4072–4081.
249. Terp, G. E., Cruciani, G., Christensen, I. T., and Jorgensen, F. S. (2002) Structural differences of matrix metalloproteinases with potential implications for inhibitor selectivity examined by the GRID/CPCA approach. *J. Med. Chem.* **45**, 2675–2684.
250. Ji, H., Li, H., Flinspach, M., Poulos, T. L., and Silverman, R. B. (2003) Computer modeling of selective regions in the active site of nitric oxide synthases: implication for the design of isoform-selective inhibitors. *J. Med. Chem.* **46**, 5700–5711.
251. Naumann, T. and Matter, H. (2002) Structural classification of protein kinases using 3D molecular interaction field analysis of their ligand binding sites: target family landscapes. *J. Med. Chem.* **45**, 2366–2378.
252. Myshkin, E. and Wang, B. (2003) Chemometrical classification of ephrin ligands and Eph kinases using GRID/CPCA approach. *J. Chem. Inf. Comput. Sci.* **43**, 1004–1010.
253. Kurz, M., Brachvogel, V., Matter, H., Stengelin, S., Thuring, H., and Kramer, W. (2003) Insights into the bile acid transportation system: the human ileal lipid-binding protein-cholyltaurine complex and its comparison with homologous structures. *Proteins* **50**, 312–328.
254. Doytchinova, I. A., Guan, P., and Flower, D. R. (2004) Identifiying human MHC supertypes using bioinformatic methods. *J. Immunol.* **172**, 4314–4323.
255. Joseph-McCarthy, D., Hogle, J. M., and Karplus, M. (1997) Use of the multiple copy simultaneous search (MCSS) method to design a new class of picornavirus capsid binding drugs. *Proteins* **29**, 32–58.
256. Miranker, A. and Karplus, M. (1991) Functionality maps of binding sites: a multiple copy simultaneous search method. *Proteins* **11**, 29–34.
257. Miranker, A. and Karplus, M. (1995) An automated method for dynamic ligand design. *Proteins* **23**, 472–490.

258. Stultz, C. M. and Karplus, M. (2000) Dynamic ligand design and combinatorial optimization: designing inhibitors to endothiapepsin. *Proteins* **40,** 258–289.

259. Stultz, C. M. and Karplus, M. (1999) MCSS functionality maps for a flexible protein. *Proteins* **37,** 512–529.

260. Gohlke, H., Hendlich, M., and Klebe, G. (2000) Predicting binding modes, binding affinities and 'hot spots' for protein–ligand complexes using a knowledge-based scoring function. *Perspect. Drug Discov. Des.* **20,** 115–144.

261. Ringe, D. and Mattos, C. (1999) Analysis of the binding surfaces of proteins. *Med. Res. Rev.* **19,** 321–331.

262. English, A. C., Done, S. H., Caves, L. S., Groom, C. R., and Hubbard, R. E. (1999) Locating interaction sites on proteins: the crystal structure of thermolysin soaked in 2% to 100% isopropanol. *Proteins* **37,** 628–640.

263. English, A. C., Groom, C. R., and Hubbard, R. E. (2001) Experimental and computational mapping of the binding surface of a crystalline protein. *Protein Eng.* **14,** 47–59.

264. Byerly, D. W., McElroy, C. A., and Foster, M. P. (2002) Mapping the surface of Escherichia coli peptide deformylase by NMR with organic solvents. *Protein Sci.* **11,** 1850–1853.

265. Joseph-McCarthy, D., Fedorov, A. A., and Almo, S. C. (1996) Comparison of experimental and computational functional group mapping of an RNase A structure: implications for computer-aided drug design. *Protein Eng.* **9,** 773–780.

266. Klebe, G. (1994) The use of composite crystal-field environments in molecular recognition and the de novo design of protein ligands. *J. Mol. Biol.* **237,** 212–235.

267. Boehm, H. J. (1992) The computer program LUDI: a new method for the de novo design of enzyme inhibitors. *J. Comput. Aided Mol. Des.* **6,** 61–78.

268. Boehm, H. J. (1992) LUDI: rule-based automatic design of new substituents for enzyme inhibitor leads. *J. Comput. Aided Mol. Des.* **6,** 593–606.

269. Verdonk, M. L., Cole, J. C., and Taylor, R. (1999) SUPERSTAR: a knowledge based approach for identifying interaction sites in proteins. *J. Mol. Biol.* **289,** 1093–1108.

270. Verdonk, M. L., Cole, J. C., Watson, P., Gillet, V., and Willett, P. (2001) SUPERSTAR: improved knowledge-based interaction fields for protein binding sites. *J. Mol. Biol.* **307,** 841–859.

271. Laskowski, R. A, Thornton, J. M., Humblet, C., and Singh, J. (1996) X-SITE: use of empirically derived atomic packing preferences to identify favourable interaction regions in the binding sites of proteins. *J. Mol. Biol.* **259,** 175–201.

272. Bliznyuk, A. A. and Gready, J. E. (1998) Identification and energetic ranking of possible docking sites for pterin on dihydrofolate reductase. *J. Comput. Aided Mol. Des.* **12,** 325–333.

273. Bliznyuk, A. A. and Gready, J. E. (1999) Simple method for locating possible ligand binding sites on protein surfaces. *J. Comput. Chem.* **20,** 983–988.

274. Ruppert, J., Welch, W., and Jain, A. N. (1997) Automatic identification and representation of protein binding sites for molecular docking. *Protein Sci.* **6,** 524–533.

275. Radmer, R. J. and Kollman, P. A. (1998) The application of three approximate free energy calculations methods to structure based ligand design: trypsin and its complex with inhibitors. *J. Comput. Aided Mol. Des.* **12,** 215–227.

276. Pearlman, D. A. and Charifson, P. S. (2001) Improved scoring of ligand-protein interactions using OWFEG free energy grids. *J. Med. Chem.* **44,** 502–511.

277. Shoichet, B. K. and Kuntz, I. D. (1993) Matching chemistry and shape in molecular docking. *Protein Eng.* **6,** 223–232.

278. Goodsell, D. S., Morris, G. M., and Olson, A. J. (1996) Docking of flexible ligands: applications of autodock. *J. Mol. Recognit.* **9,** 1–5.

279. Rarey, M., Kramer, B., Lengauer, T., and Klebe, G. (1996) Predicting receptor-ligand interactions by an incremental construction algorithm. *J. Mol. Biol.* **261,** 470–489.

280. Shoichet, B. K., Stroud, R. M., Santi, D. V., Kuntz, I. D., and Perry, K. M. (1993) Structure-based discovery of inhibitors of thymidylate synthase. *Science* **259,** 1445–1450.

281. Burkhard, P., Taylor, P., and Walkinshaw, M. D. (1998) An example of a protein ligand found by database mining: description of the docking method and its verification by a 2.3 A X-ray structure of a thrombin-ligand complex. *J. Mol. Biol.* **277,** 449–466.

282. Janin, J. (1995) Elusive affinities. *Proteins Biol.* **21,** 30–39.

283. Tokarski, J. and Hopfinger, A. J. (1997) Constructing protein models for ligand-receptor binding thermodynamic simulations. *J. Chem. Inf. Comput. Sci.* **37,** 779–791.

284. Horvath, D. (1997) A virtual screening approach applied to the search for trypanothione reductase inhibitors. *J. Med. Chem.* **40,** 2412–2423.

285. Lipinski, C. A. (2000) Drug-like properties and the causes of poor solubility and poor permeability. *J. Pharmacol. Toxicol. Methods* **44,** 235–249.

286. Wenlock, M. C., Austin, R. P., Barton, P., Davis, A. M., and Leeson, P. D. (2003) A comparison of physiochemical property profiles of development and marketed oral drugs. *J. Med. Chem.* **46,** 1250–1256.

287. Bissantz, C., Bernard, P., Hibert, M., and Rognan, D. (2003) Protein-based virtual screening of chemical databases. II. Are homology models of G-protein coupled receptors suitable targets? *Proteins* **50,** 5–25.

288. Evers, A. and Klebe, G. (2004) Ligand-supported homology modeling of G-protein-coupled receptor sites: models sufficient for successful virtual screening. *Angew Chem. Int. Ed. Engl.* **43,** 248–251.

289. Bostrom, J. (2001) Reproducing the conformations of protein-bound ligands: a critical evaluation of several popular conformational searching tools. *J. Comput. Aided Mol. Des.* **15,** 1137–1152.

290. Bostrom, J., Greenwood, J. R., and Gottfries, J. (2003) Assessing the performance of OMEGA with respect to retrieving bioactive conformations. *J. Mol. Graph. Model* **21,** 449–462.

291. Anderson, A. C., O'Neil, R. H., Surti, T. S., and Stroud, R. M. (2001) Approaches to solving the rigid receptor problem by identifying a minimal set of flexible residues during ligand docking. *Chem. Biol.* **8,** 445–457.

292. Leach, A. R. (1994) Ligand docking to proteins with discrete side-chain flexibility. *J. Mol. Biol.* **235,** 345–356.

293. Lawrence, M. C. and Davis, P. C. (1992) CLIX: a search algorithm for finding novel ligands capable of binding proteins of known three-dimensional structure. *Proteins* **12,** 31–41.

294. Glick, M., Grant, G. H., and Richards, W. G. (2002) Docking of flexible molecules using multiscale ligand representations. *J. Med. Chem.* **45,** 4639–4646.

295. Glick, M., Robinson, D. D., Grant, G. H., and Richards, W. G. (2002) Identification of ligand binding sites on proteins using a multi-scale approach. *J. Am. Chem. Soc.* **124,** 2337–2344.

296. Gohlke, H. and Klebe, G. (2001) Statistical potentials and scoring functions applied to protein-ligand binding. *Curr. Opin. Struct. Biol.* **11,** 231–235.

297. Morris, G. M., Goodsell, D. S., Huey, R., and Olson, A. J. (1996) Distributed automated docking of flexible ligands to proteins: parallel applications of AUTODOCK 2.4. *J. Comput. Aided Mol. Des.* **10,** 293–304.

298. Morris, G. M., Goodsell, D. S., Halliday, R. S., et al. (1998) Automated docking using a Lamarckian genetic algorithm and an empirical binding free energy function. *J. Comput. Chem.* **19,** 1639–1662.

299. Totrov, M. and Abagyan, R. (2001) Protein-ligand docking as an energy optimization problem, in *Drug-Receptor Thermodynamics: Introduction and Applications* (Raffa, R. B., ed.), Wiley, Chichester, UK, 603–624.

300. Meng, E. C., Shoichet, B. K., and Kuntz, I. D. (1992) Automated docking with grid-based energy evaluation. *J. Comput. Chem.* **13,** 505–523.

301. Ewing, T. J., Makino, S., Skillman, A. G., and Kuntz, I. D. (2001) DOCK 4.0: search strategies for automated molecular docking of flexible molecule databases. *J. Comput. Aided Mol. Des.* **15,** 411–428.

302. Trosset, J. Y. and Scheraga, H. A. (1999) PRODOCK: software package for protein modeling and docking. *J. Comput. Chem.* **20,** 412–427.

303. Bohm, H. J. (1994) The development of a simple empirical scoring function to estimate the binding constant for a protein-ligand complex of known three-dimensional structure. *J. Comput. Aided Mol. Des.* **8,** 243–256.

304. Bohm, H. J. (1998) Prediction of binding constants of protein ligands: a fast method for the prioritization of hits obtained from de novo design or 3D database search programs. *J. Comput. Aided Mol. Des.* **12,** 309–323.

305. Eldridge, M. D., Murray, C. W., Auton, T. R., Paolini, G. V., and Mee, R. P. (1997) Empirical scoring functions: I. The development of a fast empirical scoring function to estimate the binding affinity of ligands in receptor complexes. *J. Comput. Aided Mol. Des.* **11,** 425–445.

306. Jones, G., Willett, P., Glen, R. C., Leach, A. R., and Taylor, R. (1997) Development and validation of a genetic algorithm for flexible docking. *J. Mol. Biol.* **267,** 727–748.

307. Aqvist, J., Medina, C., and Samuelsson, J. E. (1994) A new method for predicting binding affinity in computer-aided drug design. *Protein Eng.* **7,** 385–391.

308. Rognan, D., Lauemoller, S. L., Holm, A., Buus, S., and Tschinke, V. (1999) Predicting binding affinities of protein ligands from three-dimensional models: application to peptide binding to class I major histocompatibility proteins. *J. Med. Chem.* **42,** 4650–4658.

309. Logean, A., Sette, A., and Rognan, D. (2001) Customized versus universal scoring functions: application to class I MHC-peptide binding free energy predictions. *Bioorg. Med. Chem. Lett.* **11,** 675–679.

310. McMartin, C. and Bohacek, R. S. (1995) Flexible matching of test ligands to a 3D pharmacophore using a molecular superposition force field: comparison of predicted and experimental conformations of inhibitors of three enzymes. *J. Comput. Aided Mol. Des.* **9,** 237–250.

311. Kasper, P., Christen, P., and Gehring, H. (2000) Empirical calculation of the relative free energies of peptide binding to the molecular chaperone DnaK. *Proteins* **40,** 185–192.

312. Head, R. D., Smythe, M. L., Oprea, T. I., et al. (1996) VALIDATE—a new method for the receptor-based prediction of binding affinities of novel ligands. *J. Am. Chem. Soc.* **118,** 3959–3969.

313. Vedani, A., Zbinden, P., and Snyder, J. P. (1993) Pseudo-receptor modelling: a new concept for the three-dimensional construction of receptor binding sites. *J. Receptor Res.* **13,** 163–177.

314. Zbinden, P., Dobler, M., Folkers, G., and Vedani, A. (1998) PRGEN—pseudoreceptor modelling using receptor-mediated ligand alignment and pharmacophore equilibration. *Quant. Struct.-Activity Relationships* **17,** 122–130.

315. Nobeli, I., Mitchell, J. B. O., Alex, A., and Thornton, J. M. (2001) Evaluation of a knowledge-based potential of mean force for scoring docked protein-ligand complexes. *J. Comput. Chem.* **22,** 673–688.

316. Davies, E. K. and Richards, W. G. (2002) The potential of internet computing for drug discovery. *Drug Discov. Today* **7**, S99–S103.

317. Richards, W. G. (2002) Virtual screening using grid computing: the screensaver project. *Nat. Rev. Drug Discov.* **1**, 551–555.

318. So, S. S. and Karplus, M. (1999) Comparative study of ligand-receptor complex binding affinity prediction methods based on glycogen phosphorylase inhibitors. *J. Comput. Aided Mol. Des.* **13**, 243–258.

319. Charifson, P. S., Corkery, J. J., Murcko, M. A., and Walters, W. P. (1999) Consensus scoring: a method for obtaining improved hit rates from docking databases of three-dimensional structures into proteins. *J. Med. Chem.* **42**, 5100–5109.

320. Gehlhaar, D. K., Verkhivker, G. M., Rejto, P. A., et al. (1995) Molecular recognition of the inhibitor AG-1343 by HIV-1 protease: conformationally flexible docking by evolutionary programming. *Chem. Biol.* **2**, 317–324.

321. Stahl, M. and Rarey, M. (2001) Detailed analysis of scoring functions for virtual screening. *J. Med. Chem.* **44**, 1035–1042.

322. Terp, G. E., Johansen, B. N., Christensen, I. T., and Jorgensen, F. S. (2001) A new concept for multidimensional selection of ligand conformations (MultiSelect) and multidimensional scoring (MultiScore) of protein-ligand binding affinities. *J. Med. Chem.* **44**, 2333–2343.

323. Froloff, N., Windemuth, A., and Honig, B. (1997) On the calculation of binding free energies using continuum methods: application to MHC class I protein-peptide interactions. *Protein Sci.* **6**, 1293–1301.

324. Hoffmann, D., Kramer, B., Washio, T., Steinmetzer, T., Rarey, M., and Lengauer, T. (1999) Two-stage method for protein-ligand docking. *J. Med. Chem.* **42**, 4422–4433.

325. Polticelli, F., Ascenzi, P., Bolognesi, M., and Honig, B. (1999) Structural determinants of trypsin affinity and specificity for cationic inhibitors. *Protein Sci.* **8**, 2621–2629.

326. Zou, X., Sun, Y., and Kuntz, I. D. (1999) Inclusion of solvation in ligand binding free energy calculations using the generalized-born model. *J. Am. Chem. Soc.* **121**, 8033–8043.

327. Still, W. C., Tempczyk, A., Hawley, R. C., and Hendrickson, T. (1990) Semianalytical treatment of solvation for molecular mechanics and dynamics. *J. Am. Chem. Soc.* **112**, 6127–6129.

328. Kollman, P. A., Massova, I., Reyes, C., et al. (2000) Calculating structures and free energies of complex molecules: combining molecular mechanics and continuum models. *Acc. Chem. Res.* **33**, 889–897.

329. Gouda, H., Kuntz, I. D., Case, D. A., and Kollman, P. A. (2003) Free energy calculations for theophylline binding to an RNA aptamer: comparison of MM-PBSA and thermodynamic integration methods. *Biopolymers* **68**, 16–34.

330. Srinivasan, J., Cheatham, T. E. III, Cieplak, P., Kollman, P. A., and Case, D. A. (1998) Continuum solvent studies of the stability of DNA, RNA, and phosphoramidate-DNA helices. *J. Am. Chem. Soc.* **120**, 9401–9409.

331. Zhang, W., Hou, T., Qiao, X., and Xu, X. (2003) Parameters for the generalized born model consistent with RESP atomic partial charge assignment protocol. *J. Phys. Chem. B.* **107**, 9071–9078.

332. Rosenfeld, R., Zheng, Q., Vajda, S., and DeLisi, C. (1995) Flexible docking of peptides to class I major-histocompatibility-complex receptors. *Genet. Anal.* **12**, 1–21.

333. Sezerman, U., Vajda, S., and DeLisi, C. (1996) Free energy mapping of class I MHC molecules and structural determination of bound peptides. *Protein Sci.* **5**, 1272–1281.

334. Vasmatzis, G., Zhang, C., Cornette, J. L., and DeLisi, C. (1996) Computational determination of side chain specificity for pockets in class I MHC molecules. *Mol. Immunol.* **33**, 1231–1239.

335. Zhang, C., Cornette, J. L., and Delisi, C. (1997) Consistency in structural energetics of protein folding and peptide recognition. *Protein Sci.* **6**, 1057–1064.

336. Weng, Z. and DeLisi, C. (1998) Toward a predictive understanding of molecular recognition. *Immunol. Rev.* **163**, 251–266.

337. Rognan, D., Reddehase, M. J., Koszinowski, U. H., and Folkers, G. (1992) Molecular modeling of an antigenic complex between a viral peptide and a class I major histocompatibility glycoprotein. *Proteins* **13**, 70–85.

338. Rognan, D., Zimmermann, N., Jung, G., and Folkers, G. (1992) Molecular dynamics study of a complex between the human histocompatibility antigen HLA-A2 and the IMP58-66 nonapeptide from influenza virus matrix protein. *Eur. J. Biochem.* **208**, 101–113.

339. Rognan, D., Scapozza, L., Folkers, G., and Daser, A. (1994) Molecular dynamics simulation of MHC-peptide complexes as a tool for predicting potential T cell epitopes. *Biochemistry* **33**, 11,476–11,485.

340. Kern, P., Brunne, R. M., Rognan, D., and Folkers, G. (1996) A pseudo-particle approach for studying protein-ligand models truncated to their active sites. *Biopolymers* **38**, 619–637.

341. Rognan, D., Krebs, S., Kuonen, O., Lamas, J. R., Lopez de Castro, J. A., and Folkers, G. (1997) Fine specificity of antigen binding to two class I major histocompatibility proteins B*2705 and B*2703) differing in a single amino acid residue. *J. Comput. Aided Mol. Des.* **11**, 463–478.

342. Krebs, S., Rognan, D., and Lopez de Castro, J. A. (1999) Long-range effects in protein—ligand interactions mediate peptide specificity in the human major histocompatibilty antigen HLA-B27 (B*2701). *Protein Sci.* **8**, 1393–1399.

343. Rognan, D., Scapozza, L., Folkers, G., and Daser, A. (1995) Rational design of nonnatural peptides as high-affinity ligands for the HLA-B*2705 human leukocyte antigen. *Proc. Natl. Acad. Sci. USA* **92**, 753–757.

344. Krebs, S. and Rognan, D. (1998) From peptides to peptidomimetics: design of nonpeptide ligands for major histocompatibility proteins. *Pharm. Acta Helv.* **73**, 173–181.

345. Dedier, S., Krebs, S., Lamas, J. R., et al. (1999) Structure-based design of nonnatural ligands for the HLA-B27 protein. *J. Recept. Signal Transduct. Res.* **19**, 645–657.

346. Caflisch, A., Niederer, P., and Anliker, M. (1992) Monte Carlo docking of oligopeptides to proteins. *Proteins* **13**, 223–230.

347. Lim, J. S., Kim, S., Lee, H. G., Lee, K. Y., Kwon, T. J., and Kim, K. (1996) Selection of peptides that bind to the HLA-A2.1 molecule by molecular modelling. *Mol. Immunol.* **33**, 221–230.

348. Androulakis, I. P., Nayak, N. N., Ierapetritou, M. G., Monos, D. S., and Floudas, C. A. (1997) A predictive method for the evaluation of peptide binding in pocket 1 of HLA-DRB1 via global minimization of energy interactions. *Proteins* **29**, 87–102.

349. Toh, H., Kamikawaji, N., Tana, T., Muta, S., Sasazuki, T., and Kuhara, S. (2000) Magnitude of structural changes of the T-cell receptor binding regions determine the strength of T-cell antagonism: molecular dynamics simulations of HLA-DR4 (DRB1*0405) complexed with analogue peptide. *Protein Eng.* **13**, 423–429.

350. Wan, S., Coveney, P., and Flower, D. R. (2004) Large scale molecular dynamics simulations of HLA-A*0201 complexed with a tumour-specific antigenic peptide: can the alpha-3 and beta-2M domains be neglected? *J. Comp. Chem.* **25**, 1803–1813.

351. Grueneberg, S., Wendt, B., and Klebe, G. (2001) Subnanomolar inhibitors from computer screening: a model study using human carbonic anhydrase II. *Angew. Chem. Int. Ed.* **40**, 389–393.

352. Boehm, H. J., Boehringer, M., Bur, D., et al. (2000) Novel inhibitors of DNA gyrase: 3D structure based biased needle screening, hit validation by biophysical methods, and 3D guided optimization. A promising alternative to random screening. *J. Med. Chem.* **43,** 2664–2674.

353. Berman, H. M., Battistuz, T., Bhat, T. N., et al. (2002) The Protein Data Bank. *Acta Crystallogr. D Biol. Crystallogr.* **58,** 899–907.

354. Bourne, P. E., Addess, K. J., Bluhm, W. F., et al. (2004) The distribution and query systems of the RCSB Protein Data Bank. *Nucleic Acids Res.* **32,** D223–D225.

355. Orengo, C. A., Pearl, F. M., Bray, J. E., et al. (1999) The CATH database provides insights into protein structure/function relationships. *Nucleic Acids Res.* **27,** 275–279.

356. Pearl, F., Todd, A. E., Bray, J. E., et al. (2000) Using the CATH domain database to assign structures and functions to the genome sequences. *Biochem. Soc. Trans.* **28,** 269–275.

357. Andreeva, A., Howorth, D., Brenner, S. E., Hubbard, T. J., Chothia, C., and Murzin, A. G. (2004) SCOP database in 2004: refinements integrate structure and sequence family data. *Nucleic Acids Res.* **32,** D226–D229.

358. Bruno, I. J., Cole, J. C., Lommerse, J. P., Rowland, R. S., Taylor, R., and Verdonk, M. L. (1997) ISOSTAR: a library of information about nonbonded interactions. *J. Comput. Aided Mol. Des.* **11,** 525–537.

359. Gunther, J., Bergner, A., Hendlich, M., and Klebe, G. (2003) Utilising structural knowledge in drug design strategies: applications using Relibase. *J. Mol. Biol.* **326,** 621–636.

360. Hendlich, M., Bergner, A., Gunther, J., and Klebe, G. (2003) Relibase: design and development of a database for comprehensive analysis of protein-ligand interactions. *J. Mol. Biol.* **326,** 607–620.

361. Schmitt, S., Kuhn, D., and Klebe, G. (2002) A new method to detect related function among proteins independent of sequence and fold homology. *J. Mol. Biol.* **323,** 387–406.

362. Schmitt, S., Hendlich, M., and Klebe, G. (2001) From structure to function: a new approach to detect functional similarity among proteins independent from sequence and fold homology. *Angew. Chem. Int. Ed.* **40,** 3141–3144.

363. Kinoshita, K., Furui, J., and Nakamura, H. (2002) Identification of protein functions from a molecular surface database, eF-site. *J. Struct. Funct. Genomics* **2,** 9–22.

364. Boutselakis, H., Dimitropoulos, D., Fillon, J., et al. (2003) E-MSD: the European Bioinformatics Institute Macromolecular Structure Database. *Nucleic Acids Res.* **31,** 458–462.

365. Ferre, F., Ausiello, G., Zanzoni, A., and Helmer-Citterich, M. (2004) SURFACE: a database of protein surface regions for functional annotation. *Nucleic Acids Res.* **32,** D240–D244.

366. Porter, C. T., Bartlett, G. J., and Thornton, J. M. (2004) The Catalytic Site Atlas: a resource of catalytic sites and residues identified in enzymes using structural data. *Nucleic Acids Res.* **32,** D129–D133.

367. Stuart, A. C., Ilyin, V. A., and Sali, A. (2002) LigBase: a database of families of aligned ligand binding sites in known protein sequences and structures. *Bioinformatics* **18,** 200–201.

368. Bava, K. A., Gromiha, M. M., Uedaira, H., Kitajima, K., and Sarai, A. (2004) ProTherm, version 4.0: thermodynamic database for proteins and mutants. *Nucleic Acids Res.* **32,** D120–D121.

369. Chen, X., Lin, Y., Liu, M., and Gilson, M. K. (2002) The Binding Database: data management and interface design. *Bioinformatics* **18,** 130–139.

370. Blythe, M. J., Doytchinova, I. A., and Flower, D. R. (2002) JenPep: a database of quantitative functional peptide data for immunology. *Bioinformatics* **18,** 434–439.

371. McSparron, H., Blythe, M. J., Zygouri, C., Doytchinova, I. A., and Flower, D. R. (2003) JenPep: a novel computational information resource for immunobiology and vaccinology. *J. Chem. Inf. Comput. Sci.* **43,** 1276–1287.

372. Salwinski, L., Miller, C. S., Smith, A. J., Pettit, F. K., Bowie, J. U., and Eisenberg, D. (2004) The Database of Interacting Proteins: 2004 update. *Nucleic Acids Res.* **32,** D449–D451.
373. Hermjakob, H., Montecchi-Palazzi, L., Lewington, C., et al. (2004) IntAct: an open source molecular interaction database. *Nucleic Acids Res.* **32,** D452–D455.
374. Clark, D. E., Murray, C. W., and Li, J. (1997) Current issues in de novo molecular design, in *Reviews in Computational Chemistry* (Lipkowitz, K. B. and Boyd, D. B., eds.), Wiley-VCH, New York, pp. 67–125.

13

In Silico Protein Design

Fitting Sequence Onto Structure

Bassil I. Dahiyat

Summary

In the last 10 yr, efforts have begun to combine the goals and approaches of computational molecular design and protein sequence analysis to provide tools for the rational mutagenesis and functional modification of proteins. These approaches use analysis of the three-dimensional structure of a protein to guide the selection of appropriate amino acid sequences to create desired properties or functions. The convergence of low-cost, high-speed computers, a tremendous increase in protein structure information, and a growing understanding of the forces that control protein structure has resulted in dramatic advances in the ability to control protein function and structure and to create the first truly artificial proteins. Various academic software packages have been developed for *in silico* protein design. The methods for selecting the protein structure, defining the portion to be designed, and choosing the input parameters for the software are described in this chapter.

Key Words: Protein design; molecular modeling; computational design; protein engineering; *de novo* protein design; protein stabilization; inverse protein folding; protein stability; protein function design.

1. Introduction

In the early 1980s, Pabo *(1)* introduced the concept of screening protein sequences for their compatibility with a protein structure as a way of designing novel proteins. This idea is called inverse protein folding. The approach starts with a target protein three-dimensional structure and attempts to find sequences that will fold into this structure. By contrast, protein folding attempts to predict the structure into which a particular sequence will fold. A key point of inverse protein folding is the large degeneracy of solutions; a particular protein structure will have an enormous number of sequences that are compatible with it, potentially providing a large set of proteins with different properties that nevertheless take the same fold and perform the same function. This

From: *Methods in Molecular Biology, vol. 316: Bioinformatics and Drug Discovery*
Edited by: R. S. Larson © Humana Press Inc., Totowa, NJ

degeneracy makes inverse folding a much more tractable problem than protein folding, for which the single conformation of a polypeptide has to be found from the vast number of possible chain configurations. Therefore, a complete solution of the inverse folding problem is not necessary because even a small subset of sequence solutions can produce improved proteins. Although discovery of the complete set of sequences for a protein structure is not necessary to design proteins, finding more sequences offers a broader set of protein properties and likely will enhance the performance of the protein against the design goal. Mutagenesis to manipulate protein properties has been undertaken since the creation of tools for molecular cloning, but only in recent years has the inverse protein-folding approach to protein design been tested *(2–4)*. This chapter describes the methods of *in silico* protein design and discusses the practical scope for its use as a generic tool for protein optimization.

The process outline for *in silico* protein design consists of four steps:

1. Defining the design goal in a structural biology context.
2. Defining the structural and conformational variation that will be tested.
3. Applying scoring functions to differentiate the possible sequences.
4. Searching the sequence diversity defined in **steps 1** and **2** for the optimally scoring sequences.

Figure 1 illustrates this process and also points out the critical role that experimental testing of designed sequences plays, both in validating novel sequences and in improving the design methodology. Although feedback from laboratory experiments is necessary for testing designed sequences, it has also been pivotal in development of design methods over the last decade by allowing for the accurate parameterization of potential functions, and the improvement of sequence search techniques.

The first two steps of the process are the role of the user, and although they rely on execution of the particular software package, the strategy for design changes little. All of the *in silico* design packages are based on the same principles and operate very similarly. Some design tasks are more suited to particular software, but availability of the software is more important; there are no commercially available packages, and all *in silico* design software is in a state of continual development in academic laboratories (*see* **Subheading 2.3.**). The methods described in this chapter focus on those aspects that are controlled by the software user attempting to design a protein, and some aspects of the various software packages are described to assist in selecting a particular package.

2. Methods

The following methods outline how to set up *in silico* design calculations by covering design goal translation into desired structural perturbations, definition of the specific conformational and compositional diversity, and selection of the appropriate software package.

2.1. Design Goal Definition

A protein design goal is usually a change in property, such as increased stability, or a modulation of function, such as heightened signaling potency. The first step for *in silico* design is relating this goal to a structural change. Simple examples are increas-

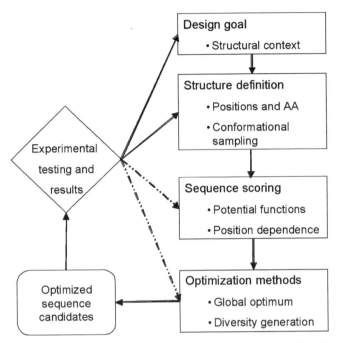

Fig. 1. *In silico* protein design process flow. The functional design goal defines a region of the protein to be manipulated, as well as a molecular context for the calculation such as receptor or substrate complexes. The structure definition provides the details of the residue positions, types of amino acids (AA), and the conformational variation considered for each side chain. Sequence scoring is done by calculating side-chain interaction energies using the potential functions specified for each region of the protein. The sequences with the best combination of interaction energies are then generated, followed by experimental testing. The success or failure of the designed sequences is used not only to improve the particular protein design, but also to improve the scoring functions and performance of optimization methods.

ing the hydrophilicity of the protein surface to increase its solubility, or creating a more selective receptor interaction by modifying the receptor-contacting residues. The structural strategy for design often draws heavily on insights from protein mutagenesis and biophysical work on protein structure function, and often *in silico* design simply allows the more comprehensive, more rapid, and more successful mutagenesis of a protein. However, new frontiers, such as creating completely new protein folds, are possible, (5) or introducing novel activities into a protein (6,7).

2.1.1. Structural Data

One of the challenges in creating effective protein design strategies is the variable, and sometimes limited, structural data available for the protein of interest. The quality of a structural model has a large impact on translation of the design goal into sequence positions and amino acid diversity to be tested; poor structural quality or lack of data on protein structure–function relationships makes it difficult to predict where a protein can be modified or even what structural features need to be changed. For example, lack of knowledge of the binding site of a hormone can make it impossible to modify its surface residues to improve solubility without disrupting its binding function. In addition, the level of information on the structural context for the design is often poor; for example, there are rarely structures of complexes between a protein of interest and its receptor, or an enzyme with a substrate bound. This structural context serves as important inputs to design software and can drive sequence selection. Limitations in the quality of structural information challenge designers to select the appropriate structural regions and perturbation to the protein structure that will give a successful design. A number of approaches have been tried to overcome this issue, but operator skill is still the most important factor. An experienced designer can anticipate the inaccuracies that might arise from imperfect structural information and set up the design calculations to modify features of the structure that can be modeled more accurately or, alternatively, to avoid situations in which there is too little information to proceed.

Aside from selecting design problems that have high-quality structural information and structure–function data, there are two general approaches to dealing with low-quality structure–function and structure data: designing multiple protein sequences to, in effect, check multiple hypotheses for how the structure might be designed *(8)*; or using information from homologous proteins to limit the amino acids considered, thereby reducing the chance of error in the calculation. If designing multiple sequences, two to three amino acid substitutions per position often need to be tested to provide a reasonable chance of success. For 5 positions that results in on the order of 10^2 sequences; for 10 positions, 10^4 sequences; and for 15 positions, 10^6 sequences (*see* **Note 1**). This approach is workable for small structural regions, such as surface hydrophobic patches of four or five residues that are being redesigned, or for problems for which protein expression and experimental testing are very scalable, such as an enzyme optimization in which a genetic selection assay can be used to test 10^6 sequences. Homology information is most useful when large sets of homologous proteins are available to generate probabilities of amino acid occurrences at each position in the homology family. The most commonly occurring amino acids are then selected as the diversity (*see* **Subheading 2.2.2.1.**) at each position of the design.

2.1.2. Stability Design

Historically, the first design goals for automated protein design were improvement of physical properties, such as stability and solubility *(9,10)*. This choice was largely driven by the use of molecular mechanics scoring functions that modeled energetic interactions of amino acids, and that tried to find sequence arrangements that minimized sequence energy on the protein backbone structure. Although not a prediction of free energy of folding of a protein, this energy minimization approach was expected to, and in fact did, find sequences that fit better on the protein backbone than the wild-type sequence and, hence, resulted in more stable structures. The fitness of a sequence for a structure is correlated to, although not identical to, the stability of the protein; a key difference is that the design algorithm would need to consider whether the optimized

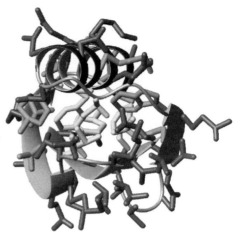

Core residues
Surface residues
Boundary residues

Fig. 2. Core (light gray), boundary (dark gray), and surface (medium gray) residues in protein G β1 (Protein Data Bank identifier 1gb1). Region classification was by buried surface area calculations.

sequence, although more stable on the target structure, would actually take a different fold and confound the design altogether.

2.1.2.1. CORE AND BOUNDARY REGION

A variety of structural strategies are used to stabilize a protein. One of the most successful is redesigning the hydrophobic core, which has been used to create stabilized nonnative versions of proteins from numerous structural families (*11–14*). The hydrophobic core is typically selected to avoid modifying active sites or receptor-binding sites, which are typically solvent exposed, and to increase the overall folding stability of the protein by increasing the hydrophobic surface buried in the core and optimizing steric interactions. Core redesigns are typically well behaved and do not result in modification of the protein backbone structure because of the tight steric constraints on sequences. Expanding the region of design outward from the core, into the boundary region between the core and the surface of the protein, has the potential for burial of significantly more hydrophobic surface because of the greater flexibility of amino acid side chains in the boundary, allowing more ways to pack and bury residues and to find stabilizing interactions (**Fig. 2**). This approach has been used to create highly stable proteins (*10,15*), but the terms in the scoring function must be balanced carefully to avoid creating the potential for nonspecific interactions that can dominate the desired interactions (*14*). This imbalance, possible because of the increased flexibility in the boundary region, leads to poorly ordered proteins with ill-defined structures.

2.1.2.2. SURFACE REGION

Designs of the hydrophilic surface of proteins have also been successful at improving physical properties; however, such designs must avoid disrupting functional interactions or catalytic sites, which typically occur at the surface. Improved solubility can often be achieved by redesign of hydrophobic residues exposed on the protein surface, replacing them with more soluble amino acids. Simple substitution with charged residues, such as lysine or glutamic acid, however, is not always successful and can lead to nonspecific aggregation or destabilization of the protein fold. Selection of a design region that encompasses the hydrophobic surface residues and includes proximal positions, or selection of clusters with multiple hydrophobic residues, typically provides greater enhancement of solubility while preserving structure and, indeed, often enhancing stability *(9,16)*. Design of a region allows the algorithms to balance the solvation, hydrogen bond, and coulombic and steric forces; too much hydrophilicity can disrupt local structure and often optimal designs have amphipathic or small charged residues. Further, consideration of the secondary structure propensity of residues can often create stabilizing designs on the surface, such as finding Thr substitutions in β sheets *(17)*. *In silico* designs, whether in the core or surface regions or a combination, are very successful at optimizing stability because they perform simultaneous optimization of multiple interacting residues and, hence, allow the addition of many small contributions to enhanced stability.

2.1.3. Functional Designs

In silico design goals have expanded beyond stability and have included enzyme catalysis, ligand-binding affinity, receptor selectivity, and pharmacokinetics. These are widely varied goals, but the first step in defining the design strategy is similar. Either a small structural region that mediates the function, such as an enzyme active site, is selected or a large region, perhaps the entire protein, is selected to allow allosteric or indirect structural modifications to affect function. Sometimes large regions are selected because the functional site is not known, other times because indirect perturbations are desired. It is possible to use both approaches simultaneously, but in any case the local design vs large area strategies have very different structural change goals.

2.1.3.1. LOCAL DESIGNS AT FUNCTIONAL SITE

Local designs at functional sites have two general strategies. One is to preserve the critical structural features of the site, such as ligand-binding residues, while creating adjacent sequence diversity to modify protein performance. This strategy is used to modify an existing function, such as changing the substrate specificity of an enzyme *(8)*. The other strategy brings new amino acids into a specific functional geometry, such as a catalytic triad, to create altogether new functions by fixing the new side-chain arrangements and reengineering the surrounding residues *(18–21)*. The inverse folding approach to protein design ensures that any new amino acid sequences designed in these local areas will conserve the structure of the protein and the local functional area. This explicit preservation of structure allows focused designs to make unexpected and nonconservative changes in the sequence at a functional site and, hence, large changes in function with little risk of making mutations that ablate function. This ability to modify directly the most conserved regions of a protein is in stark contrast to random mutagenesis and evolution, which conserve residues in a functional site to avoid destroying the function. Controlling structure is pivotal for designs that attempt to create new functional sites and has enabled the *de novo* design of sensors and enzymes *(20,22,23)*. One difference in strategy between *de novo* designs and functional site modification is that *de novo* designs use highly detailed models of the desired functional site and target a very specific structural arrangement, whereas site reengineering typically does not have as much detailed structural information. For example, an enzyme structure with substrate bound might not be available. Therefore, several modifications that preserve the overall structure of the site would be sampled without a specific structural goal. Then experimental testing of the candidates would be used to find the best designs.

2.1.3.2. LARGE STRUCTURAL REGION DESIGNS

Local designs are attempted when the functional site is clear even if complete detail is not available. In many cases, there is no information about what part of the structure is involved directly in activity. In particular, designs involving protein–protein interactions often have no information about what residues are involved in binding. In such cases, a large region, or perhaps the entire protein, is selected for design and broad diversity is generated over a large part of the structure. Typical approaches are to redesign the surface and adjacent boundary and core residues on a particular face of the protein suspected to be important *(12,24)*. Alternatively, the entire protein surface can be designed to assist in deducing where the functional site is while simultaneously optimizing binding, by experimentally testing a large number of the designs. These large-region designs act by the same mechanism as local designs: nonconservative diversity that still preserves protein structure is created at multiple sites so that major improvements in protein function are created without the risk of loss of function. The size of the calculation can become a limiting factor, however, when the design region is more than 50 residues, with both scoring function and optimization calculations becoming intractable. Several approaches are used to control the calculation size, such as limiting how many amino acids are considered at each position, but the most important factor is limiting the number of positions, so that there is always a balance between trying to engage allosteric mechanisms and having practical design calculations. Typically, assumptions are made about which regions of the protein are least likely to impact function or are most prone to deleterious changes, and those parts are left out of the design. Furthermore, large, indirect design calculations can require experimental testing of a large number of proteins, a very expensive proposition. A common approach is to select a subset of the best designed sequences that cover a diverse set of amino acid sequence changes, and test those sequences to build a structure–function relationship that guides additional experimental testing.

2.1.3.3. COMBINING LOCAL AND LARGE-REGION DESIGNS IN PRACTICE

An interesting example of the combination of local site design and global sequence diversity design is the engineering of dominant negative variants of tumor necrosis factor (TNF)-α *(24)*, an important cytokine in inflammation and autoimmune disease. The design goal was to create variants of TNF-α that are incapable of binding receptor but are still capable of trimerizing with other TNF-α molecules, thereby creating a dominant negative agent that could be used as a therapeutic. In this case, a structure of the ligand was available, and the structure of a homologous protein bound to its receptor was also available. The overall arrangement of the homology model of the ligand–receptor complex was supported by mutagenesis data, but the presence of long, flexible loops that had significantly different sequences between the homologous protein and TNF-α made the details of the local structure suspect. Further, the ligand–receptor interface targeted for disruption was largely overlapping with the TNF-α-TNF-α contacts that control trimerization. A large-region design was first undertaken along the whole of the ligand–receptor interface, an area more than 30 residues, and mutations that disrupted receptor interactions but preserved trimerization were found. The degree of receptor-binding disruption was insufficient to create potent dominant negatives, however, and a second phase of design that focused on sites identified in the first phase was done. These sites were designed with more amino acid diversity and with greater inclusion of adjacent residues that were left out of the first phase. Additional dominant negative variants were found that when combined created potent inhibitors. This design shows how initial large-region design can be used to allow more detailed calculations of manageable size in order to explore more sequence diversity and find superior performance.

2.2. Structural and Conformational Description

Following definition of the design goal and selection of a structural strategy, the protein structure and the amino acid diversity that will be considered in the design must be defined quantitatively. The detailed structural description is an absolutely critical step of the design and usually determines the success or failure of the design more strongly than the details of the computational algorithms used. Because there are presently no completely general objective methods for performing structure analysis and position/ amino acid assignment, operator care is important in successful protein design.

2.2.1. Selection of Backbone Scaffold Structure

The backbone structure is selected for the most accurate and complete representation of the region being modeled. The primary consideration is the quality of the structure in the design region. For example, if backbone or side-chain atoms are missing or temperature factors are very high, then the model is not representative of the true situation and is likely to impact design results negatively. In addition, structures with atomic resolution data result in superior designs because lower resolution means that atomic coordinates are only weakly guided by experimental constraints. The most common issue in backbone selection, however, is the lack of a three-dimensional structure for the protein of interest, resulting in the need to construct a homology model from a related structure. Advances in homology modeling and the explosion in the number of publicly available structures has mitigated this issue in recent years, and adequate models can typically be made from structures with as little as 50% sequence identity (*see* **Note 2**). Sequence conservation in the design region is more important than overall identity, and low-homology regions such as loops or receptor-binding sites can lead to inaccurate structure models and poor design performance, whereas highly conserved motifs such as cysteine knots or four-helix bundles can offer good structural models with as low as 25% identity. The underlying model parameter that determines design accuracy is the deviation of the model structure from the true structure. A protein design study that systematically perturbed the backbone coordinates of a structure demonstrated that deviations less than 1.25 Å from the true structure did not degrade sequence designs, but greater than 1.5 Å had a severe effect *(11)*. Although no quantitative correlation between sequence identity and structure deviation is known, these results generally correlate with the successful use of homology models in protein design.

2.2.2. Position and Identity of Side-Chains

Once a structure for the protein backbone has been decided, there are two major tasks in describing the protein structure and sequence diversity for design calculations: selecting the region of protein to design at the level of individual amino acid positions, and defining the amino acid diversity that needs to be sampled. Selecting the structural positions to be designed, of course, is determined by the structural analysis of the design strategy, but inclusion of specific residues particularly on the boundaries of the design region can be ambiguous. The amino acids that are considered typically differ at the different positions in the design and are determined by the structural and functional role played by each residue. Limiting amino acid diversity from the full repertoire of 20 commonly occurring ones is desirable for two reasons: to reduce the number of sequence combinations that must be considered during calculations and to avoid presenting amino acids in contexts in which limitations in the scoring functions might result in improper selection. In addition, the number of conformational states that will be tested for each amino acid must be decided; too few will reduce accuracy and too many will increase calculation time.

2.2.2.1. ASSIGNMENT OF AMINO ACID SET

Rules for deciding the amino acid identities to be considered in protein design should be simple, general, and objective. The most common approach taken is to assign amino acid sets based on whether a position is buried in the core of the protein, exposed on the surface, or in the boundary between the two (**Table 1**). The rationale is that these structural regions are each dominated by residues of particular types: the core is predominantly hydrophobic and the surface is predominantly hydrophilic, while the boundary has both types of amino acid. Taking the simplest implementation of a core/surface/boundary approach, there would be 8 hydrophobic amino acids at each core position, 10 hydrophilic amino acids at each surface position, and 17 amino acids at the boundary positions (alanine is considered in both core and surface groups) (**Table 1**). Of course, there are exceptions to these simple polarity rules in many proteins with either buried polar residues or exposed nonpolar residues. Often, to account for these situations we include the exceptional amino acid in the set for that position, and possibly similar residues; for example, a buried glutamine residue could be added to the hydrophobic amino acid set, plus glutamic acid and asparagine. Additionally, homology-guided amino acid set selection is also used (*see* **Subheading 2.1.1.**).

Other refinements of the basic considerations for amino acid diversity selection are used to improve design accuracy or to create particular functionality. A common modification to improve the stability of core designs is to eliminate methionine from buried

Table 1
Typical Amino Acid Sets

Amino acid set	Typical use
AVLIFYW(M)	Hydrophobic core or binding patches (eliminate M for lower entropy loss)
AVLF	Minimal hydrophobic set to limit design size
ASTHDNEQKR	Hydrophilic surface region
SEQK	Minimal hydrophilic set to limit design size
AVLIFYWMSTHDNEQKR	Boundary regions, functional sites, core
AVLFSEQK	Minimal boundary set to limit design size
GND	Unusual backbone conformation, e.g., positive backbone ϕ angle
EQKR(N)	Helical surface positions, for maximal stability (N for amino-terminal capping)
TYQ	β Sheet surface positions, for maximal stability

core amino acid sets. Methionine is the only hydrophobic residue that has more than two rotatable side-chain dihedral angles and, therefore, loses the most entropy when buried in the core. Elimination of methionine also speeds calculations. At times, amino acid sets are selected in order to stabilize a secondary structure, such as picking amino acids with high α-helix propensities (lysine, arginine, or glutamate) for helical regions *(9)*. Secondary structure biasing is only useful for surface designs, because the effects of structural propensity are overwhelmed by tertiary structure packing in protein cores. A very common modification to standard amino acid sets is to add functionality, such as nonpolar residues to create a surface receptor-binding patch or specific hydrogen bond donors to match to a ligand's binding interface. In these cases, analysis of the particular structural situation is used to guide a selection of an amino acid group. Three amino acids, proline, glycine, and cysteine, are not used except in specific cases in which their unusual properties are needed. Glycine, the only residue without an α carbon, has a high degree of backbone flexibility and is used when extreme backbone dihedral angles are needed, such as positive ϕ angles. Proline, by contrast, is very inflexible and is used to terminate helical structures or to control backbone turn conformations. Cysteine is used to create disulfide crosslinks, metal ligation sites, or, more recently, to introduce nonnative chemical modification handles into specific locations in the protein.

2.2.2.2. Residue Position Definition of Design Region

Selection of most structural positions to include in a design is quantitative. In the case of functional designs, it is usually based on distance from the putative functional site, and in the case of region designs (e.g., core or surface regions), it is usually based on the fraction of a residue surface area that is buried from solvent. Distance criteria are typically defined by measuring the distance between side-chain heavy atoms in the functional site to side-chain heavy atoms in the backbone model structure of the surrounding protein. Alternatively, α carbon to α carbon or β carbon to β carbon distances are used, although there are no data on which of these definitions are best. Cutoff magnitudes of 4.5–5.5 Å select the first shell of residues around a site and result in 10–15 residues being selected. Ambiguity arises, however, because the side-chain placements in the model structure are sometimes not predictive of those required for function and, therefore, can be improperly left out or included by the strict application of distance criteria. Similarly, calculations of solvent-accessible surface area of side chains usually assign residue positions unequivocally to the core or surface, but the somewhat arbitrary thresholds used (typically >90% buried is core, <50% buried is surface, and others are boundary) can lead to assignments that do not properly reflect the structural disposition of residues *(14)*. In these difficult cases, subjective analysis is necessary, and design success depends on the experience of the user in understanding the behavior of the design algorithm (*see* **Note 3**).

An objective criterion that is based solely on the backbone atom coordinates has been proposed *(17)*. Calculations of a solvent-accessible pseudosurface of the protein using just C α atoms and a large pseudosolvent probe were done to define a metric for solvent accessibility independent of side-chain identity and conformation. The C α to C β vector directions for each residue were calculated and the distances along this vector from the C α and C β atoms to the pseudosurface were used to determine whether a residue was in the core, surface, or boundary region. The specific distance criteria were derived by comparing predictions for core or surface identity with calculations of solvent-accessible area in complete protein structures, and as such, the criteria do not have meaningful physical interpretations. This technique has been used successfully and is an example of a less subjective methodology.

2.2.2.3. Amino Acid Conformational Diversity: Rotamer Set Assignment

Definition of the conformational diversity that will be tested for amino acids is the final component in defining the structural model. Because *in silico* design models the interactions of amino acids at atomic resolution, a detailed conformational description that defines the position of each atom in the side chain is required. Therefore, each possible configuration of each amino acid side chain, defined by the torsion angles of the rotatable bonds (χ angles), must be considered when testing the goodness of fit of each sequence. Detailed surveys of the conformations of side chains in the Protein Data Bank have generated lists of common side-chain conformations, which, unsurprisingly, follow standard noneclipsed conformations of small organic molecules *(25,26)*. Leucine for example, can take three possible states (60°, −60°, and 180°) for each of its two rotatable bonds ($\chi 1$ and $\chi 2$), resulting in 3 × 3, or 9, possible conformations. These discrete conformations are called rotamers and are grouped into rotamer libraries. The true conformational diversity of a protein, however, is continuous, not a set of discrete rotamers, which has led to the use of expanded rotamer sets in which each rotamer has multiple additional rotamers with small angle deviations generated. For example, the 60° leucine rotamer would have a 50° and a 70° rotamer generated. This would lead to 9 × 9, or 81, possible leucine conformations to consider, which is a considerable expansion of the number of computations but often significantly improves design performance by reducing the deviation of the model from the actual states that occur in the protein.

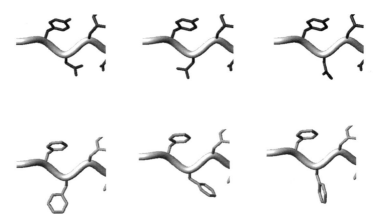

Fig. 3. Examples of different conformations of different rotamers for phenylalanine demonstrating dramatically different positioning of rigid aromatic ring arising from rotations about χ angles.

Note that bond and bond angle stretches are not considered, nor are the rotations of methyl groups.

Expansion of the rotamer set to improve the sampling of side-chain conformations is important to improve the accuracy of the model, but the benefit is more pronounced in some structural regions, allowing the selective use of rotamer expansion of certain positions to minimize computational cost. Most *in silico* design software packages allow control of this aspect of the rotamer library but limit selection to a set of predefined options. Core packing benefits significantly from the small changes in side-chain conformation that come from expanded rotamer libraries because of the dominant role that the very stiff steric force plays in defining protein cores. Rotamer expansion is especially critical for limiting spurious clashes of aromatic residues (phenylalanine, tyrosine, and trytophan) because of the large rigid ring structure that can move several angstroms from minor deviations in rotamer angle (**Fig. 3**). Surface residues are much less dependent on rotamer expansion because of the much lower packing density on the protein surface and the softer nature of the energetic terms that control exposed residues, such as electrostatics and polar solvation. Limiting or eliminating rotamer expansion for surface positions is therefore typical, because many hydrophilic residues are large and have three or four rotatable bonds, such as lysine and arginine, so rotamer expansion would cause an explosion in the number of conformations that must be considered. Boundary residues are, unfortunately, impacted strongly by steric constraints but also have hydrophilic residues playing a key role. Therefore, calculations that include boundary residues often require the use of expanded rotamer sets for hydrophilic residues, and the number of amino acid types and residue positions must be limited, or different calculations must be combined (*see* **Subheading 2.1.3.3.**), in order to prevent enormous problem sizes and impractical calculation times. This costly approach is necessary because inaccurate conformational modeling for boundary residues can result in spurious amino acid selection that destabilizes the protein. A common tactic to limit the size of expanded rotamer sets for hydrophilic residues is to expand only the first two χ angles, leaving the distal rotatable bonds unexpanded.

2.3. In Silico *Design Software Packages*

Several software packages have been developed for protein design. Each has been used in multiple successful designs and has mostly overlapping functionality because all were developed as general design tools. The most well-known packages are ORBIT *(2,17,27)*, DEZYMER/RECEPTORDESIGN *(4,19,23)*, and RosettaDesign *(28)*. No software packages are commercially available; therefore, access is via direct contact with the authors of the packages at their academic institutions. These three *in silico* design software packages share very similar approaches and can be used in similar ways. In particular, the strategies in **Subheading 2.1.** and **2.2.** are applicable. Because all packages are undergoing continuing development and are constantly in flux, it is impossible to provide detailed instructions on their operation, even though they all operate on the same underlying principles. Although all are general tools, they have been used and optimized by their authors for particular problems: DEZYMER/RECEPTOR DESIGN has been very successful at *de novo* enzyme and substrate binding design, RosettaDesign has been used for *de novo* backbone and sequence design, and ORBIT has been used for stability design and for improvement of binding affinity.

In silico design software has two main components: calculation of amino acid interaction energy based on the conformational diversity and positions specified by the user, and searching of the defined sequences for those with the best scores. Little user control is afforded over the optimization routines in design software; therefore, no specification by the user is required. The scoring functions used are also mostly defined but do have some elements of user control, primarily in selecting which terms of the potential function, each modeling a particular physical force, are used. It is not recommended that the user manipulate the quantitative parameters of the potentials, such as van der Waals radii or partial charge values. These parameters all impact each other and their values have been balanced by laborious trial and error, like most potential functions, and therefore should be viewed as a self-consistent set.

2.3.1. Selection of Potential Function Terms

The structural region that is being designed is the main factor in selecting potential function components. The general principle is to use the terms appropriate for a region and not to include other terms when not necessary, because additional terms can add essentially random error to the calculation (*see* **Note 4**). The software packages mentioned in **Subheading 2.3.** all have developed potential functions that attempt to deal with this issue by selecting parameter values to minimize these possible errors or by allowing for selection of different potential functions at different positions. Core regions are dominated by steric forces, with a contribution from hydrophobic solvation, because nearly all residues are hydrophobic in the core. Electrostatics and hydrogen bonding are usually not necessary in the core and, therefore, should be eliminated unless hydrophilic amino acids are being considered, which is rare. Similarly, surface residues are not typically modeled using hydrophobic solvation because of the high conformational flexibility of these residues and their highly polar nature. Electrostatics and hydrogen bonding are critical, with sterics playing a less crucial role in scoring sequences. Boundary residues again pose a problem, because they can be buried or exposed, depending on the rotamer in question, and therefore usually require all potential function terms because both polar and nonpolar residues are considered.

3. Notes

1. The combinatorial definition of the sequences that can arise during protein design is a central feature to the problem. The number of amino acids possible at each position is multiplied by the number possible at every other position. If each position has 5 possible amino acids, then a 10-position calculation has 10^7 possible sequences, 15 positions have 10^{10} possible sequences, and 20 positions have 10^{13} possible sequences. Therefore, control of the number of positions is the most important factor in limiting the size of the problem and, hence, the speed of the calculation. Current software packages can readily deal with problems of approx 50 amino acids on single central processing unit servers, and new optimization methods are now allowing problems of 100 or more positions to be considered on multiprocessor machines.

2. Homology modeling methods in both commercial and academic software have been used effectively in protein design, but several pitfalls need to be avoided. First, flexible loop regions are extremely difficult to model and often do not provide reasonable results. These regions often lack a fixed structure and therefore are not good candidates for design. Second, regions of low sequence identity can make the overall sequence identity appear too low for accurate modeling; however, if the design region has good identity (>70%), then a successful design is usually possible. Finally, energy relaxation of the final structure, typically via conjugate gradient energy minimization, is important because residual strain in the packing or electrostatic energies can create very high energies in design calculations.

3. An important tactic to limit the negative impact of the somewhat arbitrary exclusion of a residue position from the design is to allow some positions on the boundary of the design to change conformation but to keep their identity fixed at the wild-type amino acid. This approach allows flexibility in the conformational sampling of the design region, generally improves accuracy, and increases the problem size only modestly. Usually, all residues that contact a significant portion of any designed residue are modeled with this conformational flexibility.

4. Development of accurate scoring functions was crucial to enable *in silico* protein design. Scoring functions are used to calculate the fitness of a sequence for the structure relative to the other possible sequences being considered for the design. The goal is not to determine an absolute energy for a sequence, which is a very difficult task, but, rather, to differentiate accurately and rapidly among the usually very large number of alternatives. Although the scoring functions in use today have been successful in a number of design problems, including enzyme function, stability enhancement, and binding, there is still a need for improvements in sequence scoring accuracy.

   A significant decision in scoring function development was the emphasis on using biophysical potential functions, rather than informatics or sequence-based functions. The primary advantage of a biophysical strategy is that it is unbiased and not limited by which protein structures happen to have been studied, or which sequences are present in a database. Biophysical potentials, such as steric interactions, electrostatics, and solvation, are the same no matter which protein structure or function is being considered. This independence from bias to known sequences and structures is crucial because there is no guarantee that a new functional property or new structure is best achieved by sequences that are related to natural proteins. In addition, methods based on sequence informatics are likely not to be applicable to proteins that fall outside of the information data set. Of course, the challenge in achieving the benefits of using biophysical potential functions is in accurately modeling the highly complex and interrelated physical forces that govern protein structure.

The dominant forces are steric interactions usually modeled by van der Waals potentials, solvation usually modeled by surface area-based atomic solvation potentials, electrostatic interactions usually modeled with a coulombic potential, and hydrogen bonding usually modeled by specific potentials to account for polar hydrogen interactions. The forms of these potential functions are very similar to standard molecular mechanics functions used in force fields such as CHARMM, AMBER, or DRIEDING. Protein design algorithms rebalance the emphasis of these forces, however, and often simplify the functional forms. Simplification of the functional forms allows more rapid calculation, a key issue in protein design, as well as simplified interpretation; the more complex functional forms are usually not more accurate at scoring sequences and can be seen as a source of "noise" in interpreting results. The rebalancing of forces is driven by the need to differentiate accurately among the many sequence choices that fit best in the protein structure, and the lack of a need to calculate absolute energies. The inherent inaccuracies of the energy models, especially for electrostatic energies, are such that an attempt at calculation of absolute energy is rife with random error when viewed over the entire sequence set being considered. Therefore, a rebalancing that tunes down the contribution of the electrostatic terms in particular creates more accurate results.

References

1. Pabo, C. (1983) Molecular technology: designing proteins and peptides. *Nature* **301,** 200.
2. Dahiyat, B. I. and Mayo, S. L. (1996) Protein design automation. *Protein Sci.* **5,** 895–903.
3. Desjarlais, J. R. and Handel, T. M. (1995) De novo design of the hydrophobic cores of proteins. *Protein Sci.* **4,** 2006–2018.
4. Hellinga, H. W. and Richards, F. M. (1994) Optimal sequence selection in proteins of known structure by simulated evolution. *Proc. Natl. Acad. Sci. USA* **91,** 5803–5807.
5. Kuhlman, B., Dantas, G., Ireton, G. C., Varani, G., Stoddard, B. L., and Baker, D. (2003) Design of a novel globular protein fold with atomic-level accuracy. *Science* **302,** 1364–1368.
6. Marvin, J. S., Corcoran, E. E., Hattangadi, N. A., Zhang, J. V., Gere, S. A., and Hellinga, H. W. (1997) The rational design of allosteric interactions in a monomeric protein and its applications to the construction of biosensors. *Proc. Natl. Acad. Sci. USA* **94,** 4366–4371.
7. Marvin, J. S. and Hellinga, H. W. (2001) Conversion of a maltose receptor into a zinc biosensor by computational design. *Proc. Natl. Acad. Sci. USA* **98,** 4955–4960.
8. Hayes, R. J., Bentzien, J., Ary, M. L., et al. (2002) Combining computational and experimental screening for rapid optimization of protein properties. *Proc. Natl. Acad. Sci. USA* **99,** 15,926–15,931.
9. Dahiyat, B. I., Gordon, D. B., and Mayo, S. L. (1997) Automated design of the surface positions of protein helices. *Protein Sci.* **6,** 1333–1337.
10. Malakauskas, S. M. and Mayo, S. L. (1998) Design, structure and stability of a hyperthermophilic protein variant. *Nat. Struct. Biol.* **5,** 470–475.

11. Su, A. and Mayo, S. L. (1997) Coupling backbone flexibility and amino acid sequence selection in protein design. *Protein Sci.* **6,** 1701–1707.

12. Luo, P., Hayes, R. J., Chan, C., et al. (2002) Development of a cytokine analog with enhanced stability using computational ultrahigh throughput screening. *Protein Sci.* **11,** 1218–1226.

13. Filikov, A. V., Hayes, R. J., Luo, P., et al. (2002) Computational stabilization of human growth hormone. *Protein Sci.* **11,** 1452–1461.

14. Dahiyat, B. I. and Mayo, S. L. (1997) Probing the role of packing specificity in protein design. *Proc. Natl. Acad. Sci. USA* **94,** 10,172–10,177.

15. Marshall, S. A. and Mayo, S. L. (2001) Achieving stability and conformational specificity in designed proteins via binary patterning. *J. Mol. Biol.* **305,** 619–631.

16. Marshall, S. A., Morgan, C. S., and Mayo, S. L. (2002) Electrostatics significantly affect the stability of designed homeodomain variants. *J. Mol. Biol.* **316,** 189–199.

17. Dahiyat, B. I. and Mayo, S. L. (1997) De novo protein design: fully automated sequence selection. *Science* **278,** 82–87.

18. Hellinga, H. W. and Richards, F. M. (1991) Construction of new ligand binding sites in proteins of known structure. I. Computer-aided modeling of sites with pre-defined geometry. *J. Mol. Biol.* **222,** 763–785.

19. Hellinga, H. W., Caradonna, J. P., and Richards, F. M. (1991) Construction of new ligand binding sites in proteins of known structure. II. Grafting of a buried transition metal binding site into Escherichia coli thioredoxin. *J. Mol. Biol.* **222,** 787–803.

20. Dwyer, M. A., Looger, L. L., and Hellinga, H. W. (2004) Computational design of a biologically active enzyme. *Science* **304,** 1967–1971.

21. Bolon, D. N. and Mayo, S. L. (2001) Enzyme-like proteins by computational design. *Proc. Natl. Acad. Sci. USA* **98,** 14,274–14,279.

22. Dwyer, M. A., Looger, L. L., and Hellinga, H. W. (2003) Computational design of a Zn2+ receptor that controls bacterial gene expression. *Proc. Natl. Acad. Sci. USA* **100,** 11,255–11,260.

23. Looger, L. L., Dwyer, M. A., Smith, J. J., and Hellinga, H. W. (2003) Computational design of receptor and sensor proteins with novel functions. *Nature* **423,** 185–190.

24. Steed, P. M., Tansey, M. G., Zalevsky, J., et al. (2003) Inactivation of TNF signaling by rationally designed dominant-negative TNF variants. *Science* **301,** 1895–1898.

25. Ponder, J. W. and Richards, F. M. (1987) Tertiary templates for proteins: use of packing criteria in the enumeration of allowed sequences for different structural classes. *J. Mol. Biol.* **193,** 775–791.

26. Dunbrack, R. L. Jr. and Karplus, M. (1993) Backbone-dependent rotamer library for proteins: application to side-chain prediction. *J. Mol. Biol.* **230,** 543–574.

27. Ross, S. A., Sarisky, C. A., Su, A., and Mayo, S. L. (2001) Designed protein G core variants fold to native-like structures: sequence selection by ORBIT tolerates variation in backbone specification. *Protein Sci.* **10,** 450–454.

28. Kuhlman, B. and Baker, D. (2000) Native protein sequences are close to optimal for their structures. *Proc. Natl. Acad. Sci. USA* **97,** 10,383–10,388.

14

Chemical Database Preparation
for Compound Acquisition or Virtual Screening

Cristian G. Bologa, Marius M. Olah, and Tudor I. Oprea

Summary

Virtual and high-throughput screening are time-saving techniques that have been successfully applied to identify novel chemotypes in biologically active molecules. Both methods require the ability to aptly handle large numbers of chemicals prior to an experiment or acquisition. We describe a step-by-step preparation procedure for handling large collections of existing or virtual compounds prior to virtual screening or acquisition.

Key Words: Cheminformatics; drug discovery; high-throughput screening; leadlikeness; property filtering; unwanted structures; virtual screening.

1. Introduction

Recently established (*1,2*), virtual screening is regarded as a complement to bioactivity screening (*3,4*). The aim of virtual screening is to sift through a vast amount of compounds, in order to identify rapidly structures of interest for biological screening. Its experimental counterpart, high-throughput screening (HTS) is also aimed at sifting through a large amount of structures, based (often) on single-point, single-experiment results. Both procedures rely on the ability to process, using cheminformatics tools, a large number of structures (*5*). However, post-HTS analyses (*6*) are often clouded by the presence of reactive species or optically interfering components (which can be the result of sample degradation) in biochemical assays (*7*) and the tendency of chemicals to aggregate (*8*) or turn up as frequent hitters (*9*). Computational filters geared to remove "unwanted" molecular species are now in place and are discussed in **Section 3**. The progression *HTS hits => HTS actives => lead series => drug candidate => launched drug* has shifted the focus from good-quality candidate drugs to good-quality leads (*10*). A set of simple property filters known as the "rule of five" (Ro5) (*11*) is implemented in the pharmaceutical industry to restrict small-molecule synthesis in the property space defined by ClogP (octanol/water partition coefficient), molecular weight, HDO

From: *Methods in Molecular Biology, vol. 316: Bioinformatics and Drug Discovery*
Edited by: R. S. Larson © Humana Press Inc., Totowa, NJ

(number of hydrogen bond donors), and HAC (number of hydrogen bond acceptors). The property distribution of chemical and drug databases in the Ro5 space is well characterized *(12)*. Many library design programs based on combinatorial chemistry or compound acquisition are now Ro5 compliant. Smaller compounds are easier to optimize *(13)* toward the *drug candidate* status, and leadlikeness has become an established concept in drug discovery *(14)*. Here we discuss compound databases in the context of both "unwanted structure" removal *(7)* and property (leadlike) filtering *(14)*. However, the responsibility of implementing such criteria in database evaluation resides with the end user and should be regarded as context dependent. Whether for compound acquisition for HTS, or in preparation for a virtual screen, there is a clear need for database cleanup and preparation. What follows is a step-by-step procedure on how an existing or commercial collection of compounds should be processed prior to virtual screening or acquisition. Its emphasis is on software from Daylight (www.daylight.com/), Open Eye (www.eyesopen.com/), and MESA (www.mesaac.com). Similar software is available from Optive Research (www.optive.com; Optive products are also available from Tripos, at www.tripos.com), Accelrys (www.accelrys.com/), Tripos (www.tripos.com), SciTegic (http://scitegic.com), and Chemical ComputingGroup(www.chemcomp.com/).

2. Materials

1. Software to convert chemical structures based on standard file formats (e.g., SDF, mol2) into canonical isomeric SMILES *(15,16)*, or equivalent representations of chemical structures (e.g., **refs.** *17* and *18*).
2. Software to handle canonical isomeric SMILES (or equivalent) and provide chemical fingerprints, e.g., Daylight *(19)*, Unity *(20)*, Mesa Analytics and Computing *(21)*, Barnard Chemical Information (*[22]*; *see also* www.bci.gb.com/clusteranalysis.html), MDL Keys *[23]*; *see also* www.mdli.com/), or Chemical Computing Group's MOE *(24)*.
3. Software to compute chemical properties from structures; e.g., to calculate the octanol/water partition coefficient, LogP *(25)* with CLogP *(26)*, KowWIN *(27)*, or ALogPS (*[28]*; *see also* http://146.107.217.178/lab/alogps/index.html) among many LogP predictors.
4. Software to cluster chemical structures from fingerprints or from computed properties *(29–32)*.
5. Software to convert SMILES (or equivalent) into appropriate three-dimensional (3D)–coordinate systems using CONCORD (www.optive.com or www.tripos.com), CORINA (available from Molecular Networks GmbH, www.mol-net.de/), OMEGA (www.eyesopen.com/).
6. Software to appropriately handle D-optimal design based on multidimensional spaces, e.g., MODDE 7 from Umetrics (www.umetrics.com/).

3. Methods

3.1. Assembling the Collection(s)

In time, and often via merges and acquisitions, large pharmaceutical companies have acquired compound collections, *Reals (14),* that contain a significant number of molecules, including marketed drugs and other high-activity compounds. The *Reals* are, by themselves, a valuable resource that is routinely screened against novel targets. One can argue that these collections reflect the chemistry used to address targets from the past, and that novel targets require novel chemistry, because yesterday's chemistry is by now overpatented. These arguments do not exclude these molecules from being considered for either HTS or virtual screening. By the same token, such collections of structures must include existing sets of commercially available chemicals, or *Tangibles*—termed this way because one can conceivably acquire them or synthesize them in-house using tractable chemistry *(14)*. Thus, any collection prepared for virtual or HTS would sample both the in-house and the "external" chemical spaces. In addition to the *Reals* and the *Tangibles*, one can also define the *Virtuals*—an extremely large set of molecules (10^{60}–10^{200}) that cannot all be made, at least with current chemistry, but that can essentially be used as "resource" for virtual screening.

Having appropriate informatics systems to access these virtual and existing compounds via fingerprints, two-dimensional (2D) or 3D descriptors, or other measured or computed property spaces is key to the screening strategy. The largest collection of *Virtuals* and *Tangibles* is represented by the ChemNavigator database *(33)*. As of April 2005, this database contained more than 21 million samples, representing more than 13 million unique chemicals. This database is available on a subscription basis. If access fees for this database are an issue, one can download other collections from chemical vendors over the Internet; some are given in **Table 1**. ChemNavigator offers compounds from more than 154 companies; therefore, the list in **Table 1** is far from exhaustive. The virtual space alternative is best represented by the ChemSpace™ technology, a patented database/software approach from Tripos (www.tripos.com) that routinely explores 10^{14}–10^{15} *Virtuals* *(34)*. ChemSpace is only available on a collaborative basis.

3.2. Cleaning Up the Collection

There is no "perfect" chemical database, unless it contains rather simple (e.g., NaCl, H_2O) or a rather small number of molecules. The user needs to spend a significant effort in cleaning up the collection, whether it includes *Virtuals, Reals*, or *Tangibles*. Some sites, such as ChemNavigator *(33)*, provide their own solution to this problem. We prefer FILTER (*see* **Note 1**), a program available from OpenEye *(35)*, although you can "wash" your collection in MOE (*see* www.chemcomp.com/) or pass it through SciTegic's Pipeline Pilot (http://scitegic.com/). Regardless of the method used, the user needs to make some early decisions regarding the collection's "makeup." One obvious suggestion is to remove "unwanted" chemical structures, such as those depicted in **Fig. 1**.

3.2.1. Removing Garbage From the Collection

Split covalent salts, remove small fragments (salts), and normalize charges. This is clearly an instance in which the user is confronted with multiple choices. For typical pharmaceutical screening, it is advisable to remove unwanted structures, such as those depicted in **Fig. 1**. One should always consider "unwanted" structures in context; for example, a large number of antineoplastic agents would be considered as "reactive species" according to **Fig. 1**. Furthermore, the vast majority of flavor compounds are monofunctional aldehydes. Therefore, when seeking actives in oncology or in flavor science, substructure filters need to be reevaluated.

Table 1
Examples of Company Databases Available for Purchase

Company name	Web address	Number of compounds	Description
4SC	www.4sc.de/	5,000,000	Virtual library; small-molecule drug candidates
ACB BLOCKS	www.acbblocks.com/acb/bblocks.html	90,000	Building blocks for combinatorial chemistry
Advanced ChemTech	http://triton.peptide.com/index.php	18,000	OmniProbeTM: peptide libraries; 8000 tripeptide, 10,000 tetrapeptide
Advanced SynTech	www.advsyntech.com/omnicore.htm	170,000	Targeted libraries: protease, protein kinase, GPCR, steroid mimetics, antimicrobials
Ambinter	http://ourworld.compuserve.com/homepages/ambinter/Mole.htm	1,750,000	Combinatorial and parallel chemistry, building blocks, HTS
Asinex	www.asinex.com/prod/index.html	150,000	Platinum collection: drug-like compounds
Asinex		250,000	Gold collection: drug-like compounds
Asinex		5009	Targeted libraries: GPCR (16 different targets)
Asinex		4307	Kinase-targeted library (11 targets)
Asinex		1629	Ion-channel targeted (4 targets)
Asinex		2987	Protease-targeted library (5 targets)
Asinex		1,200,000	Combinatorial constructor
BioFocus	www.biofocus.com/pages/drug_discovery.mhtml	100,000	Diverse primary screening compounds
BioFocus		~16,000	SoftFocus: kinase target-directed libraries
BioFocus		~10,000	SoftFocus: GPCR target-directed libraries
CEREP	www.cerep.fr/cerep/users/pages/Products Services/Odyssey.asp	>16,000	Odyssey II library: diverse and unique discovery library; more than 350 chemical families
CEREP		5000	GPCR-focused library (21 targets)
Chemical Diversity Labs, Inc.	www.chemdiv.com/discovery/downloads/	>750,000	Leadlike compounds for bioscreening
ChemStar	www.chemstar.ru/page4.htm	60,260	High-quality organic compounds for screening
ChemStar		>500,000	Virtual database of organic compounds
COMBI-BLOCKS	www.combi-blocks.com/	908	Combinatorial building blocks
ComGenex	www.comgenex.hu/cgi-bin/inside.php?in=products&l_id=compound	260,000	"Pharma relevant", discrete structures for multitarget screening purposes

Supplier	Website	Number	Description
ComGenex		240	GPCR library
ComGenex		2000	Cytotoxic discovery library: very toxic compounds suitable for anticancer and antiviral discovery research
ComGenex		5000	Low-Tox MeDiverse: druglike, diverse, nontoxic discovery library
ComGenex		10,000	MeDiverse Natural: natural product–like compounds
EMC microcollection	www.microcollections.de/catalogue_compounds.htm#	30,000	Highly diverse combinatorial compound collections for lead discovery
InterBioScreen	www.ibscreen.com/products.shtml	350,000	Synthetic compounds
InterBioScreen		40,000	Natural compounds
Maybridge plc	www.maybridge.com/html/m_company.htm	60,000	Organic druglike compounds
Maybridge plc		13,000	Building blocks
MicroSource Discovery Systems, Inc.	www.msdiscovery.com/download.html	2000	GenPlus: collection of known bioactive compounds
			NatProd: collection of pure natural products
Nanosyn	www.nanosyn.com/thankyou.shtml	46,715	Pharma library
Nanosyn		18,613	Explore library
Pharmacopeia Drug Discovery, Inc.	www.pharmacopeia.com/dcs/order_form.html	N/A	Targeted library: GPCR and kinase
Polyphor	www.polyphor.com/	15,000	Diverse general screening library
Sigma-Aldrich	http://www.sigmaaldrich.com/Area_of_Interest/Chemistry/Drug_Discovery/Assay_Dev_and_Screening/Compound_Libraries/Screening_Compounds.html	90,000	Diverse library of drug-like compounds, selected based on Lipinski's Rule of Five
Specs	www.specs.net/	240,000	Diverse library
Specs		10,000	World Diversity Set: pre-plateled library
Specs		6000	Building blocks
Specs		500	Natural products (diverse and unique)
TimTec	www.timtec.net/	>160,000	Compound libraries and building blocks
Tranzyme® Pharma	www.tranzyme.com/drug_discovery.html	25,000	HitCREATE library: macrocycles library
Tripos	www.tripos.com/sciTech/researchCollab/chemCompLib/IqCompound/index.html	80,000	LeadQuest compound libraries

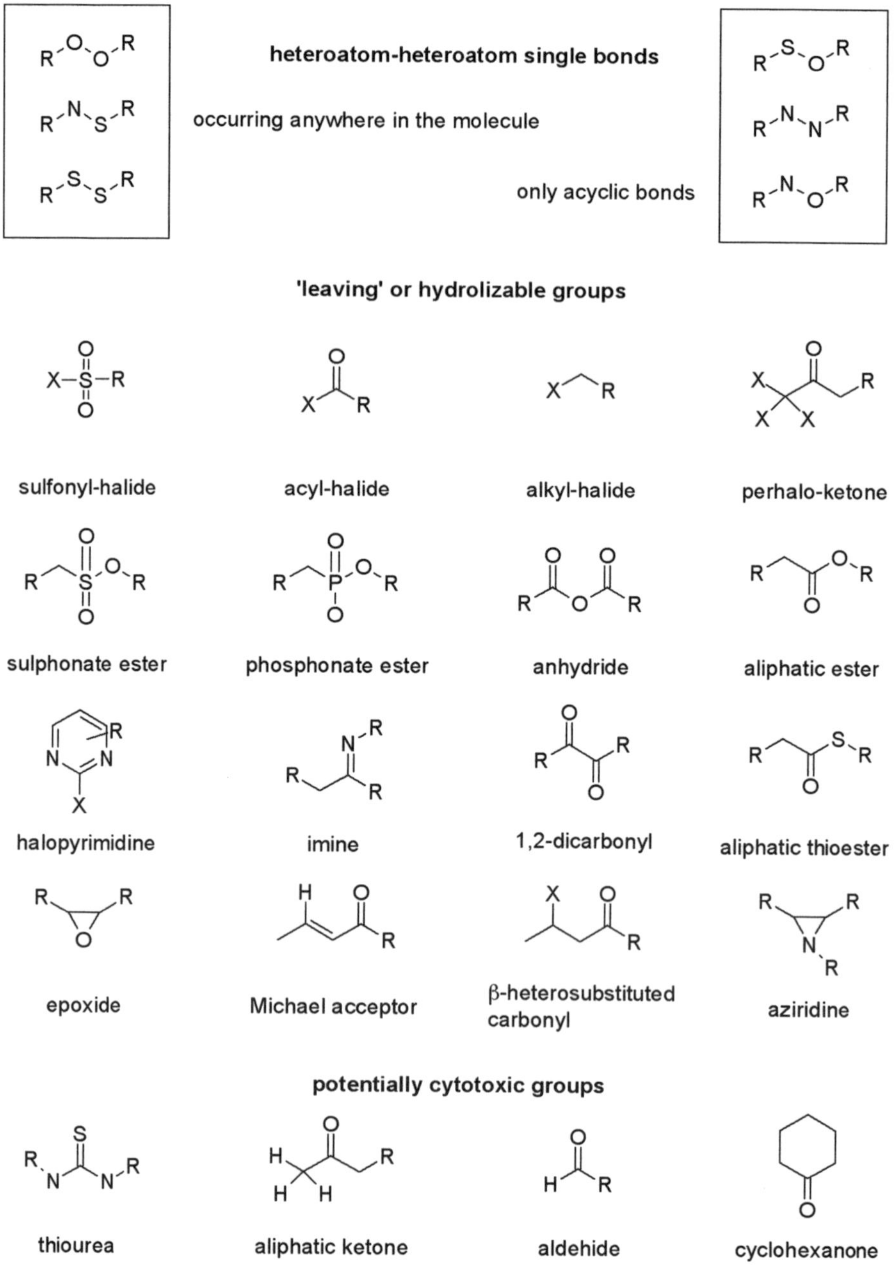

heteroatom-heteroatom single bonds

occurring anywhere in the molecule

only acyclic bonds

'leaving' or hydrolizable groups

sulfonyl-halide

acyl-halide

alkyl-halide

perhalo-ketone

sulphonate ester

phosphonate ester

anhydride

aliphatic ester

halopyrimidine

imine

1,2-dicarbonyl

aliphatic thioester

epoxide

Michael acceptor

β-heterosubstituted carbonyl

aziridine

potentially cytotoxic groups

thiourea

aliphatic ketone

aldehide

cyclohexanone

Fig. 1. Examples of chemical substructures that can cause interference with biochemical assays under high-throughput screening conditions.

3.2.2. Verifying Integrity of Molecular Structure

To be correctly understood and processed by computer, the structures must be entered in a "computer-friendly" format, which is not necessarily "human friendly." A significant amount of "wrong" molecules appear *(36)* because of incorrectly drawn chiral centers, conformers, bridge compounds, and so forth. This can become a significant source of errors in structure–activity relationship studies *(37,38)*. Because visual inspection for all the structures is not an option in really large collections, one has to use an automated procedure for detection (and perhaps correction) of some of the wrong entries. If specialized software for this operation, such as *CheD (39)*, is not available, good results in detecting errors can be achieved after converting the original structural files (usually in SDF format) into SMILES using two or more conversion tools (e.g., Daylight *mol2smi*, OpenEye *babel2*), followed by canonicalization (Daylight's *cansmi*), and then by comparing the resulting SMILES. The number of errors differs significantly among chemical vendors, ranging from under 0.05 to 10%, or higher. A totally automated method for error detection and removal of faulty structures needs to be implemented prior to large-scale screening of any collection, be it *Reals* or *Virtuals*.

3.2.3. Generation of Unique, Normalized SMILES

Once canonical SMILES are derived, one should store just unique SMILES by verifying structure identity while ignoring compound IDs or molnames. If the *Virtuals* or *Tangibles* are compiled from a large number of software vendors, there is a good chance that this will clean up 50% or more of the starting collection. At this step, it is advisable to use a list of "preferred" or "trusted" vendors first. Such lists are developed with time, so first-time users must take some risks in this step. Whenever the budget is limited, a script to keep low-price structures can be used.

3.3. Filtering for Lead-Likeness

After cleanup, the collection can be processed to remove compounds that do not have leadlike properties *(7,13,14)*. Compounds that pass this filter—between 10 and 80%, depending on the source of the compounds in the collection—are prioritized for screening. It is advisable to cluster (*see* **Subheading 3.7.**) the remaining "nonleadlike" set and to include a representative set of these compounds (up to 30%), because they are likely to capture additional chemotypes. It remains the responsibility of the end user to apply, or discard, the leadlike concept, or to adjust the parameters prior to acquiring/screening compounds. Our suggestions for exclusions according to leadlikeness are as follows:

- More than four rings.
- More than three fused aromatic rings (avoid polyaromatic rings, because they are likely to be processed by cytochrome P450 enzymes and yield epoxides and other carcinogens).
- HDO more than 4; HDO ≤ 5 is one of the Ro5 criteria, but 80% of drugs have HDO less than 3 *(12)*.
- More than four halogens, except fluorine (avoid "pesticides"). A notable exception is the crop-protectant business; in such situations, the collection must be processed with entirely different criteria.
- More than two CF3 groups (avoid highly halogenated molecules).

The "unwanted" list is likely to reflect a "cultural bias" that is particular to each company. For example, companies active in contraceptive research (e.g., Organon and Wyeth) might regard steroids favorably at this stage, whereas other companies might want to actively exclude them from the collection at an early stage. Similar arguments could be made, e.g., for the lactam nucleus (penicillins, cephalosporins) and peptides. An additional step may include removal of known frequent hitters *(8)* or promiscuous binders *(9)*, and the removal of compounds that contain fragments responsible for cytotoxicity (*see* **Fig. 1**).

The collection could be regarded as an initial step, in which manipulation occurs only *once* prior to all (virtual) screens (*see* **Note 2**), assuming that targets are similar and that the drug discovery projects have similar goals, such as orally available drugs that should not penetrate the blood–brain barrier. However, the screening set may be just the *Tangibles* subset. The collection may therefore require different processing criteria for different targets and discovery goals; targets located in the lung require a different pharmacokinetic profile, e.g., for inhalation therapy, compared with targets located in the urinary tract that may require good aqueous solubility at pH = 5.0, or on the skin (LogP between 5 and 7 is ideal for such topical agents). Such biases should be introduced as much as possible at the property filtering stage, because they reduce the size of the chemical space that needs to be sampled.

3.4. Searching for Similarity If Known Active Molecules are Available

Whenever high-activity molecules are available from the literature, from patents or in-house data, the user is advised to perform a similarity search on the entire *Virtuals* or *Tangibles* for similar molecules (*see* **Subheading 3.7.**), and to seek actively to include them in the (virtual) screening subset, even though they might have been removed during the previous steps. These molecules should serve as positive controls; that is, they should be retrieved at the end of the virtual or HTS as "hits," if the similarity principle holds.

3.5. Exploring Alternative Structures

The user should seek alternative structures by modifying *(40)* the canonical isomeric SMILES, because these may occur in solution or at the ligand-receptor interface:

- Tautomerism, which shifts one hydrogen along a path of alternating single/double bonds, mostly involving nitrogen and oxygen (e.g., imidazole).
- Acid/base equilibria, which explore different protonation states by assigning formal charges to those chemical moieties that are likely to be charged (e.g., phosphate or guanidine) and by assigning charges to some of those moieties that are likely to be charged under different microenvironmental conditions ("chargeable" moieties such as tetrazole and aliphatic amine).
- Exploration of alternate structures whenever chiral centers are not specified (Daylight's *chirality,* OpenEye's *flipper)*—because 3D structure conversion from SMILES in such cases does not "explode" all possible states. Another example is pseudochiral centers such as pyramidal ("flappy") nitrogen inversions that explore noncharged, nonaromatic, pseudochiral nitrogens (three substituents), because these are easily interconverted into three dimensions.

Exploring alternative structures is advisable prior to processing any collection with computational means, such as for diversity analysis (*see* **Note 3**). The results will influence any "buy" decision, as well as the results of any virtual screen.

3.6. Generating 3D Structures

Perhaps more important for virtual screening, but equally relevant for selection methods using 3D-based chemical descriptors, is the effort of exploring one or more conformers per molecule. For example, in virtual screening, one or multiple conformers per molecule are needed. Some docking software, such as FRED *(41)*, can generate the 3D structures from SMILES prior to the actual docking step. Other docking programs require a separate 3D conversion step *(42)*, such as using CONCORD (www. optive.com or www.tripos.com) or CORINA (www.mol-net.de). OpenEye's SZYBKL (www.eyesopen.com) has integrated force-field and solvation models, allowing the user to explore multiple conformational spaces. Other conformational "exploders" are also available: Catalyst (www.accelrys.com/), Confort (www.optive.com or www.tripos.com) and OMEGA (www.eyesopen.com). To address the missing or improper chirality information, CONCORD is now coupled with StereoPlex (www.optive.com or www.tripos. com), a software that makes "educated guesses" about the chiral centers that require systematic 3D exploration.

3.7. Selecting Chemical Structure Representatives

Screening compounds that are similar to known actives increases the likelihood of finding new active compounds, but it may not lead to different chemotypes, a highly desirable situation in the industrial context. The severity of this situation is increased if the original actives are covered by third-party patents or if the lead chemotype is toxic. Sometimes, the processed collection may simply be too large to be evaluated in detail, or even to be submitted to a virtual screen. In such cases, a strategy based on clustering and perhaps on statistical molecular design (SMD) is a better alternative, compared to random selection. Clustering methods aim at grouping molecules into "families" (clusters) of related structures that are perceived—at a given resolution— to be different from other chemical families. With clustering, the end user has the ability to select one or more representatives from each family. SMD methods aim at sampling various areas of chemical space and selecting representatives from each area. Some software is designed to select compounds from multidimensional spaces, such as Library Explorer *(43)*, which is based on the BCUT metric *(44,45)*. The outcome of the selection is likely to be influenced by several factors, as discussed next.

3.7.1. Chemical Descriptors

Chemical descriptors are used to encode chemical structures and properties of compounds: 2D/3D binary fingerprints or counts of different substructural features, or perhaps (computed) physicochemical properties (e.g., molecular weight, CLogP, HDO, HAC), as well as other types of steric, electronic, electrostatic, topological, or hydrogen-bonding descriptors. The choice of what descriptors to use, and in what context, depends on the size of the collection, the software and hardware available, as well as the time constraints given for a particular selection process.

3.7.2. Similarity (Dissimilarity) Measure

Chemical similarity is used to quantify the "distance" between a pair of compounds (dissimilarity, or 1 − similarity), or how related the two compounds are (similarity). The basic tenet of chemical similarity is that molecules exhibiting similar features are expected to have similar biological activity *(46)*. Similarity is, by definition, related to a particular framework: that of a descriptor system (a metric by which to judge similarity), as well as that of an object, or class of objects, reference point with which objects can be compared is needed *(47)*. Similarity depends on the choice of molecular descriptors *(48)*, the choice of the weighting scheme(s), and the similarity coefficient itself. The coefficient is typically based on Tanimoto's symmetric distance-between-patterns *(49)*, and on Tversky's asymmetric contrast model *(50)*. Multiple types of methods are available for evaluation of chemical similarity *(46,51–54*; *see* **Note 4**).

3.7.3. Clustering Algorithms

Clustering algorithms can be classified using many criteria and also implemented in different ways *(29–32)*. Hierarchical clustering methods have been traditionally used to a greater extent, in part owing to computational simplicity. More recently, chemical structure classifications are examining nonhierarchical methods. In practice, the individual choice of different factors (descriptors, similarity measure, clustering algorithm) depends also on the hardware and software resources available, the size and diversity of the collection that must be clustered, and not ultimately on the user experience in producing a useful classification that has the ability to predict property values. We prefer Mesa's clustering method *(31)* for its ability to provide assymetric clustering and to deal with the "false singletons" (borderline compounds that are often assigned to one of at least two equally distant chemical families).

3.7.4. Statistical Molecular Design

SMD can be applied to rationally select collection representatives, as illustrated for building block selection in combinatorial synthesis planning *(55)*. Various methods for experimental design *(56)*, such as fractional factorial or composite design, can be applied for sampling large solution spaces, particularly if only a rather small screening deck can be investigated in the first round.

3.8. Assembling List of Compounds for Acquisition or Virtual Screening

Once provided with an output from one or several methods for compound selection, the now-selected collection representatives are *almost* ready to be submitted for acquisition or for virtual screening. The end user is encouraged to allow nonleadlike molecules (i.e., molecules that violate one or several criteria outlined in **Subheading 3.3.**) to be reentered into the candidate pool. An additional random, perhaps nonleadlike selection (up to 30%) can, and should, be entered in the final list of compounds. This does not imply that random selection is more successful compared to rational methods, or that criteria for rational selection ought to be taken lightly. However, since serendipity has played a major role in drug discovery *(57)*, one should allow a certain degree of randomness in the final selection. If randomly selected compounds are included, the final list of compounds should be verified, once more, for uniqueness—to avoid screening duplicates.

4. Notes

1. In its current implementation, FILTER rewrites the canonical (Daylight) SMILES. One cannot restore the canonical format post-FILTER by redirecting the output via *cansmi,* because canonicalization using OELib (pre-OEChem product from OpenEye)–generated SMILES can be erroneous for some structures. Instead, the user is advised to restore the original, canonical Daylight SMILES from the input file (pre-FILTER). Future OEChem-based versions of FILTER may not require this procedure.
2. For virtual screening, it is also advisable to eliminate molecules that contain more than nine connected single bonds not in ring or more than eight connected unsubstituted single bonds not in ring; and macrocycles with more than 22 atoms in a ring or macrocycles with more than 14 flexible bonds, because high flexibility has been shown to decrease the accuracy of the docking procedure *(58).*
3. If alternative structures are not explored prior to virtual screening, the method will explore only a limited state of the "parent" compounds. These changes are likely to occur in reality, because the receptor and the solvent environment, or simple Brownian motion will influence the particular 3D and chemical state(s) that the parent molecule is sampling. Their combinatorial explosion needs to be, within limits, explored at the SMILES level before the 3D structure generation step.
4. If the 3D structure of the bioactive conformation is available (e.g., an active ligand crystallized in the target binding site), then the user should perform both a 3D similarity search and a 2D-based one, because they are likely to yield different results. Including representatives from both searches is preferred.

Conclusion

The procedure described herein can be summarized as follows:

1. Assemble the collection starting from in-house and on-line databases.
2. Clean up the collection by removing "garbage," verifying structural integrity, and making sure that only unique structures are screened.
3. Perform property filtering to remove unwanted structures based on substructures, property profiling, or various scoring schemes; the collection can become the virtual screening set at this stage, or it can be further subdivided in a target- and project-dependent manner.
4. Use similarity to given actives to seek compounds with related properties.
5. Explore the possible stereoisomers, tautomers, and protonation states.
6. Generate the 3D structures in preparation for virtual screening, or for computation of 3D descriptors.
7. Use clustering or SMD to select compound representatives for acquisition.
8. Add a random subset to the final list of compounds. The final list can now be submitted for compound acquisition or virtual screening.

Acknowledgment

These studies were supported in part by New Mexico Tobacco Settlement funds.

References

1. Horvath, D. (1997) A virtual screening approach applied to the search for trypanothione reductase inhibitors. *J. Med. Chem.* **40,** 2412–2423.
2. Walters, W. P., Stahl, M. T., and Murcko, M. A. (1998) Virtual screening—an overview. *Drug Discov. Today* **3,** 160–178.
3. Mestres, J. (2002) Virtual screening: a real screening complement to high-throughput screening. *Biochem. Soc. Trans.* **30,** 797–799.
4. Oprea, T. I. and Matter, H. (2004) Integrating virtual screening in lead discovery. *Curr. Opin. Chem. Biol.* **8,** 349–358.
5. Oprea, T. I., Li, J., Muresan, S., and Mattes, K. C. (2003) High throughput and virtual screening: choosing the appropriate leads, in *EuroQSAR 2002—Designing Drugs and Crop Protectants: Processes, Problems and Solutions* (Ford, M., Livingstone, D., Dearden, J., and Van de Waterbeemd, H., eds.), Blackwell Publishing, New York, pp. 40–47.
6. Oprea, T. I., Bologa, C. G., Edwards, B. S., Prossnitz, E. A., and Sklar, L. A. (2005) Post-HTS analysis: an empirical compound prioritization scheme. *J. Biomol. Screen.* **10,** in press.
7. Rishton, G. (2003) Nonleadlikeness and leadlikeness in biochemical screening. *Drug Discov. Today* **8,** 86–96.
8. McGovern, S. L., Caselli, E., Grigorieff, N., and Shoichet, B. K. (2002) A common mechanism underlying promiscuous inhibitors from virtual and high-throughput screening. *J. Med. Chem.* **45,** 1712–1722.
9. Roche, O., Schneider, P., Zuegge, J., et al. (2002) Development of a virtual screening method for identification of "frequent hitters" in compound libraries. *J. Med. Chem.* **45,** 137–142.
10. Oprea, T. I. (2002) Lead structure searching: Are we looking for the appropriate properties? *J. Comput.-Aided Mol. Des.* **16,** 325–334.
11. Lipinski, C. A., Lombardo, F., Dominy, B. W., and Feeney, P. J. (1997) Experimental and computational approaches to estimate solubility and permeability in drug discovery and development settings. *Adv. Drug Deliv. Rev.* **23,** 3–25.
12. Oprea, T. I. (2000) Property distribution of drug-related chemical databases. *J. Comput.-Aided Mol. Des.* **14,** 251–264.
13. Teague, S. J., Davis, A. M., Leeson, P. D., and Oprea, T. I. (1999) The design of leadlike combinatorial libraries. *Angew. Chem. Int. Ed. 38,* 3743–3748; German version: *Angew. Chem.* **111,** 3962–3967.
14. Hann, M. M. and Oprea, T. I. (2004) Pursuing the leadlikeness concept in pharmaceutical research. *Curr. Opin. Chem. Biol.* **8,** 255–263.
15. Weininger, D. (1988) SMILES, a chemical language and information system. 1. Introduction to methodology and encoding rules. *J. Chem. Inf. Comput. Sci.* **28,** 31–36.
16. Daylight Toolkit v4.81, Daylight Chemical Information Systems, www.daylight.com/.
17. OEChem Toolkit v1.3, Openeye Scientific Software, www.eyesopen.com/.
18. Open Babel, http://openbabel.sourceforge.net/.
19. Smi2fp_ascii, Daylight Chemical Information Systems, www.daylight.com/.
20. UNITY® 4.4.2, Tripos, www.tripos.com/.
21. MACCSKeys320Generator, Mesa Analytics and Computing LLC, www.mesaac.com/.
22. Barnard, J. M. and Downs, G. M. (1997) Chemical fragment generation and clustering software. *J. Chem. Inf. Comput. Sci.* **37,** 141, 142.
23. Durant, J. L., Leland, B. A., Henry, D. R., and Nourse, J. G. (2002) Reoptimization of MDL keys for use in drug discovery. *J. Chem. Inf. Comput. Sci.* **42,** 1273–1280.
24. MOE: The Molecular Operating Environment from Chemical Computing Group Inc., www.chemcomp.com/.

25. Leo, A. (1993) Calculating log P_{oct} from structures. *Chem. Rev.* **93,** 1281–1306.
26. CLogP 4.0, BioByte Corporation, www.biobyte.com/.
27. EPI Suite v3.11, U.S. Environmental Protection Agency, www.epa.gov/.
28. Tetko, I. V. and Tanchuk, V. Y. (2002) Application of associative neural networks for prediction of lipophilicity in ALogPS 2.1 program. *J. Chem. Inf. Comput. Sci.* **42,** 1136–1145.
29. Barnard clustering, Virtual Computational Chemistry Laboratory, www.bci.gb.com/cluster analysis.html.
30. Cluster Package, Daylight Chemical Information Systems, www.daylight.com/.
31. Measures, Mesa Analytics and Computing LLC, www.mesaac.com/.
32. ChemoMine Consultancy, www.chemomine.co.uk/.
33. iResearch™ Library, ChemNavigator, Inc., www.chemnavigator.com/cnc/products/IRL.asp.
34. Andrews, K. M. and Cramer, R. D. (2000) Toward general methods of targeted library design: topomer shape similarity searching with diverse structures as queries. *J. Med. Chem.* **43,** 1723–1740.
35. FILTER 2.1, OpenEye Scientific Software, www.eyesopen.com/products/applications/filter.html.
36. Olah, M., Mracec, M., Ostopovici, L., et al. (2004) WOMBAT: World of Molecular Bioactivity, in *Cheminformatics in Drug Discovery* (Oprea, T. I., ed.), Wiley-VCH, New York, pp. 223–239.
37. Coats, E. A. (1998) The CoMFA steroids as a benchmark dataset for development of 3D-QSAR methods, in *3D QSAR in Drug Design. Volume 3. Recent Advances* (Kubinyi, H., Folkers, G., and Martin, Y. C., eds.), Kluwer/ESCOM, Dordrecht, The Netherlands, pp. 199–213.
38. Oprea, T. I., Olah, M., Ostopovici, L., Rad, R., and Mracec, M. (2003) On the propagation of errors in the QSAR literature, in *EuroQSAR 2002—Designing Drugs and Crop Protectants: Processes, Problems and Solutions* (Ford, M., Livingstone, D., Dearden, J., and Van de Waterbeemd, H., eds.), Blackwell Publishing, New York, pp. 314–315.
39. Chem DB, Chemical database management software, TimTec Inc., http://software.timtec.net/ched.htm.
40. Kenny, P. W. and Sadowski, J. (2004) Structure modification in chemical databases, in *Cheminformatics in Drug Discovery* (Oprea, T. I., ed.), Wiley-VCH, New York, in press.
41. FRED, OpenEye Scientific Software, www.eyesopen.com/products/applications/fred.html.
42. Sadowski, J. and Gasteiger, J. (1993) From atoms and bonds to three-dimensional atomic coordinates: automatic model builders. *Chem. Rev.* **93,** 2567–2581.
43. LibraryExplorer, Optive Research Inc., www.optive.com/productDetailLibraryExplorer.do.
44. Pearlman, R. S. (1996) Novel Software Tools for Addressing Chemical Diversity. Network Science, http://netsci.org/Science/Combichem/feature08.html.
45. Pearlman, R. S. and Smith, K. M. (1998) Novel software tools for chemical diversity. *Perspect. Drug Discov.* **9–11,** 339–353.
46. Johnson, M. A. and Maggiora, G. M. (1990) *Concepts and Applications of Molecular Similarity,* Wiley-VCH, New York.
47. Oprea, T. I. (2002) Chemical space navigation in lead discovery. *Curr. Opin. Chem. Biol.* **6,** 384–389.
48. Todeschini, R. and Consonni, V. (2002) *Handbook of Molecular Descriptors,* WileyVCH, Weinheim, Germany.
49. Tanimoto, T. T. (1961) Non-linear model for a computer assisted medical diagnostic procedure. *Trans. NY Acad. Sci. Ser.* **2(23),** 576–580.
50. Tversky, A. (1977) Features of similarity. *Psychol. Rev.* **84,** 327–352.

51. Willett, P. (1987) *Similarity and Clustering Techniques in Chemical Information Systems,* Research Studies Press, Letchworth, England.
52. Willett, P. (2000) Chemoinformatics—similarity and diversity in chemical libraries. *Curr. Opin. Biotechnol.* **11,** 85–88.
53. Lewis, R. A., Pickett, S. D., and Clark, D. E. (2000) Computer-aided molecular diversity analysis and combinatorial library design. *Rev. Comput. Chem.* **16,** 1–51.
54. Martin, Y. C. (2001) Diverse viewpoints on computational aspects of molecular diversity. *J. Comb. Chem.* **3,** 231–250.
55. Linusson, A., Gottfries, J., Lindgren, F., and Wold, S. (2000) Statistical molecular design of building blocks for combinatorial chemistry. *J. Med. Chem.* **43,** 1320–1328.
56. Eriksson, L., Johansson, E., Kettaneh-Wold, N., Wikstrom, C., and Wold, S. (2000) *Design of Experiments: Principles and Applications,* Umetrics Academy, Umea, Sweden.
57. Kubinyi, H. (1999) Chance favors the prepared mind—from serendipity to rational drug design. *J. Rec. Signal Transd. Res.* **19,** *15–39.*
58. Bostrom, J., Norrby, P.-O., and Liljefors, T. (1998) Conformational energy penalties of protein-bound ligands. *J. Comput.-Aided Mol. Des.* **12,** 383–396.

15

Bioinformatics Platform Development

From Gene to Lead Compound

**Alexis S. Ivanov, Alexander V. Veselovsky,
Alexander V. Dubanov, and Vladlen S. Skvortsov**

Summary

In the past 10 yr, the field of bioinformatics has been characterized by the mapping of many genomes. These efforts have stimulated explosive development of novel bioinformatics and experimental approaches to predict the functions and metabolic role of the new proteins. The main application of the work is to search, validate, and prioritize new targets for designing a new generation of drugs. Modern computer and experimental methods for discovery of new lead compounds have also expanded and integrated into the process referred to as rational drug design. They are directed to accelerate and optimize the drug discovery process using experimental and virtual (computer-aided drug discovery) methods. Recently, these methods and approaches have merged into a "from gene to lead" platform that includes the processes from new target discovery through obtaining highly effective lead compounds. This chapter describes the strategies as employed by the "From Gene to Lead" platform, including the major computer and experimental approaches and their interrelationship. The latter part of the chapter contains some examples of the steps required for implementing this platform.

Key Words: Rational drug design; bioinformatics; lead compound; computer-aided drug discovery; target discovery; database mining; target validation; structure-based drug design; ligand-based drug design; *de novo* design.

1. Introduction

The pipeline of drug discovery from idea to market consists of seven basic steps: disease selection, target selection, lead compound identification, lead optimization, preclinical trial evaluation, clinical trials, and drug manufacturing. For a long time, the principle sources of compounds for experimental testing were living organisms (plants, animals, microorganisms) and "classic" chemical synthesis. During experimental testing, most of the compounds were rejected as unpromising owing to the absence

From: *Methods in Molecular Biology, vol. 316: Bioinformatics and Drug Discovery*
Edited by: R. S. Larson © Humana Press Inc., Totowa, NJ

of or low requested activity, the existence of toxicity or carcinogenity, the complexity of synthesis, and so on. As a result, only one of several hundred thousand examined compounds would become a drug and be available in the pharmaceutical market. Thus, the time it takes new drugs to be developed may reach up to 12–15 yr at a total cost of $800 million *(1,2)*. The reduction of time- and money-consuming final stages of the drug discovery pipeline (clinical trials and drug manufacturing) is practically impossible owing to strict state standards and laws. Therefore, main efforts to increase the efficiency of drug development are directed at the earlier stages of lead discovery and optimization.

During the past 10 yr, researchers in the lead discovery area paid special attention to modern approaches such as computer sciences, i.e., bioinformatics integrated with new experimental methods, frequently called "rational drug design." This methodology is directed at accelerating and optimizing the discovery of new biologically active compounds suitable as drug candidates (lead compounds). It includes two approaches: experimental and virtual (computer-aided drug discovery [CADD]). Extensive genome decoding of various organisms, including human, has also allowed bioinformatics approaches to predict several new potential targets.

Recently these methods and approaches have merged into a "from gene to lead" platform that covers the principle part of the pipeline from new target discovery to obtaining highly effective lead compounds that can be tested in preclinical and clinical trials (**Fig. 1**). Several steps of this platform include computer modeling, virtual screening, and properties predictions that decrease time- and money-consuming steps. For instance, CADD methods can reduce the amount of compounds that are synthesized and tested by up to two orders of magnitude. Nonetheless, these approaches cannot completely replace the real experiments. The purpose of computer methods is to generate highly probable hypotheses about new targets and/or ligands that must be tested later in direct experiments.

This chapter describes the main strategies and methods of a from gene to lead platform, employing computer and experimental approaches at different steps and in a complementary manner. The last part of the chapter contains specific examples of the steps in implementing this platform.

2. Materials

2.1. Genomic and Protein Databases

For automated target selection various databases can be employed:

1. Databases with primary genomic data (complete genomes, plasmids, and protein sequences): National Center for Biotechnology Information (NCBI) GenBank *(3)*, EBI-EMBL *(4)*, DNA Databank of Japan (DDBJ) *(5)*.
2. Databases with annotated protein sequences, such as Swiss-Prot and TrEMBL *(6)* and Protein Information Resource (PIR) *(7)*.
3. Databases with results of cross-genome comparisons, such as COG/KOG (Clusters of Orthologous groups of proteins) *(8)* and Kyoto Encyclopedia of Genes and Genomes (KEGG) orthologies *(9)*.

391

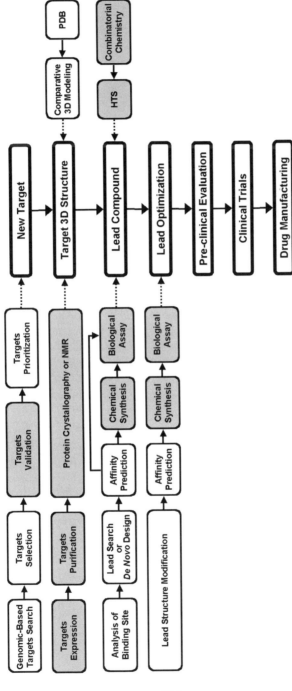

Fig. 1. General pipeline of target-based drug design and main steps of platform "From Gene to Lead." The experimental steps are highlighted in gray.

4. Databases containing information on protein families and protein classification, such as Pfam and SUPFAM *(10)*, and TIGRFAMs *(11)*.
5. Web services for cross-genome analysis (including tools for antimicrobial target selection), such as TIGR Comprehensive Microbial Resource (CMR) *(12)* and Microbial Genome Database for Comparative Analysis (MBGD) *(13)*.
6. Databases on protein–protein interactions (both experimental and predicted data), such as DIP *(14)*, BIND *(15)*, InterDom *(16)*, and FusionDB *(17)*.
7. Databases on metabolic and regulatory pathways, such as KEGG *(9)* and PathDB *(18)*.
8. Databases with protein three-dimensional (3D) structures, such as Protein Data Bank (PDB) *(19)* and satellite databases and their recompilations, e.g., PDB-REPRDB *(20)*.
9. Integrated resources such as PEDANT *(21)*.

Complete information on currently available collections of databases on the Internet can be obtained from special issues of *Nuclear Acid Research (22)*. A list of databases suitable for novel antimicrobial target selection is provided in **ref. 23**.

2.2. Molecular Databases

It is crucial to have access to some databases that hold different structures of macromolecules and small compounds. The spatial structures of proteins are principally collected in PDB *(19)*. There are numerous different databases with structures of small compounds. The crystallographic structures are collected in Cambridge Structural Database *(24)*. This database is currently the largest, unique collection of experimental data on 3D structures of small compounds (about 300,000). Its enormous size, however, has at least two weaknesses. First, it contains numerous structures that are not attractive for drug design (e.g., organometallic compounds). Second, many compounds that are not factual and must be synthesized are present. These compounds require considerable effort to synthesize. Pharmaceutical companies often prefer to use their own corporative databases, collected from different open and corporate sources. Other molecular databases are commercially available ones, such as NCI *(25)*, MDDR *(26)*, and CMC *(27)*. The main disadvantage of these databases is that they have been extensively analyzed, so the chance of finding new lead compounds is very low. In practice, it is more convenient to use specialized databases that collect the structures of commercially available samples of small compounds from different chemical classes. These samples can be promptly purchased for experimental testing and using such databases precludes chemical synthesis. Examples of such databases are ASINEX *(28)*, ChemBridge *(29)*, and MayBridge *(30)*. In some cases, these databases can be replaced with personal databases holding virtual structures of compounds generated by a special computer program, such as CombiFlexX from the SYBYL suite *(31)*.

2.3. Software and Hardware

Automated target selection for novel antimicrobial agents can be performed with the help of specialized software tools:

1. "Homegrown" software developed by academic researchers in accordance with their particular target selection tasks. This approach is characteristic of the earlier phase of automated target selection methods *(32,33)*.

2. Commercial software and databases designed for solution of routine bioinformatics tasks. For example, GeneData Phylosopher suite *(34)* contains the module for antimicrobial target selection.
3. Custom scenarios (scripts, macros) that were written in interpretative programming languages (e.g., Perl *[35]* or Python *[36]*) using free libraries, classes, and functions for bioinformatics data processing *(37)*, such as BioPerl *(38)* and BioPython *(39)*. From our point of view, this approach is more preferable because target selection may be performed in strict accordance with project requirements. All calculations and target search can be performed both locally and by using Web services, such as Entrez Utilities *(40)* and NCBI BLAST *(41)*. These services offer a good alternative to commercial software because they provide considerable flexibility in comparison to many approaches.
4. Web services for cross-genome analyses, such as Comprehensive Microbial Resource *(12)*. These services are mainly demonstrative but can be used for preliminary target searches.

Many cross-genome analyses can be carried out locally in cases in which unpublished genomes are utilized in target selection. CADD requires various methods of calculation by using specialized software and highly effective hardware. Recent CADD investigations frequently employ multiprocessor servers and graphical stations under UNIX management. Currently, PC clusters under LINUX are becoming more and more popular for such calculation. Two major commercial software suites, SYBYL from Tripos *(31)* and Insight II and Quanta from Accelrys *(42)*, are suitable for CADD, implementing nearly complete processing of drug design. We prefer to use SYBYL, and this chapter is based on using the different modules from this suite (*see* **Note 1**). For some local purposes, we also use several cheap academic programs, such as AMBER *(43)*, and shareware or freeware programs (e.g., GROMACS *[44]*, a very popular program for molecular dynamics simulation).

3. Methods

3.1. Genome-Based Antiinfective Target Selection

3.1.1. Bioinformatics Approaches in Genome-Based Target Selection

Automated target selection is usually used as the first step in novel anti-infective agent design, because most of the feature requirements for the target protein in pathogenic microbes can be easily formalized. These requirements can be deduced from desired features of "ideal" antiinfective drug (*see* **Table 1**) *(33,45)*. In accordance with the modern concept of target selection, all proteins encoded by target microbial genomes should be examined for fitness to these requirements and the best candidates can be selected as potential targets.

Target selection is usually divided into two steps: preliminary automated potential target search, and the final manual target selection based on the data about protein function. The first step reduces the number of potential targets from thousands (typical bacterial genome coding about 1500–4000 proteins) to about 10–20 put on the preliminary hit list. In the second step, the perspective potential targets are selected and prioritized. We recommend using step-by-step selection *(33)* instead of the scoring scheme

Table 1
Requirements of "Ideal" Antimicrobial Agent and Its Target

Drug	Target
Biomedical requirements	
Effective suppression of growth and reproduction of micro-organism	Important for growth and reproduction
Lethality to pathogen	Essential for survival
Definite antimicrobial spectrum	Occurs in all target microbial species and strains
Selectivity: minimal host toxicity	Absent in host (human)
Selectivity: minimal alteration of normal microflora	Absent in host's (human) symbiont bacteria
Low risk of resistance	Conserved in all target strains
Technological requirements	
Target-based CADD	Available 3D structure
Definite mechanism of action	Known function

CADD, computer-aided drug discovery.

(32) because the significance of several criteria may vary in different studies. We believe that serial semiautomated selection makes procedures more manageable.

3.1.2. Main Criteria of Target Selection for Antimicrobial Agents

3.1.2.1. SPECTRUM AND SELECTIVITY

Every protein in a microbial genome can be estimated for its compliance to the requested biomedical requirements by examining homologous proteins (genes) in genomes of other organisms. Usually one microbial genome (the most extensively studied) from the microbial group of interest is selected as the target genome, while other genomes are divided into genomes in which the presence of the target (or its homologs) is favorable. The contents of this group (different strains of target species and other pathogenic species) reflect the requirements for the desired antimicrobial spectrum of a new drug and genomes in which the presence of the target (or its homologs) is unfavorable, and the contents of this group (human and other mammalian genomes, genomes of human symbiont bacteria) reflect the requirements for selectivity of a new drug. The proteins from target genome that have homologs from the first group and not from the second group are selected as potential targets.

Cross-genome homology maps may be utilized for target selection in accordance with the required spectrum and selectivity of a new drug. The use of gene orthology databases seems to be optimal *(23)*. However, detection of similar proteins in different species cannot guarantee their identical drug specificity. There is no effective automated approach for overcoming this difficulty, because potential drug-binding sites are not yet determined at the stage of target selection.

3.1.2.2. 3D Structure of Target

At present the most rational way to find the lead compound for a drug with a novel mechanism of action is structure-based drug design (SBDD) using the 3D structure of a new target. Naturally, spatial structure of the target protein (solved experimentally or modeled) should be available. The possibility of homology modeling of the 3D structure of a target depends on the availability of close homologs (templates) with known 3D structures in PDB. Not less than 40% sequence identity of target and template proteins is required for successful homology modeling (*see* **Subheading 3.3.**). It was shown previously that the presence in PDB of the 3D structure of a target or close homolog is a very strict requirement, which can eliminate the bulk of targets meeting other requirements *(33)*. In this case the resulting hit list will contain potential targets that have already been studied (or its homologs) for different reasons. On the other hand, such selection makes subsequent computational and experimental steps simpler, faster, and more cost-effective, because the main methods and rules of expression, purification, crystallization, and so on have already been developed.

All criteria related to the spectrum, selectivity, and 3D structure of a target are well formalized. They can be estimated directly from the sequence similarity. Therefore, these criteria are used for automated screening in the first step of target selection.

3.1.2.3. Protein–Protein Interactions

Much attention is focused on the development of novel antimicrobial drugs acting as inhibitors of protein–protein interactions *(46,47)*. Protein–protein interfaces are more conserved than enzymes' active sites and other functional elements of protein structures. Therefore, it is possible to decrease significantly the risk of drug resistance caused by target protein mutations. It is expected that it is more preferable to select enzymes acting in homo- or hetero-oligomeric forms as target. Mutations in the interface areas of oligomeric complexes seem unlikely because two correlated mutations must occur in order for the mutant complex to survive. Nevertheless, such improbable correlated mutations apparently take place in molecular evolution, and this phenomenon was proposed for prediction of probable protein-protein interactions *(48)*.

Many tools are now available for computational analysis of protein–protein interactions as a first step of target selection. Examination of interacting proteins is based on the results of cross-genome analysis and includes old established as well as completely new approaches:

1. *Annotation by similarity*: Several proteins from the target organism may exhibit significant similarities with proteins involved in complex formation in other organisms. The majority of annotations indicating that a protein is involved in a protein–protein complex were obtained in this manner.
2. *Phylogenetic patterns (genomic profiles, cooccurrence)*: The use of phylogenetic patterns for finding the proteins involved in a common pathway or complex (i.e., functionally linked proteins) is based on a suggestion that such proteins are jointly present or absent in several organisms. Phylogenetic pattern describes an occurrence of a particular protein in several organisms. If two or more proteins have identical phylogenetic patterns, it can be suggested that these proteins are functionally linked *(48,49)*. This approach provides only general information about functional dependencies between proteins and not discovered putative complexes.

3. *Chromosome neighbors*: If in several genomes the genes coding particular proteins are neighbors on the chromosome DNA sequence, these proteins tend to be functionally linked *(23,49)*. For example, it was shown that this method correctly identifies functional links among eight enzymes involved in the pathway of arginine biosynthesis in *Mycobacterium tuberculosis (23)*. This method is considered to be more useful for prokaryoteic genome analysis, in which operons are common; however, it can also be applied for eukaryotic genomes *(7,49)*.

4. *Domain fusion ("Rosetta Stone")*: Analysis of fused domains is based on the suggestion that evolution results in fusion of neighboring functionally linked protein-coding genes. The reverse situation is also possible: it has been suggested that two or more proteins in one organism are functionally linked (most likely forming complex) and correspond to different domains of a single polypeptide chain in other species *(48,49)*.

5. *Correlated mutations*: If a particular pair of residues in separate proteins is important for protein-protein complex formation, cases of correlated mutations of these residues are expected. For example, if a negative-charged residue (−) in one protein interacts with a positive-charge residue (+) in another protein, the change of the first residue to (positive) should be correlated with the change of the second residue to (negative). Therefore, the prediction of complex formation may be based on finding examples of such mutations *(48)*.

6. *Interacting domains (sequence signatures)*: Sequence motifs of interacting domains can be found in annotated proteins. The likelihood of interaction between every pair of motif can be used to find the interacting pairs between other proteins in which these motifs are present *(48)*. Several of the aforementioned methods (Chromosome neighbors, Domain fusion, and Correlated mutations) can predict the formation of heterooligomeric complexes. The finding of interacting domains may also suggest the formation of homooligomeric complexes. However, prediction of homo-oligomers is mostly done by sequence similarity.

The results of these methods employed for the analysis of several genomes are available via the Internet (*see* **Subheading 2.1.**).

The methods just discussed usually produce false-positive and negative-results. To improve the reliability of predictions, it is recommended that these methods be employed simultaneously *(49–53)*. The incompleteness of genome sequencing and errors in gene recognition also may result in wrong predictions of protein–protein interactions. The current state of the art requires that the results of computational prediction of protein–protein interactions be experimentally validated.

3.1.2.4. Final Target Selection and Prioritization

Currently, the crucial step of final target selection and prioritization in modern drug development requires considerable manual effort. Computation of probable expenses and some not-well-formalized criteria are used at this step. In addition, protein function and its metabolic role are principally considered. Enzymes of cell wall components, vitamin biosynthesis, and proteins involved in transcription and/or translation are preferable. Enzymes that catalyze "key" reactions are also preferable, whereas structural transport proteins and enzymes from alternative metabolic pathways are not preferable *(32)*. The presence of mammalian enzyme with the same function as the target but with different sequence may increase the complexity of selective drug creation.

From a technological point of view, the water-soluble proteins are more preferable than membrane-bound ones. In the case of a published genome, the information about probable protein solubility and intracellular localization may also be found in annotated protein databases (*see* **Subheading 2.1.**). There are also some approaches for predicting a protein's intracellular localization. The three principle approaches for predicting a protein's subcellular localization are as follows *(48,54)*:

1. Direct prediction from sequence similarity with already annotated proteins;
2. Prediction using phylogeny (based on conception of the cell components' evolution);
3. Prediction based on recognition of the sorting signal sequence motifs.

The third approach is the most accurate, but knowledge on sorting signals is not complete. The combination of these approaches should be the optimal strategy *(48)*. Recently, high-throughput approaches for experimental target validation have been developed. These technologies make it possible to validate approx 10% of proteins encoded by typical bacterial genomes *(55)*.

3.2. Experimental Technologies for Target Validation

Currently, the number of known targets that respond to the action of known drugs approaches several hundred, while the number of new perspective targets that can be retrieved from genomic information is reaching the thousands. In this context, it is very difficult to choose optimal targets. In the pharmaceutical and biotech industries, this selection is vital to the reduction in cost and time needed to produce a drug *(56)*. Expensive failures might be avoided as early as possible by using experimental target validation—the process of deciding whether a probable target protein can be used for designing new drugs. Thus, target validation is currently the bottleneck of "from gene to lead" platform implementation. It is important to note that final target selection defines all subsequent phases of the platform. When several targets are selected, the project will be divided into several independent projects with a proportional increase in total expenses. Thus, the main task of target validation is a maximal reduction in the number of potential targets (at least to 10) and obtainment of additional information for target prioritization. The existing experimental techniques for target validation are diverse and range from in vitro approaches to animal models. It is stipulated by novelty of the given problem, which solution is only at the beginning. The final choice of the "right" or "best" target can be made by the researchers once the target's implementation has proven successful and feasible.

3.2.1. Proteomic Methods

It is quite reasonable to utilize proteomic methods *(57–61)* for tentative target validation with the task of eliminating the "wrong" proteins, meaning those that do not meet the right criteria.

3.2.1.1. Examination of Target Expression

Initially, researchers must check whether the proteins of interest selected by genome-driven methods are expressed in the target organism. For this purpose, standard proteomic analysis has been used (**Fig. 2**). When researchers propose the creation of a new antimicrobial agent with an extended spectrum of action, it is necessary to examine the expression of target proteins in all representatives of the selected micro-organism's group.

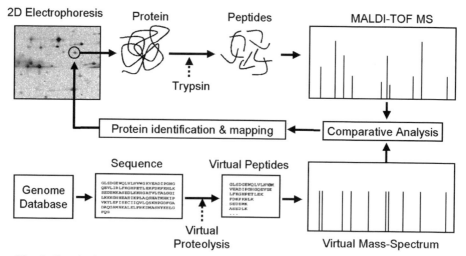

Fig. 2. Standard proteomic analysis flow chart. MALDI-TOF MS, matrix-assisted laser desorption ionization time-of-flight mass spectrometry.

3.2.1.2. EXAMINATION OF TARGET EXPRESSION IN DIFFERENT STRAINS

Researchers should obtain proteomic maps for different strains of all target microorganisms and perform comparative analysis. If a variation in target expression is detected, such a protein can be rejected from the list of potential targets for the reason of possible drug resistance.

3.2.1.3. ANALYSIS OF PROTEIN–PROTEIN INTERACTIONS

Currently, the perspective of creating novel drugs that act on the level of molecular ensembles has been discussed *(47)*. More frequently, the inhibitors of protein-protein interactions, especially the inhibitors of dimerization, have been considered *(46,62)*. Now the newest proteomic methods for analysis of protein–protein interactions can give some functional description of protein-protein interaction *(63–65)*. Using such information as a basis, researchers can select proteins in molecular complexes as new potential targets *(66)*.

3.2.2. Genomic Methods of Target Validation

Further validation of targets, successfully passed through proteomic examination, can be accomplished by using different genomic methods *(66–69)*. The majority of such approaches are based on one common idea—to verify the functional importance of potential targets by stopping their expression at the different steps of the pathway "from gene to protein" (**Fig. 3**). Certainly, genomic methods of blocking protein expression are more preferable in fast-growing cells. In species in which the potential targets have long half-lives and are renewed slowly, the methods of direct protein inactivation are more subjective (*see* **Subheading 3.2.3.**).

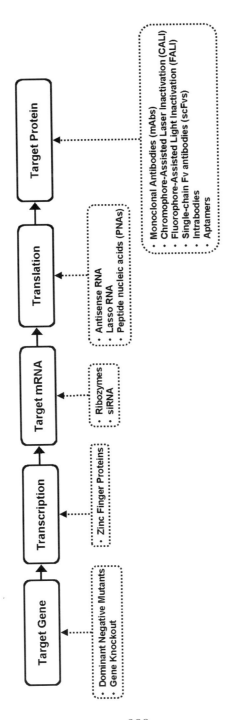

Fig. 3. Genomic methods of target validation.

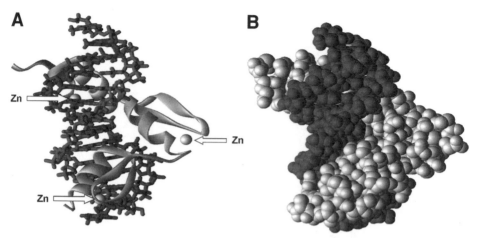

Fig. 4. Zinc-finger protein–DNA recognition. A designed consensus zinc-finger protein (in white) bound to DNA (in gray), available from Protein Data Bank (PDB) (PDB index 1MEY), is shown *(73)*. (**A**) Schematic representation of complex; (**B**) Van der Waals representation.

3.2.2.1. TARGET GENE INACTIVATION

3.2.2.1.1. Dominant Negative Mutants. The Dominant Negative Mutant approach is based on engineering of such mutations that eliminate protein function and also inhibit the function of simultaneously expressed wild-type protein *(70)*. Dominant negative mutants have already provided the understanding of molecular mechanisms of some protein families' action, such as hormones and growth factors. This method tends to be most effective for proteins that need to assemble into multimers to be functional.

3.2.2.1.2. Gene Knockout. A genetically engineered mutant organism that carries one or more genes whose function has been completely eliminated (a "null allele") can be produced. Knockouts (KOs) are mostly directed at learning about a gene that has been sequenced but has an unknown or incompletely known function *(69,71)*. Researchers draw inferences from how the KO differs from individuals in which the gene of interest has not been made inoperative.

3.2.2.2. Transcription Suppression: Zinc-Finger Proteins. Zinc-finger proteins belong to the group of transcription factors and constitute the largest individual family of proteins (>1000 sequences) *(72)*. Zinc-finger proteins are characterized by a short, two-stranded antiparalled β-sheet followed by an α-helix. Two pairs of conserved histidine and cysteine in the α-helix and second β-strand coordinate a single zinc ion. Proteins contain multiple fingers that wrap round the DNA in a spiral manner (**Fig. 4**). Fingers insert the α-helix in the major groove with a high level of recognition between the helix and DNA. The selectivity of these proteins can be changed by mutations in finger amino acid positions 1, 2, 3, and 6 relative to the start of α-helix *(74–76)* and by adjusting the number of fingers. Using zinc-finger engineering methods, researchers are able to produce different zinc-finger transcription factors that specifically regulate any given gene of interest. These features allow the use of zinc-finger proteins for target validation.

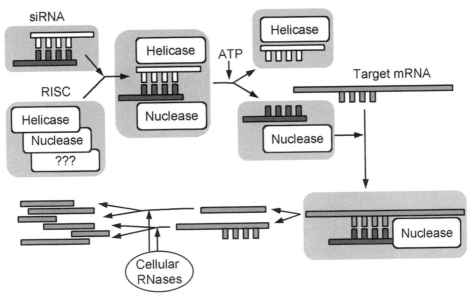

Fig. 5. Action of small, interfering RNA on mRNA. ATP, adenosine triphosphate.

3.2.2.3. DESTRUCTION OF TARGET mRNA

3.2.2.3.1. Ribozymes. Ribozymes are specific RNA molecules (oligonucleotides) that can catalyze specific biochemical reactions without the need for ancillary proteins. Natural ribozyme-catalyzed reactions may be either intramolecular (autocatalytic), such as self-splicing or self-cleaving, or intermolecular, using RNA or DNA as substrates *(77)*. Numerous ribozyme motifs have been found in nature, and additional catalytic motifs have been identified via in vitro selection *(78)*. Hammerhead motif (the smallest naturally occurring ribozyme motif) can be engineered and chemically synthesized to serve as a highly active agent of mRNA destruction *(79)*. Such artificial ribozymes are a useful tool for selective inhibition of specific mRNAs *(80)*. Broad applications of this approach in target validation are currently being discussed *(81,82)*.

3.2.2.3.2. Small Interfering RNAs. RNA interference is a revolutionary new discovery of the last 10 yr *(83,84)*. This effect is based on the action of small interfering RNAs (siRNAs) and presents the phenomenon of certain genes becoming silent. siRNAs are double-chain RNAs composed of about 20 bases *(85)*. The nucleotides of opposite chains of siRNAs are paired according to the same laws of complementarity as DNA chains in chromosomes. In addition, the boundaries of each siRNA chain always contain two unpaired nucleotides. The principle of siRNA action is shown in **Fig.'5**. When siRNA occurs in the cell, it binds with two enzymes (helicase and nuclease), forming the so-called RNA-induced silencing complex. As the result of helicase action, the chains of siRNA untwist and break up. Then the chain with bound nuclease interacts with the complement site of the target mRNA, allowing nuclease to cut the last target mRNA. After that the parts of mRNA are eliminated by the action of other cellular RNases.

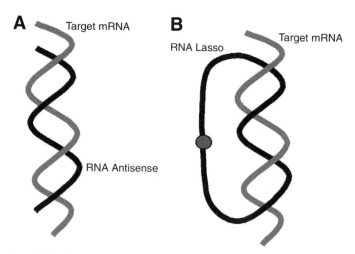

Fig. 6. Principle of binding (**A**) antisense RNA and (**B**) RNA Lasso.

Thus, the main specialty of siRNA is to knock down target gene expression effectively and with high specificity. The use of siRNA makes it possible to validate targets in a wide variety of cell types in culture in a cost-effective fashion. For these purposes, chemically synthesized siRNA duplexes as well as expression vectors encoding siRNAs can be utilized.

3.2.2.4. TRANSLATION SUPPRESSION

3.2.2.4.1. Antisense RNA. Antisense RNAs are oligonucleotides (about 20 bases long) that are complementary to a portion of target mRNAs and repress the expression of certain genes *(86,87)*. Antisense binds to the mRNA and forms a DNA-like double-helix complex (**Fig. 6A**). It prevents the reading of information from mRNA and, hence, stops the synthesis of encoded protein. After this gene has been knocked out, the functional effects of the gene can be studied. Using recombinant DNA methods, some synthetic genes coding antisense RNAs can be brought into the organism. Thus, antisense RNA can be utilized for experimental validation of potential target proteins *(88–95)*.

3.2.2.4.2. RNA Lasso. In cells the duplex RNAs, including antisense/mRNA complexes, are destroyed quickly by RNases. Alternatively, antisense can be displaced by the helicase-like action of the ribosome during translation. As a result, the effect of antisense action can be short. SomaGenic has created a gene-targeting approach, called the RNA Lasso *(96)*, based on special antisense RNAs forming very stable complexes with mRNA, since the ends of this molecule can form the knot (**Fig. 6B**). Thus, RNA Lasso may be a good choice for experimental target validation.

3.2.2.4.3. Peptide Nucleic Acids. Peptide nucleic acids (PNA) is an alternative to antisense technology, i.e., artificial oligonucleotides analogously based on polyamide backbone (such as peptides) with attached bases *(97–100)*. PNAs hybridize to DNA and RNA with high efficiency like conventional antisense and form highly stable PNA/DNA and PNA/RNA duplexes that are more resistant to enzyme degradation and nontoxic *(101,102)*. Homopyrimidine PNAs and PNAs with a high ratio of pyrimidine/purine can bind to DNA or RNA, forming highly stable triple helices *(103)*. Therefore, PNAs can be a good substitution for antisense RNA in target validation *(104)*.

3.2.3. Inactivation of Target Proteins

3.2.3.1. MONOCLONAL ANTIBODIES

The use of monoclonal antibodies (MAbs) is one of the oldest approaches to targeting proteins. It is known that antibodies can interact with target proteins with high specificity *(105)*. Unfortunately, only about 0.5% of target proteins to which they bind become functionally inactive in bacteria *(85,106)*. Therefore, new technologies based on a combination of recombinant antibodies that have high specificity and affinity against their targets coupled with neutralizing agents have been recently developed. For example, a new method of using MAbs coupled with a chromophore group for irreversible inactivation of target proteins with laser irradiation uptake is described next *(85)*.

3.2.3.2. CHROMOPHORE-ASSISTED LASER INACTIVATION

The approach of chromophore-assisted laser inactivation (CALI) is based on a linked complex of target-specific MAbs with chromophore (usually malachite green). This complex can interact with target protein and inactivate it by photochemical reaction initiated by laser irradiation. Depending on the type of chromophore, the average radius of target damage is about 15–40 Å *(107)*. This is sufficient for inactivation of target proteins or single subunits within multimeric protein complexes but excludes effects on neighboring proteins. CALI allows the conversion of more than 90% of the antibodies into real inhibitory tools *(85)*. Initially, CALI was used to study cell-surface phenomena by inactivating the functions of single proteins on living cells *(108)*, and later it was used to assay protein function both in vivo and in vitro *(109)*.

3.2.3.3. FLUOROPHORE-ASSISTED LIGHT INACTIVATION

The fluorophore-assisted light inactivation (FALI) method *(110)*, which uses labeled MAbs to target light-initiated destruction of the protein of interest, is analogous to CALI. FALI uses coherent or diffuse light targeted by fluorescein-labeled probes. The half-maximal radius of damage is approx 40 Å. The advantage of FALI is simultaneous irradiation of multiwell plates; thus, it can be utilized in proteomics for high-throughput screening (HTS) *(111)*.

3.2.3.4. SINGLE-CHAIN FV ANTIBODIES

Single-chain Fv antibodies (scFvs) are rather small single-chain polypeptides (six times smaller than intact MAbs) engineered from two regions of Fab fragment of common antibodies *(112,113)*. The heavy and light variable regions are joined by a flexible linker (e.g., Gly) sufficiently long to join the two domains (**Fig. 7**). The most popular way to obtain scFvs is through phage display libraries *(114)* or by cloning in hybridoma cells *(115)*. The main advantages of scFvs over intact MAbs and Fab fragments are their homogeneous, small size (about 30 kDa) and the absence of Fc domains, which makes them more penetrating, less immunogenic responsive, and less capable of binding to

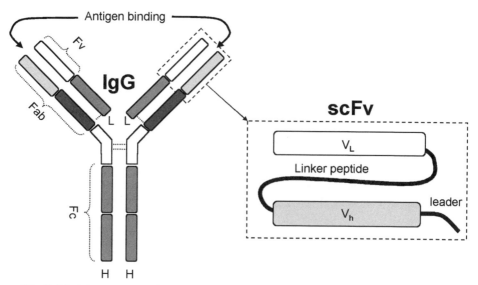

Fig. 7. Modular structure of IgG and single-chain Fv antibody. Immunoglobulins are composed of two identical light (L) chains and two identical heavy (H) chains. Light chains are composed of one constant and one variable domain, and heavy chains are composed of three constant and one variable domain. The heavy chains are covalently linked to the hinge region, and the light chains are covalently linked to the heavy chain. The variable domains of both H and L compose the antigen-binding part of the molecule, termed Fv.

Fc receptors distributed on normal cells. Thus, scFvs are a potentially useful substitution for MAbs in all target validation approaches based on MAbs.

3.2.3.5. INTRABODIES

Recent advances in antibody engineering have raised the possibility of encoding genes for the antigen-binding domain and expressing them as intracellular antibodies. In fact, scFvs can be expressed within cells and directed against target proteins *(116–119)*. Intrabodies can interfere with and inhibit intracellular processes in several ways, such as inhibiting the function of proteins directly and interfering with protein–protein interactions or target-specific domains of the protein. These features make intrabodies a great potential tool for target validation *(120)*.

3.2.3.6. APTAMERS

Aptamers are synthetic RNA or DNA oligonucleotides (5–25 kDa), which are capable of highly specific binding to a wide variety of target proteins *(121,122)*. They generally show an affinity in the nanomolar range and a high specificity of target recognition *(123)*. In contrast to antibodies conventionally selected in animals, aptamers are generated by an in vitro selection process and can be directed against almost every target, including nonimmunogenic targets, against which conventional antibodies cannot be raised *(124)*. They can be synthesized in vitro in a random combinatorial library (up to

A **B**

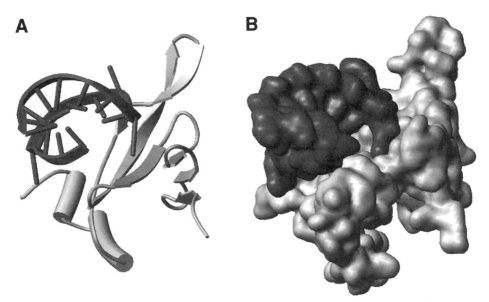

Fig. 8. Complex of capsid protein (in white) from Bacteriophage MS2 with RNA aptamer (in gray), available from Protein Data Bank (PDB) (PDB index 5MSF) *(125)*. (**A**) Schematic representation of complex; (**B**) solvent surface representation.

10^{15} different molecules), rapidly isolated, and replicated by polymerase chain reaction. The unique advantage of aptamers is the rapid automated generation of sophisticated ligands against any targets. No immunogenicity or toxicity of aptamers was observed. Their chemical stability and high inhibitory potential meet the criteria of a multifunctional tool for the validation of targets *(122)*. Aptamers have proven to be effective ligands for modulating the function of endogenous cellular proteins in their natural environment. They mimic the effect of a small-molecule drug in terms of binding and inactivating target protein (**Fig. 8**). Some approaches have been developed to use aptamers for the validation of potential drug targets in disease models. Currently, aptamers and RNA interference are often used jointly, because these two technologies are highly complementary. siRNAs can reduce the amount of target protein by decreasing the mRNA concentration, and aptamers act directly at the protein level and can be utilized to inactivate stable proteins with a slow biological turnover. The features of aptamers make them very useful for lead identification, which links target validation with drug discovery *(122,126)*. Thus, aptamer technology can be exploited to address the functional prioritization of potential drug targets and can accelerate small-molecule lead identification.

3.2.4. High-Throughput Technologies for Protein Target Search and Validation

In the last decade, many pharmaceutical companies focused on developing new high-throughput technologies for searching new drug targets and their validation, based on automatic multiparallel processes and analysis *(127,128)*. Robotic systems are capable of handling thousands of compounds per day. Many genomic, proteomic, and other methods have been applied to high-throughput target validation approaches for studies of novel potential targets retrieved from the whole genome. Such applications often focus on "loss-of-function" tactics *(129)*. Amid different approaches that provide high-throughput and systematic drug target validation and gene function discovery, the most popular are proteomics analysis *(130)*; transgenic KOs *(131)*; siRNA-based methods *(132)*; antisense technology *(133)*; aptamers *(122,126)*, which can link the process of target validation directly with the search for lead compounds by HTS; CALI; and FALI *(109–111)*. Recently, the newest approaches utilizing DNA microarrays, DNA chips, and microfluidic device technologies are revolutionizing screening for target validation and lead discovery in the pharmaceutical industry *(134–138)*; these topics are considered elsewhere in this book (*see* **Chapters 2–4** and **7**).

3.2.5. Target Validation In Vivo

Among different approaches to target validation, in vivo methods should not be neglected. Recent advances in genomics research have shown that small, multicellular organisms, such as nematodes, fruitflies, and zebra fish share a high percentage of human disease genes. Thus, diverse animal models (from invertebrates to humanized mice) can be used for in vivo target validation directed at the different types of human diseases *(139)*. These include transgenic and KO systems based on mice *(140–142)*; zebra fish (*Danio rerio*) *(143,144)*; nematodes (roundworms) *(145)*, including the well-known *Caenorhabditis elegans* *(146,147)*; fruitfly (*Drosophila melanogaster*) *(148)*; mouse-based platform VITA (Validation In Vivo of Targets and Assays for Anti-infectives) *(149, 150)*; and target validation in parasitic organisms *(151)*.

3.3. 3D Structure of Target

It is apparent that the detailed 3D structure of a selected target plays a key role in SBDD. These data can be obtained by utilizing experimental and/or bioinformatics methods.

3.3.1. Experimental Approaches

Two basic methods of protein 3D investigation are X-ray crystallography *(152)* and multidimensional nuclear magnetic resonance (NMR) *(153)*. The main steps of these experimental approaches need to obtain the necessary quantity of pure native protein (**Fig. 1**). The majority of solved protein 3D structures are stored in PDB *(19)* and access is free. As of June 2004, PDB held more than 26,000 structures (about 22,000 solved by X-ray diffraction and about 4000 by NMR). Most of these structures are those of self-same proteins (different mutants and complexes with diverse ligands). Thus, the number of unique protein structures is only about 6000. Recent genomic explorations have radically increased the number of known protein sequences. Modern methods of protein 3D investigation (X-ray crystallography and NMR) cannot keep pace with sequence determination. Moreover, both approaches are suitable mainly for water-soluble proteins and, in addition, NMR cannot solve 3D structures of proteins larger than 30,000 Daltons. At the same time, up to 40% of proteins in living organisms are membrane bound *(154)*. Nowadays only tens of membrane-bound protein structures are available from PDB because of the existing problems with their expression and crystallization *(155)*. The deficiency of known 3D structures therefore forces the researcher to use computer 3D modeling.

3.3.2. 3D Modeling

Presently only one method of target 3D modeling is suitable for SBDD. It is homology modeling (also known as comparative modeling), based on sequence and structural similarity between a model protein and its homologs with known 3D structures (templates) *(156)*. Currently, some computer programs provide the tools for knowledge-based homology modeling of protein structure (e.g., SYBYL *[31]*, Insight II *[42]*, Quanta *[42]*, Modeller *[157]*). We prefer to use SYBYL software (Tripos), and this chapter is based on using Composer *(158)* from the SYBYL suite *(31)*.

3.3.2.1. CRITERIA FOR PROTEIN HOMOLOGY MODELING

Large-scale Internet-based experiments called CASP (critical assessment of protein structure prediction) *(159,160)* have shown that the accuracy of homology modeling strongly depends on the similarity between the sequences of the model and the template. As a rule, the model is supposed to be good if the modeled sequence is more than 40% identical to the template. In cases of sequence identity less than 30%, the major factor that limits the use of this approach is the alignment problem. The fraction of incorrectly aligned residues may reach 20%. This number rises sharply with further decreases in sequence similarity. The low sequence identity limits the usefulness of homology modeling, because no current modeling technique can compensate for the errors coming from an incorrect input alignment.

3.3.2.2. MAIN STEPS OF PROTEIN HOMOLOGY MODELING (*SEE* FIG. 9)

The main steps of protein homology modeling are as follows:

1. Find homology proteins with known 3D structure in PDB. PDB is scanned for sequences similar to the model sequence.
2. Identify "seed residues" based on sequence homology. Seeds are only used for an initial structural alignment, and some errors or mismatches can be tolerated in the next step. For this reason, it is not necessary to spend a lot of time on this step.
3. Generate structural alignment using seed residues for determination of structurally conserved regions (SCRs). Composer uses seeds to generate the optimal structural alignment for the set of homologs. Only 3D coordinates of Cα atoms of residues are used to fit the structures to each other. If there are only two known homologs, fitting becomes a straightforward least-squares procedure. For three or more structures, multiple fitting is accomplished by performing a series of pairwise weighted least-squares fits. This determines SCRs and derives an average structure of the conserved regions to use in constructing the model protein.
4. Determine model SCRs. The procedure of pair sequence alignment for modeling and the best homolog (template) is used to determine of model SCRs.
5. Construct model SCRs. The framework structure produced at the previous stage represents the overall 3D structure of the conserved regions of the protein family, but it lacks real protein geometry because it is an average structure. The "Build SCRs" operation of

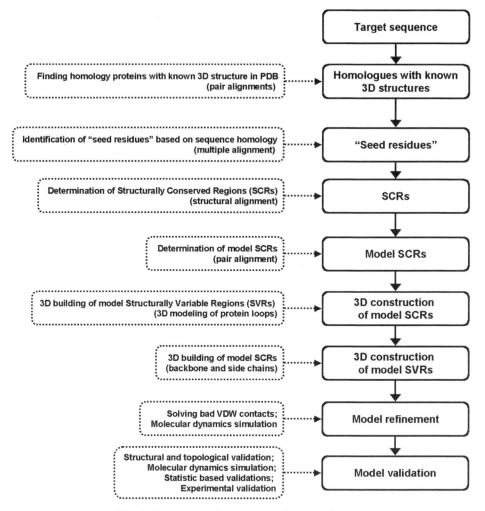

Fig. 9. Main steps of protein homology modeling.

Composer program (Sybyl) creates the backbone of each SCR in the model by fitting a fragment from one of the known homologs to the appropriate region of the framework structure. Then a knowledge-based approach is used to determine the side-chain conformations, taking into account the backbone secondary structure and the side chains at the corresponding residues in each of the homologs. Rule Database is used for this purpose.

6. Construct structurally variable regions of the model using loops from homologous or the general protein database. The "Add Loops" operation completes the protein model by constructing the structurally variable regions (loop regions). For each loop, the Composer program tries to find fragments of the known structures that are compatible with the rest of the model. Then, the program uses sequence information to find the best single fragment to be used in the final model. If any homolog of the known structure has a loop of the same length in the corresponding region as a model, then this fragment is a good choice.

Alternative approaches include finding fragments whose geometry is compatible with the geometry of the conserved regions flanking the loop in the model, and using geometric and sequence information to select the best loop fragment. Modeling the extended loops requires additional expert analysis and selection of suitable loops from the sets retrieved from PDB. The mutual position and interaction of neighbor loops, as well as all known experimental data about target structure, must be taken into account (*see* **Note 2**).

7. Refine the model. The model structure should be improved by solving bad Van der Waals contacts, and by passing the procedures of energy minimization and molecular dynamics simulation.

3.3.2.3. MODEL VALIDATION

The steps to model validation are as follows:

1. *Structural and topological model validation*: The model is examined on the absence of the following mismatches:
   a. The exposure of hydrophobic residues to the solvent.
   b. The presence of charged or polar side chains in the model interior.
   c. The positive free energy of solvation and so on.
2. *Molecular dynamics simulation*: The model is tested for the fold and secondary structure stability during molecular dynamics simulation in water.
3. *Statistics-based model validations*: Various programs based on statistical data from PDB can be used.
   a. ProCheck *(161)* inspects the model structure using Ramachandran plots.
   b. ProTable *(162)* is one of the modules from SYBYL *(31)* and was designed to analyze the protein structure quality by various criteria (e.g., geometry and stereochemistry, solvent-accessible surface area, conformations of side chains, backbone, secondary structures); ProTable can be used as an analytical tool for 3D visualization of all calculated parameters.
   c. MatchMaker, also a SYBYL module *(163)* is based on the approach known as "inverse folding" and can check the relative correctness of a protein model, by determining its compatibility with sequence.
   d. WHAT IF *(164)* checks the correspondence of model parameters to statistical data, such as bond angles and lengths, buried hydrogen bond donor, peptide plane flip, side-chain conformation and planarity, proline puckering, packing quality, side-chain rotamer, symmetry, torsion angles, water clusters, and atomic occupancy.
   e. Prosa II *(165)* allows control of protein structure quality.
   f. Profiles-3D *(166)* searches for databases of 3D profiles, looking for compatibility using environmental classification of amino acids, and the model can be compared to its own sequence to evaluate its quality.
4. *Model validation by experimental data*: Some indirect experimental data (e.g., chemical modifications of surface residues, protease action sites, point mutations, antigenic determinants) can be used for model verification: partial spectroscopic evidence, mapping surface structure.

3.4. Strategy of CADD

Once a target is selected, CADD can be initiated. CADD methods are used only when the 3D structure of a target or sets of known ligands to the target are available. Otherwise, only experimental methods can be employed. The main experimental methods are combinatorial chemistry *(167)* and HTS *(168,169)*. Identifying new compounds by computer methods consists of several steps: (1) target structure analysis and finding the binding site, (2) prediction of lead compounds and their experimental testing, (3) optimization of lead structure with further experimental testing, and (4) preclinical evaluation and clinical trials (**Fig. 10**). The purpose of CADD is to generate hypotheses about probable new ligands and their interaction with targets. However, these approaches cannot replace the experimental tests. Therefore, each step of CADD has to be finished with experimental testing of selected compounds. All steps of computer prediction can be repeated several times if negative results in the previous steps are obtained. If predicted lead compounds are inactive, a second cycle of computer modeling will be carried out taking into account the obtained negative results, i.e., using another molecular database for mining, remodeling pharmacophore or quantitative structure–activity relationships (QSAR) models, conducting additional analysis of the structure of the active site (checking the ability of conformational change during ligand interaction, involving water molecules in ligand binding, and so on). If the predicted lead compound is identified, active optimization reiteration of the process for activity should be carried out. Eventually, the set of related compounds with selected lead structure should be synthesized and tested for biological (pharmacological) activity. If the optimized structures of the lead compound exhibit high activity, preclinical tests (for activity in vivo, toxicity, carcinogenity, and so on) can be performed. Further cycles of computer structure optimization for improvement of pharmacokinetic properties (absorption, distribution, metabolism, and excretion [ADME]) *(170)* are also possible. It is considered that CADD can reduce the amount of compounds that need to be synthesized and tested for biological activity up to two orders. Thus, it is capable of decreasing time-consuming and financial expenses for the development of drugs.

The key point of the choice of CADD methods is the availability of a 3D structure of the target. The accessibility of target structure allows one to employ the methods consolidated in group SBDD ("direct methods"). In this case, compounds with properties complementary to the target surface can be designed, based on the knowledge of properties and features of the spatial structure of the target. If target 3D structure remains unknown, another group of methods, ligand-based drug design (LBDD) ("indirect methods"), should be applied. Under these circumstances, analysis of a set of known ligands is carried out to reveal their common essential properties correlated with biological activity (*see* **Note 3**). The first successful result of SBDD was obtained with creation of the antihypertensive drug captopril, based on the 3D structure of carboxypeptidase A *(171)*.

3.4.1. Structure-Based Drug Design

The first step of SBDD consists of analysis of the 3D structure of a target and definition of its ligand-binding site. If the spatial structure of the complex of a target with known ligand (substrate or competitive inhibitor) is available, the binding site is known empirically. Alternatively, a putative binding site must be identified. This problem can be approached in several ways. The rough approach determines the cavities in the protein structure and assumes that the longest, biggest cavity is the active site. A more elegant approach searches for key amino acids involved in catalysis (e.g., a triad of

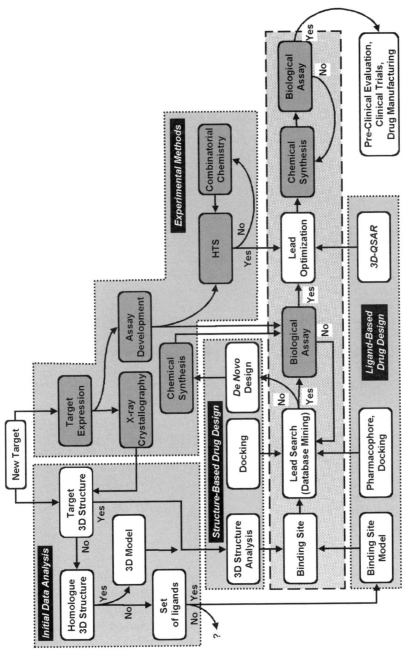

Fig. 10. General strategy of computer-assisted drug discovery.

411

serine proteases) or cofactor, and the neighbor region is assumed to be the binding site. However, the problem of uncertainty of spatial position of ligand in the active site still remains. Docking of the known substrates and/or inhibitors to the whole surface of an enzyme is the optimal approach for predicting a binding site based on using the position of docked ligands *(172)* (see **Subheading 3.4.3.**).

A popular strategy for searching for new lead structures is virtual screening of small compounds in molecular databases (database mining). This approach is based on the assumption that compounds with requested activity were synthesized earlier, but not tested for this activity. Presently, the data on several million structures of small compounds are collected in different databases (*see* **Subheading 2.2.**). The main method for database mining is molecular docking of small compounds into the binding site of target. Several docking programs have been developed (*see* **Subheading 3.4.3.**). They allow fast screening of databases containing large numbers of small compounds. All docking programs generate hypotheses about probable spatial positions of ligands in the active site of a target macromolecule. Assessment of these hypotheses is carried out by using different types of scoring functions (e.g., binding energy, area of contacting surfaces) (*see* **Subheading 3.4.4.**). Based on scoring results, the compounds with the best correspondence to the binding site structure and properties are selected *(173)*. The obvious advantage of this method is its high rate of obtaining results and ability to test the numerous compounds. However, this approach is usually unable to discover compounds with high activity (the researcher should not expect to find any "hit" with a dissociation constant better than 10^{-4}). If database mining for lead compounds was unsuccessful, *de novo* design methods can be employed. Several programs of ligand *de novo* design have been developed (*see* **Subheading 3.4.5.**).

The efficiency of ligand binding with a target is estimated by values of virtual binding energy (*see* **Subheading 3.4.4.**). The major problem with all methods of SBDD is the inability to predict the real binding energy and convert its calculated values into experimentally determined parameters (K_d, IC_{50}, K_i, and so on). Although in several cases a reasonable correlation between structure and interaction energy was found for some sets of compounds, these relationships are not generally transferable from one protein system to another *(174)*. If the lead compound with required activity has been discovered or designed, it can be utilized for increasing activity by structural modifications. The lead compound structure can be optimized with the same *de novo* methods (*see* **Subheading 3.4.5.**). These methods are also employed in the next step of preclinical evaluation for decreasing side effects and optimization of pharmacokinetic properties.

3.4.2. Ligand-Based Drug Design

LBDD methods are applied when the spatial structure of a target macromolecule is unknown and it is not possible to design its reliable model. LBDD methods are based on the analysis of sets of known ligands with the requested biological activity. Because the structure of a binding site is unknown, it is necessary to design models that reproduce the character features of the target in the binding site. There are two major approaches: the pharmacophore model *(175,176)* and various types of the "pseudoreceptor" model *(177–180)*. The pharmacophore model consists of a set of points in space with certain attributed properties and distances between them. These points and their positions define the binding of given groups of ligands with target. The pseudoreceptor models describe mainly the geometrical shape of a binding site in the spatial structure of the target.

In the first step of LBDD, as well as of SBDD, it is preferable to start with lead searching using molecular database mining. The pharmacophore models or various models of the cavity of the binding site can be used for this purpose. Database mining using a pharmacophore model assumes the selection of such structures that contain a set of chemical groups satisfying pharmacophore points. Another method of database mining uses molecular docking of small compounds from a database into the model of spatial structure of the binding site. When a target pharmacophore model contains only a few pharmacophore points, the outcome of the database mining using such a pharmacophore model may be a huge number of possible hit compounds that must be tested experimentally. In this case, methods of database mining with the model of binding site cavity are preferable.

For prediction of a requested activity of "hits" found in databases, as well as for lead structure optimization, the methods of QSAR are used. The classic QSAR method is based on the regression analysis of the relationship between the biological activity of a set of homolog compounds and their description with various descriptors. The correlation equations of this relationship predict the activity of new analogs from the same homology group *(181)*. At present, the method of 3D-QSAR is widely used. Special methods for description of 3D distribution of ligand properties (i.e., comparative molecular fields analysis [CoMFA] and comparative molecular similarity indices analysis [CoMSIA]), are also applied *(182,183)*. This approach characterizes the steric, electrostatic, and hydrophobic regions around molecules.

Recently, 3D-QSAR models have been designed for the subsequent prediction of the activity of compounds found in molecular databases or designed *de novo* even when target 3D structure is known *(184,185)*. This approach is used because of significant difficulties in converting calculated virtual binding energies into real values (K_d, K_i, IC_{50}, and so on).

3.4.3. Database Mining for New Leads

There are three main groups of methods for database mining:

1. Searching by similarity or existence the required two-dimensional (2D) patterns.
2. Database mining using the pharmacophore model.
3. Database mining by molecular docking.

The first group of methods, searching by similarity, is frequently built-in tools of a database's interface, such as ISIS/BASE (MDL) *(186)*, UNITY® (Tripos) *(187)*, and Quest (CSD) *(24)*. The second group of methods, using the pharmacophore model, can select structures that contain a set of chemical groups satisfying pharmacophore points. DOCK *(188,189)* and FlexX *(190)*, which utilize the molecular docking procedure, are the frequently used programs from the third group. Many investigators employ their own docking programs, such as the program DockSearch, for fast geometrical docking developed in our laboratory *(191)*.

Before starting a docking procedure, several preliminary operations must be done. The main one is preprocessing of the database (forming a reduced sample from the database) by retrieving compounds based on some principles, such as the allowed range of molecular weight, absence or existence of specific chemical groups, and physicochemical properties of compounds (e.g., hydrophobicity, solubility, permeability). Some of these properties can be calculated using numerous programs (SLIPPER *[192]*, DISCON *[193]*, BALPS *[193]*, and so on). Other preliminary operations are the generation of 3D structures of compounds (e.g., databases with commercially available samples of small compounds usually contain only 2D structures), the generation of their conformers, and energy optimization of structures. The conversion of structures from 2D into 3D form can be done by various programs, such as CORINA *(194,195)* and Concord *(196,197)*. Generation of conformers, which can be fulfilled by special programs, such as Confort *(198)* and CONFLEX *(199)*, is used for database updating when subsequent mining will be carried out using pharmacophore models or a program of "rigid" docking, such as DOCK *(188,189)* or DockSearch *(191)*. Database mining allows the selection of compounds with requested activity, but probably the value of activity will be low. However, these compounds can be used for further optimization of structure for increasing activity or as structural blocks for *de novo* design.

3.4.4. Prediction of Affinity

Prediction of ligand affinity is a very important step in SBDD, yet current methodologies are indefinite and complex. The majority of docking programs have their own procedures for estimation of affinity, but these values are very coarse, owing to the need to increase the speed of the docking procedure. Thus, independent methods are preferred. The popular methods for prediction of ligand affinity are based on scoring functions that use statistical relationships between numerous descriptors, which are calculated from known 3D structures of protein–ligand complexes, and the corresponding experimental data on affinity *(200–203)*. A high rate of prediction and independence of type of target is appealing. Examples of such scoring function are Validate *(204)*, SCORE *(204)*, and NNC *(205)*. These methods were developed for a wide range of protein-ligand complexes. It is important to note that the scoring functions, which have been optimized for strict targets, are always preferable owing to the increase in prediction reliability. Another approach is simultaneous employment of some fast scoring functions, such with the CScore program from the SYBYL suite *(206)*. In this program, four different scoring functions are calculated with subsequent selection of compounds based on summarized rating.

The most precise method for predicting the affinity is certainly free energy perturbation (FEP) *(207)*. Unfortunately, its execution requires large-scale computations. This method provides precise prediction of affinity in the case of a set of homologous compounds, whereas for heterogeneous sets the predictions are often ambiguous. The Gibbs program from the AMBER suite *(43)* is an example of the FEP method. Thus, the process of affinity prediction consists of serial scoring steps (from rough to precise prediction) directed to decrease the number of probable hits step-by-step:

1. Preliminary selection of hypothetic complexes during the docking procedure.

2. Estimation of affinity by fast scoring functions.
3. Affinity prediction by precise scoring functions.
4. Affinity prediction of complexes using molecular dynamics simulation and FEP methods.

The number of such steps depends on the size of the set of compounds that must be experimentally tested.

3.4.5. Modification of Lead Compounds and De Novo Design

Methods for modification of lead compounds and *de novo* design are employed to increase activity, to improve the physicochemical and pharmacokinetic properties of leads, and to decrease side effects. If database mining does not identify the lead compound, these methods remain the single way for further investigation. The advantage of these methods is their ability to design compounds with high affinity, and their disadvantage is the necessity of chemical synthesis of designed compounds. The popular programs of *de novo* design are LUDI *(208)*, CLIX *(209)*, CAVEAT *(210)*, and LeapFrog *(211)*. They all share similar principles that consist of virtual modeling of new molecules, and optimization of their structures and their spatial position in the active site. The first step of ligand design in these programs begins with searching the specific groups capable of participating in noncovalent interactions with the target macromolecule. The next step is to select the linkers for composition of these groups in one structure. Simultaneously conformation of designed ligands and their spatial positions are then optimized. Binding energy is estimated after each step of design, and the compounds with the highest values of energy are selected for further optimization. The program LeapFrog has three alternatives for structure modification:

1. Mode "Guide" updates the structures by the procedures of addition, deletion, replacement, cyclization of chemical groups, and so on, which are determined by the investigator.
2. Mode "Optimize" automatically generates the numerous modifications of lead compound with subsequent selection by their scoring function.
3. Mode "Dream" generates the lead structures *de novo* without any starting ligand structure.

As in previous cases, the next step in these approaches is the prediction of affinity by various methods (*see* **Subheading 3.4.4.**).

3.4.6. Prediction of Pharmacokinetic Properties

In addition, several programs can be used to predict various ADME properties that must be tested later during preclinical evaluation to determine whether a hit from a screening process is suitable for further development as a therapeutic agent *(170)*. Such prediction systems can be used for both selection of compounds for experimental testing for requested activity and prediction of possible side effects (e.g., toxicity, carcinogenity). These systems identify unwanted negative properties of the developing new drugs at the earliest stages. The program PASS is a very good example of such a system *(212)*.

3.5. Experimental Testing of Probable Lead Compounds

One of the crucial rate-limiting steps is experimental testing of probable lead compounds ("hits"). Many different in vitro and in vivo bioassays can be utilized for this purpose, depending on the type and function of target protein. The SBDD approach

Mycobacterium tuberculosis H37Rv

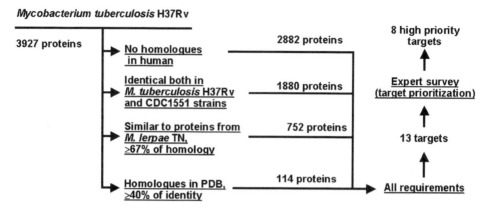

Fig. 11. Target selection in genome of *Mycobacterium tuberculosis* H37Rv *(33)*.

gives a list of hits obtained by virtual screening (database mining by molecular docking) or constructed *de novo*. All these hits are scored using calculated parameters such as geometric complementarity, areas of contact surfaces, and binding energy (in relative units). Thus, SBDD is oriented on discovery of hits selectively interacting and forming the complex with a target based on steric and energetic reasons. No direct information can be obtained at this stage of SBDD about possible modulation of target function. Thus, in the first step of experimental testing of hits, it is preferable to use a simple in vitro assay, which can directly measure the interaction of testing small compounds with target protein. From our point of view, the optical biosensor analyzers Biacore 3000 *(213)* or Biacore S51 *(214)* are the perfect instruments for the initial evaluation of hits and conversion into lead compounds. These instruments are specifically designed for rapid and efficient high-throughput assessment of intermolecular interactions using nonlabel surface plasmon resonance technology *(215,216)*, enabling interactions to be studied in near-native states. These instruments can detect the interaction of small ligands (>200 Daltons) with immobilized target protein, record the real-time binding kinetics, and determine the affinity and specificity of the interaction. Optical biosensor assays are therefore adequate for preliminary experimental evaluation of hits.

3.6. Examples of Passing Execution of Some Bioinformatics Steps of Platform "From Gene to Lead"

3.6.1. Target Selection in Genome of M. Tuberculosis

Recently, we have used bioinformatics approaches for predicting new potential targets for antitubercular agents *(33)*. GenMesh *(33)* was applied to the genome of *M. tuberculosis* H37Rv and compared by BLAST *(217)* with (1) the genome of *M. tuberculosis* CDC1551, (2) the genome of *Mycobacterium leprae*, (3) all known human proteins, and (4) proteins from PDB. Filtration of proteins encoded by the mycobacterial genome was carried out as shown in **Fig. 11**. A preliminary hit list of targets is shown in **Table 2**. This set was analyzed in detail. Target prioritization, based on probable protein functions, was also carried out. As a result, only eight proteins were selected as poten-

Table 2
Potential Targets Found in Genome of *Mycobacterium tuberculosis* H37Rv

Target no.	Gene	Target protein
1.	*infA*	Translation initiation factor IF-1
2.	*hupB*	Histone-like protein
3.	*rpoA*	DNA-directed RNA polymerase (transcriptase) α-chain
4.	*rpsD*	30S ribosomal protein S4
5.	*rpsE*	30S ribosomal protein S5
6.	*rpsH*	30S ribosomal protein S8
7.	*bfrA*	Bacterioferritin
8.	*kdtB*	Phosphopantetheine adenylyltransferase
9.	*glcB*	Malate synthase G
10.	*purE*	Phosphoribosylaminoimidazole carboxylase catalytic subunit
11.	*ruvA*	Holliday junction DNA helicase
12.	*trpB*	Tryptophan synthase β-chain
13.	*mscL*	Large-conductance mechanosensitive channel

tial targets. Their genes are *rpoA, rpsD, rpsE, prsH, kdtB, ruvA,* and *kdtB*. Later, two of them were also found by other investigators (by both experimental and computational studies) as potential targets for wide-spectrum antibacterial agents: phosphopantetheine adenylyltransferase *kdtB (218)* and Holliday junction DNA helicase *ruvA (55)*.

Recently, we have also developed capabilities to identify targets for antibacterial agents with a wide spectrum, including mycobacteria, but without influencing normal human microflora. The genomes of *B. subtilis, E. coli* K12, and *Bifidium longum* NCC2705 represent human symbiont bacteria. The target selection flow chart is shown in **Fig. 12A**. The preliminary target list consists of 41 proteins. Therefore, it can be suggested that a drug with a relatively wide antibacterial spectrum and without effect on human symbiont bacteria can be designed.

It is known that antifungal azoles are active against *M. tuberculosis*, first of all owing to the targets' similarity. Therefore, we have also attempted to find mutual targets for *Mycobacteria* and fungi. *Saccharomyces cerevisiae* genome was used as the model genome of pathogenic fungi. A target selection flow chart is shown in **Fig. 12B**. The preliminary target list consists of 14 proteins. Therefore, there are several targets that can be used for both antitubercular and antifungal drug design. However, there was no intersection between two sets of targets obtained in two searches, as shown in **Fig. 12**.

3.6.2. 3D Modeling of Cytochrome P450 1A2 and Database Mining for New Leads Using Docking Procedure

The main task of this work was the modeling of 3D structure of cytochrome P450 1A2 (CYP1A2) and searching for new inhibitors by database mining *(219)*.

3.6.2.1. METHODS

All calculations were carried out using molecular modeling software suite SYBYL *(31)*, HINT® *(220,221)*, and the original molecular docking program DockSearch *(191)*

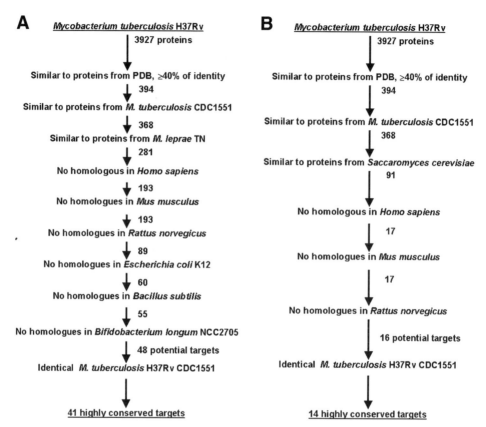

Fig. 12. Target selection in *Mycobacterium tuberculosis* H37Rv using broadened set of genomes for analysis. (**A**) Selection of targets for antibacterial agents with a wide spectrum. (**B**) Selection of mutual targets for *Mycobacterium* and fungi.

running on an SGI workstation. For mining, the databases Maybridge *(30)*, ASINEX *(28)*, and CMC *(27)*, which contain commercially available compounds, were used.

3.6.2.2. MODELING

The model of CYP1A2 was constructed by using the COMPOSER program from SYBYL based on homology with P450s with known 3D structures available from PDB. The obtained model was optimized using an energy minimization procedure. The model was verified using special software, PROCHECK *(161)*.

Attention was primarily focused on modeling the active site. To optimize the active site's structure, two models of CYP1A2 complexes with characteristic substrates (caffeine and 7-ethoxyresorufin) were designed. These complexes were optimized by molecular dynamics simulation in water.

3.6.2.3. Prediction of Affinity

Models of 24 CYP1A2 complexes with 24 known ligands and with known corresponding K_d values were designed using DockSearch and the LeapFrog program from SYBYL. A 3D-QSAR model with good predictive force was created based on these complexes.

3.6.2.4. Database Preprocessing

The integral database was compiled from three databases with commercially available compounds. To test the efficiency of mining, 204 known CYP1A2 ligands were included as the internal control.

3.6.2.5. Searching for New Ligands for CYP1A2 by Database Mining

Database mining was carried out in three steps: (1) the program DockSearch was used to generate hypotheses about ligand positions in the active site of CYP1A2; (2) the structures of hypothetical molecular complexes were adjusted using the LeapFrog program by energy optimization of protein-ligand binding; and (3) K_d values were estimated using a 3D-QSAR equation. The final hit list contained 185 from the control group of 204 known ligands (about 90%), which points to the high efficiency of mining. An example of affinity prediction for some known ligands is given in **Table 3**. As the result of database mining, 52 new potential ligands of CYP1A2 were selected for further purchasing and experimental testing.

3.6.3. Monoamine Oxidases:
Lead Searching When 3D Structure of Target is Unknown

As it was mentioned in **Subheading 3.4.2.**, when the target's 3D structure is not known, the main method of lead compound searching is molecular database mining with a pharmacophore model. However, when such a model is too simple (consists of few pharmacophore points), the use of this method leads to selection of a large number of potential hits that must be experimentally tested. In this case, it is possible to employ another approach based on searching the lead compounds in molecular databases by the docking procedure with the model of binding site cavity. As an example, we give here the results of using this method to search for new monoamine oxidase (MAO) A inhibitors. The pharmacophore model of this enzyme consists of only two points (aromatic ring with nearby heteroatom). We designed the model of active site reflecting geometrical features of the ligand-binding cavity (called "mold") using superposition of effective competitive inhibitors from a variety of chemical types *(180)*. The mold was used for molecular database mining to search for new MAO A inhibitors. The molecular database, which contained about 8000 commercially available small compounds, was precompiled by the generation of all possible conformers for all compounds and gave about 50,000 structures. All these structures were docked into the mold of MAO A. As a result of this step, about 7000 conformers able to fit in the binding cavity were selected. The next step was prediction of MAO A inhibitory activity for selected structures using 3D-QSAR with CoMFA models of MAO A. Then, the four top compounds

Table 3
Affinity Prediction for Some Known Ligands of CYP1A2

Name	Structure	K_d (μM)	
		Predicted	Experimental
Substrates			
Paracetamol (acetaminophen)		3000	3430
Zileuton		200	340
7-Ethoxycoumarin		20	21
Inhibitors			
2-Ethynylnaphthalene		30	26
α-Naphthoflavone		0.5	0.013
Mirtazapine		30	159
Lomefloxacin		400	1230

Table 4
Results of Experimental Testing of Inhibitory Activity (IC$_{50}$, µM) for MAO A and MAO B of Selected Compounds

Database index	Structure	MAO A	MAO B
BAS 0318949		316	>>100
BAS 0355758		>100	>>100
BAS 0370811		160	>>100
BAS 0442467		79	>>100

MAO, monoamine oxidase.

with highest predicted inhibitory activity were tested in direct experiments (**Table 4**). All compounds exhibited selective MAO A inhibition. The best of them had an IC$_{50}$ of about 80 µM. Although the inhibitory activity of these lead compounds was not high, their structures may be used in the next step for subsequent optimization by CADD methods.

4. Notes

1. For some limited purposes, other commercial programs can also be used, such as Hyper Chem (*222*) and programs by ACD (*223*).
2. A novel method of *de novo* design can be used for loop building (*224,225*), but this also requires careful expert judgment and structure refinement using energy minimization and molecular dynamics simulation.
3. It is possible to use SBDD when an accurate 3D model of target protein can be designed by homology 3D modeling (*226,227*) (*see* **Subheading 3.3.2.**). Such models also can be used to search for new ligands (*219,228,229*).

References

1. Lohse, M. J. (1998) The future of pharmacology. *Trends Pharmacol. Sci.* **19**, 198–200.
2. Borchardt, J. K. (2001) New drug development costs now average $802 million. *Alchemist* **6**. (www.chemweb.com/alchem/articles/1005928853806.html). Accessed on 12/6/2004.
3. National Center for Biotechnology Information, www.ncbi.nlm.nih.gov.
4. Kulikova, T., Aldebert, P., Althorpe, N., et al. (2004) The EMBL Nucleotide Sequence Database. *Nucleic Acids Res.* **32(database issue)**, D27–D30. (www.ebi.ac.uk/embl).
5. DNA Data Bank of Japan, www.ddbj.nig.ac.jp.
6. Boeckmann, B., Bairoch, A., Apweiler, R., et al. (2003) The SWISS-PROT protein knowledgebase and its supplement TrEMBL in 2003. *Nucleic Acids Res.* **31**, 365–370 (www.expasy.org/sprot).
7. Wu, C. H., Huang, H., Yeh, L.-S. L., and Barker, W. C. (2003) Protein family classification and functional annotation. *Comput. Biol. Chem.* **27**, 37–47 (http://pir.georgetown.edu)
8. Tatusov, R. L., Fedorova, N. D., Jackson, J. D., et al. (2003) The COG database: an updated version includes eukaryotes. *BMC Bioinfor.* **4**, 41.
9. Kanehisa, M., Goto, S., Kawashima, S., Okuno, Y., and Hattori, M. (2004) The KEGG resource for deciphering the genome. *Nucleic Acids Res.* **32(database issue)**, D277–D280.
10. Pandit, S. B., Bhadra, R., Gowri, V. S., Balaji, S., Anand, B., and Srinivasan, N. (2004) SUPFAM: a database of sequence superfamilies of protein domains. *BMC Bioinf.* **5**, 28–32. (www.sanger.ac.uk/Software/Pfam/).
11. Haft, D. H., Selengut, J. D., and White, O. (2003) The TIGRFAMs database of protein families. *Nucleic Acids Res.* **31**, 371–373 (www.tigr.org/TIGRFAMs/).
12. Peterson, J. D., Umayam, L. A., Dickinson, T., Hickey, E. K., and White, O. (2001) The comprehensive microbial resource. *Nucleic Acids Res.* **29**, 123–125 (www.tigr.org/CMR).
13. Uchiyama, I. (2003) MBGD: microbial genome database for comparative analysis. *Nucleic Acids Res.* **31**, 58–62 (http://mbgd.genome.ad.jp).
14. Xenarios, I., Salwinski, L., Duan, X. J., Higney, P., Kim, S. M., and Eisenberg, D. (2002) DIP, the Database of Interacting Proteins: a research tool for studying cellular networks of protein interactions. *Nucleic Acids Res.* **30**, 303–305 (http://dip.doe-mbi.ucla.edu).
15. Bader, G. D., Betel, D., and Hogue, C. W. (2003) BIND: the Biomolecular Interaction Network Database. *Nucleic Acids Res.* **31**, 248–250 (http://bind.ca).
16. Ng, S. K., Zhang, Z., and Tan, S. H. (2003) Integrative approach for computationally inferring protein domain interactions. *Bioinformatics* **19**, 923–929 (http://interdom.lit.org.sg).
17. Suhre, K. and Claverie, J.-M. (2004) FusionDB: a database for in-depth analysis of prokaryotic gene fusion events. *Nucleic Acids Res.* **32(database issue)**, D273–D276 (http://igs-server.cnrs-mrs.fr/FusionDB/).
18. NCGR, National Center for Genome Resources, www.ncgr.org/pathdb/.
19. Berman, H. M., Westbrook, J., Feng, Z., et al. (2000) The Protein Data Bank. *Nucleic Acids Res.* **28**, 235–242 (www.rcsb.org/pdb).
20. Noguchi, T. and Akiyama, Y. (2003) PDB-REPRDB: a database of representative protein chains from the Protein Data Bank (PDB) in 2003. *Nucleic Acids Res.* **31**, 492, 493 (http://mbs.crbc.jp/pdbreprdb-cgi/reprdb_menu.pl).
21. Frishman, D., Mokrejs, M., Kosykh, D., et al. (2003) The PEDANT genome database. *Nucleic Acids Res.* **31**, 207–211 (http://pedant.gsf.de).
22. Galperin, M. Y. (2004) The Molecular Biology Database Collection: 2004 update. *Nucleic Acids Res.* **32(database issue)**, D3–D22.

23. Freiberg, C. (2001) Novel computation methods in anti-microbial target identification. *Drug Discov. Today* **6**, S72–S80.
24. Allen, F. H. (2002) The Cambridge Structural Database: a quarter of a million crystal structures and rising. *Acta Crystallogr.* **B58**, 380–388 (www.ccdc.cam.ac.uk).
25. National Cancer Institute: Pure Chemicals Repository, www.dtp.nci.nih.gov/branches/dscb/repo_open.html.
26. MDL Drug Data Report, MDL Information Systems, www.mdl.com.
27. Comprehensive Medicinal Chemistry, MDL Information Systems, www.mdl.com.
28. ASINEX Ltd., www.asinex.com.
29. ChemBridge Corporation, www.chembridge.com.
30. Maybridge, www.maybridge.com.
31. SYBYL 6.7.1, Tripos Inc., www.tripos.com.
32. Spaltmann, F., Blunck, M., and Ziegelbauer, K. (1999) Computer-aided target selection-prioritizing targets for antifungal drug discovery. *Drug Discov. Today* **4**, 17–26.
33. Dubanov, A. V., Ivanov, A. S., and Archakov, A. I. (2001) Computer searching of new targets for antimicrobial drugs based on comparative analysis of genomes. *Vopr. Med. Khim.* **47**, 353–367 (in Russian).
34. Genedatar, www.genedata.com.
35. The Perl Directory, www.perl.org.
36. Python, www.python.org.
37. Mangalam, H. (2002) The Bio* toolkits—a brief overview. *Brief Bioinform.* **3**, 296–302.
38. Bioperl, www.bioperl.org.
39. Biopython, www.biopython.org.
40. Entrez Programming Utilities, www.ncbi.nlm.nih.gov/entrez/query/static/eutils_help.html.
41. BLAST, www.ncbi.nlm.nih.gov/BLAST/Doc/urlapi.html.
42. Accelrys, www.accelrys.com.
43. Case, D. A., Darden, T. A., Cheatham, T. E. III, et al. (2004) AMBER 8, University of California, San Francisco (http://amber.scripps.edu).
44. Berendsen, H. J. C., van der Spoel, D., and van Drunen, R. (1995) GROMACS: A message-passing parallel molecular dynamics implementation. *Comp. Phys. Commun.* **91**, 43–56 (www.gromacs.org).
45. Allsop, A. E. (1998) New antibiotic discovery, novel screens, novel targets and impact of microbial genomics. *Curr. Opin. Microbiol.* **1**, 530–534.
46. Veselovsky, A. V., Ivanov, Y. D., Ivanov, A. S., Archakov, A. I., Lewi, P., and Janssen, P. (2002) Protein-protein interactions: mechanisms and modification by drugs. *J. Mol. Recognit.* **15**, 405–422.
47. Archakov, A. I., Govorun, V. M., Dubanov, A. V., et al. (2003) Protein-protein interactions as a target for drugs in proteomics. *Proteomics* **3**, 380–391.
48. Rost, B., Liu, J., Wrzeszczynski, K. O., and Ofran, Y. (2003) Automatic prediction of protein fuction. *Cell. Mol. Life Sci.* **60**, 2637–2650.
49. Eisenberg, D., Marcotte, E. M., Xenarios, I., and Yeates, T. O. (2000) Protein function in the post-genomic era. *Nature* 2000 **405**, 823–826.
50. Butte A. J. and Kohane I. S. (2000) Mutual information relevance networks: functional genomic clustering using pairwise entropy measurements. *Pac. Symp. Biocomput.* **5**, 415–426.
51. Yanai, I. and DeLisi, C. (2002) The society of genes: networks of functional links between genes from comparative genomics. *Genome Biol.* **3**, research0064/12 (http://genomebiology.com/content/pdg/gb-2002-3-11-research0064.pdf).

52. Jansen, R., Lan, N., Qian, J., and Gerstein, M. (2002) Integration of genomic datasets to predict protein complexes in yeast. *J. Struct. Funct. Genomics* **2,** 71–81.
53. Jansen, R., Yu, H., Greenbaum, D., et al. (2003) A Bayesian networks approach for predicting protein-protein interactions from genomic data. *Science* **302,** 449–453.
54. Marcotte, E. M., Xenarios, I., van Der Bliek, A. M., and Eisenberg D. (2000) Localizing proteins in the cell from their phylogenetic profiles. *Proc. Natl. Acad. Sci. USA* **97,** 12,115–12,120.
55. Thanassi, J. A., Hartman-Neumann, S. L., Dougherty, T. J., Dougherty, B. A., and Pucci, M. J. (2002) Identification of 113 conserved essential genes using a high-throughput gene disruption system in Streptococcus pneumoniae. *Nucleic Acids Res.* **30,** 3152–3162.
56. Boguslavsky, J. (2002) Target validation: finding a needle in a haystack. *Drug Discov. Dev.* **5,** 41–48.
57. Lau, A. T., He, Q. Y., and Chiu, J. F. (2003) Proteomic technology and its biomedical application. *Acta Biochim. Biophys. Sinica* **35,** 965–975.
58. Walgren, J. L. and Thompson, D. C. (2004) Application of proteomic technologies in the drug development process. *Toxicol. Lett.* **149,** 377–385.
59. Cooper, R. A. and Carucci, D. J. (2004) Proteomic approaches to studying drug targets and resistance in Plasmodium. *Curr. Drug Targets Infect. Disord.* **4,** 41–51.
60. Flory, M. R. and Aebersold, R. (2003) Proteomic approaches for the identification of cell cycle-related drug targets. *Prog. Cell. Cycle Res.* **5,** 167–171.
61. Lopez, M. F. (1998) Proteomic databases: roadmaps for drug discovery. *Am. Clin. Lab.* **17,** 16–18.
62. Jones, S. and Thornton, J. M. (1995) Protein-protein interactions: a review of protein dimer structures. *Prog. Biophys. Mol. Biol.* **63,** 31–65.
63. Wilkinson, K. D. (2004) Quantitative analysis of protein-protein interactions. *Methods Mol. Biol.* **261,** 15–32.
64. Nedelkov, D. and Nelson, R. W. (2003) Delineating protein-protein interactions via biomolecular interaction analysis-mass spectrometry. *J. Mol. Recognit.* **16,** 9–14.
65. Strosberg, A. D. (2002) Protein interaction mapping for target validation: the need for an integrated combinatory process involving complementary approaches. *Curr. Opin. Mol. Ther.* **4,** 594–600.
66. Pillutla, R. C., Goldstein, N. I., Blume, A. J., and Fisher, P. B. (2002) Target validation and drug discovery using genomic and protein-protein interaction technologies. *Expert Opin. Ther. Targets* **6,** 517–531.
67. Butcher, S. P. (2003) Target discovery and validation in the post-genomic era. *Neurochem. Res.* **28,** 367–371.
68. Williams, M. (2003) Target validation. *Curr. Opin. Pharmacol.* **3,** 571–577.
69. Cowman, A. F. and Crabb, B. S. (2003) Functional genomics: identifying drug targets for parasitic diseases. *Trends Parasitol.* **19,** 538–543.
70. Sheppard, D. (1994) Dominant negative mutants: tools for the study of protein function in vitro and in vivo. *Am. J. Respir. Cell. Mol. Biol.* **11,** 1–6.
71. Homanics, G. E., Quinlan, J. J., Mihalek, R., and Firestone, L. L. (1998) Genetic dissection of the molecular target(s) of anesthetics with the gene knockout approach in mice. *Toxicol. Lett.* **100–101,** 301–307.
72. Luscombe, N. M., Austin, S. E., Berman, H. M., and Thornton, J. M. (2000) An overview of the structures of protein-DNA complexes. *Genome Biol.* **1,** reviews 001.1–001.10 (http://genomebiology.com/content/pdf/gb-2000-1-1-reviews001.pdf).

73. Kim, C. A. and Berg, J. M. (1996) A 2.2 A resolution crystal structure of a designed zinc finger protein bound to DNA. *Nat. Struct. Biol.* **3**, 940–945.

74. Jacobs, G. H. (1992) Determination of the base recognition positions of zinc finger from sequence-analysis. *EMBO J.* **11**, 4507–4517.

75. Pavletich, N. P. and Pabo, C. O. (1991) Zinc finger-DNA recognition: crystal structure of a Zif268-DNA complex at 2.1A. *Science* **252**, 809–817.

76. Suzuki, M., Gerstein, M. B., and Yagi, N. (1994) Stereochemical basis of DNA recognition by Zn fingers. *Nucleic Acids Res.* **22**, 3397–3405.

77. Cech, T. R. (1992) Ribozyme engineering. *Curr. Opin. Struct. Biol.* **2**, 605–609.

78. Breaker, R. R. (1997) In vitro selection of catalytic polynucleotides. *Chem. Rev.* **97**, 371–390.

79. Usman, N., Beigelman, L., and McSwiggen, J. A. (1996) Hammerhead ribozyme engineering. *Curr. Opin. Struct. Biol.* **6**, 527–533.

80. Uhlenbeck, O. C. (1987) A small catalytic oligoribonucleotide. *Nature* **328**, 596–600.

81. Jarvis, T. C., Bouhana, K. S., Lesch, M. E., et al. (2000) Ribozymes as tools for therapeutic target validation in arthritis. *J. Immunol.* **165**, 493–498.

82. Goodchild, J. (2002) Hammerhead ribozymes for target validation. *Expert Opin. Ther. Targets* **6**, 235–247.

83. Lehner, B., Fraser, A. G., and Sanderson, C. M. (2004) Technique review: how to use RNA interference. *Brief Funct. Genomic Proteomic* **3**, 68–83.

84. Jain, K. K. (2004) RNAi and siRNA in target validation. *Drug Discov. Today* **9**, 307–309.

85. Henning, S. W. and Beste, G. (2002) Loss-function strategies in drug target validation. *Curr. Drug Discov.* **5**, 17–21.

86. Baker, B. F. and Monia, B. P. (1999) Novel mechanisms for antisense mediated regulation of gene expression. *Biochim. Biophys. Acta* **1489**, 3–18.

87. Inouye, M. (1988) Antisense RNA: its functions and applications in gene regulation—a review. *Gene* **72**, 25–34.

88. Ravichandran, L. V., Dean, N. M., and Marcusson, E. G. (2004) Use of antisense oligonucleotides in functional genomics and target validation. *Oligonucleotides* **14**, 49–64.

89. Ji, Y., Yin, D., Fox, B., Holmes, D. J., Payne, D., and Rosenberg, M. (2004) Validation of antibacterial mechanism of action using regulated antisense RNA expression in Staphylococcus aureus. *FEMS Microbiol. Lett.* **231**, 177–184.

90. Lavery, K. S. and King, T. H. (2003) Antisense and RNAi: powerful tools in drug target discovery and validation. *Curr. Opin. Drug Discov. Dev.* **6**, 561–569.

91. Taylor, M. F. (2001) Target validation and functional analyses using antisense oligonucleotides. *Expert Opin. Ther. Targets* **5**, 297–301.

92. Dean, N. M. (2001) Functional genomics and target validation approaches using antisense oligonucleotide technology. *Curr. Opin. Biotechnol.* **12**, 622–625.

93. Koller, E., Gaarde, W. A., and Monia, B. P. (2000) Elucidating cell signaling mechanisms using antisense technology. *Trends Pharmacol. Sci.* **21**, 142–148.

94. Bennett, C. F. and Cowsert, L. M. (1999) Application of antisense oligonucleotides for gene functionalization and target validation. *Curr. Opin. Mol. Ther.* **1**, 359–371.

95. Ho, S. P. and Hartig, P. R. (1999) Antisense oligonucleotides for target validation in the CNS. *Curr. Opin. Mol. Ther.* **1**, 336–343.

96. Somagenics, www.somagenics.com/platform.html.

97. Pellestor, F. and Paulasova, P. (2004) The peptide nucleic acids, efficient tools for molecular diagnosis (review). *Int. J. Mol. Med.* **13**, 521–525.

 98. Gambari, R. (2001) Peptide-nucleic acids (PNAs): a tool for the development of gene expression modifiers. *Curr. Pharm. Des.* **7,** 1839–1862.
 99. Demidov, V. V. (2002) PNA comes of age: from infancy to maturity. *Drug Discov. Today* **7,** 153–155.
100. Ganesh, K. N. and Nielsen, P. E. (2000) Peptide nucleic acids: analogs and derivatives. *Curr. Organic Chem.* **4,** 916–928.
101. Winters, T. A. (2000) Gene targeting agents, new opportunities for rational drug development. *Curr. Opin. Mol. Ther.* **2,** 670–681.
102. Nielsen, P. E. (2000) Antisense peptide nucleic acids. *Curr. Opin. Mol. Ther.* **2,** 282–287.
103. Demidov, V. V. and Frank-Kamenetskii, M. D. (2001) Sequence-specific targeting of duplex DNA by peptide nucleic acids via triplex strand invasion. *Methods* **23,** 108–122.
104. Ray, A. and Norden, B. (2000) Peptide nucleic acid (PNA): its medical and biotechnological applications and promise for the future. *FASEB J.* **14,** 1041–1060.
105. Banker, D. D. (2001) Monoclonal antibodies: a review. *Indian J. Med. Sci.* **55,** 651–654.
106. Peet, N. P. (2003) What constitutes target validation? *Targets* **2,** 125–127.
107. Liao, J. C., Roider, J., and Jay, D. G. (1994) Chromophore-assisted laser inactivation of proteins is mediated by the photogeneration of free radicals. *Proc. Natl. Acad. Sci. USA* **91,** 2659–2663.
108. Jay, D. G. (1988) Selective destruction of protein function by chromophore-assisted laser inactivation. *Proc. Natl. Acad. Sci. USA* **85,** 5454–5458.
109. Niewohner, J., Rubenwolf, S., Meyer, E., and Rudert, F. (2001) Laser-mediated protein inactivation for target validation. *Am. Genomic/Proteomic Technol.* **4,** 28–33. (http://www.iscpubs.com/articles/agpt/g0108nie.pdf).
110. Eustace, B. K. and Jay, D. G. (2003) Fluorophore-assisted light inactivation for multiplex analysis of protein function in cellular processes. *Methods Enzymol.* **360,** 649–660.
111. Beck, S., Sakurai, T., Eustace, B. K., Beste, G., Schier, R., Rudert, F., and Jay, D. G. (2002) Fluorophore-assisted light inactivation: a high-throughput tool for direct target validation of proteins. *Proteomics* **2,** 247–255.
112. Bradbury, A. (2003) scFvs and beyond. *Drug Discov. Today* **8,** 737–739.
113. Chowdhury, P. S. and Vasmatzis, G. (2003) Engineering scFvs for improved stability. *Methods Mol. Biol.* **207,** 237–254.
114. van Wyngaardt, W., Malatji, T., Mashau, C., et al. (2004) A large semi-synthetic single-chain Fv phage display library based on chicken immunoglobulin genes. *BMC Biotechnol.* **4,** 6.
115. Toleikis, L., Broders, O., and Dubel, S. (2004) Cloning single-chain antibody fragments (scFv) from hybridoma cells. *Methods Mol. Med.* **94,** 447–458.
116. Tanaka, T., Lobato, M. N., and Rabbitts, T. H. (2003) Single domain intracellular antibodies: a minimal fragment for direct in vivo selection of antigen-specific intrabodies. *J. Mol. Biol.* **331,** 1109–1120.
117. Donini, M., Morea, V., Desiderio, A., et al. (2003) Engineering stable cytoplasmic intrabodies with designed specificity. *J. Mol. Biol.* **330,** 323–332.
118. Cohen, P. A. (2002) Intrabodies: targeting scFv expression to eukaryotic intracellular compartments. *Methods Mol. Biol.* **178,** 367–378.
119. Marasco, W. A. (1997) Intrabodies: turning the humoral immune system outside in for intracellular immunization. *Gene Ther.* **4,** 11–15.
120. Mundt, K. E. (2002) Intrabodies—valuable tools for target validation. Selection procedures for the use of intrabodies in functional genomics. Reprinted from *Eur. Pharm. Contractor* Winter 2001 issue. Samedan Ltd. Tech. ed. **10,** 1–5. (http://www.esbatech.com/pr/publications/ebr_preview.pdf).

121. Rimmele, M. (2003) Nucleic acid aptamers as tools and drugs: recent developments. *Chembiochemistry* **4**, 963–971.
122. Burgstaller, P., Girod, A., and Blind, M. (2002) Aptamers as tools for target prioritization and lead identification. *Drug Discov. Today* **7**, 1221–1228.
123. Toulme, J. J., Di Primo, C., and Boucard, D. (2004) Regulating eukaryotic gene expression with aptamers. *FEBS Lett.* **567**, 55–62.
124. Ulrich, H., Martins, A. H., and Pesquero, J. B. (2004) RNA and DNA aptamers in cytomics analysis. *Cytometry* **59A**, 220–231.
125. Convery, M. A., Rowsell, S., Stonehouse, N. J., et al. (1998) Crystal structure of an RNA aptamer-protein complex at 2.8 A resolution. *Nat. Struct. Biol.* **5**, 133–139.
126. Burgstaller, P., Jenne, A., and Blind, M. (2002) Aptamers and aptazymes: accelerating small molecule drug discovery. *Curr. Opin. Drug Discov. Dev.* **5**, 690–700.
127. Kubinyi, H. (2002) High throughput in drug discovery. *Drug Discov. Today* **7**, 707–709.
128. Ilag, L. L., Ng, J. H., Beste, G., and Henning, S. W. (2002) Emerging high-throughput drug target validation technologies. *Drug Discov. Today* **7**, S136–S142.
129. Hardy, L. W. and Peet, N. P. (2004) The multiple orthogonal tools approach to define molecular causation in the validation of druggable targets. *Drug Discov. Today* **9**, 117–126.
130. Flook, P. K., Yan, L., and Szalma, S. (2003) Target validation through high throughput proteomics analysis. *Targets* **2**, 217–223.
131. Harris, S. (2001) Transgenic knockouts as part of high-throughput, evidence-based target selection and validation strategies. *Drug Discov. Today* **6**, 628–636.
132. Xin, H., Bernal, A., Amato, F. A., et al. (2004) High-throughput siRNA-based functional target validation. *J. Biomol. Screen.* **9**, 286–293.
133. Taylor, M. F., Wiederholt, K., and Sverdrup, F. (1999) Antisense oligonucleotides: a systematic high-throughput approach to target validation and gene function determination. *Drug Discov. Today* **4**, 562–567.
134. Sinibaldi, R. (2004) Gene expression analysis and R&D. *Drug Discov. World* **5**, 37–43.
135. Sundberg, S. A., Chow, A., Nikiforov, T., and Wada, H. G. (2000) Microchip-based systems for target validation and HTS. *Drug Discov. Today* **5**, 92–103.
136. Huels, C., Muellner, S., Meyer, H. E., and Cahill, D. J. (2002) The impact of protein biochips and microarrays on the drug development process. *Drug Discov. Today* **7**, S119–S124.
137. Barsky, V., Perov, A., Tokalov, S., et al. (2002) Fluorescence data analysis on gel-based biochips. *J. Biomol. Screen.* **7**, 247–257.
138. Rubina, A. Y., Dementieva, E. I., Stomakhin, A. A., et al. (2003) Hydrogel-based protein microchips: manufacturing, properties, and applications. *Biotechniques* **34**, 1008–1022.
139. Matthews, D. and Kopczynski, J. (2001) Using model-system genetics for drug-based target discovery. *Drug Discov. Today* **6**, 141–149.
140. Tornell, J. and Snaith, M. (2002) Transgenic systems in drug discovery: from target identification to humanized mice. *Drug Discov. Today* **7**, 461–470.
141. Abuin, A., Holt, K. H., Platt, K. A., Sands, A. T., and Zambrowicz, B. P. (2002) Full-speed mammalian genetics: in vivo target validation in the drug discovery process. *Trends Biotechnol.* **20**, 36–42.
142. Russ, A., Stumm, G., Augustin, M., Sedlmeir, R., Wattler, S., and Nehls, M. (2002) Random mutagenesis in the mouse as a toll in drug discovery. *Drug Discov. Today* **7**, 1175–1183.
143. Rubinstein, A. L. (2003) Zebrafish: from disease modeling to drug discovery. *Curr. Opin. Drug Discov. Devel.* **6**, 218–223.
144. Sumanas, S. and Lin, S. (2004) Zebrafish as a model system for drug target screening and validation. *Drug Discov. Today Targets* **3**, 89–96.

145. Sommer, R. J. (2000) Comparative genetics: a third model nematode species. *Curr. Biol.* **10,** R879–R881.

146. Sternberg, P. W. and Han, M. (1998) Genetics of RAS signaling in *C. elegans. Trends Genet.* **14,** 466–472.

147. Lee, J., Nam, S., Hwang, S. B., et al. (2004) Functional genomic approaches using the nematode Caenorhabditis elegans as a model system. *J. Biochem. Mol. Biol.* **37,** 107–113.

148. Wassarman, D. A., Therrien, M., and Rubin, G. M. (1995) The Ras signaling pathway in *Drosophila. Curr. Opin. Genet. Dev.* **5,** 44–50.

149. VITA (Validation In Vivo of Targets and Assays for Antiinfectives) technology (www.cubist.com/ar2000text/discovery.html).

150. Chopra, I. (2000) New drugs for the superbugs. *Microbiol. Today* **27,** 4–6.

151. Jackson, L. K. and Phillips, M. A. (2002) Target validation for drug discovery in parasitic organisms. *Curr. Top. Med. Chem.* **2,** 425–438.

152. Carter, C. W. Jr. and Sweet, R. M. (eds.) (2003) *Methods in Enzymology. Volume 368: Macromolecular Crystallography, Part C,* Academic, San Diego.

153. Downing, A. K. (2004) *Protein NMR Techniques,* 2nd ed. Humana, Totowa, NJ.

154. Wallin, E. and Von Heijne, G. (1998) Genome-wide analysis of integral membrane proteins from eubacterial, archaean, and eukaryotic organisms. *Protein Sci.* **7,** 1029–1038.

155. Grisshammer, R. and Tate, C. G. (1995) Overexpression of integral membrane proteins for structural studies. *Q. Rev. Biophys.* **28,** 315–422.

156. Eswar, N., John, B., Mirkovic, N., et al. (2003) Tools for comparative protein structure modeling and analysis. *Nucleic Acids Res.* **31,** 3375–3380.

157. Fiser, A. and Sali, A. (2003) Modeller: generation and refinement of homology-based protein structure models. *Methods Enzymol.* **374,** 461–491.

158. Topham, C. M., Thomas, P., Overington, J. P., Johnson, M. S., Eisenmenger, F., and Blundell, T. L. (1990) An assessment of COMPOSER: a rule-based approach to modelling protein structure. *Biochem. Soc. Symp.* **57,** 1–9.

159. Protein Structure Prediction Center, http://predictioncenter.llnl.gov.

160. Moult, J., Fidelis, K., Zemla, A., and Hubbard, T. (2003) Critical assessment of methods of protein structure prediction (CASP)-round V. *Proteins* **53(Suppl. 6),** 334–339.

161. Laskowski, R. A., MacArthur, M. W., Moss, D. S., and Thornton, J. M. (1993) PROCHECK: a program to check the stereochemical quality of protein structures. *J. Appl. Crystallogr.* **26,** 283–291 (www.biochem.ucl.ac.uk/~roman/procheck/procheck.html).

162. Protable. www.tripos.com/sciTech/inSilicoDisc/media/LITCTR/PROTABLE.PDF.

163. Godzik, A., Kolinski, A., and Skolnick, J. (1993) De novo and inverse folding predictions of protein structure and dynamics. *J. Comput. Aided Mol. Des.* **7,** 397–438 (www.tripos.com/admin/LitCtr/matchmaker.pdf).

164. Vriend, G. (1990) WHAT IF: a molecular modeling and drug design program. *J. Mol. Graph.* **8,** 52–56 (cmbi.kun.nl/whatif/).

165. Sippl, M. J. (1993) Recognition of errors in three-dimensional structures of proteins. *Proteins* **17,** 355–362 (http://smft.www.came.sbg.ac.at/came-frames/prosa.html).

166. Luthy, R., Bowie, J. U., and Eisenberg, D. (1992) Assessment of protein models with three-dimensional profiles. *Nature* **356,** 83–85 (www.accelrys.com/products/datasheets/i2_profiles_3d_data.pdf).

167. Myers, P. L. (1997) Will combinatorial chemistry deliver real medicines? *Curr. Opin. Biotechnol.* **8,** 701–707.

168. Fernandes, P. B. (1998) Technological advances in high-throughput screening. *Curr. Opin. Chem. Biol.* **2,** 597–603.
169. Entzeroth, M. (2003) Emerging trends in high-throughput screening. *Curr. Opin. Pharmacol.* **3,** 522–529.
170. Clark, D. E. and Pickett, S. D. (2000) Computational methods for the prediction of "drug-likeness." *Drug Discov. Today* **5,** 49–58.
171. Kubinyi, H. (1998) Structure-based design of enzyme inhibitors and receptor ligands. *Curr. Opin. Drug Discov. Dev.* **1,** 4–15.
172. Ivanov, A. S., Dubanov, A. V., Skvortsov, V. S., and Archakov, A. I. (2002) Computer aided drug design based on structure of macromolecular target: I. Search and description of ligand binding site in target protein. *Vopr. Med. Khim.* **48,** 304–315 (in Russian).
173. Hoffmann, D., Kramer, B., Washio, T., Steinmetzer, T., Rarey, M., and Lengauer, T. (1999) Two-stage method for protein-ligand docking. *J. Med. Chem.* **42,** 4422–4433.
174. Hubbard, R. E. (1997) Can drugs be designed? *Curr. Opin. Biotechol.* **8,** 696–700.
175. Flohr, S., Kurz, M., Kostenis, E., Brkovich, A., Fournier, A., and Klabunde. T. (2002) Identification of nonpeptidic urotensin II receptor antagonists by virtual screening based on a pharmacophore model derived from structure-activity relationships and nuclear magnetic resonance studies on urotensin II. *J. Med. Chem.* **45,** 1799–1805.
176. Ghose, A. K. and Wendoloski, J. J. (1998) Pharmacophore modeling: methods, experimental verification and applications, in *Perspectives in Drug Discovery and Design,* vol. 9–11, pp. 253–271.
177. Kettmann, V. and Holtje, H.-D. (1998) Mapping of the benzothiazepine binding site on the calcium channel. *Quant. Struct.-Act. Relat.* **17,** 91–101.
178. Zbinden, P., Dobler, M., Folkers, G., and Vedani, A. (1998) PrGen: pseudoreceptor modeling using receptor-mediated ligand alignment and pharmacophore equilibration. *Quant. Struct.-Act. Relat.* **17,** 122–129.
179. Schleifer, K.-J. (2000) Pseudoreceptor model for ryanodine derivatives at calcium release channels. *J. Comput.-Aided Mol. Des.* **14,** 467–475.
180. Veselovsky, A. V., Tikhonova, O. V., Skvortsov, V. S., Medvedev, A. E., and Ivanov, A. S. (2001) An approach for visualization of active site of enzymes with unknown three-dimensional structures. *QSAR SAR Environ. Res.* **12,** 345–358.
181. Kubinyi, H. (1994) Variable selection in QSAR studies. I. An evolutionary algorithm. *Quant. Struct.-Act. Relat.* **13,** 285–294.
182. Kim, K. H. (1995) Comparative molecular field analysis (CoMFA), in *Molecular Simulation and Drug Design* (Dean, P. M., ed.), Blackie Academic & Professional, London, UK, pp. 291–331.
183. Cramer, R. D. III, Petterson, D. E., and Bunce, J. D. (1988) Comparative molecular field analysis (CoMFA). 1. Effect of share on binding of steroids to carrier proteins. *J. Am. Chem. Soc.* **110,** 5959–5967.
184. Sippl, W. (2000) Receptor-based 3D QSAR analysis of estrogen receptor ligands—merging the accuracy of receptor-based alignments with the computational efficiency of ligand-based methods. *J. Comput.-Aided Mol. Des.* **14,** 559–572.
185. Sippl, W., Contreras, J.-M., Parrot, I., Rival, Y. M., and Wermuth, C. G. (2001) Structure-based 3D QSAR and design of novel acetylcholineesterase inhibitors. *J. Comput.-Aided Mol. Des.* **15,** 395–410.
186. MDL Information Systems, www.mdl.com.
187. UNITY® 4.4.2 Tripos Inc., www.tripos.com.

188. Kuntz, I. D., Blaney, J. M., Oatley, S. J., Landridge, R., and Ferrin, T. E. (1982) A geometric approach to macromolecule-ligand interactions. *J. Mol. Biol.* **161,** 269–288.

189. Ewing, T. J. A., Makino, S., Skillman, A. G., and Kuntz, I. D. (2001) DOCK 4.0: Search strategies for automated molecular docking of flexible molecule databases. *J. Comput.-Aided Mol. Des.* **15,** 411–428.

190. BioSolveIT GmbH, www.biosolveit.de.

191. DockSearch. http://Imgdd.ibmh.msk.su/lab/docksearch.

192. Raevsky, O. A., Trepalin, S. V., Trepalina, E. P., Gerasimenko, V. A., and Raevskaja, O. E. (2002) SLIPPER-2001—software for predicting molecular properties on the basis of physicochemical descriptors and structural similarity. *J. Chem. Inf. Comput. Sci.* **42,** 540–549.

193. Raevsky, O. A., Schaper, K.-J., van de Waterbeemd, H., and McFarland, J. W. (2000) Hydrogen bond contributions to properties and activities of chemicals and drugs, in *Molecular Modelling and Prediction of Bioactivity* (Gundertofe, K. and Jorgensen, F., eds.), Kluwer Academic/Plenum, New York, pp. 221–227.

194. CORINA, www2.chemie.uni-erlangen.de/software/corina.

195. Molecular Networks GmbH, www.mol-net.de.

196. Pearlman, R. S. (1987) Rapid generation of high quality approximate 3-dimension molecular structures. *Chem. Des. Auto. News* **2,** 1–7.

197. Pearlman, R.S. "Concord User's Manual," distributed by Tripos Inc., www.tripos.com.

198. Pearlman, R. S. and Balducci, R. (1998) Confort: a novel algorithm for conformational analysis. *National Meeting of the American Chemical Society,* New Orleans. (http://www.tripos.com/sciTech/inSilicoDisc/media/LITCTR/CONFORT.PDF).

199. CONFLEX Corporation, www.conflex.us.

200. Jones, G., Willett, P., Glen, R., Leach, A. R., and Taylor, R. (1997) Development and validation of a genetic algorithm for flexible docking. *J. Mol. Biol.* **267,** 727–748.

201. Muegge, I. and Martin, Y. C. (1999) A general and fast scoring function for protein-ligand interactions: a simplified potential approach. *J. Med. Chem.* **42,** 791–804.

202. Ewing, T. J. A. and Kuntz, I. D. (1996) Critical evaluation of search algorithms for automated molecular docking and database screening. *J. Comp. Chem.* **18,** 1175–1189 (http://dock.compbio.ucsf.edu).

203. Eldridge, M. D., Murray, C. W., Auton, T. R., Paolini, G. V., and Mee, R. P. (1997) Empirical scoring functions: I. The development of a fast empirical scoring function to estimate the binding affinity of ligands in receptor complexes. *J. Comput.-Aided Mol. Des.* **11,** 425–445.

204. Wang, R., Liu, L., Lai, L., and Tang, Y. (1998) SCORE: A new empirical method for estimating the binding affinity of a protein-ligand complex. *J. Mol. Model.* **4,** 379–394.

205. Krepets, V. V., Belkina, N. V., Skvortsov, V. S., and Ivanov, A. S. (2000) Prediction of binding affinities for protein-ligand complexes by using non-linear models. *Vopr. Med. Chim.* **46,** 462–474 (in Russian).

206. Clark, R. D., Strizhev, A., Leonard, J. M., Blake, J. F., and Matthew, J. B. (2002) Consensus scoring for ligand/protein interactions. *J. Mol. Graph. Model.* **20,** 281–295.

207. Pearlman, D. A. and Rao, B. G. (1998) Free energy calculations: methods and applications, in *Encyclopedia of Computational Chemistry* (von Schleyer, P. R., Allinger, N. L., Clark, T., Gasteiger, J., Kollman, P. A., and Schaefer, H. F. III, eds.), John Wiley, Chichester, UK, pp. 1036–1061.

208. Bohm, H. J. (1992) The computer program LUDI: a new method for the de novo design of enzyme inhibitors. *J. Comput.-Aided. Mol. Des.* **6,** 61–78.

209. Lawrence, M. C. and David, P. C. (1992) CLIX: a search algorithm for finding novel ligands capable of binding protein of known three-dimensional structure. *Proteins: Struct. Funct. Genet.* **12,** 31–41.
210. Bartlett, P. A., Shea, G. T., Telfer, S. J., and Waterman, S. (1989) CAVEAT: a program to facilitate the structure-derived design of biologically active molecules, in *Molecular Recognition in Chemical and Biological Problems*, vol. 78 (Roberts, S. M., ed.), Royal Chemistry Society, London, UK, pp. 182–196.
211. LeapFrog: SYBYL® 6.9.2, www.tripos.com/sciTech/inSilicoDisc/media/LITCTR/LEAP FROG.PDF.
212. Poroikov, V. V., Filimonov, D. A., Borodina, Yu. V., Lagunin, A. A., and Kos, A. (2000) Robustness of biological activity predicting by computer program PASS for noncongeneric sets of chemical compounds. *J. Chem. Inf. Comput. Sci.* **40,** 1349–1355 (www.ibmh.msk. su/PASS/).
213. Biacore 3000 preprint (www.biacore.com/lifesciences/products/systems_overview/3000/ system_information/index.html).
214. Biacore S51 preprint (www.biacore.com/lifesciences/products/systems_overview/s51/ system_information/index.html).
215. Nagata, K. and Handa, H. (eds.). (2000) *Real-Time Analysis of Biomolecular Interactions: Applications of Biacore*, Springer-Verlag, Tokyo.
216. Rich, R. L. and Myszka, D. G. (2000) Advances in surface plasmon resonance biosensor analysis. *Curr. Opin. Biotechnol.* **11,** 54–61.
217. Altschul, S. F., Madden, T. L., Schaffer, A. A., Zhang, J., Zhang, Z., Miller, W., and Lipman, D. J. (1997) Gapped BLAST and PSI-BLAST: a new generation of protein database search programs. *Nucleic Acids Res.* **25,** 3389–3402.
218. Freiberg, C., Wieland, B., Spaltmann, F., Ehlert, K., Brotz, H., and Labischinski, H. (2001) Identification of novel essential Escherichia coli genes conserved among pathogenic bacteria. *J. Mol. Microbiol. Biotechnol.* **3,** 483–489.
219. Belkina, N. V., Skvortsov, V. S., Ivanov, A. S., and Archakov, A. I. (1998) Modeling of a three-dimensional structure of cytochrome P-450 1A2 and search for its new ligands. *Vopr. Med. Khim.* **44,** 464–473 (in Russian).
220. Kellogg, G. E., Semus, S. F., and Abraham, D. J. (1991) HINT—A new method of empirical hydrophobic field calculation for CoMFA. *J. Comput.-Aided Mol. Des.* **5,** 545–552.
221. HINT® (Hydropathic INTeractions), www.edusoft-lc.com/hint/.
222. HyperChem, www.hyper.com/products/.
223. Advanced Chemistry Development (ACD), www.acdlabs.com/products.
224. Schonbrun, J., Wedemeyer, W. J., and Baker, D. (2002) Protein structure prediction in 2002. *Curr. Opin. Struct. Biol.* **12,** 348–354.
225. Fiser, A., Do, R. K., and Sali, A. (2000) Modeling of loops in protein structures. *Protein Sci.* **9,** 1753–1773.
226. Ooms, F. (2000) Molecular modeling and computer aided drug design: examples of their applications in medicinal chemistry. *Curr. Med. Chem.* **7,** 141–158.
227. Amzel, L. M. (1998) Structure-based drug design. *Curr. Opin. Biotechnol.* **9,** 366–369.
228. Yamamoto, K., Masuno, H., Choi, M., et al. (2000) Three-dimensional modeling of and ligand docking to vitamin D receptor ligand binding domain. *Proc. Natl. Acad. Sci. USA* **97,** 1467–1472.
229. Vangrevelinghe, E., Zimmermann, K., Schoepfer, J., Portmann, R., Fabbro, D., and Furet, P. (2003) Discovery of a potent and selective protein kinase CK2 inhibitor by high-throughput docking. *J. Med. Chem.* **46,** 2656–2662.

Index

433